VIRAL INFECTIONS OF THE NERVOUS SYSTEM

Second Edition

Viral Infections of the Nervous System

Second Edition

Richard T. Johnson, M.D.

Professor of Neurology, Microbiology, and Neuroscience
The Johns Hopkins University School of Medicine
Joint Appointment
The Department of Molecular Microbiology and Immunology
The Johns Hopkins University School of Public Health and Hygiene
Neurologist
The Johns Hopkins Hospital
Baltimore, Maryland
and
Director
National Neuroscience Institute of Singapore

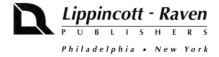

Lippincott - Raven
PUBLISHERS

Philadelphia • New York

Acquisitions Editor: Mark Placito
Manufacturing Manager: Dennis Teston
Production Manager: Robert Pancotti
Production Editor: Emily Harkavy
Cover Designer: Ox Company, Inc.
Indexer: Keith Shostak
Compositor: Lippincott–Raven Desktop Division
Printer: Maple Press
Art rendered by Jennifer Smith

Printed in the United States of America

9 8 7 6 5 4 3 2 1

Library of Congress Cataloging-in-Publication Data

Johnson, Richard T. (Richard Tidball), 1931–
    Viral infections of the nervous system   /   Richard T. Johnson.—2nd ed.
      p.   cm.
    Includes bibliographical references and index.
    ISBN 0-7817-1440-0
    1, Neurovirology.   2. Nervous system—Infections.   3. Virus diseases.   I. Title.
    [DNLM: 1. Virus Diseases.   2. Nervous System Diseases.   WC 540
    J68v 1998]
    RC359.5.J64   1998
DNLM/DLC
For Library of Congress   97-52761
                                                        CIP

Contents

Preface to First Edition   ix

Preface   xi

Acknowledgments   xiii

Part I: GENERAL PRINCIPLES   1

1. Historical Background   3

2. Viruses and Virus-Cell Interactions   11
    Nature of Viruses   11
    Virus-Cell Interactions   23
    Virus-Virus Interactions   27
    Effects of Virus Replication on Cells   29

3. Pathogenesis of Central Nervous System Infections   35
    Experimental Approaches   36
    Entry of Viruses   38
    Pathways of Neuroinvasion   40
    Neurotropism   53
    Neurovirulence   56

4. Immune Responses   61
    Anatomy of the Immune System   62
    Immune Responses to Viruses   68
    Immune Responses in the CNS   76
    Virus Clearance from the CNS   82

Part II: ACUTE NEUROLOGICAL DISEASES   85

5. Meningitis, Encephalitis, and Poliomyelitis   87
    General Considerations   88
    Enteroviruses   93
    Mumps Virus   100
    Adenoviruses   102

Parvovirus 104
Arenaviruses 105
Filoviruses 109
Arboviruses 109
Differential Diagnosis 125

6. Herpesvirus Infections 133
   Latency 136
   Herpes Simplex Viruses 137
   Varicella-Zoster Virus 151
   Epstein-Barr Virus 160
   Cytomegalovirus 164
   Human Herpesviruses 6 and 7 167

7. Rabies 169

8. Postinfectious Demyelinating Diseases 181
   Considerations of Mechanisms 182
   Postinfectious Encephalomyelitis 192
   Guillain-Barré Syndrome 202

9. Other Postviral Syndromes 211
   Virus-Induced Encephalopathy 212
   Reye's Syndrome 212
   Postpolio Syndrome 216
   Chronic Fatigue Syndrome 220

Part III: CHRONIC NEUROLOGICAL DISEASES 225

10. Chronic Inflammatory and Demyelinating Diseases 227
    Mechanisms of Virus Persistence in the CNS 228
    Subacute Sclerosing Panencephalitis 231
    Progressive Rubella Panencephalitis 239
    Progressive Multifocal Leukoencephalopathy 241
    Possible Viral Cause of Multiple Sclerosis 248
    Possible Viral Causes of Other Chronic
    Inflammatory Diseases 258

11. Retroviruses 265
    Nature of Retroviruses 267
    Human T-cell Lymphotropic Viruses 268
    Neurological Diseases of Animal Retroviruses 277

12. Human Immunodeficiency Virus 287
    Human Immunodeficiency Virus Infections 288

Neurological Diseases 294
Pathogenesis of Neurological Diseases 302
Treatment 311

13. Viral Infections of the Developing Nervous System 315
Pathogenesis of Fetal Infections 316
Fetal and Neonatal Infections in Humans 319
Viral Teratogenesis in Animals 339

14. Degenerative Diseases and Prions 349
Scrapie 350
Kuru 353
Creutzfeldt-Jakob Disease 356
Bovine Spongiform Encephalopathy 364
Possible Viral Causes of Human Degenerative Diseases 368

Part IV: OTHER PERSPECTIVES 375

15. Cerebral Tumors 377
Pathogenesis of Cell Transformation by Viruses 379
Experimental Production of Cerebral Tumors 380
Evidence for Viruses in Human Brain Tumors 383

16. Neurovirology Afield 387
Retinitis 388
Labyrinthitis 394
Myositis 402
Vasculitis 405

17. Prevention and Therapy 411
Environmental Control 412
Vaccines 414
Antiviral Drugs 418

18. Postscripts 423
In Defense of the White Mouse 424
Koch's Postulates Revisited 426
Emerging Viral Infections 429

References 437

Subject Index 511

Preface to First Edition

Twenty-two years ago, when I left the Department of Virus Diseases at Walter Reed Army Institute of Research for residency training in neurology and neuropathology, my colleagues were bewildered because clinician-virologists were expected to practice pediatrics or, at least, internal medicine. Three years later, when I left the Massachusetts General Hospital to return to virology at the Australian National University, my clinical mentors were dismayed that a neurologist would abandon promising areas of neurological research to return to such an irrelevant discipline. Events of the past 15 years seem to have justified my decisions. Experiments with viruses have produced a remarkable spectrum of neurological diseases; slow infections of man have proved to be primarily neurological diseases; interest in viral infections of the nervous system has burgeoned. I hasten to add, however, that my decisions were not made because of foresight, but because the policies of National Institutes of Health training programs allowed indulgence in tangentially related interests and because I was, and am, intrigued by neurological diseases and by viruses.

This book has been written with a clinical audience in mind. Nevertheless, I hope it also will be useful to some basic microbiologists and neurobiologists because it is not a compendium of methods for the diagnosis and treatment of specific disease syndromes. Those aspects of viral infections are discussed in traditional texts. Instead, this book emphasizes the biology of nervous-system infections based on the premise that only an understanding of mechanisms can lead to rational and innovative diagnosis and therapy. In the past few years, developments in molecular biology and animal virology have converged, and this happy union is beginning to have an impact on clinical medicine. Biochemical identification of the early protein secreted by cells infected with herpes simplex virus should allow the development of an immunoassay for the early diagnosis of herpetic encephalitis. Advances in viral genetics are permitting meaningful definitions of neurovirulence and should, in the future, lead to the rational construction of vaccines; further knowledge of the transcription and translation of viral proteins and replication of nucleic acids will allow us to tailor chemotherapeutic tools that can block virus replication without destroying the host cell.

After four introductory chapters on general principles, different clinical syndromes and diseases are discussed in what seems to be a logical order because it follows my own sojourns. I began in virology with studies of diagnosis and epidemiology of acute viral infections of the nervous system during the late

1950s, followed by studies of the pathogenesis of experimental herpes, rabies, and arbovirus infections in the early 1960s. During attempts to induce postinfectious encephalomyelitis, I stumbled inadvertently into viral teratology in the late 1960s, and currently my laboratory is studying persistent infections with conventional viruses, with occasional deviations into cerebral tumors and infections of the retina, inner ear, and muscle.

A book focusing solely on the more glamorous area of slow infections might seem more timely, but I think it better to strip some of the mystique from this area by putting these infections into a general context. Under the right circumstances, many viruses have the capacity to persist with or without chronic disease, and chronic disease can evolve with or without persistent infection. A separation of slow infections from acute, latent, or persistent infections is increasingly difficult. The exceptions are the spongiform encephalopathy agents, which appear to be inherently slow. Although I visited New Guinea in the early 1960s and have closely followed the work of my friends in this area, I have always maintained a "scrapie-free" laboratory. Therefore, this area I discuss as an outsider. Some "scrapieologists" have voiced irritation with conventional virologists, like myself, who address their field in standard virological terminology. However, until they can better clarify the nature of their strange agents, I have included them tentatively as "viruses" and have discussed them as such, albeit as an interested onlooker who admires their patience but does not share it.

This is a candidly personal book. It not only follows my own sequence of interests, but also expresses many personal opinions and relies heavily on examples drawn from my own studies and those of my co-workers, past and present. This does not necessarily mean that I regard these studies as better—just more familiar.

Baltimore, 1982

Preface

Fifteen years is far too long a lag for a second edition of a book in a swiftly moving field. The changes in neurovirology over this time have been remarkable: some could have been anticipated, but some have been unimaginable. Evolution of new enteroviruses and influenza viruses, recovery of new herpesviruses and a human parvovirus, first encounters with zoonotic agents such as hantaviruses and arenaviruses, and wider spread of filoviruses might all have been foreseen. The emergence of human retroviruses as major neuropathogens and the sudden appearance of bovine spongiform encephalopathy and its probable transmission to humans were unforeseeable. Changes in technology have evolved in a similar pattern. Better means to identify and purify nucleic acids and proteins, rapid methods of sequencing, and improved immunocytochemical techniques were expected; but the development and applications of techniques using the polymerase chain reaction challenge the imagination. Who could have anticipated that the tedious methods of virus recovery in animals and cell cultures could be replaced by a rapid method whose greatest drawback is excessive sensitivity or that any method could detect agents that had never been isolated?

The first edition contained the statement that the retrovirus family included "no known human pathogens." This edition, however, includes two chapters on retroviruses and human disease, and a substantial addition on human immunodeficiency virus has been necessary in the chapter on infections of the developing nervous system. A chapter on "other" postinfectious syndromes has also been added to deal with several politically charged illnesses. The advances in virology have been so vast that I simply shortened Chapter 2 and advise readers to look at conventional texts; immunology also has made enormous strides, and Chapter 4 has been focused more selectively on CNS aspects. Nevertheless, within these chapters the new important topics of apoptosis and cytokines have been added. I also have heeded reviewers of the first edition; one admonished me for giving short shrift to the possible role of a virus in multiple sclerosis (it now may be too long) and another criticized my failure to mention schizophrenia (it now is included with appropriate skepticism). Finally, 15 years ago I told Stan Prusiner that if he convinced me that prions contained no nucleic acid, I would delete the chapter devoted to them in the second edition; he has convinced me, but with the exciting new information on Creutzfeldt-Jakob disease and bovine spongiform encephalopathy I could not bring myself to leave them out.

(Some believe there is a bit of nucleic acid in there somewhere, and that can rationalize their inclusion.)

This continues to be a very personal and opinionated book. The orientation of this edition is more international, however, but that too reflects my personal experiences since the first edition. For 10 years I, along with Baltimorean and Peruvian colleagues, worked on measles each winter in Lima; we also spent several weeks working with patients with hemorrhagic fever in Argentina; and I worked at the Armed Forces laboratory on Japanese encephalitis in Thailand in 1984. The "exotic" infectious agents are given greater coverage, not only because of their importance on other continents but also because in our shrinking global environment, all the viruses of Asia, Africa, and Latin America can find their way into any of our communities within a single incubation period. The final essay of the postscripts deals with this present and growing future danger.

Baltimore, 1997

Acknowledgments

Often in talks and papers, and again in this book, I have used the image of steps of complexity in animal virology. Virus-cell interactions, where the most sophisticated experiments have been done, constitute the first step; pathogenesis studies in animal hosts involve a higher level of complexity; epidemiological and clinical studies, although often disparaged, are at the highest level of complexity, dealing with viral ecology and animal populations. During the preparation of this book, I realized that the same image had been used previously by one of my mentors, Frank Fenner, and later I found it in earlier writings of Sir Macfarlane Burnet, one of his former teachers. We are all conglomerates of our teachers, our students, and our colleagues, including those we encounter only on the printed page. I thank them all.

I thank my early teachers in virology at Walter Reed Army Institute of Research and the Australian National University, especially Ed Buescher, Nancy Rogers, Frank Fenner, and Cedric Mims, and in neurology and neuropathology at the Massachusetts General Hospital and Cleveland Metropolitan General Hospital, particularly Raymond Adams, E. Pierson Richardson, Maurice Victor, and Betty Banker. My matchless colleagues, students, and fellows at Johns Hopkins over the past 28 years have provided the needed challenges and encouragement. To peer-review this book I called on some of those former postdoctoral fellows who are now valued colleagues—indeed, Diane Griffin is now my chairman since I retired from my chairmanship in the medical school and moved into her department in the School of Hygiene and Public Health. Other former fellows who critiqued chapters include Opendra Narayan, Henry McFarland, Howard Lipton, Larry Davis, Raymond Roos, John Greenlee, Janice Clements, Micheline McCarthy, Burk Jubelt, Patricia Coyle, Alan Seay, Peter Kennedy, Alan Jackson, Thiravat Hemachudha, William Tyor, David Irani, and Christopher Power.

Special gratitude is due for my many colleagues and longterm research partners at Universidad Peruana Cayetano Heredia and the Institute of Tropical Medicine Alexander von Humboldt in Lima; to Volker ter Muelen, my host and sponsor as a Humboldt Awardee at the Institute for Virology and Immunology in Wurzburg; to Don Burke, Charlie Hoke, and the personnel of the Armed Forces Research Institute of Medical Science in Bangkok during our work on Japanese encephalitis; and to Bruce Chesebro and his staff in the Laboratory of Persistent Viral Diseases at the Rocky Mountain Laboratories of the National Institute of

Allergy and Infectious Diseases in Hamilton, Montana, where I have been a visiting scientist for three summers and hope to return.

I am profoundly grateful for financial support from the National Institute of Neurological Disorders and Stroke of the National Institute of Health that has sustained me for over 38 years (5 years as a trainee and 34 years of uninterrupted grant support). Many years of support also has been provided the National Multiple Sclerosis Society, the United Cerebral Palsy Research and Educational Foundation, the Hamilton Roddis Foundation, the Pew Charitable Trusts, the Kroc Foundation, the Rockefeller Foundation, the Myerberg Foundation, the Amyotrophic Lateral Sclerosis Society of America, and other institutes of the National Institutes of Health.

Mark Placito and other friends at Lippincott-Raven have maintained affable but sustained pressure on me to undertake and complete this second edition. Jennifer Smith of St. Simon Island, Georgia, provided illustrations.

Sheila Garrity, my former administrative assistant and now Managing Editor of *Annals of Neurology*, has worked nights and weekends to see this project through to completion. Her devotion and loyalty have been extraordinary and deserving of very special thanks.

Fran, my wife and closest friend, has provided good-humored encouragement, unselfish gifts of time, and gentle criticisms of my English composition and attempts at humor. I dedicate this volume to her.

VIRAL INFECTIONS OF THE NERVOUS SYSTEM

Second Edition

PART I

General Principles

Neurovirology, the study of viral infections of the nervous system, has developed as an interdisciplinary field that incorporates aspects of virology, neurobiology, pathology, and immunology. Major contributions have not been dominated by one discipline. Descriptive morphological studies have broken new ground as dramatically as have studies in molecular biology; this is evident for diseases such as subacute sclerosing panencephalitis and progressive multifocal leukoencephalopathy, in which the ultrastructural observations of viruslike particles guided the direction of subsequent virologic studies.

The virologic aspects include any viruses that can infect or affect neural tissue, and thus they encompass most major families of animal viruses. The study of the anatomy and pathology of these infections must deal with the systemic infection as well as the unique aspects of neuroanatomy relevant to penetration and spread of viruses within the nervous system. The immunology of viral infections is complex. Viruses contain an array of different antigens and pose a moving target, because they amplify the antigenic load exponentially during the time that the immune responses are being marshaled. The cytokine network, so critical in stimulating and regulating immune responses, can be overstimulated, jammed, or counterfeited by viral products. Within the central nervous system, the compartmentalization of the immune responses provides a unique milieu in which to achieve viral clearance or allow persistence.

These short introductory chapters do not cover the whole of virology, pathogenesis, and immunology. In virology, coverage has not been limited to viruses that infect humans, because studies of natural and experimental viral infections of other vertebrates often are important in understanding disease mechanisms. The pathogenesis of animal disease is not exhaustively reviewed, but examples have been selected with possible relevance to human disease. Immunologic coverage is similarly limited, with emphasis on the humoral and cellular immune responses within the nervous system.

1

Historical Background

Headache roameth over the desert, blowing like the wind, …
It standeth hostile against the wayfarer, scorching him like the day,
This man it hath struck and
Like the one with heart disease he staggereth,
Like the one bereft of reason he is broken.
Mesopotamian Medical Text

This Babylonian description of Tiu, the evil spirit of headache and an attendant of the Sumerian god of pestilence, is the first known account of an association of headache and fever. The historian Sigerist (1951) speculated that it might represent the first description of meningitis or encephalitis. However, any clinician quickly will recognize that this description could apply to a variety of ailments— ailments that over the next 3,000 years remained undifferentiated under the vague category of "brain fevers."

The evidence for viral infections of the nervous system in ancient times is indirect. An Egyptian stela from the second millenium B.C. pictures a young man with a withered and shortened leg that resembles a sequela of poliomyelitis; and Hippocrates described epidemic parotitis, so neurologic complications presumably occurred. Paralytic poliomyelitis and mumps encephalitis were not described clinically, however, until the 18th century. Shingles were mentioned in premedieval writings, but their relationship to varicella and to nerve roots was not appreciated until the 19th century. Only rabies, the most dramatic of all central nervous system (CNS) infections, was clearly differentiated by the Greek and Roman physicians. Democritus's description of rabies in 500 B.C. is generally granted priority, but it is unclear whether he differentiated rabies from tetanus (Wilkinson, 1974). Aristotle, in 322 B.C., described the behavior of rabid dogs and recognized that the disease was transmitted to other animals by biting, but he specifically commented that humans were exempt. Celsus, in the first century A.D., was the first to relate hydrophobia in humans to rabies in animals. He also ascribed the disease to a "virus," using the term in its classical sense as a disease-producing vapor, like the stench arising from swamps. Oddly, he did differentiate between "viruses" in animal bites and "venoms" in snakebites.

Brain fevers and sleeping sickness were recorded during the Middle Ages, but anatomic localization of signs and differentiation of syndromes were not accomplished until the 17th century. The application of pathology and the systematization of medicine were introduced primarily by Thomas Sydenham, whose method of organizing the morass of clinical signs and symptoms into syndromes provided the basis for the great European schools of medicine that flourished during the 18th and 19th centuries. During that time, Underwood's clinical description of paralytic poliomyelitis (1787) and Hamilton's description of the neurologic complications of mumps (1790) appeared. Despite the advances made in other areas of medicine, virology and neuropathology bloomed late, and the clinical differentiation of most CNS infections had to await a technical development—a method for spinal fluid examination.

Heinrich Quinke (1842–1922) studied under Virchow and Helmholtz and spent most of his academic life on the faculty at Kiel, Germany. His name has been memorialized by eponymic association with angioneurotic edema and the ungual pulses of syphilitic aortic insufficiency, but clearly his great contribution to medicine was the development of lumbar puncture and examination of cerebrospinal fluid. During his student days, Quinke had introduced needles into the subarachnoid spaces of dogs and had found that removal of fluid caused no apparent damage. Therefore, he posited that introduction of a fine needle into a lumbar interspace in infants with hydrocephalus might relieve the pressure and save their lives (Hiller, 1953). Unfortunately, his efforts to cure hydrocephalus failed, but he exploited the technique to other ends (Quinke, 1891). In a remarkable series of studies over the next 5 years, he described the cells, protein measurements, and sugar concentrations in normal and abnormal fluid; he described diminished sugar concentration and identified bacteria in purulent meningitis, and he found the tubercle bacilli in the fibrinous pedicle in tuberculous meningitis. In 1896, he published the first description of viral meningitis and encephalitis under the title of "Ueber Meningitis serosa und verwandte Zustande." This paper described patients suffering from varied diseases, but it included descriptions of several young servant girls with a mild illness of headache and fever, increased numbers of cells and increased protein in the spinal fluid, and a benign clinical course.

This description went largely unnoticed, however, and credit for the first description of viral meningitis usually is given to a Swedish pediatrician, Arvid Wallgren (1925). He described the same syndrome as a "new" disease entity 29 years after Quinke's description, and he coined the name aseptic meningitis. Initial interest in encephalitis, its neuropathologic correlates, and its possible viral cause came with the epidemic of encephalitis lethargica. This began with von Economo's clinical and pathologic studies in 1917, but the disease mysteriously disappeared before modern virologic methods were developed. Ironically, the cause of the disease that kindled early interest in viral infections of the CNS may never be found.

ORIGINS OF VIROLOGY

The concept of contagion also developed during the 19th century and culminated with Pasteur's formulation of immunology and his development of a postexposure vaccine for rabies. However, Pasteur did not suspect that the agent of rabies was fundamentally different from other microorganisms (Wilkinson, 1974).

Virology as a distinct discipline began in botany, not in medicine. Tobacco mosaic virus was the first virus that was recovered in the laboratory and recognized as a filterable agent. This occurred in independent studies by Iwanowski in Russia and Beijerinck in Holland, and Beijerinck proposed an obligate intracellular parasitism of the virus. Soon, other infectious agents were found that passed through "bacteria-proof filters," but arguments continued as to whether they represented ultrasmall bacteria, liquid forms, toxins, or complex molecules. The visualization of viruses had to await the development of the electron microscope. The unraveling of their physical–chemical structures began with the crystallization of tobacco mosaic virus and poliovirus in the 1930s, but the molecular biologic studies were largely limited to bacteriophages until the cell culture methods of the 1950s enabled studies of nucleic acids and protein synthesis of animal viruses.

Although the nature of filterable viruses was not defined, a great deal of information about viral illnesses was accumulated during the early 20th century. The arthropod transmission of yellow fever was established in 1901, the filterable nature of rabies virus was demonstrated in 1903, and poliomyelitis was transmitted to monkeys in 1909. Although clinical virology was still limited to animal transmission studies in the early 1930s, encephalitis viruses were recovered from brain tissues of patients dying of epidemic encephalitis in Japan and St. Louis, as well as from horses with encephalitis in California and the Middle Atlantic area (western and eastern "equine" encephalitis viruses). In 1935, lymphocytic choriomeningitis virus, previously found in healthy mice, was isolated from spinal fluids of patients with meningitis, and this became the first established viral cause of aseptic meningitis. With the introduction of new methods for clinical virus isolation, including embryonated eggs in the 1930s and tissue cultures in the 1950s, the numbers of viruses found to be associated with acute neurologic diseases burgeoned and then reached a plateau (Fig. 1.1). Only a small number of new viruses have been related to acute neurologic diseases during the past 30 years. Knowledge about their pathogenesis, epidemiology, and clinical presentations has expanded, but the excitement about viruses in neurologic diseases has moved to new arenas.

VIRUSES AND CHRONIC DISEASE

Speculation and investigation concerning the possible roles of viruses in chronic diseases had progressed in different quarters for many years, but then,

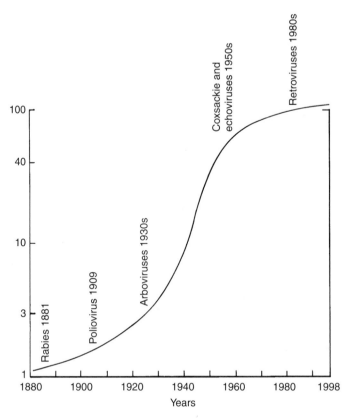

FIG. 1.1. Viruses recovered from human CNS diseases over the past century. The abrupt increase in numbers between 1950 and 1965 is evident on the logarithmic scale.

30 years ago, diverse approaches and observations seemed to coalesce abruptly. In medical research, attempts to transmit or recover viruses from chronic neurologic diseases were centered primarily in the Soviet Union. Most virologists in the United States and Western Europe were oriented toward acute epidemic viral infections, because most, like myself, had served their laboratory apprenticeships working with influenza and poliomyelitis viruses. In contrast, many Soviet virologists had been initiated with work on tick-borne encephalitis virus. This virus, first isolated by Zil'ber and his colleagues in 1937, had been associated with epilepsia partialis continua, a chronic and even progressive sequela of the acute encephalitis, and the virus has been isolated from surgically removed epileptogenic foci years after the acute encephalitis (Brody et al., 1965). Other chronic neurologic diseases, including Parkinson's disease, amyotrophic lateral sclerosis, and multiple sclerosis, were also believed to result

from persistent infections with this or other viruses. It was no accident that the first reports of possible virus recovery from multiple sclerosis (Margulis et al., 1946) and transmission of amyotrophic lateral sclerosis (Zil'ber et al., 1963) originated in the Soviet Union. Although unconfirmed, these studies stimulated others to search beyond the horizons fixed by studies of acute influenza and poliomyelitis.

The contributions of veterinary medicine and comparative pathology must not be underestimated. The term *slow infection* was coined in 1954 by Bjorn Sigurdsson at the Institute of Experimental Pathology in Iceland. He used the term in relation to several sheep diseases with long latency periods and progressive clinical courses leading to death. The prototype was scrapie, referred to in Icelandic as rida, a disease that had been recognized for 200 years and had been assumed to represent an autosomal recessive degenerative disease of the brain. The disease was transmitted between sheep by two French investigators in 1936 (Cuille and Chelle), but controversy persisted into the 1960s as to whether scrapie was an infectious disease or a genetically transmitted disease. However, the heated controversies about scrapie were not widely appreciated outside of the veterinary fraternity. Following the initial descriptions of kuru by Carleton Gajdusek and Vincent Zigas in 1957, with its strange epidemiology, progressive ataxia, and noninflammatory gray matter cell loss and vacuolization, William Hadlow (1959), a veterinarian, brought scrapie to the attention of the medical world, noting its remarkable similarities to kuru.

In December 1964, a workshop on slow, latent, and temperate infections was organized by Gajdusek and Gibbs at the National Institutes of Health (NIH). The workshop included veterinarians, pathologists, epidemiologists, immunologists, clinicians, and virologists of varied interests. Many met for the first time. One group of us had recently returned from a visit to the Soviet laboratories; the week before, at a New York City meeting, two teams of neuropathologists had reported papovavirus-like particles in the brains of patients with progressive multifocal leukoencephalopathy; and the attempts at NIH to transmit kuru and other chronic neurologic diseases to subhuman primates were under way.

There was an aura of excitement that we were on the verge of relating viruses to chronic human neurologic disease. Gajdusek and Gibbs wrote, "if even a single one of these many syndromes of unknown etiology can be traced to a virus or virus–gene interactions—we shall win a significant advance in our understanding of diseases of the human brain." The next year, filamentous particles were described in subacute sclerosing panencephalitis (Boutielle et al., 1965). In 1966, kuru was transmitted (Gajdusek et al., 1966). In 1968, Creutzfeldt–Jakob disease was transmitted (Gibbs et al., 1968). In 1969, measles virus was recovered from patients with subacute sclerosing panencephalitis (Horta-Barbosa et al., 1969). In 1971, viruses were recovered from progressive multifocal leukoencephalopathy (Padgett et al., 1971). These advances gave promise to the possible relation of viruses to common chronic neurologic diseases, such as multiple sclerosis, amyotrophic lateral sclerosis, Parkinson's disease, Alzheimer's disease, and schizophrenia. Over the subsequent two decades, however, only progressive rubella panencephalitis was added to the list. The next and unexpected challenge among slow infections was from a new virus with an unprecedented array of clinical syndromes related to that single virus.

RETROVIRUSES

Since 1980, four retroviruses have been related to human disease: human T-cell lymphotropic virus (HTLV) types I and II and human immunodeficiency virus (HIV) types 1 and 2. Each of these viruses has been associated with neurologic diseases. HTLV-I has been linked to tropical spastic paraparesis, a chronic myelopathy, and HTLV-I has been related tenuously to polymyositis. In contrast, HIV-1 and 2 have been associated with a variety of diseases of the CNS, peripheral nervous system, and muscle.

Retrospective studies of autopsies have documented sporadic deaths from the acquired immunodeficiency syndrome (AIDS) in the 1960s, but the disease was not recognized until 1981 (Blattner, 1991). The subsequent spread of this infection throughout the world has been unprecedented in modern times. Over 4 million have developed AIDS and over 21 million are currently infected with HIV (Piot, 1996). Since the majority of those infected incur infection of the CNS early and since the majority of those with CNS infection will eventually develop neurologic disease, HIV has become the most prevalent CNS infection in the world and about 10 million of those currently infected may develop neurologic diseases during the next decade.

From a historical perspective, the spread of HIV in human populations came at a fortuitous time. Markers for hematopoietic cells had been developed, and growth factors had been defined to enable their cultivation; extensive knowledge of the molecular biology of retroviruses had been gained through cancer research; and some insights into the pathogenesis of animal disease had been accumulated through studies of lentiviruses in ungulates as possible models for multiple sclerosis. Had the epidemic occurred a decade or two earlier, it is hard to imagine the frustrations that would have arisen in trying to recover a virus, in explaining the immunodeficiency, or in mounting efforts in prevention or treatment. Instead, the progress in understanding AIDS has been unparalleled—the virus was recovered within 2 years of the description of the disease; 2 years later, sequencing of the virus was completed, the complex replication cycle was largely defined, the major modes and determinants of human-to-human spread were clarified, and animal models were discovered; an effective antiviral drug was developed, tested, and licensed by 1987; and, by 1988, several candidate vaccines were in initial stages of testing. Despite these accomplishments, the spread of HIV continues, but stemming the epidemic requires modifying human behavior—a challenge beyond the scope of this book.

SUPPLEMENTARY BIBLIOGRAPHY

Evans AS. *Causation and disease: a chronological journey.* New York: Plenum Publishing, 1993.
Gajdusek DC, Gibbs CJ, Alpers M. *Slow latent and temperate virus infections.* NINDB monograph 2. Washington, DC: US Government Printing Office, 1965.
Hughes SS. *The virus: a history of the concept.* New York: Science History Publications, 1977.

2

Viruses and Virus–Cell Interactions

Alive or dead is a stupid question, because it does not exhaust the possibilities. Our general notion of the structure of the universe leads us to expect that we shall meet with things that are not so alive as a sunflower, and not so dead as a brick.

A.E. Boycott,
The Transition from Live to Dead:
The Nature of Filterable Viruses,
presidential address, Royal Society of Medicine, 1928

Over the past generations, Boycott's prediction has proved correct. It has been shown that viruses contain genetic information encoded in nucleic acids and that this genome is enmeshed within a protective protein coating, but other hallmarks of life are missing. Despite the knowledge of structure and chemical composition of many viruses, the arguments of whether viruses were alive or dead and whether or not they were microorganisms continued—albeit, at a more sophisticated level. Lwoff (1957), emphasizing the presence of only a single nucleic acid in viruses, their lack of organelles or a nucleus, their inability to grow or undergo binary fission, and their lack of any system for energy production, concluded that viruses are not microorganisms and that they are not alive. His conclusion was simply that "viruses are viruses." On the other hand, Luria and associates (1978) defended the vitality of viruses and took the position that genetic perpetuation is the very essence of life.

NATURE OF VIRUSES

Viruses can be defined as "entities whose genomes are elements of nucleic acid that replicate inside living cells using the cellular synthetic machinery and causing the synthesis of specialized elements that can transfer the viral genome to other cells" (Luria et al., 1978). The definition of a virus is no longer dependent on size, lack of a cell wall, or morphology. Viruses contain only one species of nucleic acid. Initially it was assumed this must be DNA to allow for replication, but the majority of animal viruses contain a genome of single-stranded

RNA. Thus, viruses have modes of transmission of genetic information that are unique in biology. Furthermore, some viruses have proved to have single-stranded DNA, others double-stranded RNA, and others RNA that can be reverse transcribed to DNA, so virology is rife with exceptions to the Watson–Crick model of double-helical DNA replication.

Structures of Viruses

The nucleic acid and protective coats of viruses can be arranged in a variety of structural forms. The two major basic configurations are spherical and helical (Fig. 2.1). In the former, the nucleic acid is surrounded by a shell of repeated polypeptide structural units that are grouped into morphological units termed

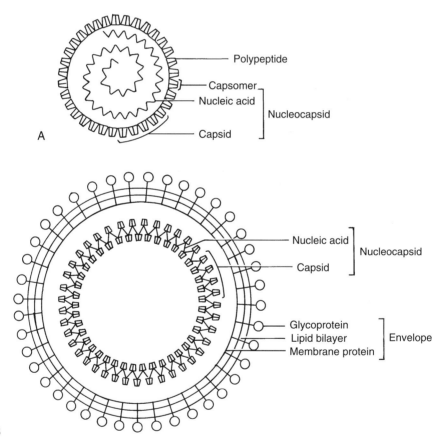

FIG. 2.1. Diagrams of the structures of a nonenveloped icosahedral virus **(A)** and an enveloped virus with helical nucleocapsid structure **(B)**. Most viruses have additional core proteins, associated with the nucleic acid in the icosahedral virus and with the nucleocapsid in the helical virus. (Adapted from Caspar et al., 1962.)

capsomers that can be seen with the electron microscope. This shell or capsid usually takes the form of an icosahedron (isometric polyhedron) with faces of repeating subunits arranged in precisely defined triangular patterns. In the helical configuration, the nucleic acid is interwoven among repeated capsid proteins stacked like a spiral staircase in defined patterns to form tubules. Orthomyxoviruses and paramyxoviruses, rhabdoviruses, bunyaviruses, filoviruses, arenaviruses, and coronaviruses are constructed in this form, but each has a distinctive length, width and periodicity.

In either spherical or helical configuration, the nucleic acid and its capsid together form the virus nucleocapsid. This nucleocapsid may or may not be enclosed by an envelope. Many icosahedral viruses and all known helical animal viruses have envelopes. The envelope usually is added as the virus buds through a lipid bilayer membrane of the host cell in which host proteins have been replaced by viral proteins. The envelope proteins extending out from the lipid envelope usually are glycosylated. The viral membrane proteins serve as receptor-binding sites, activate fusion, and may facilitate virus release by receptor destruction. With the exception of the large and complex poxviruses, the lipids and carbohydrates of enveloped viruses are of cellular origin and, therefore, are characteristic of the species and cell type of the host cell.

The term *virion* is used to describe the mature particle. In the case of nonenveloped animal viruses, the virion is the polyhedral nucleocapsid. In the case of enveloped viruses, the virion refers to the enveloped nucleocapsid. The term *virus* embraces not just the virion but all phases in the virus life cycle (Caspar et al., 1962). Thus, a cell containing only the viral nucleic acid can be said to be virus infected. These definitions explain why the tubular structures seen in subacute sclerosing panencephalitis are referred to as viruses or as nucleocapsids but not as virions, because measles virus in its final form is enveloped. Conversely, the papovavirus nucleocapsids seen in the oligodendrocytes of patients with progressive multifocal leukoencephalopathy can be called virions, because papovaviruses in their final form have no envelopes.

Virion morphology can be studied by electron microscopy, using primarily two methods: shadow casting, in which an opaque material is vaporized and angled in order to cast images of the virus shape; and negative staining, in which a suspension of virus is dried with phosphotungstic acid or uranyl acetate so that the various angular faces of the virus will become visible. With these two methods, the numbers of faces and angles and the capsomeric structure have been determined. This structural detail cannot be seen in transmission electron micrographs of infected cells or tissues. Consequently, definitive virus identification within cells often is not possible. Many ultrastructural alterations within cells may resemble viruses. Ribosomes in damaged cells can form pseudocrystalline patterns resembling picornavirus arrays (Byers, 1966); glycogen particles or reticulosomes can be confused with papovaviruses (Carter et al., 1972); cytoplasmic rod-shaped tubular bodies of endothelial cells (Kirk and Hutchinson, 1978) and the marginization of nuclear chromatin can assume filamentous configurations simulating paramyxovirus nucleocapsids. Conversely, the absence of morphologically identifiable particles in cells or tissues does not constitute substantive evidence against the presence of a virus.

Classification of Viruses

Virus taxonomy has been beset with debate. Logically, viruses should be catalogued according to nucleic acid content, nucleocapsid structure, type of envelope, and other structural and chemical properties (Gibbs et al., 1966), but the traditional haphazard terminology is too firmly entrenched to be readily displaced by logical taxonomy. Some viruses have names that were given to describe their resultant diseases, which were recognized and named long before the viruses were discovered (e.g., smallpox, yellow fever, rabies, and mumps). Other names describe the pathologic changes associated with the infection (e.g., poliomyelitis and lymphocytic choriomeningitis). Still other names have been devised to reflect the cytopathic effects seen in tissue cultures (e.g., foamy viruses) or to reflect ultrastructural features (e.g., arenaviruses, whose envelopes contain granules resembling sand, filamentous filoviruses, and togaviruses, which have neatly uniform envelopes). Other names refer to the anatomic site of the original or most frequent isolation (e.g., adenovirus, enterovirus, and rhinovirus) or refer to the geographic site of first recovery (an honored tradition with arthropod-borne and zoonotic viruses that has given us such colorful names as Guanarito, Semliki Forest, Bunyamwera, Cache Valley, and Sixgun City).

Perhaps our fascination with the origins of names in virology has spawned this resistance to the adoption of cryptograms or a Latin binomial system similar to that used in bacteriology. A case in point concerns the original recovery of new enteroviruses during clinical poliovirus investigations. Dalldorf recovered the first such viruses from mice inoculated with stool material from paralyzed children being studied for concurrent poliovirus infections. In retrospect, he wrote, "Coxsackie is the name of an old Hudson River town and a family of viruses. The virus was named for the town because they were first recognized there and because we knew too little about the diseases they caused to venture a descriptive name" (Dalldorf, 1952). Soon after that, cell culture methods were introduced for the isolation of polioviruses from stools, and another group of viruses made themselves known. Initially, these viruses, which confused and complicated poliovirus studies, were referred to informally among laboratories as "the little bastards." When a more suitable name was needed for publication purposes, the pseudonym orphans was proposed, invoking the justification that they were "viruses in search of disease." This was later expanded to the name enteric cytopathogenic human orphans, or ECHOs, now echoviruses.

Classification into families and genuses continues to rely heavily on ultrastructural morphology, the genomic composition (e.g., RNA or DNA, positive-sense or negative-sense RNA, segmented nucleic acid), and strategies of replication. Sequence data might seem a better taxonomic criterion at first view, but the hijacking of host genes by viruses (and *vice versa*) and recombinants among viruses lead to complexities in making phylogenetic conclusions (Murphy, 1996). The International Committee on Taxonomy of Viruses has most recently classi-fied viruses into 71 families, 11 subfamilies, 164 genera, and over 4,000 member viruses (Murphy et al., 1994); 24 families contain viruses that infect humans, and the majority of those contain members that affect the nervous system.

The DNA viruses that are discussed in this volume are divided into six fami-lies (Table 2.1), and the RNA viruses can be divided into 12 families (Table 2.2). Each family, in general, has a common size and structure (Fig. 2.2). Some agents, such as the subacute spongiform encephalopathy agents or prions, are as yet so ill-defined structurally and biochemically that they defy classification (Murphy et al., 1994). Indeed, they are probably not viruses under our current definitions.

Virus Cultivation and Quantitation

The cultivation of viruses requires the use of living cells. The cellular systems used include animals, embryonated eggs, and cell cultures.

Early virus isolations and quantitations used a variety of animals. A white mouse bred for susceptibility to a variety of human viruses became the standard laboratory host in virology during the 1920s and 1930s, and newborn mice remain the most sensitive detectors of some viruses (e.g., arboviruses). Work on the subacute spongiform encephalopathy agents continues to rely on animals, because the cultivation and quantification of these agents in cell cultures still are not possible. Hamsters have proved uniquely useful in studies of virus-induced tumors and cerebral malformation because of the remarkable immaturity of the brain of newborn hamsters born after a gestation period of only 15 days.

Embryonated eggs were introduced for virus isolation and cultivation by Goodpasture and his colleagues in 1931. The different embryonic membranes of the egg that enclose the amniotic cavity, allantoic cavity, and yolk sac and the chorioallantoic membrane provide sites for growth of most of the poxviruses and herpesviruses, mumps virus, and influenza viruses. Although eggs seldom are used now for virus recovery, they still constitute an economical and efficient host for the cultivation of orthomyxoviruses and some paramyxoviruses.

The introduction of cell cultures had a singular impact on virology. Vaccinia virus had been propagated in cell cultures in 1913 (Steinhardt et al., 1913), but general application of cell culture methods was not possible until the advent of antibiotics. In 1949, Enders, Weller, and Robbins reported the growth of poliomyelitis virus in human embryonic cell culture, and cell cultures quickly became the predominant method in both diagnostic and investigative virology. When cells of animal tissues are dispersed and placed in flasks with specific medium and serum, a heterogeneous monolayer culture develops with multiple cell types. These *primary cell cultures* can be subcultured several times, but with an increasing overgrowth of fibroblasts. Human embryonic fibroblasts and other

TABLE 2.1. *Major DNA viruses*

Family Genus Examples that infect humans	Virion diameter (nm)	NA[a]	Enveloped	Distinguishing features
Poxviridae *Orthopoxvirus* Variola (smallpox) virus Vaccinia virus	200 × 300	ds	+	Large complex brick-shaped virion with helical nucleocapsid and lateral bodies; virions contain many enzymes and over 30 proteins; cause exanthemata
Herpesviridae *Simplexvirus* Herpes simplex virus, type 1 Herpes simplex virus, type 2 *Varicellovirus* Varicella–zoster virus *Cytomegalovirus* Human cytomegalovirus *Lymphocryptovirus* Epstein–Barr virus *Roseolovirus* Human herpesvirus 6 Human herpesvirus 7	120–200	ds	+	Large complex spherical or amorphic virion; commonly latent in host
Adenoviridae *Mastadenovirus* Human adenovirus, types 1–49	70–90	ds	–	Icosahedral virion with projecting spikes; associated primarily with respiratory disease in humans, but can cause neoplastic transformation in other species
Papovaviridae *Papillomavirus* Wart viruses *Polymavirus* Simian virus 40 JC virus BK virus	45–55	ds	–	Icosahedral virion with supercoded circular DNA; most types cause neoplastic transformation of cells
Hepadnaviridae *Orthohepadnavirus* Hepatitis B	40–48	ds with ss region	+	Envelope contains surface antigen hepatitis B retroid DNA step in replication
Parvoviridae *Erythrovirus* Human parvovirus B19	18–26	ss	–	Icosahedral virion; palindromic ends of DNA; DNA replicates only in cells in S phase of DNA synthesis or with aid of helper virus

[a]NA, nucleic acid; ds, double stranded; ss, single stranded.

TABLE 2.2. *Major RNA viruses*

Family Genus Examples that infect humans[a]	Virion diameter (nm)	NA[b]	Enveloped	Distinguishing features
Paramyxoviridae *Paramyxovirus* Human parainfluenza viruses 1 and 3 *Rubulavirus* Mumps virus Human parainfluenza viruses 2 and 4 *Morbillivirus* Measles virus *Pneumovirus* Human respiratory syncytial virus	150–300	ss – sense	+	Large pleomorphic virions with helical nucleocapsid; respiratory infections in humans with systemic spread
Orthomyxoviridae *Influenzavirus* Influenza viruses A, B, and C	80–120	ss – sense segmented (7–8)	+	Associated primarily with respiratory diseases in humans
Rhabdoviridae *Lyssavirus* Rabies virus *Vesiculovirus* Vesicular stomatitis virus	70–85 × 180	ss – sense	+	Internal helical structure RNA and bullet-shaped envelope
Filovividae *Filovirus* Ebola virus Marburg virus	80 × 1,000	ss – sense	+	Long filamentous forms up to 14,000-nm length, sometimes branched or curled
Bunyaviridae *Bunyavirus* California encephalitis virus La Crosse virus Jamestown Canyon virus Snowshoe hare virus Tahyna virus Inkoo virus Cache Valley virus Tensaw virus *Phlebovirus* Rift Valley fever virus *Nairovirus* Crimean–Congo hemorrhagic fever virus *Hantavirus* Hantaviruses	80 × 120	ss – sense segmented (3)	+	Helical nucleocapsids Formerly group C arboviruses Hantaviruses not arthropod-borne

TABLE 2.2. *Continued*

Family Genus Examples that infect humans[a]	Virion diameter (nm)	NA[b]	Enveloped	Distinguishing features
Arenaviridae *Arenavirus* Lymphocytic choriomeningitis virus Lassa virus Junin virus Machupo virus Guanarito virus Sabiá virus	50–300	ss – sense segmented (2)	+	Pleomorphic virions (often shaped like red cells) with helical nucleocapsid; containing granules that are host-cell ribosomes. Chronic rodent infections
Retroviridae *Oncovirus* (HTLV-BLV)[c] Human T-cell lymphotropic viruses I and II *Lentivirus* Human immunodeficiency viruses 1 and 2 *Spumavirus* Human isolates (no known pathogens)	80–100	ss + sense	+	Virions unique with diploid nucleic acid (two identical RNA molecules bonded into 70S RNA by small host RNA), reverse transcriptase, and retroid DNA step in replication
Coronaviridae *Coronavirus* Several human serotypes	80–220	ss + sense	+	Helical nucleocapsid with envelope containing drumstick projections; cause human respiratory diseases
Reoviridae *Orthoreovirus* Reoviruses 1–3 *Coltivirus* Colorado tick fever virus *Rotavirus* Group A and B human rotoviruses	60–80	ds + sense segmented (10)	–	Icosahedral virions with unique two capsid shells; RNA in 10–12 double strands Diarrhea in infants
Togaviridae *Alphavirus* Eastern encephalitis virus Western encephalitis virus Venezuelan equine encephalitis virus *Rubivirus* Rubella virus	70	ss + sense	+	Small icosahedral capsids Alpha and flaviviruses are former group A and B arboviruses: over 200 types are transmitted by and replicate in hematophagous vectors; each has limited geographic distribution

TABLE 2.2. *Continued*

Family Genus Examples that infect humans[a]	Virion diameter (nm)	NA[b]	Enveloped	Distinguishing features
Flaviviridae	45–60	ss + sense	+	
Flavirus				
St. Louis encephalitis virus				
Japanese encephalitis virus				
Murray Valley encephalitis virus				
Tick-borne encephalitis viruses				
Yellow fever virus				
Dengue viruses				
Pestivirus				
No human pathogens				
Genus unnamed				
Hepatitis C virus				
Picornaviridae	28–30	ss + sense	–	Small icosahedral virions
Enterovirus				Common enteric pathogens
Polioviruses 1–3				that may cause CNS,
Coxsackie viruses A 1–22, A 24, B 1–6				cardiac, or respiratory
Human echoviruses 1–7, 9, 11–27, 29–33				disease
Human enteroviruses 68–71				
Cardiovirus				
Encephalomyocarditis virus				
Rhinovirus				
Human rhinoviruses 1–100				
Hepatovirus				
Hepatitis A virus				

[a]Borna virus remains unclassified. Although a negative-sense single-stranded RNA virus, it has other features that suggest it will be in a new family once structure is better defined.
[b]NA, nucleic acid; ds, double stranded; ss, single stranded.
[c]HTLV-BLV, human T-cell lymphotrophic virus–bovine leukemia virus.

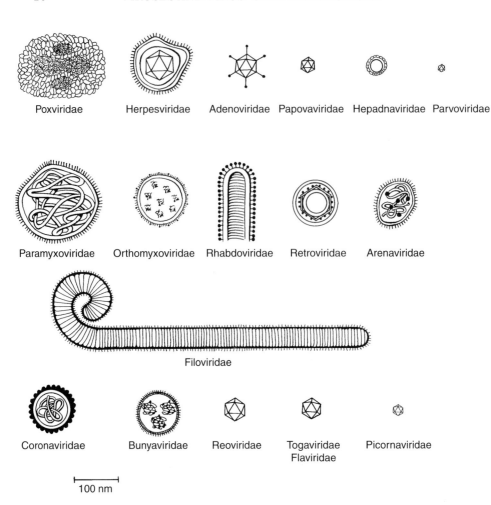

FIG. 2.2. Diagrams of shapes and relative sizes of major animal virus families. Icosahedral and helical structures of nucleocapsids are shown within enveloped viruses. Poxviruses have a complex structure with a biconcave DNA-containing nucleoid and two dense lateral bodies. Herpesviruses have a dense irregular layer of matrix protein on the inner surface of the envelope. Adenoviruses are nonenveloped viruses with characteristic elongated fibrous projections. Rhabdoviruses have a unique bullet-shaped envelope. Filoviruses resemble elongated rhabdoviruses, often circled at end. Arenaviruses are characterized by dense granules that are host cell ribosomes. Coronaviruses are characterized by the teardrop configuration of envelope glycoproteins. [Adapted from White and Fenner (1994).]

undifferentiated cells are now widely used, because they can be maintained *in vitro* through as many as 100 subcultivations before dying. These cultures maintain their original chromosome numbers and are called *diploid cell strains*. *Cell lines* consist of "immortal" cells that can be subcultured indefinitely. These cells are not diploid and usually are derived from tumors, such as the HeLa cells, or from animal cells that presumably are transformed by endogenous viruses.

Explant or organ cultures are prepared from tissue slices or fragments rather than from dispersed cells. In explant cultures of brain, neurons may persist in the central fragment, and an outgrowth of astrocytes and epithelial cells will develop. When early fetal brain is explanted, neuron and oligodendrocyte precursor cells can be identified migrating out over a rug of the astrocytes and epithelial cells (Oster-Granite and Herndon, 1978). Explant cultures have been useful for recovering viruses that are highly cell associated and for growing viruses that have fastidious requirements of cellular susceptibility. For example, the recovery of measles virus from patients with subacute sclerosing panencephalitis was successful by explanting cells from brain tissue from biopsies or autopsies, with subsequent coculture with other cells. The original isolations of the JC virus from progressive multifocal leukoencephalopathy necessitated the use of human embryonic brain explant cultures in which spongioblasts develop; these cells productively produce the virus, and these cells are not maintained in dispersed or subcultured neural cells.

Quantitation

Virus may be detected or quantitated by two general methods: (a) growth of virus and measurement of infectious units, or (b) detection and quantitation of particles, proteins, or genomes. Tissue suspensions, body fluids, or cell culture homogenates can be inoculated into animals or cell cultures in tenfold dilutions, which yields an assessment of a 50% virus-effect dose whether it be a 50% lethal dose (LD_{50}) in animals or a 50% cytopathic effect (or 50% tissue culture dose, TCD_{50}) in cell cultures. Plaquing of viruses under agar can give more precise quantitation of the number of infectious plaque-forming units (PFU). In addition, surviving animals can be challenged with lethal doses of virus to calculate a 50% infectious dose (ID_{50}), which is of interest if the amount of virus required to infect is less than the amount needed to kill or cause disease.

Methods that do not assay a biologic effect must be regarded with caution and not misinterpreted to imply amount of infectivity. Some viruses produce an envelope glycoprotein that hemagglutinates red blood cells; quantitation of hemagglutinin in embryonated egg or cell culture fluids measures the amount of protein and indirectly implies the limit of infectivity in limiting dilutions. The number of viral particles has little relationship to infectivity in many infections, because many noninfectious particles may be generated. A virus preparation that by direct electron-microscopic count may have 10^{10} particles per milliliter may contain only 10^8 TCD_{50} or PFU and 10^5 mouse LD_{50}. Many particles may be noninfectious, and in many indicator systems more than one infectious particle is necessary to produce an effect. Therefore, comparisons must use the same method of quantification.

Hybridization

Molecular hybridization or nucleic acid hybridization is a method for detecting and quantitating the viral nucleic acid. This method employs the interaction of a single-stranded polynucleotide chain with a complementary base sequence to form a double strand. Hybridization of RNA with RNA, RNA with DNA, or DNA with DNA is possible, depending on the reagents and the virus being studied. A radioactive or enzyme-labeled "probe" is made from a single-stranded polynucleotide, and this probe can be reacted in solution to detect the presence of complementary viral strands, which will form double-stranded polynucleotides, or it can be reacted with tissue, followed by autoradiography or immunocytochemistry (*in situ* hybridization) to determine the cellular localization of viral genomes or viral messenger RNA. Many variations of nucleic acid hybridization have been developed, so that it can be used to determine not only the presence of viral nucleic acid or messenger RNA but also the number of copies of the genome, whether the entire genome or only part of the genome is present, and, with *in situ* hybridization, which cells in tissues harbor the genome or messages.

Polymerase Chain Reaction

Polymerase chain reaction (PCR) is a method derived from molecular genetics that has amazing sensitivity. Optimally, a single molecule of DNA can be amplified and detected in a specimen. To examine for RNA, complementary DNA (cDNA) is generated with a reverse transcriptase. Four components are required in the reaction: (a) the specimen containing the DNA or cDNA to be examined; (b) short synthetic oligonucleotide primers, one complementary to each strand of the DNA and lying on opposite ends of the region to be amplified; (c) an excess of nucleotide triphosphate molecules for synthesizing DNA; and (d) a DNA polymerase, whose natural function is to repair or replace DNA, to catalyze the generation of the complementary strands. The use of DNA polymerase from thermophilic bacteria recovered from hot springs has allowed multiple rounds of synthesis and automation. Each cycle of amplification has three brief temperature steps: (a) heating to denature the complementary strands of deoxynucleotide, (b) physiologic temperatures for extension, and (c) a brief cycle of cooling for reannealing of complementary strands. A segment defined in length by the two primers is amplified geometrically. To determine the number of molecules in the original specimen, serial dilution of known quantities of the same fragment of DNA with a defined deletion or insertion can be added to the multiple aliquots of the original specimens before the cycling begins. These yield fragments of a shorter or longer length and the number of molecules of DNA or RNA per unit of tissue or fluid can be determined by comparison with the control. This can be done directly from homogenates of infected brain or spinal cord (Johnson et al., 1996).

With this method, primers can be synthesized complementary to common sequences of enteroviruses to screen for many viruses simultaneously or complementary to unique sequences that will differentiate between herpes simplex viruses, types 1 and 2. Sequences of a genetically heterogeneous virus such as human immunodeficiency virus (HIV) can be obtained directly from tissues, avoiding the selection of strains by *in vitro* cell culture systems. Furthermore, *in situ* PCR can be performed on tissue sections to localize single molecules of viral nucleic acid to individual cells, and double staining is feasible to identify definitely the cell type containing viral DNA or RNA.

These methods are so exquisitely sensitive that they pose many pitfalls. The temperatures of the reactions need to be set for maximal stringency. The quality and specificity of the primers are critical to avoid amplification of extraneous segments of DNA or to target a region of sequence variability without failing to detect the target DNA. Contamination of specimens by medical or laboratory personnel, or cross-contamination from a prior positive specimen, is a constant concern. If tissue blocks have touched or been touched by the same ungloved hands, cross-contamination is possible. *In situ* PCR is beset with even greater problems of nonspecific binding, drying of sections, and inexplicable artifacts. Results must be interpreted cautiously. A positive signal for Epstein–Barr, cytomegalovirus, or human herpesvirus 6 in tissue or spinal fluid may represent nothing more than a passing single mononuclear cell with a latent viral gene, and HIV in a neonate's blood might represent the contamination of a single maternal cell.

VIRUS–CELL INTERACTIONS

Viral parasitism differs from bacterial or animal parasitism in that it occurs at the biochemical level (the virus uses host enzyme systems and enzyme products for viral synthesis) and at the genetic level (there may be destruction or incapacitation of the host genome or alteration of host genes by the insertion of viral genes). Some understanding of the mechanisms of virus replication in the single cell is helpful before addressing the more complex issues of virus replication in animals.

The basic steps in the virus–cell infectious cycle are: (a) adsorption or attachment of the virus to the cell cytoplasmic membrane, (b) penetration of viral material and uncoating of the nucleic acid within the cell, (c) transcription and translation of early proteins, (d) replication of the viral nucleic acid, (e) transcription and translation of late proteins, and (f) assembly and release of mature virions (Fig. 2.3). The multiplication cycle time in permissive cell cultures ranges from 6 hours for picornaviruses to 48 hours for adenoviruses, papo-

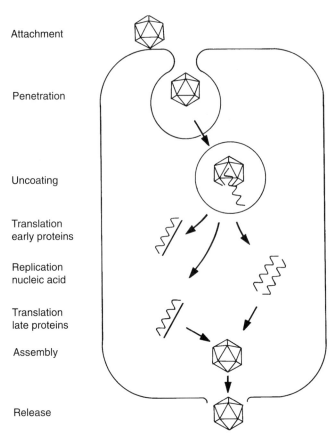

FIG. 2.3. Diagram of the infectious cycle in the host cell. Shown is a naked icosahedral virus that penetrates by endopinocytosis. Nucleic acids are represented by *wavy lines* and polypeptides by *straight lines*. The positions of the host cell nucleus and cytoplasm have been eliminated, because different viruses replicate nucleic acids and assemble in different locations.

vaviruses, and some herpesviruses. This period between inoculation and the first detection of progeny virus is referred to as the *eclipse period*.

Attachment

Viruses have no inherent mobility, and therefore their contact with cells depends on Brownian movement or passive transport by host cells or fluids. However, random contact does not often lead to adsorption; for some viruses, attachment occurs only about once in 10,000 contacts. This finding alone indicates that there are specific sites for binding on both the virus and the cell surface. A single polypeptide of the virus surface generally functions as the virus antireceptor or ligand, but it may have several domains, each of which reacts with a different receptor. Enveloped viruses have glycoproteins extending from the envelope, one of which serves to attach the virus to a receptor site. For example, some spikes of paramyxoviruses are composed of a hemagglutinin glycoprotein that determines attachment, and the others are composed of a fusion glycoprotein that determines penetration.

The specificity of cell receptor sites is an important factor in determining species specificity, tissue tropism, and the selective vulnerability of selective cell populations (Norkin, 1995; Holmes, 1997). Some viruses share common receptors; for example, the three polioviruses appear to adsorb to the same poliovirus receptor. A selection of viruses and receptors relevant to nervous system infections is presented in Table 2.3. It is clear that these are receptors that serve other functions and they have been usurped by the virus. Indeed, selective mutational pressure to adapt to new receptors may be a factor in selective survival of mutants, just as it is to avoid neutralization by antibody.

Excessive focus on receptors as *the* determinant of cell and species susceptibility is misdirected. Many viruses use several receptors; for example, rabies virus injected into muscle appears to use the acetylcholine receptor, but, when injected into skin, the virus moves up sensory axons to dorsal root ganglia neurons with the virus evidently utilizing an alternate receptor. Some viruses use more than one receptor to determine ease of cellular infection; for example, in addition to CD4, HIV uses secondary chemokine receptors on macrophage and T-cell lines (Weiss, 1996). Pharmacologic and physiologic studies of receptors promote the idea that attachment sets off a chain of predictable events. Indeed, absorption does not necessarily lead to cell entry or determine the ability to replicate and assemble progeny virus. For example, mouse cells transfected

TABLE 2.3. *Putative receptors for some viruses of neurologic interest*

Family	Virus	Receptor
Herpesviridae	Herpes simplex virus	Heparan sulfate
	Epstein–Barr virus	CD21 (CR2 receptor)
	Cytomegalovirus	Heparan sulfate
		β_2-Microglobulin/MHC 1
Parvoviridae	B19	Erythrocyte pantigen (globoside)
Myxoviridae	Influenza A, B	Sialic acid residues
	Measles	CD46
		Moesin
Rhabdoviridae	Rabies	Acetylcholine receptor
		Gangliosides
		Phospholipids
Retroviridae	HIV-1	CD4
Picornaviridae	Polioviruses	Immunoglobulin superfamily
	Echoviruses 1 and 8	Integrin VLA-2

MHC, major histocompatibility complex; VLA, viruslike antigen.

with human poliovirus receptors will replicate human polioviruses (Selinka et al., 1991), but mouse cells transfected with the CD4 receptor will not replicate HIV.

Extrapolating from cell culture phenomena to animal host infection is similarly unreliable. The susceptibility of neuroblastoma cells and oligodendrocytes in culture does not imply that neurons and oligodendrocytes can be infected *in vivo*. The observation 45 years ago that primate kidney cells, which are not infected by polioviruses *in vivo*, can be infected after they dedifferentiate in culture opened the way to the development of the poliovirus vaccine, but this classic finding also should serve as a contemporary reminder that cells in culture may not reflect the susceptibility of analogous cells within the host.

Penetration and Uncoating

Attachment does not necessarily lead to virus entry into the cell. Penetration is energy dependent and involves two general pathways: (a) surface fusion between viral envelope and the cell plasma membrane or (b) receptor-mediated endocytosis.

The envelopes of paramyxoviruses, retroviruses, and herpesviruses by the action of a surface glycoprotein can fuse with cytoplasmic membranes and release the viral nucleocapsid directly into the cytoplasm. Other enveloped viruses and most naked virions enter by endocytosis: A clathrin-coated invagination develops and engulfs the virion into an endosome. The pH drop induces conformational changes in virion proteins, allowing fusion of the envelope to the endosome membrane or lysis of endosomal membranes (Knipe, 1996). A modified form of penetration and uncoating occurs with picornaviruses. On adsorption, one of the capsid proteins is lost, the capsid loses structural integrity, and the particle is translocated across the plasma membrane.

Translation, Transcription, and Replication

Replication of most DNA viruses involves familiar mechanisms, with transcription of mRNA from DNA and replication of DNA. The double-stranded DNA viruses that replicate in the nucleus (papovaviruses, adenoviruses, and herpesviruses) can use enzymes of the host cell for DNA synthesis and mRNA transcription but often encode proteins that regulate and enhance virus replication. Cytoplasmic replication by DNA poxviruses involves establishing a relatively autonomous virus factory within the cell cytoplasm. Single-stranded DNA viruses require generation of a complementary strand and double-stranded DNA in the cell nucleus; for autonomous parvoviruses, this necessitates the cell being in the S phase of mitosis.

The RNA viruses use a variety of unique strategies in replication. Cells cannot synthesize messenger RNA from an RNA genome. Therefore, positive-sense RNA of picornaviruses, flaviviruses, and togaviruses serves as messenger RNA;

the negative-sense RNA of other RNA viruses must carry an RNA-dependent RNA polymerase in the virion. The single-stranded RNA of retroviruses has only one, but singularly unique, function—to be the template for viral DNA. This requires an RNA-dependent DNA polymerase within the virion. In every case, however, there is complex control of both cellular and viral transcription and translation in the direction of virus-coded proteins. Protein synthesis takes place in the pirated cytoplasmic host cell polyribosomes that read viral messenger RNA. All viruses encode proteins for three functions: (a) to ensure the replication of the viral genome, (b) to package the genome into a virion, and (c) to alter the structure and/or function of the host cell (Roizman and Palese, 1996).

In addition to structural proteins and virion-associated enzymes, other proteins include regulatory proteins that modulate cellular and viral genes, oncogene proteins and inactivators of cellular tumor-suppressor proteins, and virokines. Virokines are a recently recognized class of proteins encoded by large DNA viruses and retroviruses that sabotage host defenses. They include inhibitors of T-cell and antibody-mediated cytotoxicity, inhibitors of cytokines and the complement cascade, and proteins that mimic cytokines (see Chapter 4).

Assembly and Release

The virions of adenoviruses, papovaviruses, and parvoviruses are assembled in the nucleus; therefore, the structural proteins synthesized in the cytoplasm are transported to the nucleus for construction of the capsid, and cell lysis is usually needed for virus release. The herpesvirus nucleocapsid, with additional surface proteins, acquires its envelope by passing through the virus-modified nuclear membrane into cisterna of the cytoplasmic reticulum or vesicles, which can carry virus to the cell surface.

Picornaviruses and reoviruses are assembled in the cytoplasm and released by cell lysis. The enveloped RNA viruses acquire envelopes by budding through modified cell membranes at the plasma membrane (paramyxoviruses, orthomyxoviruses, alphaviruses, rhabdoviruses, and retroviruses) or into cytoplasmic cisternae (coronaviruses, bunyaviruses, and flaviviruses) with intravesicular delivery to the plasma membrane for release by exocytosis. After assembly of the icosahedral or helical nucleocapsid, the nucleocapsids align along cell membranes at sites in the cell lipid bilayer of virus-coded glycoproteins. Budding can occur without disrupting the integrity of the host cell and may show striking polarity, with budding only on the exterior surface of the epithelial cells, such as influenza virus, or vasolaterally from vascular endothelial cell, such as murine leukemia virus (see Chapter 11).

VIRUS–VIRUS INTERACTIONS

During the infectious cycle, errors occur in replication and assemblage of particles, and these mutant or defective particles, in turn, may interact with standard virus. The number of defective virus particles formed depends on the specific virus, the host cell type, and the multiplicity of the infection. These defective particles may be hollow capsids lacking the nucleic acid, or they may have mutational defects or partial deletions of the nucleic acids. Interactions can also occur between homologous standard viruses or between two different viruses that infect a cell at the same time.

Interference

The simplest form of interference occurs when noninfectious particles or fragments of envelopes occupy receptor sites and block the attachment of infectious virus. Alternatively, if two viruses have the same receptor site (e.g., polioviruses) or adjacent sites for attachment, one can interfere with infection by the other or may destroy receptor sites as myxoviruses do. Interference can also occur within the cell when viruses compete for the same site or enzyme. For example, when cells are infected with increasingly higher multiplicities of influenza virus, there is a paradoxical decrease in the amount of infectious virus released. Instead, increasing numbers of defective particles are released, and these defectives specifically lack the longest of the segmented genes. Apparently, when the cell is flooded with templates, there is competition for RNA polymerase or replicase, and the segment that takes the longest time to replicate is disadvantaged.

A specific type of defective particle that lacks a segment of the nucleic acid is called a *defective interfering particle*. By definition, these particles (a) contain all normal structural proteins, (b) lack a portion of the viral nucleic acid, (c) cannot reproduce without the presence of the complete or standard virus, and (d) interfere with the replication of the standard virus. An infection giving rise to a large number of defective interfering particles is dampened by their interference, but because of the resultant decline in standard virus particles that act as helpers, defective interfering particles decline, allowing recrudescence of standard virus. Studies with defective interfering particles in cell culture have demonstrated chronic or cycling infections, which have been proposed as models for relapsing–remitting diseases (Huang, 1973). However, this phenomenon has not been observed in natural disease. Indeed, both competition for receptor sites or enzymes and generation of defective interfering particles are seen with high multiplicities of infection in cell cultures, and the dilutional factors *in vivo* may trivialize their impact in animal infections.

Mutation, Complementation, and Recombination

The almost explosive rate of virus replication leads to frequent mutations, and this is particularly true of RNA viruses in which there is a lack of "proofreading" by the polymerase. RNA replication leads to a 10,000-fold greater rate of infidelity in base-pair matching than in DNA replication. Viruses with mutations have served as valuable tools in understanding the molecular biology of virus replication, particularly the use of conditional lethal mutants that grow only at certain temperature or other specific culture conditions. With mutants representing each function site, a map of the genome can be constructed, and functions can be assigned to specific genes and the resultant polypeptides. Although conditional lethals probably are not important in natural disease states, nonconditional lethal mutations are. Many RNA viruses vary over time, with new strains leading to new outbreaks of disease (e.g., the new strains of enteroviruses). In persistent infections, mutations can evolve within the host that allow escape from antibody neutralization or resistance to antiviral drugs (e.g., the evolution of neutralization escape mutants in animal lentiviruses and drug-resistant strains of HIV).

Interactions between different viruses occur in the case of recombination and complementation. In recombination, segments of nucleic acid are exchanged between two viruses coinfecting a cell. Reoviruses, bunyaviruses, arenaviruses, and influenza viruses, with segmented nucleic acids, recombine by simple reassortment. Exploiting this phenomenon of recombination or reassortment, an entire catalogue of reoviruses has been made, and specific functions have been assigned to specific genes and their protein products. Reassortment may be important in the natural history of influenza viruses, where the reassortment of influenza viruses of humans and animals, particularly ducks, may give rise to new pandemic strains of influenza (Laver and Webster, 1979; Kilbourne, 1991). Recombination does occur among viruses with nonsegmented genomes; for example, western encephalitis virus appears to be a recombinant between eastern encephalitis virus and a Sindbis-like virus (Hahn et al., 1988).

Complementation occurs in a dual infection when one virus codes for a gene product required for the growth of another virus. This occurs in defective interfering particle infections. Complementation also is required for growth of the nonautonomous parvoviruses where the host cell must be coinfected with a helper virus to provide enzymes necessary for DNA synthesis.

Evolution of mutants may be important in some instances, such as subacute sclerosing panencephalitis, in which the measles virus recovered from brain shows many mutations in the matrix protein and glycoproteins crucial to the enveloping and release of measles virus. Conversely, it must be remembered that, in chronic infections, mutants tend to accumulate, and the finding of defective particles, temperature-sensitive mutants, and other aberrant particles may be an epiphenomenon reflecting the degeneracy of persistent infection rather than a clue to the mechanisms of its initiation or maintenance (see Chapter 10).

EFFECTS OF VIRUS REPLICATION ON CELLS

The process of virus replication can have various effects on the host cell. It may lead to disruption of the integrity of the plasma membrane of the cell, an inhibition or acceleration of its growth rate, transformation into a cell lacking contact inhibition, fusion with neighboring cells, alteration of the antigenic composition of its cytoplasmic membrane, or triggering of the cellular suicide program or apoptosis. Furthermore, many of these effects can occur without completion of the infectious cycle. Simple attachment of viruses can, in some cases, disrupt cytoplasmic membranes, causing cell lysis. In a majority of cases, cell transformation takes place without the transcription of all viral proteins and without assembly or release of virus particles. In addition to acute cytopathic or cytocidal effects and cell transformation, many viruses cause noncytopathic infections.

Cytopathic Cytolytic Effects

Lysis of the host cell is not the inevitable consequence of virus infection. Insect and plant viruses can distend and rupture the host cell, but animal viruses never constitute more than a small percentage of the host cell mass, and the normal cell pool of amino acids and nucleotides can easily fulfill the demands of the viral genes. To induce cell lysis, specific proteins are synthesized, since in some infections the virus life cycle depends on cell rupture for release of virions. The abrupt shutoff of RNA and protein synthesis and DNA replication in host cells is directed by early proteins of some viruses, leading to cell necrosis. Viral proteins may be toxic, as exemplified by the fiber protein of adenoviruses that can lyse cells. Destructive mechanisms may be set in motion before completion of the infectious cycle. Thus, the host cell may be doomed before it has assembled or released a single infectious virus particle.

Inclusions represent cytopathic changes in cells that historically were of great importance when diagnoses of infections relied largely on histologic studies. Virus inclusions can represent actual crystalline arrays of viral particles, as in the nuclear inclusions in papovavirus, adenovirus, and reovirus infections. The cytoplasmic inclusions in rabies and poxvirus infections represent virus factories; they are amorphous masses of viral proteins with virus particles around the periphery. The nuclear inclusions of measles virus infections contain accumulations of viral nucleoprotein. In contrast, the classic Cowdry type A intranuclear inclusions of herpesvirus infections are late degenerative changes in the nucleus, with alteration of nuclear chromatin; they show little correlation with the localization of the herpesvirus cores or virions within the cell.

Transformation

Transformation of cells in cell culture is recognized by the loss of normal morphology, the piling up of cells, the ability of cells to grow in serum-free medium or semisolid medium, and the immortality of cells (their ability to be trypsinized and subcultured indefinitely). Sugar and other nutrients are more rapidly transported across the plasma membrane, and new surface antigens appear that may be coded by virus or host. Transformed cells often produce tumors when transplanted into appropriate animal hosts. The most basic alteration in the transformed host cell is the loss of normal contact inhibition, the phenomenon that normal cells, once they reach confluency, stop dividing.

Virus transformation of cells usually depends on the integration of viral DNA into host cell DNA or on episomal maintenance of virus DNA in the nucleus as a plasmidlike entity. This can occur in specific cells from specific species with the viral DNA or a portion of the viral DNA of papovaviruses, adenoviruses, or herpesviruses, or with the copy DNA of some retroviruses. Since cell mitosis facilitates integration, mitotic activity is an important determinant for viral transformation, in contrast to transformation by chemical carcinogens (zur Hausen, 1980). With the DNA viruses, transformation occurs in cells that do not produce infectious virus or recognizable virus structures. In some retrovirus infections, however, a cell may be transformed and may produce infectious progeny virus concurrently. This phenomenon leads to the confusing terminology of permissive and nonpermissive infections. Permissive means that the cell produces progeny virus; nonpermissive (not to be confused with insusceptible) means that virus has infected the cell and may direct synthesis of some viral proteins but does not produce infectious progeny virus.

Moderate or Noncytopathic Effects

Infections of cells with some viruses may continue over long periods of time with little or no interference with normal cell functions. Rabies virus causes noncytopathic infection in cell cultures, and, indeed, very little cell death may be evident in rabies in animals. Rubella virus also causes a noncytopathic infection in most susceptible cell cultures, but this infection alters cells by inhibiting mitosis, so that the rate of turnover is slowed. Paramyxoviruses do not abruptly shut down cell protein synthesis and DNA synthesis, but, over time, chronically disrupt cell functions.

One of the most interesting of the noncytopathic viruses that alter cell function is lymphocytic choriomeningitis virus. This virus grows in cell culture, and, indeed, in its natural host, the fetally infected mouse, with no cytopathic effects. However, cultures of persistently infected neuroblastoma cells, despite normal morphology, growth rates, and protein synthesis, show markedly reduced synthesis of acetylcholine, choline acetyltransferase, and acetylcholine esterases (Oldstone et al., 1977). Thus, these "normal" cells show selective inhibition of the synthesis of particular proteins that has been termed "luxury function," although *in vivo* the ability of neural cells to synthesize such transmitters or enzymes can hardly be considered a luxury. Indeed, congenitally infected mice are runts, and immunocytochemical studies show noncytopathic infection of the cells of the anterior pituitary that generate growth hormone. Growth hormone levels are reduced, so these animals are pituitary dwarfs with histologically normal pituitary glands (Oldstone et al., 1982). Similarly, noncytopathic infections of mouse neuroblastoma–glioma hybrid cells with rabies virus have been shown to affect receptor function selectively, with impaired responses to prostaglandins and preservation of responses to acetylcholine (Koschel and Halbach, 1979). Persistent infection of rat glioma cells with canine distemper virus reduces β-adrenergic receptors to 50% of normal levels (Koschel and Muenzel, 1980). Cell culture studies of this type suggest *in vitro* correlates in which marked specific neural dysfunction might occur without neuropathologic abnormalities.

In a variety of infections, such as noncytopathic infections with paramyxoviruses or lymphocytic choriomeningitis virus, virus-coded proteins are inserted into the host cell's plasma membrane. Although these proteins may not interfere with cell growth or division, in the intact host they represent foreign antigens and may make the cell the victim of immune lysis by antibody and complement or the victim of attack from cytotoxic T cells. In these cases, the infection is noncytopathic, and the cell lysis is immune mediated, a subject to be expanded in Chapter 4.

Apoptosis

Apoptosis, also called programmed cell death or self-directed cellular suicide, is an active process of cell dissolution that is triggered during embryonic development, normal tissue turnover, hormone-induced atrophy, and immunocyte clone deletion, and by cytokines of the tumor necrosis factor family, cytotoxic T-cell killing, radiation damage, and some viral infections, as well as many other circumstances (Arends and Wyllie, 1991; Thompson, 1995). Each hour, millions of our cells condense, form into apoptotic bodies, and are phagocytosed by neighboring cells or tissue macrophages without evoking an inflammatory response. This programmed cell death can be differentiated from cellular necrosis by morphological and metabolic criteria (Table 2.4). Furthermore, apoptosis usually occurs throughout tissues, whereas necrosis is focal.

Apoptosis has special relevance to CNS development and degeneration. During development of the nervous system, 50% or more of many types of neurons die soon after forming synaptic connections. This sculpturing presumably assures that neurons that project to inappropriate targets are eliminated, that all target cells become innervated, and that the number of neurons is appropriately matched to the number of target cells. Apoptosis in development represents a default response of isolated cells (Raff et al., 1993). Conversely, in the mature nervous system where neuronal turnover and replacement does not occur, the ever-present cell death effector molecules must be inhibited (Steller, 1995). In part, this protection is provided by *death-suppressor genes* such as bcl-2, first identified as an oncogene (Bredesen, 1995).

Many viruses encode proteins that interact with the pathways regulating apoptosis. Unscheduled DNA synthesis seems to activate cellular p53 and p53-

TABLE 2.4. *Comparisons of apoptosis and necrosis*

	Apoptosis[a]	Necrosis
Morphology		
Cell	Reduced size	Enlarged
Nucleus	Condensation of chromatin along nuclear membrane Nucleolar disintegration	Pyknosis
Cytoplasm	Organelles compacted Smooth endoplasmic reticulum dilate Vacuoles form	Mitochondrial swelling Dispersion of elements into extracellular space
Membrane	Smooth surface Blebs on cell surface	Membranes permeable and rupture
Inflammation	Phagocytosis of membrane-bound apoptotic bodies	Release of cytoplasmic components induces inflammatory response
Chemical changes		
Cell	Density increases	Density decreases
Nucleus	Chromatin cleaved at internucleosomal sites by endonucleases	Degeneration not dependent on cellular mechanisms
Cytoplasm	Modest or no increase in Ca Transglutaminase cross-links cytosolic proteins Glycan groups exposed on cytoplasmic membrane	Massive influx of Ca

[a]Determined by "ladder" of DNA fragments on gel electrophoresis, detected in tissue by typical electron-microscopic changes in cell nuclei, or enzymatic staining techniques to detect cleaved DNA (TUNEL staining) (Gold et al., 1994).

dependent apoptosis. Therefore, most DNA viruses have proteins that inactivate p53, simulate bcl-2, or in other ways inhibit apoptosis (Teodora and Branton, 1997). On the other hand, herpesviruses, parvoviruses, orthomyxoviruses and paramyxoviruses, retroviruses, reoviruses, alphaviruses, and picornaviruses can induce apoptosis (Lewis et al., 1996; Rodgers et al., 1997). The possible implications of virus-induced apoptosis in the nervous system have only recently been addressed, particularly in the model system of Sindbis virus encephalitis in mice and the clinical disorder of HIV-associated encephalopathy in humans. The susceptibility to acute fatal encephalitis with Sindbis virus drops abruptly over 1-million-fold in the first week of life (Johnson et al., 1972). Cells *in vitro* are killed by Sindbis virus by apoptosis, and transfection of cultured cells with bcl-2 prevents cell death and leads to persistent infection (Levine et al., 1993). Morphological evidence of apoptosis correlates with infection and is directly related to mortality (Lewis et al., 1996). This suggests that the activation of genes to suppress apoptosis with maturation of the nervous system also suppress virus-induced apoptosis and may be a major determinant of age-dependent susceptibility to this form of encephalitis and in establishment of persistent infection.

This shifts from cell culture phenomena to the more complex issues of the pathogenesis of nervous system infections.

SUPPLEMENTARY BIBLIOGRAPHY

Fields BN, Knipe DM, Howley PM, eds. *Fields virology,* 3rd ed. New York: Raven Press, 1996.
White DO, Fenner FJ. *Medical virology,* 4th ed. San Diego: Academic Press, 1994.

3

Pathogenesis of CNS Infections

In animal virology . . . the great advances of the past decade have come from the application of the methods of molecular biology to the study of animal viruses and their interactions with animal cells. Of course this encompasses only a limited segment of animal virology, for animals are complex and integrated assemblages of many different kinds of cells and animal virology involves the study of events at the level of organism and of population as well as the level of cell. However, animal virology at the cellular level is ripe for investigation by the precise physicochemical approach of the molecular biologist; at higher levels of complexity we are still faced with baffling problems for which adequate experimental approaches are only just being developed.

Frank Fenner

Modern Trends in Animal Virology, lecture to the Australia–New Zealand Association for the Advancement of Science, 1967

The structural and genetic simplicity of viruses provided ideal grist for the development of molecular biology. However, the origins of virology were in pathology, with the goal of understanding disease. To address the problems of disease, we must return to pathology and consider both the viruses and the terrain in which they replicate and spread. The virus–cell interactions learned in cell culture systems are applicable in this transition, but virus–host interactions rise to a higher level of complexity confounded by a mosaic of cells of varied susceptibilities and by a myriad of host defense mechanisms.

Different cells within the animal, even within a given organ, may have different virus-receptor sites and greater or lesser capacity to replicate or release virus. Furthermore, virus replication may have different effects on different host cells and thus lead to varied clinical manifestations or pathologic changes. For example, even though the mechanisms of replication and cell lysis are the same, poliovirus infections of the gastrointestinal tract cause little, if any, disease, whereas poliovirus infections of the motor neurons cause paralysis. The susceptibility to and the effects of viral infections may vary for different cell populations in the same tissue. This is exemplified in progressive multifocal leukoencephalopathy, in which neurons appear to be insusceptible to papovavirus infections, oligodendrocytes are permissively infected and lysed causing demyelinating lesions, and astrocytes produce only small amounts of virus and develop bizarre configurations and abnormal mitotic figures suggestive of transformation.

The defenses of the host that may prevent or inhibit infection are also complex, not only in the specific cellular and humoral immune responses but also in responses such as the infected cell's release of interferon or other cytokines. Phagocytic macrophages monitor the respiratory, gastrointestinal, and subcutaneous areas, and their ingestion of viral particles may inactivate viruses in addition to delivering the viral antigens to the regional lymph nodes for initiation of specific immune responses (Mims, 1964). Nonspecific host defenses also may play important roles: for example, fever, which can inactivate thermolabile viruses; populations of insusceptible cells, which may form anatomic barriers to virus spread; the ciliary activity of the respiratory tract, which actively sweeps particles outward; and gastric acid and bile, which inactivate most viruses.

Compared with the prevalence of viral infections, viral CNS diseases are uncommon. This fact is not explained by the scarcity of CNS pathogens, because viral meningitis and encephalitis usually are caused by common viruses that frequently infect humans. Viral infections of the CNS are less dependent on encounter with a potentially neuropathogenic agent than on some breach in the usual barriers that normally exclude viruses from invading and infecting susceptible cells of the CNS. In this chapter, we consider how viruses enter the body, the pathways of invasion of the CNS, the possible mechanisms of spread within the CNS and selective vulnerability of neural cells, and the mechanisms of neurovirulence. In this regard, it is essential to define a few terms that are used:

Neuroinvasiveness: the ability to gain access to the nervous system
Neurotropism: the ability to infect neural cells (neuronotropism means infections specifically of neurons)
Neurovirulence: the ability to cause disease

EXPERIMENTAL APPROACHES

The spread of virus, the activation of host defenses, and indeed the outcome of infection may be largely determined during the incubation period—that interval of good health between encounter with the virus and onset of clinical symptoms or signs. Early clinical observations of natural infections of humans and experimental infections in animals provided data on the length of the incubation period and the mode of onset of disease, but almost no insight into the events during this critical period. Histologic studies of fatal human and animal infections failed to yield much information, because the disease at death generally is too widespread to enable reconstruction of its evolution. In the 19th century, rabies virus became the first virus employed in experimental studies of pathogenesis. Amputation of limbs and cutting of peripheral nerves were performed at intervals after distal inoculation to determine the rate of virus spread and to determine whether the virus moved along nerves.

Goodpasture, in the 1920s, with limited tools and techniques, attempted to follow the cellular progression of infection during the incubation period. He collected tissues for histologic examination at regular intervals during the incubation period. He was also lucky: rabies and polioviruses, the other experimental agents of the period, leave little histologic evidence of extraneural infection, but he chose herpes simplex virus, whose characteristic inclusion bodies leave footprints of the infection. Thus, through careful sequential histologic observations, Goodpasture made remarkable conclusions on viral spread within nerves (Johnson, 1993a).

A further approach to unraveling the pathogenesis of infection is to quantitate virus in different organs at regular intervals. Fenner (1949) pioneered this method in his classic studies of ectromelia virus infections of mice. By dissecting animals at intervals during the incubation period and assaying virus content in different organs, growth curves for the virus and the sequence of organs involved can be plotted. In the face of substantial viremia, however, virus in organs may only reflect blood-borne virus in transit (Johnson, 1965b; Albrecht, 1968). Indeed, the phagocytic cells of the liver that clear the viremia can concentrate virus, and so a disproportionately high level will give the appearance that the liver is infected when in fact no virus has replicated in any hepatic cells (Mims, 1964). Furthermore, the method does not determine which cells are involved. For example, virus growth in the brain cannot be interpreted as neuronal infection or even as infection of parenchymal cells, because large quantities of virus may be found in infections limited to meningeal or ependymal cells (Johnson, 1968).

Immunocytochemistry has enabled the localization of viral infection at a cellular level. Fluorescent antibody staining of viral antigens and cell markers initially provided a simple and practical method. Enzymatic amplification of signal has increased the sensitivity of immunocytochemistry and, in many cases, made possible the localization of viral proteins in archival material in paraffin-embedded blocks. Antigens specific to cell types, such as glial fibrillary acidic protein as a marker for astrocytes, can definitively identify specific cell types, and this is of particular value in examining CNS tissue. *In situ* hybridization can localize viral nucleic acids, and the new development of *in situ* polymerase chain reaction enables the identification of segments of a single molecule of DNA or cDNA to be localized. Double and triple labeling have opened the feasibility of identifying viral nucleic acids in cells whose identity is defined by specific markers and determining with monoclonal antibodies which proteins are being translated.

Because the study of pathogenesis relies on tracking the spread of viral infection during an asymptomatic time preceding disease, as well as during disease, few data have been collected in human infections. From experimental studies, however, analogies can be made to probable counterparts in human disease, particularly if the studies use the same route of virus entry as in the natural infection. There has been some controversy regarding optimal simulacra: some investigators argue that studies of a related animal virus in a natural host animal yields greater insight into human disease, whereas others champion the use of a human virus in an animal that is not a natural host for the virus. For example, in studies designed to clarify the pathogenesis of subacute sclerosing panencephalitis, some workers have studied chronic canine distemper encephalitis in dogs (a related virus causing a similar disease in its natural host), whereas others have investigated measles virus in laboratory rodents (the causal human virus in an unnatural host). Both approaches can provide useful information that can ultimately be applied in studies of human tissues.

ENTRY OF VIRUSES

The body presents formidable barriers to the entry of viruses from the environment, whether by direct contact, respiratory droplets, or contamination of food or water (Table 3.1). The most extensive barrier is the skin, because the intact epidermis is covered by the stratum corneum, a layer of dead keratinized cells that will not support virus growth. Therefore, penetration of virus through the skin requires that this barrier be broached by a bite (such as the bite of an infected arthropod or animal) or by mechanical manipulations (such as in intentional vaccination, by unknowing transfusion of infected blood, or by the sullied needle of a drug abuser).

In contrast, naked viable cells are exposed on the mucous membranes of the respiratory, gastrointestinal, and genitourinary tracts, and these are the major portals of entry for viruses. If the host has had previous contact with a given virus, however, these membranes may be coated with secretory immunoglobulins (immunoglobulin A) that neutralize the virus. The respiratory tract is covered by mucous film, and the constant beating of cilia moves this mucous film outward, sweeping viral particles, along with other particulate matter, away from the epithelial cells of the lower respiratory tract. This mucous film also contains mucopolysaccharides that can nonspecifically inhibit virus attachment. Even if virus in the inspired air gains access to the alveoli, the macrophages that line these cavities actively phagocytose viruses and other particles that reach the alveoli.

The gastrointestinal tract poses a harsh environment for most viruses. Stomach acidity can inactivate most swallowed viruses, enzymes throughout the gastrointestinal tract can disrupt envelopes and capsid proteins, and bile can dissociate the lipoprotein membranes of enveloped viruses. Nevertheless, some nonenveloped acid-resistant viruses, such as the enteroviruses, adenoviruses, reoviruses, and parvoviruses, are adapted to replicate within the gastrointestinal tract.

Whether virus has been injected into the subcutaneous or muscle tissue, as in rabies, or gains access to cells within the respiratory or gastrointestinal tract, as in measles and enterovirus infections, the virus must make contact with the receptor site of a susceptible cell and must make this contact prior to thermal

TABLE 3.1. *Portals of entry for viruses causing human CNS disease*

Route or entry in natural infection	Viruses
Inoculation	
Arthropod bite	Arboviruses
Animal bite	Rabies virus
	Herpesvirus simiae
Blood transfusion	Cytomegalovirus
	Hepatitis B virus
	Human immunodeficiency virus
	Human T-cell lymphotropic virus
Transplantation	Rabies virus
	Creutzfeldt–Jakob disease
Intentional	Vaccine viruses
Respiratory	
Droplet	Mumps virus
	Parainfluenza virus
	Measles virus
	Influenza virus
	Lymphocytic choriomeningitis virus
	Other arenaviruses
	Adenoviruses
	Varicella–zoster virus
Saliva	Herpes simplex virus, type 1
	Cytomegalovirus
	Epstein–Barr virus
Enteric	Enteroviruses (poliovirus, coxsackie virus, and echoviruses)
	Adenoviruses
	Hepatitis A virus
Venereal	Herpes simplex virus, type 2
	Cytomegalovirus
	Hepatitis B virus
	Human immunodeficiency virus
	Human T-cell lymphotropic virus
Transplacental	Rubella virus
	Cytomegalovirus
	Human immunodeficiency virus
	Other viruses

inactivation, degradation by phagocytes, or mechanical expulsion. Following this initial successful cellular interaction and initial replication, some viral infections remain confined to the local site of entry. For example, rhinoviruses, which replicate poorly at body temperatures, remain confined to those areas of cooler temperatures, such as the nasal mucosa and sinus mucosa; papillomaviruses remain confined to the skin and genital epithelium; and influenza viruses rarely spread beyond the epithelial cells of the respiratory tract. Other viruses routinely disseminate more widely, and most of these agents have the potential to invade the CNS.

PATHWAYS OF NEUROINVASION
The Neural Route

Virus spread to the CNS along peripheral nerves was the pathway first suggested by both clinical observations and experimental studies. In 1769, Morgagni noted that paresthesias at the site of the original bite often heralded the onset of rabies, and he postulated that "virus was not carried up the veins but up the nerves to their origins." The 19th-century experiments with rabies supported this hypothesis. Virus was recovered from the nerves in animals with experimental rabies; initial CNS infection was observed at the spinal cord level corresponding to the inoculation site; and rabies was prevented by chopping off the tails of dogs the day after distal inoculation. Subsequently, less inelegant studies showed that severing the appropriate nerve protected against disease (Nicolau and Meteiesco, 1928). Thus, the peripheral nerves appeared to be the pathway of rabies virus into the CNS.

In the 1920s, experimental studies of herpes simplex virus reinforced the idea that viruses spread to the CNS along nerves. The localized brainstem encephalitis that develops in rabbits after corneal inoculation was widely studied, and the initial histologic lesion in the ipsilateral trigeminal-root entry zone pointed to a neural pathway. Movement of the virus along the perineural spaces or lymphatics (Marinesco and Draganesco, 1923) and growth of virus in axis cylinders (Goodpasture and Teague, 1923) were postulated as mechanisms. The idea of herpesvirus replication within axons now is untenable because of the known obligatory nuclear site of replication of herpesviruses. Studies of herpes simiae and pseudorabies virus showed no replication of virus within nerve, and Sabin (1937) concluded that "virus may have to travel up the long axis cylinders to the nucleus before any increase or multiplication can occur." Indeed, axons lack the capability for protein synthesis, so replication of any virus within axoplasm is unlikely.

Early studies of poliovirus also implicated CNS invasion along nerve fibers. Bodian and Howe (1941) showed that monkeys could be infected by dipping the freshly cut end of a peripheral nerve into a virus suspension. However, if the nerve first was frozen proximally to produce degeneration of the axonal processes and their myelin sheaths without interrupting the physical continuity of the nerve, no paralysis occurred. They concluded that the axis cylinder was involved in the transmission. Because a large number of fibers had to be exposed, they suggested that viral increase "does not take place in the axon, but that the original amount which enters the axon must succeed in reaching the nerve cell body before multiplication and further spread can occur."

These studies, combined with the growing conviction that the blood–brain barrier was impervious to most, if not all, viruses, led to the doctrine of the 1930s and 1940s that all viruses spread to the CNS along peripheral or olfactory nerves (Friedemann, 1943). The mechanism, however, was disputed. Wright (1953) concluded that nerve trunks contained three conduits: the axons, the perineural lymphatics, and tissue spaces between nerve fibers (Fig. 3.1). He dis-

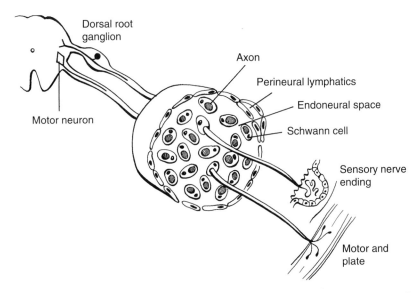

FIG. 3.1. Neural pathways for CNS infection. Virus can be taken up at sensory or motor endings and moved within axons. (Movement within endoneural space, perineural lymphatics, or by Schwann cell infection were previously proposed, but none are documented.) By retrograde interaxonal transport, viruses taken up at sensory endings will be delivered selectively to dorsal root ganglia cells and those at motor endings to motor neurons.

carded the possibility of axons as a pathway because of the viscosity of axoplasm and what was then believed to be solely centrifugal flow of axoplasm. The neural lymphatics do provide a potentially valveless access into the CNS. India-ink particles placed in the subarachnoid space collect in the arachnoid cul-de-sac at the proximal pole of the ganglia, and some diffuse through this cuff into the perineural lymphatics (Brierley, 1950). Abdominal pressure can reverse this flow, forcing particles from lymphatics into the dorsal root ganglia, but entry of particles into the subarachnoid space by this route requires nonphysiologic pressures. Therefore, Wright concluded by elimination that interspaces must be involved.

Initial fluorescent antibody studies of herpes simplex virus in mice showed a sequential infection of Schwann cells from the site of inoculation to the appropriate spinal cord segment and suggested a fourth pathway (Johnson, 1964a). However, even in those studies some observations suggested the possibility of spread within axons. First, the Schwann cell infection, as it neared the spinal cord, was limited to the dorsal root, totally sparing the anterior root, which suggests movement in sensory axons (Johnson, 1964a). Second, studies of the same virus in rabbits (Johnson and Mims, 1968) and rabies virus in mice (Johnson, 1965a) showed similar early involvement of the dorsal ganglia and root entry zones without detectable viral antigen in Schwann cells. The Schwann cell infection appeared to be "merely silent witness of centripetally moving virus" (Wildy, 1967).

Axonal Transport

Discarding Goodpasture's idea of transit within the axoplasm was premature. In addition to the slow anterograde ooze of axoplasm observed in early studies, rapid bidirectional axonal transport has been established, and virus particle size is not a restraint, because organelles as large as mitochondria are moved in these systems. Fast transport is a microtubule-based system of bidirectional movement of membranous organelles. Fast transport moves at a rate of 200 to 400 mm per day and functions to deliver products for renewal of the axolemma and synapses and to return endopinocytosed membranes and samplings of the synaptic milieu. Nerve growth factor, tetanus toxin, foreign proteins, and several viruses are picked up in these vesicles and moved to the cell body (Griffin and Watson, 1988).

By electron microscopy, herpesviruses have been shown in axoplasm within the smooth endoplasmic reticulum (Kristensson et al., 1974). Morphological studies (Baringer and Griffith, 1970) and virologic studies (Cook and Stevens, 1973) have shown arrival of herpesvirus in the dorsal root ganglia more quickly than could be explained by ascending infection of Schwann cells or slow transport. Furthermore, this spread can be prevented by freezing the nerve or by local treatment of the nerve with colchicine, a mitotic inhibitor that causes collapse of the axons and disintegration of myelin sheaths but leaves normal Schwann cells and widened endoneural spaces (Kristensson et al., 1971). Demonstration of receptors for herpes simplex virus on synaptosomes and a lack of receptor sites on cell bodies of neurons suggests that entry may be selectively confined to synapses or sensory endings, with endopinocytosis and axonal transport to the cell body (Vahlne et al., 1978).

Intramuscular injection of rabies in hamsters leads to initial replication in local muscle fibers, with virus budding on plasma membranes of myocytes. Neuromuscular and neurotendinal spindles are involved before detectable proximal spread along sensory fibers (Murphy, 1977). In another study, rabies virus was found to concentrate and bind at motor end plates before any replication could occur and to invade corresponding ipsilateral anterior horn cells within 20 hours (Watson et al., 1981). The acetylcholine receptor was implicated by these studies, but studies of intraocular infection have demonstrated spread along parasympathetic fibers, retinopetal fibers of pretectal origin, and intraocular fibers of the ophthalmic nerve, while failing to demonstrate spread along intraocular adrenergic fibers or within optic nerve (Kucera et al., 1985). This confirms that the virus can use multiple receptors but cannot gain access to all nerve terminals. Other viruses such as Borna virus show no evidence of peripheral replication, but the inoculum appears to be picked up by nerve endings (Carbone et al., 1989).

Centrifugal spread of virus within peripheral nerves is observed with a variety of viruses. After intracerebral inoculation of California encephalitis virus in mice, virus spreads down the nerves to infect intrafusal muscle fibers selectively (Johnson and Johnson, 1968a). In rabies virus infections, centrifugal spread of virus is of biologic importance, because after invasion of the CNS, centrifugal spread of virus along nerves to the salivary glands allows transmission in saliva. Removal of the lingual nerve and cranial cervical ganglia in dogs and foxes impedes the transmission of the virus to the ipsilateral salivary gland (Dean et al., 1963).

Neural Spread in Human Infection

Despite a wealth of experimental data documenting a neural pathway for virus spread, its importance in human infections is limited (Table 3.2). In rabies and B virus (herpes simiae) infections in humans, paresthesias or clinical signs often occur in the segmental level of the original bite; this suggests that virus has moved along nerves, causing segmental involvement of ganglia or spinal cord. Spread of polioviruses from the gut to the CNS via nerves remains feasible (Sabin, 1956) and is supported by studies that poliovirus can spread centripetally

TABLE 3.2. *Pathways for virus spread to the CNS*

Pathway	Experimental hosts	Natural disease of humans
Neural	Herpes simplex virus B virus Rabies virus Polioviruses Reovirus, type 3 Borna virus Scrapie agent Creutzfeldt–Jakob disease agent	B virus Rabies virus Herpes simplex virus Varicella–zoster virus
Olfactory	Herpes simplex virus Polioviruses Arboviruses Coronavirus	?Herpes simplex virus, type 1 Aerosol infections with rabies and arboviruses

Hematogenous	Herpes simplex virus
	Cytomegalovirus
	Polioviruses
	Coxsackieviruses
	Mumps virus
	Lymphocytic choriomeningitis
	  virus
	Most arboviruses
	Parvoviruses
	Reovirus, type 1
	Simian immunodeficiency virus
	Other lentiviruses and oncoviruses
		Enteroviruses (poliovirus, coxsackie
		  virus, and echoviruses)
		Cytomegaloviruses
		Epstein–Barr virus
		Mumps virus
		Measles virus
		Adenovirus
		Filoviruses
		Lymphocytic choriomeningitis virus
		Other arenaviruses
		Arboviruses
		Human immunodeficiency virus
		Human T-cell lymphotropic virus

along nerves in transgenic mice that express the poliovirus receptor (Ren and Racaniello, 1992).

In human infections with herpes simplex viruses, centripetal transport probably is crucial to the establishment of latency in trigeminal or sacral ganglia neurons and centrifugal transport to exacerbations of mucocutaneous disease. The pathogenesis of varicella–zoster virus is assumed to be similar. During the primary varicella–zoster infection (chickenpox), a viremia occurs, with infection of the skin from the blood. Virus then spreads centripetally in cutaneous nerves to the sensory ganglia, where latency develops in neurons. In some persons, virus replication is later activated, virus multiplies within the ganglia, and virus passes down the nerve and infects the dermatome of skin supplied by the ganglion; this results in the eruption of zoster or shingles (see Chapter 6).

The Olfactory Route

The isolation of poliovirus from the nasopharynx in experimentally infected monkeys probably was one of the most unfortunate observations in poliovirus research (Flexner and Lewis, 1910). For the next 30 years, the concept persisted that the olfactory mucosa provided not only a route of elimination of virus from the cerebrospinal fluid, but also the major route of entry into the CNS in natural infection. This idea dominated pathogenetic studies and led to futile trials of nasal sprays and swabs for poliomyelitis prophylaxis that delayed vaccine development (Paul, 1971). Studies of intranasal inoculation of herpes simplex virus, flaviviruses, and togaviruses in experimental animals also resulted in early infection and histologic changes in the olfactory bulbs. Inhibition of infection by cutting the olfactory tracts or chemical treatment of the olfactory mucosa strengthened the evidence for an olfactory route for CNS invasion. When the necessity of viremia in the natural cycle of arbovirus infections was recognized, the doctrine that the blood–brain barrier was impenetrable by viruses was so well entrenched that it was concluded that the viremia was needed for transport of virus from the site of inoculation to the nasal mucosa for CNS invasion (Friedemann, 1943).

Anatomy of Olfactory Spread

Several anatomic features are unique to the olfactory mucosa (Fig. 3.2). As in spinal roots, cuffs of arachnoid extend around the nerve fibers, but these cuffs pass through the cribriform plate and dura and form a cul-de-sac in direct contact with submucosal connective tissue. Carbon particles and labeled proteins in cerebrospinal fluid can diffuse through these cuffs into the lymphatic channels of the olfactory submucosa, and this diffusion is of greater magnitude than diffusion from the spinal roots into the perineural lymphatics (Knopf et al., 1995). Although lymphatic flow is centrifugal, virus growing in submucosal connective tissue can infect these arachnoidal cells and gain direct access into the subarachnoid space.

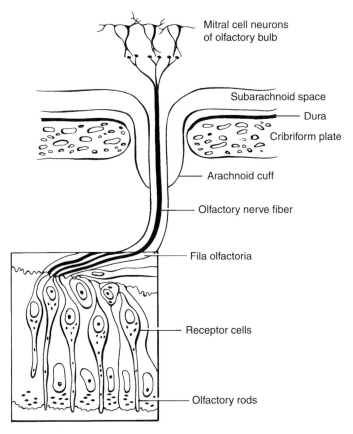

FIG. 3.2. Olfactory pathways for CNS infection. The dura is affixed to the inner table of the skull and is penetrated by the arachnoid, which forms a cuff surrounding the olfactory fibers in the nasal submucosal tissue. Receptor cells (*below*), which synapse directly with mitral cell processes in the olfactory bulb of the CNS, have rods that extend beyond the epithelium of the nasal mucosa. (Adapted from Johnson and Griffin, 1978.)

An additional unique anatomic feature of the olfactory mucosa is the extension of the apical processes of the receptor cells beyond the free surface of the epithelium as olfactory rods. These are the only neural cells whose processes synapse within the CNS and whose distal naked axons are in direct contact with the ambient environment (Fig. 3.2). When dyes are placed on the olfactory mucosa, prompt staining of the olfactory bulbs and brain is seen. When colloidal gold is placed on the olfactory mucosa, particles are taken up in pinocytotic vesicles into the cytoplasm of receptor cells. Within 30 minutes, aggregates of particles are found in the axons of the fila olfactoria and, within 1 hour, they have been transported to the olfactory bulb (De Lorenzo, 1970).

Experimental and Clinical Evidence of Olfactory Spread

Under experimental conditions, many viruses can invade the CNS directly from the olfactory mucosa. Poliovirus in the monkey has been traced from olfactory mucosa to olfactory bulbs (Bodian and Howe, 1941). Intranasal inoculation of herpes simplex virus in suckling mice has shown both infection of mucosal and submucosal cells, with extension into the subarachnoid space via the subarachnoid cuffs, and infection of endoneural cells of the olfactory fibers, resulting in the initial infection of neurons of the olfactory bulbs (Johnson, 1964a). Intranasal inoculations of Semliki Forest virus and vesicular stomatitis virus in mice have shown similar infection of mucosa, evidence of spread within nerve fibers, and early infection of cells in the olfactory bulb (Kaluza et al., 1987; Lunch et al., 1987). Aerosol infections with West Nile virus, murine hepatitis virus, and rabies virus have shown no evidence of infection of nasal mucosal cells or submucosal cells but an initial infection of olfactory bulbs that suggests that virus moves within the axons or interspaces directly from the olfactory mucosa into the CNS (Nir et al., 1965; Fischman and Schaeffer, 1971; Lavi et al., 1988). A novel route of CNS invasions was found in hamsters inoculated peripherally with St. Louis encephalitis virus: a brief and low-magnitude viremia followed with infection of the olfactory neuroepithelium and axonal transport to the olfactory bulb (Monath et al., 1983).

Although the relationship of the olfactory mucosa to the CNS provides novel anatomic arrangements that would appear to welcome virus invasion, and although experimental studies have shown that viruses can reach the CNS by invasion of the arachnoid cuff or by direct spread along receptor cell processes, there are few data to implicate this route of CNS invasion in humans. Olfactory spread of aerosols of some arboviruses and rabies virus has been suspected in several laboratory-acquired CNS infections (Nir et al., 1965; Albrecht, 1968; Winkler et al., 1973) and in the transmission of rabies in bat-infested caves where dense virus aerosols exist (Constantine, 1962). Olfactory spread of herpes simplex virus may be one explanation for the frontal and temporal localization of encephalitis in adults (Johnson and Mims, 1968), but spread along neural fibers from the trigeminal ganglia to the base of the frontal and middle fossae provides an alternative explanation (Davis and Johnson, 1979) (see Chapter 6).

The Hematogenous Route

Experimental studies and observations in humans have indicated that most viral CNS infections are acquired from the blood. The old dogma that the blood–brain barrier was impervious to viruses was based on three sets of experimental data: (a) Studies with trypan blue and other dyes showed exclusion from the CNS and led to the assumption that particulate matter would not cross the blood–brain barrier. (b) Rabies, herpes, and polioviruses can spread to the CNS via the peripheral and olfactory nerves. (c) A shorter incubation period is seen after intracerebral inoculation than after extraneural inoculation, and the incubation period after intravenous inoculation usually is equivalent to the longer incubation period following extraneural inoculation. These findings led to the assumption that intravenously injected virus was spread to some peripheral site, with subsequent movement to the brain via neural or olfactory pathways (Friedemann, 1943). This argument was formulated prior to our recognition that particles in the blood are rapidly removed by the reticuloendothelial system.

Virus particles in the blood are cleared like other colloidal particles, and the speed of removal is directly related to particle size. Thus, large viruses are cleared promptly from the bloodstream, whereas small viruses are cleared more slowly, but even the smallest arboviruses show 90% clearance in less than 1 hour (Mims, 1964). Although intravenous inoculations of vast quantities of arboviruses have been followed by almost immediate replication in the CNS (Huang and Wong, 1963), this is not comparable to natural transmission, in which small inocula are delivered and in which extraneural virus replication must occur to produce a viremia of sufficient magnitude and duration to allow CNS invasion. Under most circumstances, intravenous inoculation of virus is an inoculation of the reticuloendothelial system.

Recognition of the importance of viremia in the spread of virus to the brain began with the demonstration that a viremia preceded the invasion of the CNS in chimpanzees infected orally with polioviruses (Bodian, 1954). Current evidence indicates that most viruses grow at some extraneural site, establish a viremia by one of several mechanisms, and cross from blood to brain or cerebrospinal fluid by varied pathways (Table 3.2).

Extraneural Growth

Extraneural multiplication of viruses usually occurs first along the portal of entry. The enteroviruses, after ingestion, multiply first in the peritonsillar lymphatic cells and in Peyer's patches; infection of reticuloendothelial cells of the lamina propria of the intestine and vascular endothelial cells has also been shown by immunocytochemistry (Kanamitsu et al., 1967). Penetration from gut lumen to the lymphoid cells may be mediated by the microfold (or M) cells, which overlie Peyer's patches and transport particulate antigens (Kernéis et al., 1997). Reovirus has been shown to adhere selectively to these cells and to be transported in vesicles across to the underlying lymphoid cells (Wolf et al., 1981).

Arboviruses, after subcutaneous inoculation, usually grow in muscle and subcutaneous tissue, and the flaviviruses often replicate in endocrine glands, liver, and spleen as well (Johnson, 1965b; Albrecht, 1968). Most respiratory viruses multiply in the epithelium of the upper respiratory tract or in the alveolar cells of the lung. From these initial sites of infection, virus often is disseminated to vascular tissues, such as liver, spleen, and muscle, where multiplication augments the viremia (Johnson and Mims, 1968). The infection of vascular endothelial cells by some viruses provides an optimal opportunity to seed viruses into the blood (Johnson and Johnson, 1968a). Viruses, whether entering by way of the gut, subcutaneous tissue, or lung, are phagocytosed by macrophages that then transport the intact or degraded virus particles to the local lymphatics, where the immune response is initiated. If the local lymph node contains a population of susceptible cells, however, this defense mechanism may disadvantage the host. Virus may multiply within the lymph nodes, with progeny virus being released directly into the blood via the thoracic duct.

This initial replication of virus may or may not give prodromal symptoms before signs of the CNS infection. Mild gastrointestinal symptoms may precede paralytic poliomyelitis; respiratory symptoms may precede meningitis or encephalitis due to lymphocytic choriomeningitis virus; and severe myalgias often precede human arbovirus encephalitis, possibly because of muscle infection.

Maintenance of Viremia

Although virus released into the bloodstream is normally cleared efficiently by the reticuloendothelial system, several mechanisms subvert this clearance. Size alone aids small arboviruses and enteroviruses in sustaining a plasma viremia. Furthermore, a number of these viruses grow in vascular endothelium or lymphatic tissues, and so a high input of virus into the plasma is sustained (Johnson and Mims, 1968).

In many infections, blood-borne virus is cell associated, so that the virus is protected from the normal clearance function of the reticuloendothelial system. The orthomyxoviruses and paramyxoviruses and some arboviruses and papovaviruses adsorb to red blood cells, a property long exploited in serologic studies but useless for most virus replication schemes. Indeed, this adsorption to red cells may represent a selective genetic advantage to elude clearance from the blood. Other viruses in the blood are in white blood cells (Gresser and Lang, 1966). Measles virus can be identified in human monocytes during viremia (Esolen et al., 1993); herpesviruses, mumps virus, and retroviruses grow in human lymphocytes; and a variety of viruses are associated with leukocytes during viremias in experimental animals (Baratawidjaja et al., 1965). Transit within white cells not only protects the virus from phagocytosis by the reticuloendothelial system but also shields it from neutralization by circulating antibody or inactivation by nonspecific serum inhibitors.

Alterations in the efficiency of clearance by the reticuloendothelial system may also be an important determinant of viremia and therefore a determinant of CNS infection. Infection of the reticuloendothelial cells with viruses such as mouse hepatitis, ectromelia, or lymphocytic choriomeningitis diminishes clearance of other viruses (Gledhill et al., 1965). Particles such as thorotrast or silica injected into the blood blockade the phagocytic system and impede virus clearance (Mims, 1964; Zisman et al., 1971). The processing of virus by phagocytic cells can change with age (Johnson, 1964b) and can be influenced by genetic factors (Bang and Warwick, 1960; Goodman and Koprowski, 1962).

Invasion of the CNS

Viruses can pass from the blood into the brain or cerebrospinal fluid at several anatomic sites and by several different mechanisms. The cerebral capillaries lack fenestrations; they have tight junctions and dense membranes and are tightly packed against astrocytic footplates. The "barrier" has been equated with the tight junctions that exclude solutes, or with the limited pinocytic vesicles in cerebrovascular endothelial cells that regulate passage (Rosenblum, 1986) (Fig. 3.3). Most viruses invade the CNS across these vessels. Some infect the vascular endothelial cells of the CNS prior to infection of the adjacent glia and neu-

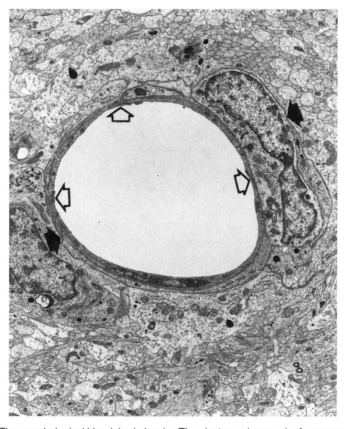

FIG. 3.3. The morphological blood–brain barrier. The electron micrograph of a precapillary arteriole in the cortex of an adult mouse shows portions of three endothelial cells that are circumferentially sealed by tight junctions (*open arrows*). The nucleus of one of the epithelial cells lies within the plane of section at the lower margin of the vessel, and there are two adjacent pericytes or perivascular macrophages (*upper right* and *lower left*); both the endothelial cells and pericytes are surrounded by and lie inside of the dense basement membrane (*filled arrow*). The foot processes of astrocytes are closely apposed to the basement membrane. ×6,850. (From Wolinsky and Johnson, 1980, with permission.)

rons (Johnson and Mims, 1968; Swarz et al., 1981). On the other hand, a number of viruses initially infect glia surrounding small intact vessels, without electron-microscopic or immunocytologic evidence of endothelial cell infection (Albrecht, 1968; Murphy and Whitfield, 1970). Transport of these viruses may occur in a manner analogous to that for ferritin particles, which cross the capillary endothelial cells in pinocytotic vesicles and are deposited in the cytoplasm of the adjacent astrocytes (Brightman, 1968).

In some infections, virus may be carried across the endothelial cells in infected leukocytes. Under normal circumstances, the traffic of lymphocytes into the CNS is limited, which may explain the infrequency of CNS infection and the need for a sustained viremia in some infections. This mechanism of invasion might be facilitated following trauma or in dual infections. Passage of virus through areas of permeability also has been postulated (Bodian, 1954), but in experimental studies no virus has been shown to cause infection preferentially related to the anatomic sites of permeability.

The structure of the blood–cerebrospinal-fluid barrier is quite different (Fig. 3.4). The vascular endothelial cells on the choroid plexus are fenestrated; they lack a dense basement membrane and are surrounded by loosely arranged stromal cells. Nevertheless, particles do not have free access to the cerebrospinal fluid, because the choroid plexus epithelial cells themselves are attached by the apical tight junctions, as are the pia-arachnoid cells that complete the barrier over the brain surface. Virus passing from blood into the stroma of the choroid plexus potentially can infect epithelial cells and seed virus directly into the cerebrospinal fluid or potentially can be transported via pinocytotic vesicles through the elongated epithelial cells. Direct seeding of virus into cerebrospinal fluid may be of particular importance in those viruses that cause widespread meningeal infections or viral meningitis. Growth of Japanese, eastern, and western encephalitis viruses in choroid plexus cells of mice has been shown by immunocytochemistry (Hamashima et al., 1959; Liu et al., 1970), but these studies failed to document that this infection preceded infection of other neural cells. Studies in hamsters of both rat virus (Lipton and Johnson, 1972) and mumps virus (Wolinsky et al., 1974) have shown a clear sequence of choroid plexus infection, followed by ependymal cell infection and then involvement of the parenchymal cells, which suggests invasion via choroid plexus. An analogous pathogenesis is implied in humans by the finding of choroid plexus and ependymal cells containing viral nucleocapsids in cerebrospinal fluid during mumps meningitis (Herndon et al., 1974).

Invasion of the CNS from blood appears to require a sequence of events involving extraneural tissues, blood, and the membranes separating the blood and brain (Fig. 3.5). This may explain why viral meningitis and encephalitis in humans are relatively rare, even though infections with viruses that have the potential to cause CNS disease are common. Along this route of infection during the incubation period, various host defense mechanisms are marshaled. The alveolar, epithelial, and subcutaneous phagocytic cells engulf and sometimes

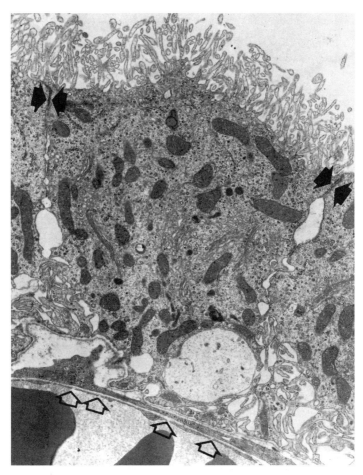

FIG. 3.4. The morphological blood–cerebrospinal-fluid barrier. The electron micrograph of the choroid plexus in an immature hamster shows the blood vessel (*below*) with portions of several red cells; the cerebrospinal fluid is *above*. The small venule has fenestrated (*open arrows*) endothelial cells. The choroid plexus epithelial cells rest on a basement membrane and have microvillous surfaces facing the spinal fluid. Apical tight junctions (*filled arrows*) between the cells form the barrier to free diffusion between serum and spinal fluid. ×13,700. (From Wolinsky and Johnson, 1980, with permission.)

inactivate virus particles; insusceptible cells in tissues pose barriers to primary and secondary multiplication; interferon is produced by infected cells; particles are cleared from the blood by the reticuloendothelial system; and the anatomic structures of the brain itself deter viruses. Presumably, only by dodging each of these barriers in sequence can virus gain access to the CNS.

The route of neuroinvasion may depend on the route of virus entry, such as experimental herpes simplex virus infections where dermal inoculation is fol-

PATHOGENESIS OF CNS INFECTIONS

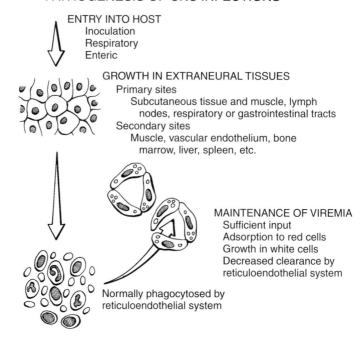

ENTRY INTO HOST
 Inoculation
 Respiratory
 Enteric

GROWTH IN EXTRANEURAL TISSUES
 Primary sites
  Subcutaneous tissue and muscle, lymph
   nodes, respiratory or gastrointestinal tracts
 Secondary sites
  Muscle, vascular endothelium, bone
   marrow, liver, spleen, etc.

MAINTENANCE OF VIREMIA
 Sufficient input
 Adsorption to red cells
 Growth in white cells
 Decreased clearance by
  reticuloendothelial system

Normally phagocytosed by
reticuloendothelial system

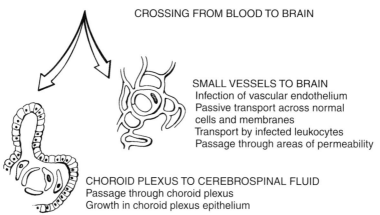

CROSSING FROM BLOOD TO BRAIN

SMALL VESSELS TO BRAIN
 Infection of vascular endothelium
 Passive transport across normal
 cells and membranes
 Transport by infected leukocytes
 Passage through areas of permeability

CHOROID PLEXUS TO CEREBROSPINAL FLUID
Passage through choroid plexus
Growth in choroid plexus epithelium

FIG. 3.5. Steps in the hematogenous spread of virus into the CNS. (Adapted from Johnson, 1974.)

lowed by neural spread to the CNS and intraperitoneal inoculation is followed by hematogenous spread (Johnson, 1964a). Route of neuroinvasion also can be virus determined by virus proteins; reovirus type 1 spreads to the mouse CNS after footpad injections via the blood, whereas reovirus type 3 spreads via axonal transport. Using recombinants of these viruses with multipartite genomes, the exchange of the S1 RNA segments coding for a single capsid protein can reverse the route of neuroinvasion (Tyler et al., 1986b).

NEUROTROPISM

Spread of Virus within the CNS

Whether virus reaches the CNS via neural, olfactory, or hematogenous routes, disease can occur only if virus spreads within the nervous system, attaches to and penetrates susceptible cells, and induces changes in those cells. Virus entering the subarachnoid space from the olfactory mucosa or from the blood across the choroid plexus is readily dispersed through the cerebrospinal fluid and thus contacts meningeal and ependymal cells throughout the neuraxis. Spread of virus through the densely packed neuropil, with its paucity of extracellular space, poses a greater theoretical problem (Fig. 3.6).

In many experimental studies, intracerebral inoculation in animals has been used but under an erroneous interpretation. Inoculations of carbon particles, horseradish peroxidase, and viruses into small laboratory rodents have shown that a particulate inoculum is not deposited within the brain or even along the needle tract. Because of the great relative pressure, particles are forced back along the needle tract, flooding the entire subarachnoid space, the perivascular spaces, the ventricles, and the central canal of the spinal cord (Jackson et al., 1987; Cifuentes et al., 1992). Inoculum also overflows into the blood (Mims, 1960). Thus, intracerebral inoculation in small animals represents a combined subarachnoid and intravenous delivery of virus.

Sequential studies in experimental animals have shown that some viruses spread within the CNS in a contiguous fashion after initial infection of meningeal or ependymal surfaces. Obvious cell-to-cell spread is not observed with the majority of viruses, however, and other mechanisms explain widespread CNS infection. Ultrastructural studies have indicated that the extracellular gaps between cells and processes in the CNS measure only 100 to 150 Å, less than the diameter of any virion (Brightman and Reese, 1969). Some viruses may move through this narrow gap, or, alternatively, they may transmit via glia, be transported along the extensive axonal and dendritic ramifications of neurons, or be actively moved by mobile leukocytes that enter the inflammatory response. Evidence to settle this question is meager, but some evidence exists for each mode of transit, and probably all are involved to greater or lesser degrees in different infections.

Arboviruses, with diameters greater than 400 Å, have been demonstrated within the intercellular gaps of the neuropil in mouse brain. The extracellular

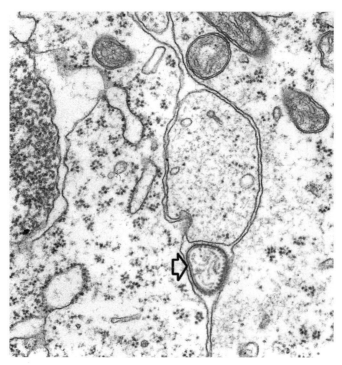

FIG. 3.6. Relationship of virus size to CNS extracellular space. A single mumps virus virion (*arrow*) is shown within the interstitial space between portions of three neurons in the hippocampal cortex of the newborn hamster. This space communicates freely with the ventricular system but restrains the movement of extracellular virus. ×47,300. (From Wolinsky and Johnson, 1980, with permission.)

spaces of the CNS may be more pliable in the intravital state than they appear to be in the rigid tissue prepared for electron microscopy (Blinzinger and Muller, 1971). The finding that hyperimmune serum can limit or arrest the progress of an existing encephalitic process due to arboviruses further indicates that viruses spread through the extracellular spaces (Albrecht, 1968).

The glia have long been suspected of forming a channel for the transport of material from blood to neurons. Inert ferritin particles, after crossing the cerebral capillaries, are found within the astrocytic footplates and subsequently in neurons (Bondareff, 1964). Similar data are not available for viruses.

Spread of virus via cytoplasmic ramifications of neurons appears important in many infections. Rabies virus, which infects only neurons, involves almost all susceptible neuronal populations within 24 hours of CNS invasion. Many of these neuron cell bodies are distant from the ependymal and meningeal surfaces and distant from one another, so that dissemination must occur by the contiguity of cell processes (Johnson, 1965a). It has been postulated that, in rabies, "passive intraneuronal movement of subviral entities must be interspersed with active viral replication at cell surfaces such that progeny virus may invade contiguous neurons or move within intercellular spaces to ultimately involve neural elements everywhere in the body" (Murphy et al., 1973a). Rabies virus normally is enveloped in the cytoplasm, but rabies virions budding from neuronal cell processes have been shown in mouse brain (Iwasaki and Clark, 1975). Herpes simplex virus normally is enveloped at the nuclear membrane, but unenveloped nucleocapsids have been demonstrated with microtubules within cytoplasmic processes in mouse brain (Schwartz and Elizan, 1975). The transit of subunits and the budding of virions at synapses may represent a mechanism for spread of enveloped viruses; this would allow rapid transport down the axon, with budding of virions against the soma of a distant but functionally linked susceptible neuron.

Our studies of human poliovirus in mice have indicated axonal spread within the CNS, because cordectomy prevents rostral or caudal spread of virus in spinal cord despite patent cerebrospinal fluid pathways. Furthermore, rates of transport increase with age, corresponding to acceleration of fast transport with age (Jubelt et al., 1980b). In humans, poliovirus-binding sites localize with synaptosomes, suggesting that similar axonal transport may occur (Brown et al., 1987b).

The agents of scrapie and Creutzfeldt–Jakob disease also spread along axonal pathways after experimental infection of mice (Liberski et al., 1990; Scott et al., 1992).

Selective Vulnerability of Cell Populations

The diverse cell populations within the CNS show variable susceptibilities to infections with different viruses. Some viruses, such as herpes simplex virus, are capable of infecting the full range of CNS cell types in multiple species. In contrast, other viruses may replicate only in ependymal and meningeal cells or only in specific neuronal populations. Furthermore, this selective vulnerability may vary from species to species or at different ages within a given species (Johnson, 1980). Such differences may explain why some viral infections of humans usually are accompanied only by meningeal signs, whereas others usually present with clinical signs of involvement of the parenchyma of the brain. Greater degrees of selectivity may explain the clinical–pathologic uniqueness of some infections. Motor nerve cells of the spinal cord seem to be selectively susceptible to poliomyelitis viruses, and this selectivity explains the clinical presentation of flaccid paralysis (Jubelt et al., 1980a). On the other hand, rabies virus, which infects only neurons, shows early localization to the neurons of the limbic system, with only relative sparing of the neocortex, and this can explain the unique clinical manifestations of the infection. Selective infection and destruction of oligodendrocytes can lead to demyelination (Weiner et al., 1973) (see Chapter 8), or infection of immature cells can lead to a wide variety of malformations (Johnson, 1972a) (see Chapter 13).

NEUROVIRULENCE

Neurovirulence is the ability of virus infection of the CNS to cause disease. The definition implies that virus is capable of invading the CNS and that CNS cells are infected. Whether or not pathologic changes and clinical disease ensue and to what extent they develop is dependent on a myriad of host factors as well as viral factors. Differences between virus strains or hosts may depend on whether different cells in the nervous system are affected, whether the virus load is different, whether there is more rapid spread of virus from cell to cell, or whether host protective factors are overcome. In some instances, replication of virus may be at the same level in the same cells, and the differential stimulation of mediators such as cytokines may determine virulence. In experimental animals, the use of recombinant viruses has identified specific proteins or noncoding regions involved in virulence. Sequence comparisons in some cases have shown point mutations at specific sites leading to single amino acid changes that alter virulence. Determinants of virulence are usually multigenic, and precisely how these molecular changes actually impact on the biology of disease still is unclear.

In experimental animals, neurovirulence of different strains of virus can be defined by comparing effects following intracerebral inoculation. Neurovirulence in human infections is difficult to assess, because the roles of neuroinvasiveness and neurotropism are difficult to sort out. The notable exceptions are human poliovirus infections where there are virulent strains known to cause paralytic human disease and oral vaccine strains that cause subclinical infections. Furthermore, these strains can be compared by a World Health Organization standard: after intraspinal inoculation of monkeys, inflammation and neuronal damage are graded and provide a numerical score of neurovirulence. The vaccine strain of type 1 virus compared with virulent viruses shows 57 nucleotide sequence differences (of 7,741 bases of the genome) leading to 21 amino acid changes. In contrast, type 3 oral vaccine virus, which has been most frequently associated with reversion to neurovirulence and paralysis in vaccinees, has only 10 point mutations resulting in 3 amino acid changes (Almond, 1987). These magnitudes of differences in attenuation may explain the more frequent reversion of the type 3 virus to cause paralysis in those exposed to vaccine strains. Paralysis due to type 1 virus after vaccine has been associated with recombinants with wild-type virus but more often with point mutations. Point mutations have been largely in the 5′ noncoding region (Evans et al., 1985; La Monica et al., 1987; Li et al., 1996). The Lansing strain of type 2 poliovirus causes paralytic disease in mice, and a nucleotide change at an analogous position causes the virus to lose its ability to replicate in mouse brain. This 5′ noncoding region is involved in protein binding and poliovirus translation (Ehrenfeld and Gebhard, 1994), and the findings suggest that the structure of this region is of critical importance for the neurovirulent phenotype (Almond, 1987). Recently, the development of transgenic mice containing the human poliovirus receptor has shown dose-dependent paralysis and rather good correlation with the results of monkey neurovirulence tests (Horie et al., 1994). These mice may provide a more accessible and economical assay system for studies of poliovirus neurovirulence.

In herpes simplex virus, a number of mutations can alter the ability of the virus to invade the nervous system, but others can attenuate virus growth in brain (Thompson et al., 1985; Chou et al., 1990). The gene coding for infected cell protein 34.5 (ICP 34.5) has been called the neurovirulence gene, and indeed mutations in this gene reduce neurovirulence while retaining normal replication and virulence in footpads (Bolovan et al., 1994). However, UL5, a component of the origin-binding complex implicated in replication of the viral genome, appears related specifically to neuronal infection; the virus without UL5 replicates in mouse brain, but predominantly in nonneuronal cells, and requires much higher inoculation doses to cause disease (Bloom and Stevens, 1994). The mutants that lack thymidine kinase also might be said to lose neurovirulence but by a different mechanism. These viruses grow well in extraneural tissues by using the cellular thymidine kinase but cannot replicate in nonreplicating neurons that lack thymidine kinase. These strains fail to replicate in murine neurons and therefore have markedly attenuated virulence when inoculated intracerebrally (Tenser et al., 1989; Tenser, 1991). It might be argued that they lost neurotropism, but indeed they are capable of infecting neurons and establishing latency even though these mutants cannot be reactivated or produce infectious progeny virus in neurons. A recent review tabulates nine different nucleotide locations on the herpes simplex virus genome that affect neurovirulence by different mechanisms (Bennett and Gilden, 1996).

Paramyxovirus and orthomyxovirus that are not normally neurovirulent in rodents have been adapted by repeated intracerebral passage to select neurovirulent strains. Wild strains of influenza, mumps, and measles virus replicate primarily in ependymal cells, whereas the neuroadapted strains of these viruses replicate in neurons (Johnson, 1968; Griffin et al., 1974; Ward, 1996). The basis of these changes is unknown in measles and in mumps viruses, but in influenza virus the neurotropic genotype is associated with changes in the neuraminidase gene (Ward, 1995).

Parallel differences in neurovirulence are seen with reoviruses in which type 1 reovirus infects ependymal cells, causing no acute clinical disease but later development of hydrocephalus similar to mumps, measles, and influenza viruses. Type 3 reovirus infects neurons and astrocytes, causing acute encephalitis similar to neuroadapted strains of these viruses. Since reovirus is a multisegmented, double-stranded RNA virus, the reassortants can be generated, and it has been shown that the S1 gene, which codes for the binding protein shifted between type 1 and type 3, reverses the specifics of neurotropism and neurovirulence (Fields, 1982; Hrdy et al., 1982). Variance within this gene can lead to infection of more restricted neuronal populations (Spriggs et al., 1983).

Very striking changes in the spread of virus leading to either focal nonlethal lesions or widespread encephalitis have been found in both rabies and Sindbis virus, and in both cases the determinant of neurovirulence has been localized to a single nucleotide. In rabies virus, an important determinant of virulence has been localized to position 333 in the glycoprotein and, although adjacent substitutions affect neutralization, only substitutions at position 333 affect pathogenicity (Seif et al., 1985). Sindbis virus normally causes acute encephalitis after intracerebral inoculation in neonatal mice, but after the first week of age a focal nonfatal encephalitis is seen. A neuroadapted strain has been developed that causes fatal encephalitis in older mice, and this has been found to depend on a single amino acid change at position 55 of the E2 surface protein gene (Tucker et al., 1993). Furthermore, evidence suggests that the development of resistance with age correlates with the protective effect of antiapoptotic cellular proteins and that the neuroadapted strains of virus with the single amino acid change in the E2 glycoprotein are neurovirulent because of their ability to kill cells despite the expression of antiapoptotic proteins such as bcl-2 (Ubol et al., 1994).

Two neurotropic murine leukemia virus strains differing only in the envelope proteins have been shown to reach similar DNA levels in brain, yet they differ markedly in induction of clinical disease (Portis et al., 1990). Differential induction of a cytokine or other neurotoxin factor has been invoked to explain this phenomenon, as it has with HIV infections in humans (Johnson et al., 1996).

It is hard to define neurovirulence between different strains of the same virus in human diseases. The frequency of paralytic disease varied between poliovirus epidemics, and this probability represented genetic variations of virus. The same variance of disease severity has been noted with other enterovirus epidemics. There has been a less well documented suggestion that neurologic complications are more frequent in certain influenza epidemics, such as the epidemic of Asian influenza of 1957. However, this could have represented a greater degree of neuroinvasiveness or a more frequent inciting of autoimmune disease. The question as to whether there are strains of HIV that produce dementia and those that do not is currently debated (see Chapter 12). Certainly, in human disease, the difference in neurovirulence between different viruses is striking (Table 3.3). For example, mumps virus is highly neuroinvasive, but its neurotropism appears limited to ependymal cells, which may account for the low level of neurovirulence. In contrast, a ubiquitous virus, such as herpes simplex virus, is thought to be relatively nonneuroinvasive, but when it does infect the CNS neurons, glial cells, pia-arachnoid, and endothelial cells are all infected and, without appropriate treatment, a 70% mortality bespeaks a very high degree of neurovirulence. The retroviruses remain the most enigmatic. Indeed, the limitation of the human T-cell lymphotropic virus I to inflammatory cells would suggest that it is not neurotropic in that it may not infect neural cells, yet it is neurovirulent. HIV infection of brain appears to be limited largely to cells of macrophage origin, but the question of how infection of perivascular macrophages, macrophages, and microglia leads to dementia is unanswered. Furthermore, early in the course of

TABLE 3.3. *Examples of neuroinvasiveness, tropism, and virulence in humans*

	Virus					
					HIV	
	Mumps	Herpes simplex	Rabies	HTLV	Early	Late
Neuroinvasive	++++	+	++++	+	+++	+
Neurotropic						
Neurons	0	+++	++++	0	0	0
Neuroglia	0	+++	0	?	?	?
Microglia	?	+++	0	0	+++	+++
Pia arachnoid/ependyma	++++	+++	0	0	0	0
Neurovirulence	+	++++	++++	++	0	+++

HTLV, human T-cell lymphotropic virus.

the long asymptomatic infection, HIV is highly neuroinvasive, with frequent infections of cells in the nervous system, but disease appears late, suggesting that the determinants of neurovirulence evolve or are uncovered only in the late stages of the infection.

SUPPLEMENTARY BIBLIOGRAPHY

Mims CA, Dimmock NJ, Nash A, Stephen J. *Mims' pathogenesis of infectious disease,* 4th ed. London: Academic Press, 1995.
Nathanson N, Ahmed R, Gonzales-Scarano F, et al. *Viral pathogenesis.* Philadelphia: Lippincott–Raven Publishers, 1997.
Roos RP, ed. *Molecular neurovirology.* Totowa, NJ: Humana Press, 1992.

4

Immune Responses

> Of the many aged people still living in the Faroes who had had measles in 1781, not one, as far as I could find out by careful inquiry, was attacked a second time. I myself saw 98 such old people, who were exempt because they had had the disease in their youth.
>
> Peter Ludwig Panum,
> *Observations Made during the Epidemic of Measles on the Faroe Islands in the Year 1846*

Several decades after Panum's observation, the term *immunity*, meaning freedom from burden or taxation, was applied to this exemption from reinfection. Yet, in his classic study of epidemic measles in an island population, Panum had documented the two salient features of immune responses: their specificity and their memory. Specificity of immune responses is now known to be conferred by surface proteins on cells of the immune system and by the variable ends of antibody molecules. Memory is conferred by specialized lymphocytes, but how this memory can be preserved for over six decades without reexposure remains a mystery.

Phylogenetically, the specialized organs and cells concerned with specific immune responses evolved with the primitive vertebrates. Less specific protective mechanisms, such as phagocytic cells that recognize and engulf foreign material, are present in invertebrates. Even prokaryotic bacterial cells have evolved mechanisms to protect against viral infections: the restriction endonucleases that cleave specific base sequences of alien DNA probably evolved to protect bacteria from infection. The evolution of complex heterogeneous immune systems in higher species is not surprising, considering the selective advantages of these systems to clear dangerous infectious agents, to protect against reinfection, and to monitor and remove material such as neoplastic cells that are identified as "nonself." These same responses, however, can be harmful to the host in the form of allergic or hypersensitivity reactions. If immune responses develop against antigens of the host, they can cause autoimmune responses.

Both humoral and cell-mediated immune responses demonstrate specificity and memory. Following encounter with an antigen (immunogen), primary immune responses follow after an interval during which specific antibody or sensitized cells are generated. If the antigen is successfully expelled, these immunoglobulins and sensitized cells quantitatively decline to lower or even undetectable concentrations. At a future time, if the same antigen is reencountered, a secondary immune response is seen that is accelerated, is of greater magnitude, and is responsive to a smaller stimulus. Secondary responses are best studied in antibody responses, but accelerated secondary responses also develop for cell-mediated immune responses (Griffin and Johnson, 1973).

The mechanism for lifelong memory is unknown. Immunoglobulins have a half-life of less than a month, and although memory cells may survive for many years, survival for half a century seems unlikely but not unthinkable. Lifelong immunity has been postulated to result from intermittent subclinical reinfection or reexposure that boosts or recalls the immune response. However, this fails to explain observations such as that by Panum, where there was no reintroduction of measles during the intervening 65-year interval. Similar observations have been made regarding long immunity without reexposure for poliomyelitis among Eskimos and for yellow fever and Rift Valley fever in the tropics. Therefore, memory cells must survive for generations, memory must be transferred vertically from non-end-stage lymphocytes to progeny, or virus or antigenic sequences must persist at some low level to maintain memory (Jamieson and Ahmed, 1989; Sprent and Tough, 1994). The latter may occur by sequestration of antigenic polypeptides by dendritic cells in lymph nodes or spleen.

Another characteristic of specific immune responses is their ability to be passively transferred. Immunity, protection, hypersensitivity, and allergy all can be transferred to a nonimmune host by inoculation of either immune serum or immunocompetent cells.

ANATOMY OF THE IMMUNE SYSTEM

The bone marrow, thymus, spleen, lymph nodes, and the lymphoid tissues of the gastrointestinal tract are the major organs of the immune system. The cellular constituents include T cells, B cells, monocytes, macrophages, dendritic cells, and endothelial cells.

Differentiation and Maturation of Cell Populations

Under the influence of the thymus, one group of lymphocytes (thymus-dependent or T cells) differentiates into a population of relatively long-lived cells that can generate cell-mediated immune responses. Under the influence of gut-associated lymphoid tissues, fetal liver, or bone marrow, other mononuclear cells develop immunoglobulin markers on their surfaces and, when stimulated by antigen, differentiate into mature B cells and plasma cells. In chickens, this differentiation is mediated by the bursa of Fabricius, which accounts for the name bursa-dependent or B cells. The T cells are more numerous in lymph nodes and thymus, B cells are more prevalent in bone marrow, and representation of T and B cells is nearly equal in the spleen.

T-cell precursors from the bone marrow migrate to the thymus, where these undifferentiated thymocytes undergo extensive proliferation and rearrangement of T-cell receptor genes. The variable portions of the T-cell receptor will be complementary to specific antigens bound to the major histocompatibility complex (MHC) of an antigen-presenting cell. In the thymus, there is a positive selection for receptors that respond to host MHC molecules and a negative selection of autoreactive receptors; this leaves a population of T cells tolerant to MHC molecules presenting self-antigens and strongly reactive toward self-MHC molecules presenting foreign antigens. In this positive and negative selection, 95% of the T cells are discarded before release into the circulation (Sprent and Tough, 1994). Further maturation goes on for several days in the blood, where populations of cells with CD4 and CD8 surface markers differentiate to the fully mature phenotype of mature but naive T cells. Those with CD4 markers include helper cells that stimulate cell-mediated immune responses (Th1) and antibody responses (Th2); those with CD8 markers include cytotoxic cells and possibly suppressor cells (Table 4.1).

B cells undergo rearrangement of the variable region of the immunoglobulin gene in the bone marrow. Clusters of genes on three different chromosomes encode the immunoglobulin (Ig) light (2) and heavy (1) chains, each with many variable gene segments. This leads to extraordinary diversity of immunoglobulins (10^8 or more *different* Ig molecules in normal serum). Selected B cells, in general, are tolerant to circulating self-antigens but not to tissue self-antigens. B cells mature further after leaving the bone marrow but retain IgM as their surface receptors until activated. B cells also serve as antigen-presenting cells for soluble antigens.

TABLE 4.1. *Mononuclear cells*

Cell type	Surface marker	Function
T	CD3 (element of T-cell receptor)	Cell-mediated immunity and regulation of B cells
T helper	CD4 (MHC class II receptor)	Effector cells and T-cell and B-cell regulation
Th1		Heighten cell-mediated immune responses
Th2		Heighten humoral immune responses
T cytotoxic	CD8 (MHC class I receptor)	Cytotoxic cells and ? suppressor cells
B	Ig CD19, and a number of activation antigens	Antibody production
NK	Fc receptors	MHC independent killing by apoptosis
Monocytes/	FC receptors	Antigen-presenting cells
macrophages	MHC class I and II	General scavengers
	C3 receptors (when activated)	Cytolytic after activation by CD4 cell
	Low levels of CD4	

Ig, immunoglobulin; MHC, major histocompatibility complex; NK, natural killer.

In young mice, the number of T cells released from the thymus is about 1×10^6 cells per day, and the number of B cells with surface IgM generated from the marrow is about 2×10^7 cells per day. In humans, about 10^{12} mononuclear cells constitute over 1% of the total body weight.

A small percentage of lymphocytes have no antigen-specific receptors (neither T-cell receptors nor surface immunoglobulins), but they do have receptors for the Fc (crystallizable fragment) of IgG. These have been referred to as null cells. This population includes the killer cells, which react with antibody on the surface of virus-infected cells in antibody-dependent cellular cytotoxicity, and the natural killer cells, which are activated by interferon and are cytotoxic for some virus-infected cells and tumor cells that do not express MHC class I.

Macrophages are the general phagocytes of the body and are the mainstays of the innate nonspecific immunity. They are derived from promonocytes in the marrow that have a common progenitor with granulocytes rather than lymphocytes. They enter the blood as monocytes. When they move into tissue compartments, they may play specialized roles, such as the Kupffer cells in the liver, the alveolar macrophage of the lung, or the microglia of the brain. They not only scavenge for foreign material, but they can process antigen and present it to lymphocytes associated with class II MHC molecules. It is this trimolecular complex of the MHC molecule, an antigenic polypeptide, and either a T-cell receptor or complex of antigen and surface immunoglobulin on a B cell that leads to activation and the clonal proliferation of specific lymphocytes. The activation, proliferation, and differentiation of T and B cells are influenced directly by soluble signaling molecules (cytokines) from T cells and macrophages.

The blood granulocytes are important in bacterial and fungal infections, but patients with agranulocytosis or granulocyte defects are not predisposed to either recurrences or heightened severity of viral infections. Although granulocytes may attend the early acute inflammatory reactions to viral infections, they have no determined function in recruiting mononuclear cells or in clearing virus.

Cellular Activation

In the recesses of the circulatory and lymphatic systems and the vast tissue spaces of the body, an antigen-presenting cell carrying the processed antigen somehow must encounter a T lymphocyte with the matching receptor, or a virion or virus-infected cell must interact with a B lymphocyte with IgM or IgD molecules specific to the antigen. This seemingly formidable search is facilitated in part by the nonrandom trafficking of nonactivated or "naive" lymphocytes and the structure of lymph nodes. Naive lymphocytes have lymph node homing receptors (adhesion molecules) on their surface, and the high-walled venular endothelium of lymphoid tissue (nodes, Peyer's patches, tonsils, and spleen) have complementary binding proteins called addressins (Butcher and Picker, 1996). A multistep sequential engagement of the lymphocyte occurs with partial adhesion and rolling, followed by firm adhesion, followed by diapedesis through the vascular endothelium. Cycles from blood through lymph nodes are made each day by each cell. The encapsulated lymph node provides a milieu that is designed for the optimum contact between macrophages and dendritic cells, which act as "professional" antigen-presenting cells, and the circulating T and B lymphocytes; the node also can maintain high concentrations of cytokines that stimulate clonal expansion of activated lymphocytes. We witness the clonal expansion and lymphocyte trapping when lymph nodes acutely increase in size (and tenderness) and when a systemic lymphopenia develops acutely in many viral infections (Doherty et al., 1992).

With activation, T cells transform to lymphoblasts that have little endoplasmic reticulum but abundant free ribosomes. These T lymphoblasts proliferate and differentiate into subsets of small CD4 and CD8 T cells that engage in inflammation, macrophage activation, cytotoxic activity, and control of T-cell and B-cell proliferation and differentiation. T helper cells (CD4+) see peptide antigens with class II MHC on the surface of macrophages, B cells, or dendritic cells and then release cytokines that may activate macrophages, enabling them to kill intracellular parasites (e.g., interferon γ), deactivate macrophages (interleukin 10), and promote T-cell proliferation and differentiation (e.g., interleukins 2 and 4) and B-cell proliferation and differentiation (e.g., interleukins 4, 5, and 6). Cytotoxic T cells (CD8+) recognize peptide antigen-associated class I MHC on the surface of infected cells and can kill them. Class I MHC molecules are present on the surface of most nucleated cells, but are most numerous on lymphoid cells and generally absent on neural cells of neuroectodermal origin. Many viruses interfere with MHC class I expression to prevent recognition of these cells.

B cells are activated by cross-linking of surface immunoglobulin receptors or interaction with T cells and begin differentiation into plasma cells with large amounts of rough endoplasmic reticulum characteristic of protein-secreting cells; immunoglobulin synthesis expands from less than 5% of protein synthesis of naive B cells to greater than 40% in plasma cells. IgM produced early is switched to IgG and IgA largely through the influence of T cells. A subpopulation of activated T and B cells persists as memory cells, but most are eliminated by apoptosis after elimination of antigen.

The primed or activated lymphocytes are altered and express different surface antigens. These include receptors of the integrin superfamily that bind preferentially, but not exclusively, to cell adhesion molecules (called CAMs) that may be expressed on the vascular endothelium of nonlymphoid tissues. Thus, once activated, cell trafficking is redirected so that these circulatory lymphocytes monitor tissue spaces and generally return to lymph nodes via the lymphatics rather than through the bloodstream (Butcher and Picker, 1996). Circulation may be tissue selective, so an activated lymphocyte may be targeted to a specific organ such as skin or intestine. Specific CNS homing molecules on lymphocytes or receptors specific to cerebrovascular endothelial cells have not yet been identified. In the CNS, cerebral vascular endothelial cells can be activated by cytokines, such as tumor necrosis factor, to increase expression of adhesion molecules (Elfont et al., 1995), and activated lymphocytes appear to enter the CNS in a nonspecific fashion (Irani and Griffin, 1996). This is probably the mechanism for the acute aseptic meningitis seen after cardiac transplantation, when OKT3 antibodies have been used as an immunosuppressant, because these antibodies cause general activation of T cells, enhancing their nonspecific entry into the nervous system (Adair et al., 1991).

Cytokine Network

Cytokines are small, soluble polypeptides produced primarily by cells of the immune system that act as intercellular signaling molecules. These molecules are potent at nanomolar or even picomolar levels, but they act transiently and at short range. Constitutive production is usually low or absent. Cytokines usually are secreted by specific cell types of mononuclear or endothelial cells (less often by fibroblasts, myoblasts, microglia and, in rare instances, astrocytes), and specific high-affinity receptors are present on the target cells' surface. In general, these molecules are not effector molecules but indirectly regulate cell proliferation, differentiation, chemoattraction, and survival.

Over 50 cytokines have been described and are variously classified by their physicochemical structure, their receptor class, or their general modes of action (Table 4.2). Cytokines are pleiotropic (act on different cell types) and pleiotypic

TABLE 4.2. *Groupings of cytokines by mode of action*

Group	Released by	Effect
Interferons	α, leukocytes β, "fibroblasts" γ, activated lymphocytes, NK cells	Interfere with virus replication; also regulate tumor growth, bone marrow maturation, and macrophage activation
Interleukins	T and B cells and macrophages (bone marrow, epithelial cells, and glial cells)	Regulate stimulation or activation of hematopoietic cells and/or upregulate or downregulate other cytokines
Chemokines	Platelets, T and B cells, macrophages, fibroblasts, endothelial cells, and possibly astrocytes	Induce leukocyte chemotaxis and activation
Tumor necrosis factors	T and B cells, monocytes, and fibroblasts	Proinflammatory but also induce apoptosis
Colony-stimulating factors	Lymphocytes and monocytes (fibroblasts and myoblasts)	Colony cell formation in bone marrow and activation of mature leukocytes
Growth factors	Mononuclear cells, fibroblasts, and many others	Stimulate cell growth and differentiation
Neural growth factors	Neural cells, salivary glands, neural cells (Schwann cells, neurons)	Differentiation and maintenance of varied neuronal populations

(act in different ways); they also tend to act in concert, thus forming a complex network. For example, proinflammatory and antiinflammatory cytokines tune up and down the inflammatory reaction at appropriate times if the dose, time of release, and balance between them are properly maintained. The complexity of this network interaction is evident in the development of subsets of T helper cells that enhance cell-mediated responses (Th1) and those that enhance antibody responses (Th2). This differentiation, in turn, depends on cytokines produced by the antigen-presenting cells. Interleukin 12 is necessary for development of the Th1 phenotype that secretes large amounts of interferon γ and interleukin 2 that regulate the cell-mediated responses. In contrast, interleukin 4 directs the T helper cell toward the Th2 phenotype that secretes interleukins 4, 5, 6, and 10 that enhance antibody responses. Infections with some viruses, such as HIV and measles virus, can disrupt this balance and lead to selective immunodeficiency (Griffin et al., 1994a; Shearer et al., 1994), and many viruses interfere directly with the production or function of cytokines.

Interferons were the first defined cytokines and were named for their interference with virus replication. They are released by many cells and bind to receptors on neighboring or distant cells to produce a virus-resistant state. As with the other cytokines, they have other functions, such as regulating tumor growth and MHC expression. Interferon γ induces cellular adhesion molecules on vascular endothelial cells.

Interleukin 1 may be produced by any nucleated cell type in response to foreign antigen, toxin, injury, or inflammation. It is a major reactant in bacterial infections mediating immunocyte activation and acute-phase responses. Interleukin 2 is produced primarily by T cells and stimulates clonal expansion of T cells. Interleukin 10 has been termed cytokine inhibitory factor because it suppresses macrophage activation by interferon γ, but is a potent B-cell growth factor. Interleukin 12 was originally termed natural killer cell stimulatory factor, but it also functions as a major regulator of interferon-γ synthesis and upregulates secretion by natural killer and T cells. Epstein–Barr virus has a region of homology with interleukin 10. It is felt this plays two roles in the pathogenesis of Epstein–Barr virus infections: first, it suppresses immunostimulatory cytokines and, second, it promotes B-cell growth, the host cell of the virus. Another class of cytokines—chemokines—primarily regulate leukocyte chemotaxis.

Some cytokines are released by neural cells or react with neural cells. Nerve growth factors are small communication polypeptides that fall into the general category of cytokines. Nerve growth factors such as brain-derived neurotrophic factor, ciliary neurotrophic factor, nerve growth factor, and neurotrophin 3 are generally released by neural cells, myocytes, or other nonlymphoid cells and act primarily on neural cells. However, other, more classic cytokines, including some interleukins, tumor necrosis factors, and vascular endothelial growth factors, can be produced by neural cells and act on the receptors of nonneural cells, whereas other cytokines are released by cells of the immune system and affect neural cells.

In the nervous system, activated microglia are the main producers of cytokines other than growth factors, although neurons and astrocytes as well as endothelial and perivascular cells have been proposed as cytokine producers. Very dramatic effects of cytokines can be seen in cultures of CNS cells. Tumor necrosis factor can lead to apoptosis of neurons and oligodendrocytes *in vitro* (Selmaj et al., 1991). In cultures of oligodendrocytes, ciliary nerve neurotrophic factor protects against tumor necrosis factor–induced apoptosis but not against complement-mediated cell necrosis (Louis et al., 1993). Tumor necrosis factor as well as interleukins 1 and 6 also have been found to alter the transendothelial cell resistance of cerebrovascular endothelial cells in culture, raising the possibility that they may have the potential to alter the blood–brain barrier *in vivo* (de Vries et al., 1996).

Cytokines do affect neural function *in vivo*, but these effects are less striking than in cultures where a single cytokine is delivered; *in vivo*, they act as a complex network. For example, interleukin 1, the major pyrogen of bacterial infections, causes fever, sleep disorders, and electroencephalogram changes presumably through action on the hypothalamus. Recent studies have found, however, a lack of receptors for interleukin 1 in the hypothalamus; apparently, interleukin 1 induces interleukin 6, for which the hypothalamus has ample receptors (Hopkins and Rothwell, 1995). Interferon also has an effect on the neural function, causing somnolence, confusion, gait disorders, and electroencephalogram abnormalities, all of which are demonstrated in patients given large doses of interferon in the treatment of tumors (Suter et al., 1984). Injection of tumor necrosis factor into rat sciatic nerves leads to endoneurial perivascular inflammation with demyelination and axonal degeneration (Redford et al., 1995).

In viral infections, cytokines play important roles. Indeed, many viruses (e.g., poxvirus, herpesvirus, adenovirus, and retroviruses) encode virokines, viral versions of cytokines and receptors that may regulate the host cytokines. Many viral infections can both increase and decrease expression of both class I and II MHC molecules via upgrading, downregulating, or binding of cytokines (Rinaldo, 1994). This may determine viral clearance or viral persistence. In viral infections of the CNS, activation of microglia leads to production of multiple cytokines; in the CNS, these cytokines may not act in the traditional role of modulatory molecules but may act as effector molecules as in the induction of neuronal apoptosis. This mechanism has been suggested in the myelopathy of human T-cell lymphotropic virus infection and the dementia with HIV infection (see Chapters 11 and 12).

IMMUNE RESPONSES TO VIRUSES

Viruses as Antigens

Technically, an immunogen is a substance that can provoke a specific immune response, and an antigen is a substance with a configuration with which antibody or T cells can react. The immunogen may have more than one reactive site, each of which is called an antigenic determinant or epitope (the site to which an antibody binds). Because most virus polypeptides are effective immunogens and antigens, the latter term is used.

Viruses code for multiple proteins, both structural and nonstructural. The amount of virus initially encountered by the host in natural transmission is very small; therefore, if the host is insusceptible to infection or if the virus is inactivated, there may be no amplification of antigens and no immune response or only a transient stimulation of IgM, a response that is not associated with the establishment of immunologic memory. In a susceptible host, however, million-fold amplifications of the antigenic mass occur during virus replication. During this amplification, phagocytosis and processing of virus-specific proteins immunize the host both to surface polypeptides and to internal and nonstructural proteins. Antibody usually is synthesized against epitopes on most or all of these constituents. Obviously, the antibodies reactive with internal or nonstructural proteins are of no importance in the neutralization or clearance of free virus. However, antibodies to internal proteins may be important in other responses and form important tools in the identification of viruses and in the diagnosis of infection.

Many variables—including the age of the host, the magnitude and site of virus replication, and the immunogenicity of the viral polypeptides—influence immune responses to viruses. Murine leukemia virus, which can be transmitted vertically with the host chromosomes (Rowe, 1972), or lymphocytic choriomeningitis virus, which may infect the ovum (Mims, 1966), may be regarded, at least in part, as "self" by the host, and thus their proteins are not regarded as antigens. Limited virus replication may lead to slow or late appearance of antibody.

Proteins and glycoproteins tend to be T-dependent antigens. Therefore, antibody responses to most viral antigens depend on T cells that act as helper cells to stimulate B-cell immunoglobulin synthesis or switch B cells from synthesis of IgM to synthesis of IgA or IgG. In the absence of T cells, no antibody response or only an IgM response occurs.

Antigens need not be exogenous. Indeed, sequestered proteins of the body, such as proteins in CNS myelin, may not be recognized as self. Inoculation of these proteins can lead to a cell-mediated immune response, with the development of experimental autoimmune encephalomyelitis (see Chapter 8). These observations have led to studies of viral antigens that have similar sequences with endogenous antigens and induce autoimmune disease by a mechanism called molecular mimicry (Oldstone et al., 1986).

Immunoglobulins

Immunoglobulins are classes of globular molecules synthesized by B lymphocytes and plasma cells. In humans, they can be divided into five types: IgG,

IgA, IgM, IgD, and IgE. IgG is present in both serum and extracellular fluid and is of major importance in virus clearance and protection from reinfection. IgA is found primarily in mucous secretions of the respiratory tract, gastrointestinal tract, saliva, tears, and breast milk, and it provides the first line of defense against virus invasion by these routes. IgM is found mainly in serum and is synthesized early in the course of infection, is more sensitive to minimal antigenic stimulation, and has a short half-life, with little, if any, memory. IgM plays a major role in the clearance of bacteremia, but its importance in clearing viremia is less certain (Table 4.3). IgD has been found as a surface marker on immature B lymphocytes, and IgE is involved in atopic reactions and asthma and probably plays a protective role in parasitic infections; neither of these two immunoglobulins plays a recognized major role in viral infections and are not considered further here.

The basic structure of immunoglobulins is a polymer of long and short polypeptide chains (Fig. 4.1). The long or heavy chains are characteristic of the immunoglobulin class and are referred to as γ, α, or μ chains. There are two classes of short or light chains: κ and λ. The short chains are the same for all classes of immunoglobulins. In humans, there are approximately twice as many antibody molecules that contain κ chains as there are those that contain λ chains.

The chains are connected with disulfide bonds. Proteolytic enzymes can cleave immunoglobulins into functionally distinct domains. Papain treatment results in two F(ab) fragments and a single Fc fragment. Pepsin will cleave the polymer at a different site, giving a single divalent fragment called $F(ab)^2$ (Fig. 4.1). The Fc fragment is involved in specialized functions, such as binding of

TABLE 4.3. *Properties of immunoglobulins important in viral infections*

	IgG	IgA	IgM
Major function	Virus clearance from extracellular spaces	Virus inactivation on mucous membrane	Virus clearance from blood
% Total immunoglobulin	80	13	6
Concentration in serum (mg/mL)	8–16	1.4–4	0.5–2
Cerebrospinal fluid–serum ratio	1/200–1/400	1/200–1/400	1/1,000
Half-life (days)	25	5	2–5
Transmission to offspring	Transplacental	Breast milk	0
Structure			
Heavy chain	$\gamma1$, $\gamma2$, $\gamma3$, $\gamma4$	$\alpha1$, $\alpha2$	μ
Light chain	κ or λ	κ or λ	κ or λ
Formula	$2\gamma + 2\kappa$ or 2λ	$2 (2\alpha + 2\kappa$ or $\lambda) + $ J chain + secretory piece	$5 (2\mu + 2\kappa$ or $\lambda) + $ J chain

Ig, immunoglobulin.

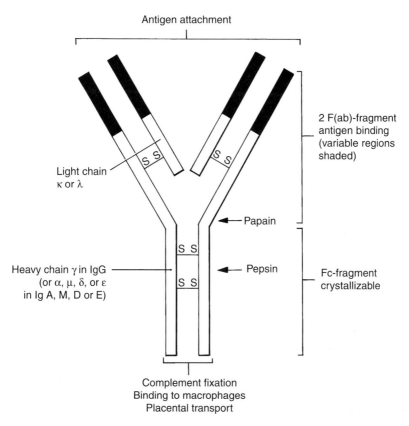

FIG. 4.1. Structure of the immunoglobulin molecule. Sulfide bonds unite light and heavy chains. Functions of the F(ab) terminus and Fc fragment and sites of cleavage by papain and pepsin are shown. This is a simplified diagram; immunoglobulin molecules have complex tertiary structures with many intricate loops.

immunoglobulin to Fc receptors on macrophages, antibody-dependent cytotoxicity, B-lymphocyte regulation, and transport across the placenta. The F(ab) fragment contains a distal sequence on each chain that determines the antigen-binding specificity (variable region).

Like IgG, IgA in the circulation consists of four peptide subunits, but on extracellular surfaces IgA is in an oligomeric form, with two such units being connected by a J chain and with an attached secretory piece. The secretory piece is synthesized in epithelial cells and is added as IgA passes through the cell to the mucosal surface and probably stabilizes the oligomer in secretions.

IgM is a polymer of five subunits, each with four peptides. This gives it a potential valence of 10 and great efficiency in aggregating antigens. As the surface immunoglobulin of unstimulated B cells, the proximity of variable regions of the same specificity facilitate cross-linkage and thus activation of B cells.

Immunoglobulin Interaction with Extracellular Virus

During viral infections, immunoglobulins can be directed against antigenic targets in two forms: either against surface components of the virion in the extracellular fluid or plasma or against host cell membranes that contain virus-coded proteins. Although these represent the same surface proteins, or glycoproteins, the effects of antibody attachment may be quite different. Antibody attachment to circulating virions usually leads to inactivation of detectable infectivity, referred to as neutralization. Neutralizing antibody may operate in three ways: (a) by coating the surface of the virion and enhancing phagocytosis, a process similar to opsonization of bacteria; (b) by preventing cellular infection by blocking attachment or penetration or enhancing the degradation of the virion within the pinocytotic vacuole; or (c) by direct virus lysis mediated through the attachment and activation of complement, which can "punch" holes in the virus envelope, similar to complement-mediated disruption of cell membranes. This activity demonstrated *in vitro* is relevant only to enveloped viruses, but it may or may not be important in inactivation of enveloped viruses *in vivo* (Iorio, 1988).

Antibody may attach to virus and continue to circulate until thermal inactivation of the virus occurs. These circulating immune complexes (antigen and antibody) are found in chronic lymphocytic choriomeningitis virus, lactic dehydrogenase virus, and retrovirus infections in mice, and in rubella virus, hepatitis B virus, Epstein–Barr virus, and cytomegalovirus infections in humans. Such immune complexes may be trapped in the glomerular basement membrane of the kidneys, but they may also be deposited in the vascular endothelium and in the choroid plexus of the CNS. In congenital chronic lymphocytic choriomeningitis virus infections in mice, the deposition of immune complexes in the renal glomeruli causes chronic glomerulonephritis, and it is this complication, rather than the chronic infection of brain and other organs, that shortens the life expectancy of carrier mice (Oldstone and Dixon, 1970). Hepatitis B antigen complexes have been implicated in vasculitis (see Chapter 16), and rubella virus complexes may play a role in the late panencephalitis that can follow fetal infection (see Chapters 10 and 13).

Even with effective antibody-mediated virus neutralization, all circulating virus may not be neutralized. This nonneutralized virus may persist, because antigen–antibody binding is a reversible phenomenon (the tightness of the fit or binding is called avidity), or the persistence may result from aggregation of virus particles, with entrapment of nonneutralized virus. Immunoglobulins are obviously most effective in clearing extracellular viruses and less effective in clearing viruses that move from cell to cell by fusion of cytoplasmic membranes.

Different Activities of Antiviral Antibodies

Different antigens of the same virus may provoke antibodies of different biologic activities, and different antibodies develop at different intervals. The categories of complement-fixing, precipitating, hemagglutination-inhibiting, and neutralizing antibodies are defined by the laboratory method of testing and are not mutually exclusive (a hemagglutination-inhibiting antibody molecule may also fix complement and neutralize virus), nor do they necessarily correlate with immunoglobulin class. IgM molecules do tend to be highly active in fixing complement, so that complement-fixing antibodies may be measurable in serum before other antibody activities. By the nature of the assay, hemagglutination-inhibiting antibodies and neutralizing antibodies usually are directed against surface proteins of the virion, and, for inexplicable reasons, antibodies that fix complement often are directed against internal components of the virus.

Not only do antibodies appear at different intervals following infection and persist for different periods of time, but the various antibodies can be useful in viral classification and diagnosis. For example, all adenoviruses contain a common antigen that elicits an antibody that fixes complement. Consequently, a complement-fixation test can be used to screen for infections by an entire family of viruses. Neutralizing antibodies against specific adenoviruses can then be used to differentiate serotypes.

Cross-reactions between antigens of related viruses also can cause confusion. For example, when a patient with no past experience with any of the group B coxsackieviruses is infected by B1 coxsackievirus, the patient will show an increase in neutralizing antibody only to that virus, and this antibody does not neutralize other group B coxsackieviruses. However, at a future date, when infected by B2 coxsackievirus, the same patient may not only develop antibody against the homologous virus but also mount an anamnestic antibody response against the previously encountered related virus. This anamnestic response can be of greater magnitude than the primary response to the infecting virus. The tendency for the domination of the immune response against the first-encountered virus of a group of related viruses is striking with the group A influenza viruses, where this phenomenon has been termed "original antigenic sin."

Complement

The complement system is comprised of a series of nine components made up of over 20 interacting serum proteins, a complex array analogous to the coagulation system. Activation by antigen–antibody reactions sets off a sequential cascade, with release of biologically active enzymes that cause histamine release from mast cells, act as chemotactic factors for polymorphonuclear cells, and induce immune adherence of the antibody–antigen complex to increase phagocytosis. The complement system also can have adverse effects—including the Arthus reaction, serum sickness, and nephrotoxic glomerulonephritis—when immune complexes activate the system.

An alternative pathway for activation of the complement system circumvents the early proteins (C1, C4, and C2) and activates the cascade at the level of the fourth component (C3). This activation does not require the presence of antibody, and the alternative pathway can be activated by some cell-wall polysac-charides and viral glycoproteins (Welsh, 1977; Hirsch et al., 1980).

The attachment of the terminal components of complement can cause circu-lar 8- to 12-nm lesions in cell membranes and osmotic lysis of the cell. Similar membrane lesions in the lipid envelopes of some viruses can cause direct viral lysis. *In vivo*, the role of complement in viral infections is varied. In mice infected with lymphocytic choriomeningitis virus, a noncytopathic infection in which disease is immune mediated, depletion of C3 protects against disease (Oldstone and Dixon, 1971). In acute viral encephalitis of mice with Sindbis virus, the effects of complement depletion are both harmful and beneficial. In decomplemented mice, viremia is prolonged and 1,000-fold more virus is repli-cated in the CNS. Complement either inactivates the enveloped virus in blood or enhances its phagocytosis or both. The prolongation of viremia may lead to greater seeding of virus in the CNS. On the other hand, the time of death from encephalitis is delayed in the complement-depleted animals, which suggests that complement-dependent cytotoxicity may hasten death from encephalitis even though the presence or absence of complement does not alter the overall mor-tality (Hirsch et al., 1978).

Immune Attack on Virus-infected Cells

The interactions of specific immune responses with virus-infected cells are complex. Immunoglobulin molecules, which can attach to extracellular virus, can prevent its attachment to subsequent host cells, augment its phagocytosis by macrophages, or cause direct virolysis mediated by complement. Immunoglob-ulins also can have varied effects when they attach to virus antigens on the cell surface: this can modulate the infection, can protect the infected cell from immune destruction, or can mediate cell destruction. The cross-linking of attached antibody molecules may lead to a consolidation of the antigen in the fluid mosaic of the cell membrane, a phenomenon called capping. Capping can then lead to extrusion of the antigen from the cell surface or endopinocytosis into the cell. It is uncertain whether this phenomenon has biologic role in dis-ease, although clearance of surface antigens could enhance virus persistence (Joseph and Oldstone, 1975). Antibody molecules can also downregulate intra-cellular virus replication by acting at the cell membrane or by entering the virus-infected cell.

Antibodies can function as intermediaries in the destruction of infected cells by complement-mediated cytotoxicity; by antibody-dependent cellular cytotoxi-city by killer cells, macrophages, or polymorphonuclear cells; and by promoting cell phagocytosis by macrophages. Cytotoxic T cells can destroy an infected cell expressing class I MHC by direct cytotoxicity without the aid of antibody (Fig. 4.2).

Many cell-mediated immune responses and interactions of T and B cells appear to be designed to destroy "foreign" cells, such as virus-infected cells.

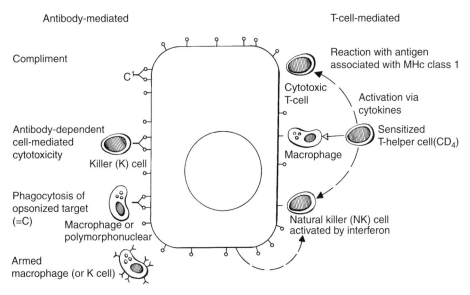

Antibody-mediated

T-cell-mediated

FIG. 4.2. Mechanisms of immune destruction of a virus-infected cell. Viral antigens are shown as projections on the infected cell. Mechanisms involving antibody are shown on the *left*, and those not involving antibody are shown on the *right*. The cytokines produced by T cells can activate macrophages, and the interferon produced by T cells or infected cells can activate natural killer cells (*arrows*).

Assuming that the cell is doomed by infection with a cytolytic virus, this attack on the infected cell hastens the release of intracellular virus to be neutralized by antibodies, or, if the full complement of virus has not been produced by the time viral proteins are incorporated into the cell surface, cell lysis can abort the infection. Alternatively, if the cell is transformed by an integrated virus genome, the cytoplasmic membrane may contain virus-coded or sequestered host antigens. This potentially neoplastic cell will be destroyed by the same mechanisms.

This complex assault of heterogeneous immune responses can be a double-edged sword. Furthermore, at various stages of the infectious process, the immune responses may have different effects: a specific response may be beneficial to the host at one time and detrimental at another. For example, in herpes simplex virus infections of mice, depletion of lymphocytes at an early stage prior to invasion of the CNS increases the incidence of CNS infection and death; if the same immunosuppression is induced after virus has invaded the CNS, the time of death is delayed (Nahmias et al., 1969). Thus, cell-mediated immunity protects against CNS invasion, but once CNS invasion occurs, the cytotoxic actions accelerate the disease. A more dramatic example is seen in noncytopathic infection of mice with lymphocytic choriomeningitis virus. When infected as fetal animals, or when mice are immunosuppressed at the time of infection, infection persists, with little, if any, abnormal function of the infected cells. If sensitized lymphoid cells from a histocompatible mouse are passively transferred to this carrier mouse, it will develop acute encephalitis and die (Cole et al., 1971).

However, no evidence has established that meningitis and encephalitis caused by the same virus in humans are immune mediated; indeed, the disease may have contrary mechanisms of pathogenesis in different hosts. The immune responses might cause disease in the mouse and abate disease in humans.

Immunopathologic viral disease refers to disease or pathologic changes in which the primary signs or symptoms or abnormalities are not mediated by the action or products of the virus genome but by cellular or humoral immune responses to those products. However, immunopathologic is an adjective of varied usage. The finding of the immunologic specificity of the inflammatory reaction in viral infection or even the presence of inflammatory cells leads some to infer immunopathologic abnormalities. The reduction in disease or pathologic findings after immunosuppression often is cited as evidence of an immunopathologic disease. However, the suppression of inflammatory infiltrates by destruction of lymphoid cells does not indicate that clinical illness or other pathologic signs result from immune responses (McFarland et al., 1972). Furthermore, some cytotoxic drugs used for immunosuppression may alter host cell susceptibility to infection, and the inhibition of virus replication by drugs is not evidence that the disease is immune mediated (Narayan et al., 1972).

IMMUNE RESPONSES IN THE CNS

The CNS is relatively isolated from systemic immune responses in the absence of disease. There appears to be no intrinsic system for antibody production; no lymphatic system in the usual sense; few, if any, phagocytic cells; lack of expression of MHC molecules on neuroectodermal cells; and cerebral capillary endothelium that binds lymphocytes poorly.

The Anatomic Barrier

Proteins and cells of blood are relatively excluded from the CNS under normal conditions by the anatomic barrier of tight junctions between capillary endothelial cells, arachnoid cells, and choroid plexus epithelial cells. Furthermore, little vesicular transport activity is seen in cerebrovascular endothelium, and few adhesion molecules are expressed. Within the CNS, free traffic between extracellular fluid and cerebrospinal fluid is assumed because of the absence of tight junctions between ventricular ependymal cells. However, the bulk flow is from extracellular space to spinal fluid, so that soluble molecules or drugs injected into the ventricles may penetrate only a few millimeters into the brain.

The immunoglobulins in normal cerebrospinal fluid are derived solely from blood (Frick and Scheid-Seydel, 1958). Spinal fluid IgG and IgA are present at about 0.2% to 0.4% of plasma levels, and IgM is present at much lower levels. In the placenta, the IgG is preferentially transmitted, and this passage depends on the Fc portion of the molecule (Spiegelberg, 1974). Passage into spinal fluid, however, appears to depend primarily on size, because F(ab) fragments enter more readily than whole IgG. Charge appears to be a secondary determinant, because more positively charged isotypes of IgG pass more readily, and synthetically charged proteins of equal size show direct correlation between entry and positive charge (Griffin and Giffels, 1982). This normal transudate of immunoglobulins may occur through the brain vasculature or across the choroid plexus.

Only small numbers of lymphocytes are found in normal cerebrospinal fluid, and these represent T cells with CD4 to CD8 ratios mirroring those of blood; B cells and polymorphonuclear cells are normally absent. Furthermore, the presence of T cells does not necessarily indicate ongoing immune monitoring of the brain parenchyma, because the itinerary of T-cell traffic may be passage from choroid plexus or arachnoid to spinal fluid to cervical lymphatics. Most T cells in spinal fluid have activation markers, in contrast to T cells in the general circulation.

Two resident neural cell types play important roles in immune responses: the pericytes (or perivascular macrophages) and the microglia. Both are of bone marrow rather than ectodermal origin but have very different life cycles, since 20% to 40% of perivascular cells turn over every 60 to 90 days while microglia are very stable and less than 1% turn over during the same interval (Hickey and Kimura, 1988; Hickey et al., 1992). The mononuclear cells of bone marrow origin enter the CNS during gestation and phagocytose fragments of the apoptotic neural cells during the process of remodeling (see Chapter 2). It is thought that the microglia persist from this population. Subsequently, they may or may not have homeostatic functions in normal adult brain, but clearly immune responses activate microglia (Perry and Gordon, 1988). With activation, they may or may not go on to become phagocytic cells (Barron, 1995). In acute encephalitis, microglial cells contribute to the nodules of neuronophagia and, in chronic encephalitis, to the "rod cell" population.

The perivascular cells are the only cells in the CNS that constitutively express MHC class II molecules and have the characteristics of "professional" antigen-presenting cells. In normal human brain, immunocytochemical stains for the major histocompatibility antigens are usually negative or weakly positive, with staining of a few meningeal macrophages, pituicytes, and the perivascular cells. Antigen is rarely detected in microglia (Sasaki and Nakazato, 1992). With activation, MHC class II antigen is rapidly upregulated in microglia. Microglia activation is also associated with release of free oxygen intermediates, nitrous oxide, proteases, arachidonic acids, quinolinic acids, and cytokines. The results of microglial activation probably can be both cytotoxic and reparative (Chao et al., 1996; Kreutzberg, 1996).

Astrocytes and cerebrovascular endothelial cells may be recruited as antigen-presenting cells and as active participants in the immune response (Frohman et al., 1989) but probably cannot activate naive T cells. These cells can be stimulated to express MHC antigens in culture, but their role *in vivo* is uncertain (Frohman et al., 1989; Mucke and Eddelston, 1993). Choroid plexus epithelium in culture also can act as antigen-presenting cells to T cells (Nathanson and Chun, 1989); the possible role of the choroid plexus in initiating immune responses and in the pathogenesis of autoimmune diseases needs better definition.

The only wandering phagocytes appear to be supraependymal cells, first identified in lizards but now recognized in mammals (Bleier and Albrecht, 1980). These cells, stretched out over the ependyma, have been shown to ingest foreign particles, including virus particles. Apparent degradation of mumps virus has been seen within secondary phagolysosomes in these cells during experimental infection (Wolinsky et al., 1974).

The route of efflux of antigens and cells from the CNS is primarily by way of the cervical lymphatics. Following intracerebral injection of radiolabeled protein, up to 47% can be traced to cervical nodes with drainage along cranial nerves, particularly the olfactory route through the cribriform plate (Cserr and Knopf, 1992; Knopf et al., 1995).

Although the brain communicates with the lymphatics, antigens in the brain can elicit humoral and fail to induce cellular immune responses. For example, myelin basic protein injected directly into the brain does not cause experimental autoimmune encephalomyelitis even though serum antibodies form against myelin basic protein. Furthermore, this sensitization is followed by an interval of resistance to the development of experimental autoimmune encephalomyelitis following peripheral inoculation of myelin basic protein with adjuvants (see Chapter 8). In some instances, even humoral responses fail. With microinjection of influenza virus into the brain or spinal fluid of mice, different responses are obtained. Influenza virus undergoes a single abortive replicative cycle in neural tissues, so that there is amplification of antigens but no spread of infection. Microinoculation of virus into the spinal fluid is followed by prompt immune response followed by prolonged production of virus-specific immunoglobulin in the spinal fluid. In contrast, after microinjection into the parenchyma of the brain, this antibody response is greatly delayed and occurs in only about half of the mice (Stevenson et al., 1997).

Inflammatory and Antibody Responses in the CNS

Most acute viral infections are associated with an inflammatory response characterized by the meningeal and perivascular accumulation of mononuclear cells. The mechanisms of the recruitment of these cells, their role in infection, and their ultimate disposition are only partially understood.

Few, if any, adhesion molecules are expressed on normal cerebral endothelial cells, but activated T cells can bind to and cross resting endothelium independent of MHC restriction, antigen, or T-cell phenotype. They traffic in the CNS for a few hours unless their antigen target is found. The effect of this local passage of activated T cells is to upregulate MHC class II antigens on microglia and to induce adhesion molecules and CD4 expression, creating "hot spots" (Hickey, 1997).

The parameters of inflammation and humoral immune responses in a nonfatal viral encephalitis have been extensively studied using Sindbis virus in mice. Following intracerebral inoculation of Sindbis virus, replication occurs in ependymal cells, followed by widespread neuronal infection and lesser infection of glial cells (Johnson et al., 1972; Jackson et al., 1987). Even though inoculation is intracerebral, the immune response is presumably initiated peripherally, probably by soluble or phagocytosed antigen being transported to the cervical lymphatics. The upregulation of class II expression on microglial cells of the brain occurs coincident with rather than prior to the beginning of the inflammatory reaction (Tyor et al., 1990). Cerebral endothelial cells can express MHC class II, but they are poor stimulators of T-cell proliferation (Pryce et al., 1989). Coincident with the onset of inflammation, cellular adhesion molecules are upregulated on vascular endothelium (Irani and Griffin, 1996). Perivascular mononuclear cell infiltration begins approximately 3 to 4 days after inoculation and reaches a maximum at 7 to 10 days.

The mononuclear cells in perivascular cuffs clearly come from a population of nondividing circulating mononuclear cells that may or may not undergo division once they cross the vascular endothelium, and prelabeling blood cells with India ink indicates that some of the small mononuclear cells contain ink, identifying them as committed macrophages prior to moving into the inflammatory response (Johnson, 1971). Immunosuppression with cyclophosphamide eliminates the inflammatory response, with prolonged virus growth in the brain, but not death. Passive transfer of cells or serum 3 days after inoculation at the time of maximum viral growth shows that the inflammatory response can be reconstituted only when animals are given virus-sensitized lymph node cells; immune serum, lymph node cells from mice immunized with other viruses, or bone marrow cells from immune mice fail to reconstitute the response, although the addition of immune or nonimmune bone marrow cells to sensitized T cells enhances the inflammatory response (McFarland et al., 1972). This clearly indicates that the induction to the inflammatory response is immunologically specific and is dependent on a population to T lymphocytes sensitized to the inoculated virus. Entry of activated cells is not antigen specific, but retention of immune cells in the CNS is (Irani and Griffin, 1996).

The spinal fluid pleocytosis is maximum on days 3 and 4 and is clearing by the time the perivascular infiltrates are maximum. Furthermore, not only do the kinetics of these inflammatory responses differ, but the constituent cells are different (Moench and Griffin, 1984). In the perivascular cuffs, the initial cells are predominantly T cells and macrophages. B cells appear in the perivascular inflammatory cuffs later, initially showing only IgM on the surface, but after approximately 10 to 14 days varied IgG isotopes and IgA are seen (Tyor et al., 1989). The early cerebrospinal fluid response contains relatively large numbers of CD4-negative and CD8-negative cells presumably representing natural killer cells along with T cells (Griffin and Hess, 1986). The ratio of CD4 to CD8 cells exceeds 4 to 1. B cells and macrophages, although plentiful in the brain, do not appear in the cerebrospinal fluid, and the cerebrospinal fluid response is largely cleared by day 7 or 8, when the perivascular reaction is maximum.

Limited parallel studies have been carried out in human infections with another arboviral infection: Japanese encephalitis virus. There are remarkable similarities to those studies with viral encephalitis in mice. In seven children who died with disease, viral antigen was limited to neurons, and the perivascular inflammatory response showed a preponderance of T cells, with only 7% to 30% of these being CD8+ cells. Inflammatory cells that invade the parenchyma are predominantly activated macrophages and a small number of the T cells. B cells enter the CNS later and remain localized to the perivascular cuff (Johnson et al., 1985a). Sequential studies of spinal fluid of 15 patients with Japanese encephalitis similarly showed a preponderance of T cells, with a greater than 4 to 1 ratio of CD4+ to CD8+ cells. B cells and macrophages were found in small numbers, but even in those patients in whom no B cells were found in spinal fluid, antibody against Japanese encephalitis virus was present. Antibody presumably was produced by B cells in the perivascular cuffs and diffused into the cerebrospinal fluid (Johnson et al., 1986).

Immunocytochemical staining of inflammatory cells in biopsied and fatal cases of herpes simplex virus encephalitis showed a preponderance of T cells, with equal proportions of CD4 and CD8 cells (Sobel et al., 1986). Similar staining of mononuclear cells in subacute sclerosing panencephalitis and postinfectious encephalomyelitis has shown a predominance of CD8 cells (Esiri et al., 1989). In lymphocytic choriomeningitis infections in mice, CD8 cells predominate in the inflammatory responses in meninges, choroid plexus, and brain and in the spinal fluid. A preponderance of CD8 cells is also evident in spinal fluid in chronic inflammatory responses in both HIV infections and subacute sclerosing panencephalitis due to measles virus.

The failure of inflammatory responses is seen in some experimental viral encephalitides, such as those caused by neuroadapted measles virus or Newcastle disease virus. Furthermore, after intracerebral inoculation of Lansing type 2 poliovirus, which infects only neurons and for which there are no known susceptible extraneural cells, no immune response can be detected; presumably, insufficient antigen is processed and delivered to the systemic circulation to stimulate an antibody response (Jubelt et al., 1980a).

During the inflammatory reaction, attenuation of the blood–brain barrier allows a transudation of serum proteins, including immunoglobulins (Fig. 4.3). Thus, with the initiation of inflammation, albumin and immunoglobulin levels increase in cerebrospinal fluid but in direct proportion to the serum levels. Once the B cell response is developed, immunoglobulins are synthesized within the CNS. These immunoglobulin-producing cells apparently differentiate from a limited number of B cells, because the immunoglobulins produced are of restricted heterogeneity. This intracerebral immunoglobulin synthesis is reflected by distortions in the spinal fluid–serum ratios of immunoglobulins, and the restricted heterogeneity is reflected by the development of oligoclonal bands

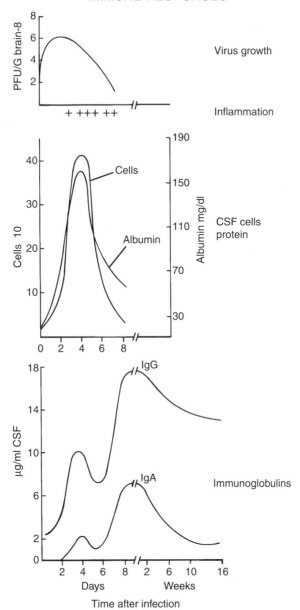

FIG. 4.3. Time course of spinal fluid changes in acute encephalitis. Nonfatal Sindbis virus encephalitis in mice after intracerebral inoculation shows maximum virus growth in brain within 1 day. The inflammatory response in the brain begins on day 3 and is maximum by days 5 and 6. The pleocytosis is maximum on days 3 and 4, and the breakdown of the blood–brain barrier, as shown by elevated cerebrospinal fluid albumin content, coincides with the pleocytosis. Concentrations of immunoglobulins show an initial rise reflecting transudation accompanying the blood–brain barrier breakdown and a late elevation indicative of intrathecal generation of IgG and IgA that persists for many weeks after the acute infection. (Adapted from Griffin, 1981.)

of IgG in spinal fluid and altered κ/λ light-chain ratios (Vandvik, 1977). Prolonged elevations of IgG and IgA are found in cerebrospinal fluid following nonfatal encephalitis even without evidence of virus persistence (Fig. 4.3).

In acute human infections, elevated concentrations of oligoclonal IgG proteins have been found 1 year after mumps virus meningitis (Vandvik et al., 1978) and for almost 4 years after herpes simplex virus encephalitis (Sköldenberg et al., 1981). After acute herpes simplex virus encephalitis, evidence for intrathecal synthesis of antibodies has continued for 2 to 43 months. This prolonged antibody synthesis in the CNS raises the probability of virus persistence and ongoing antigenic stimulation. Certainly, in known chronic human CNS infections with measles and rubella viruses, striking persistent intrathecal antibody synthesis occurs (see Chapter 10). In several experimental persistent infections of the CNS, levels of specific antibody in the cerebrospinal fluid (Griffin et al., 1978b) and brain extract (Lipton and Gonzalez-Scarano, 1978) have exceeded those in serum.

Not only plasma cells but also B memory cells can reside for extended periods in the brain. Immunocompetent cells capable of generating antibody against parainfluenza virus type 1 have been eluted from brains of mice for over 30 weeks after virus inoculation, and accelerated IgG and IgA antibody responses in cerebrospinal fluid have been shown in mice previously inoculated intracerebrally with inactivated virus (Gerhard and Koprowski, 1977; Gerhard et al., 1978). After Sindbis virus encephalitis in mice, few B cells remain, but even 1 year after infection 62% of these cells are Sindbis virus specific (Tyor et al., 1992b).

Although some immunocompetent cells may persist in perivascular or meningeal spaces for relatively long periods after acute encephalitis, the majority of inflammatory cells are cleared quite promptly. The macrophages do not appear to persist as microglial cells (Johnson, 1971), and most rod-shaped microglial cells prominent during recovery from poliovirus infections appear to have a hematogenous origin (Wolinsky et al., 1982a). Retreating lymphocytes and macrophages may cross directly back into the blood or along nerve root sleeves into extraneural lymphatic channels.

VIRUS CLEARANCE FROM THE CNS

Both antibodies and cellular immune responses are involved in the clearance of virus from the CNS. Infected cells are generally lysed by cytotoxic T cells, and extracellular virus is neutralized by antibodies. The persistence of active infections with RNA and DNA viruses depends on the infection being noncytolytic and on the evasion from immune surveillance. This evasion appears to occur primarily in two cell populations: microglia and neurons. First, lymphocytes and macrophages or brain microglia are antigen-presenting cells; cytotoxic lymphocytes, although selected during early thymic differentiation to recognize self-MHC molecules, may be preselected to not attack the antigen-presenting cells. Infection of lymphocytes also can cause immunosuppression against themselves (Oldstone and Rall, 1993). This failure of cytotoxic cells to kill antigen-presenting cells may, in part, explain the persistent microglia infection in HIV-infected individuals. Neurons are the other cell population that evades cytotoxic attack. MHC class I molecules are not constitutively expressed on glial cells in the nervous system but can be induced on astrocytes and oligodendrocytes, though not on neurons. Normal neurons do not express these recognition molecules. Even in culture, interferon γ can induce class I MHC on neurons only after they have become electrically silent, so only defunct neurons are lysed and removed (Neumann et al., 1995). Thus, neurons as a nonrenewable population presumably fail to express MHC to avoid attack by cytotoxic T cells, but this survival property makes them prone to persistent infection by nonlytic viruses (Joly et al., 1991; Mucke and Oldstone, 1992).

In Sindbis virus encephalitis in mice, antibody to specific epitopes on one of the two surface glycoproteins leads to viral clearance. This has been shown in SCID (severe combined immunodeficiency) mice that are incapable of generating antigen-specific B-cell or T-cell responses, because of a deficiency in recombination of the variable region elements of the immunoglobulin and T-cell receptor genes. These mice do not clear Sindbis virus from the brain and spinal cord, but clearance is reconstituted by transfer of immune serum, though not by immune T cells. Furthermore, complement depletion and chemical immunosuppression do not alter the ability of immune serum to terminate replication, indicating that antibody-mediated clearance occurs by mechanisms distinct from the classic antibody-dependent cell-mediated cytotoxicity or complement-dependent lysis (Levine et al., 1991). Studies suggest that the antibody inhibits intracellular viral replication, but viral RNA as detected by polymerase chain reaction persists within neurons long after apparent clearance, as determined by infectious virus recovery (Griffin et al., 1992a). These mechanisms could have important implications in a wide variety of neurologic diseases that seem to follow acute viral infections, as well as relapsing and progressive inflammatory processes.

Natural immunodeficiency states in humans indicate the importance of T-cell and B-cell responses in clearing specific viruses from the CNS (Table 4.4). B-cell deficiencies such as primary hypogammaglobulinemia in children have been

TABLE 4.4. *Persistent viral infections of CNS in humans related to immunodeficiencies*

Immune deficit	Virus
Agammaglobulinemia	Enteroviruses (polioviruses and echoviruses)
Cell-mediated immune deficiencies	Herpesviruses (varicella–zoster virus and cytomegalovirus)
	Adenovirus
	Measles virus
	Papovaviruses (JC and SV40)

associated primarily with persistent echovirus and poliovirus infections. In these children, chronic progressive CNS infections are accompanied by an intense inflammatory reaction. However, this reaction is devoid of plasma cells (Davis et al., 1977; Wilfert et al., 1977; Bodensteiner et al., 1979).

Defects in cell-mediated immunity are associated with failure to clear a variety of infections. Atypical CNS infections with herpes simplex virus, varicella–zoster virus, cytomegalovirus, adenoviruses, and measles viruses have been reported in patients with lymphoproliferative diseases, in patients receiving immunosuppressive therapy, and in patients with AIDS. These patients also are prone to have chronic inflammatory disease of the brain of unknown cause (Dayan, 1971).

Latency of viruses in neural cells, opportunistic infections of CNS in immunodeficient patients, the role of virus mutations in persistent infections, and the absence of immune responses in prion diseases are discussed in subsequent chapters.

SUPPLEMENTARY BIBLIOGRAPHY

Keane RW, Hickey WF. *Immunology of the nervous system.* New York: Oxford University Press, 1997.
Roitt I. *Essential immunology,* 8th ed. London: Blackwell Science, 1994.

PART II

Acute Neurologic Diseases

Acute viral infections cause an array of clinical neurologic syndromes, including meningitis, paralytic poliomyelitis, encephalitis, acute cerebellar ataxia, myelitis, mononeuritis, polyneuritis, and Reye's syndrome. Furthermore, each of these syndromes has been linked to multiple viruses.

Most of these illnesses represent complications of primary infections with viruses such a enteroviruses, mumps virus, lymphocytic choriomeningitis virus, or arboviruses; others can result from reactivation of a latent infection within the host, as exemplified by some herpesvirus infections. A few viruses cause distinctive clinical syndromes: for example, acute flaccid paralysis caused by polioviruses or the dermatomal rash of shingles caused by reactivation of varicella–zoster virus. However, these viruses can cause other clinical manifestations, and illnesses that simulate paralytic poliomyelitis and shingles can, on occasion, be caused by other viruses. Histopathologically, most of these diseases are characterized by focal or generalized inflammation and cell destruction; however, the postinfectious encephalomyelitis that can complicate measles and a number of other infections has distinctive demyelinating pathologic changes believed to result from an immunopathologic process. The same is true of the peripheral nerve demyelination and axonal degeneration in the Guillain–Barré syndrome. Other postinfectious syndromes are noninflammatory. Reye's syndrome, with acute cerebral edema, has been associated with diverse infections, but the pathogenetic role of the infection remains an enigma. Similarly, the role of residual neuronal stress or possible virus persistence in the postpolio syndrome is uncertain. The very existence of a biologic basis for the so-called chronic fatigue syndrome is in doubt.

5

Meningitis, Encephalitis, and Poliomyelitis

The catastrophe was dreadful: For the swelled testicles subsided suddenly the next day, the patient was seized with a most frantic delirium, the nervous system was shattered with strong convulsions, and he died raving mad the third day after.
Robert Hamilton,
An Account of a Distemper by the Common People of England Vulgarly Called the Mumps, paper to the Royal Society of Edinburgh, 1790

In this early description of the neurologic complications of mumps, Hamilton first noted an important feature missed in prior descriptions of "brain fevers"— that they are generally complications of systemic infections. Most viruses that cause acute CNS infections are common parasites of humans. Therefore, with few exceptions, viral meningitis, encephalitis, and poliomyelitis must be regarded as uncommon complications of common systemic infections. Some viruses, such as polioviruses and arthropod-borne encephalitis viruses, cause clinically significant disease only on the rare occasion when the CNS is involved; others, such as mumps virus and herpesviruses, are frequent causes of trivial diseases that can assume serious dimensions when the CNS is infected.

The viruses discussed in this chapter are the most frequent causes of aseptic meningitis, encephalitis, and paralytic poliomyelitis. Humans are the only known natural host for the human enteroviruses, mumps, adenoviruses, and parvovirus B19, and spread of infection from person to person occurs by different routes and is influenced by different environmental and social factors. Lymphocytic choriomeningitis virus and related arenaviruses are zoonotic infections and are dependent on human contacts and interactions with rodents. Filoviruses are assumed to be zoonotic infections, but their natural haunt is unknown. The arthropod-borne viruses (arboviruses) present a more complicated and intriguing pattern of population interactions; these viruses have an obligatory infectious cycle in hematophagous arthropods. Therefore, their transmission to humans depends on factors that influence mosquito or tick breeding, the susceptibility and incubation period of virus in the arthropod, the populations and movements of other vertebrates involved in the natural cycle or

87

amplification cycles of the virus, and human foresights and follies that alter our contacts with the vectors.

In considering virus epidemiology, we progress up the scale of complexity from virus–cell interactions and virus–host interactions to a level that deals with viruses within populations. We must consider not only human and animal populations, but also their behavior and interactions and the environmental factors that influence the spread and distribution of viruses between hosts.

GENERAL CONSIDERATIONS

Clinical Features

Clinical signs and symptoms of acute viral infections of the CNS depend on which neural cells are infected, and the varied cell populations of the nervous system have different susceptibilities to different viruses. If infection is limited to cells of the meninges or ependymal surfaces, clinical manifestations may be limited to headache, fever, stiff neck, and pleocytosis—or benign meningitis. If infection spreads to the parenchymal cells of the brain, in addition to signs of meningeal irritation, there may be a depression of the state of consciousness, seizures, focal neurologic deficits, or increased intracranial pressure, which define encephalitis. If signs of spinal cord disease also are present, the terms encephalomyelitis and meningoencephalomyelitis are appropriate. Some viruses selectively involve specific neural cell populations, causing more distinctive clinical signs. For example, polioviruses selectively infect and destroy anterior horn cells, resulting in the characteristic clinical findings of acute meningitis with patchy flaccid paralysis.

Viral meningitis and encephalitis are common diseases. Epidemiologic studies in Olmsted County, Minnesota, and Helsinki, Finland, have determined incidences of 10.9 to 26 per 100,000 persons per year for viral meningitis and 3.5 to 7.4 per 100,000 persons per year for encephalitis (Pönkä and Pettersson, 1982; Beghi et al., 1984; Nicolosi et al., 1986). Encephalitis is more common in children, in whom an incidence of 16.7 per 100,000 child years has been reported (Koskiniemi et al., 1991).

Viral meningitis is by definition a benign, self-limited illness. In addition to the headache, fever, and nuchal rigidity, general malaise, nausea, vomiting, drowsiness, abdominal pain, and chills are frequent. The headache often is frontal or retroorbital and may be associated with photophobia. The fever is seldom elevated above 40°C. Nuchal rigidity is usually not as severe as in bacterial meningitis and may be detected only with extreme flexion. The assumption that this syndrome represents inflammation limited to the cells covering or lining the brain has been verified in a patient with coxsackievirus B5 meningitis who died suddenly with a concurrent myocarditis. Inflammation was limited to the meninges, ependyma, and choroid plexus (Price et al., 1970).

Viral encephalitis is a more severe illness in which other signs evolve that suggest inflammation within the parenchyma of the brain. A great variability of signs is seen, and this depends, only to a limited extent, on the etiologic agent. Consciousness generally is altered; mild lethargy may progress to confusion, stupor, and coma. Focal neurologic signs usually develop, and seizures are common. Motor weakness, accentuated tendon reflexes, and extensor plantar responses often are observed. Occasionally, abnormal movements or tremors may develop. With involvement of the hypothalamic–pituitary area, hypothermia or poikilothermia, diabetes insipidus, and inappropriate antidiuretic hormone secretion are seen. Concurrent involvement of the spinal cord can lead to a superimposed flaccid paralysis, with depression of tendon reflexes and paralysis of bowel and bladder. Increased intracranial pressure is common. Pathologic studies of patients dying during the acute phase of disease usually show either diffuse or multifocal areas of inflammation in the brain that are associated with neuronal degeneration and neuronophagia. Inclusion bodies may be evident in cases due to herpesviruses, measles, or rabies; but with notable exception of herpes simplex virus encephalitis, the topography of lesions or cytopathic change are of little help in surmising the etiologic agent.

Poliomyelitis is a disease of variable severity in which clinical signs indicate selective involvement of motor neurons. The major illness may be preceded for 1 to 4 days by sore throat, gastrointestinal upset, fever, and mild headache—a prodrome referred to as the "minor illness." There is then an accentuation of fever, malaise, headache, and often vomiting. Nuchal rigidity develops. A sense of muscle stiffness with hyperreflexia and fasciculations may be evident prior to the development of asymmetric muscle weakness and corresponding tendon reflex loss. The legs are involved more often than the arms, and the bulbar musculature is affected in 10% to 15% percent of patients with paralytic disease. Cranial nerves IX and X are the most frequently involved, interfering with phonation and swallowing. Paralysis of the face, mastoid muscles, and tongue is less common, and paralysis of eye movements is very rare. Particularly in adults with bulbar poliomyelitis, involvement of the reticular formation can result in cardiorespiratory abnormalities: respiration may be atactic, sleep apnea may occur, and hypertension and arrhythmias may develop. Bladder paralysis is more common in adults. Pain and paresthesias are often experienced during the acute illness, but objective sensory loss is rare (Plum, 1956). Pathologic studies of patients dying during the acute illness show inflammation and neuronal destruction, predominantly in the anterior horns of spinal cord, bulbar motor nuclei, reticular formation, thalamus, and motor cortex. Inflammation often is prominent in the posterior horns of the spinal cord, although white matter generally is spared (Bodian, 1949). These pathologic changes are more diffuse than the clinical findings might suggest.

Etiology

Over 100 viruses have been associated with acute CNS infections. The etiologic agents vary in frequency from year to year, differ in different populations, and depend on immunization programs, exposures to animal hosts or vectors, and many other factors. Worldwide enteroviruses are the cause of a large proportion of cases of aseptic meningitis each year, although the serotypes vary from year to year. Herpes simplex virus is a major cause of severe encephalitis without evidence of geographic or temporal variation. In contrast, mumps virus has been greatly reduced as a cause of meningitis and encephalitis by immunization programs in many countries, and wild-type poliomyelitis has been eliminated from the entire Western Hemisphere. Zoonotic agents and arboviruses all show restricted geographic distributions. In many areas of Asia, Japanese encephalitis virus is the commonest cause of encephalitis and, in Sweden, tick-borne encephalitis virus causes more than half of the cases of encephalitis (Günther et al., 1997).

Data from a 10-year study at Walter Reed Army Institute of Research that are presented in Table 5.1 reflect the specific etiology of "viral" CNS syndromes (Meyer et al., 1960; Buescher et al., 1968). Although this study was completed 30 years ago, only a small number of viruses subsequently have been added as causes of aseptic meningitis and encephalitis, and no subsequent study of comparable size in the United States has achieved a comparable rate of positive laboratory diagnoses (over 60% of cases). This high rate of diagnoses can be explained by a population of military personnel and their dependents who report early for medical care and whose compliance in providing timely convalescent specimens is unknown in civilian populations. Because data obtained prior to 1959 are included, the relationship of poliomyelitis to the other syndromes is illustrated.

The syndromes of aseptic meningitis and encephalitis have diverse causes and are due to the same viruses. Thus, they represent a continuum. Nevertheless,

TABLE 5.1. *Specific etiology of "viral" CNS syndromes (1953–1963)*[a]

Agent	Aseptic meningitis	Encephalitis	Paralytic poliomyelitis	Total
Enteroviruses				
Poliovirus	56	10	179	245
Coxsackievirus A	18	3	0	21
Coxsackievirus B	148	3	1	155
Echovirus	106	4	2	112
Mumps virus	96	33	2	131
Lymphocytic choriomeningitis virus	45	20	0	65
Arboviruses	6	25	0	28
Herpes simplex virus	8	20	0	28
Leptospira	26	4	0	30
Mycobacterium tuberculosis	1	13	0	14
Others	6	11	0	17[b]
Total diagnosed (%)	516 (64)	149 (66)	184 (73)	849 (66)
Total studied	804	227	251	1,282

[a]Inclusion required the availability of both acute and convalescent-phase sera; isolation specimens were obtained in the majority but were not required for inclusion. Cases of encephalomyelitis complicating diagnosed childhood exanthems were excluded.

[b]Epstein–Barr virus (4), Rocky Mountain spotted fever (3), rubeola (3), *Mycoplasma pneumoniae* (3), influenza A2 (1), histoplasmosis (1), and coccidioidomycosis (2).

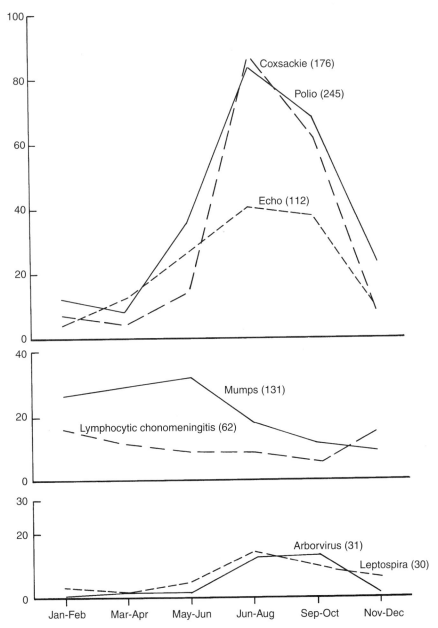

FIG. 5.1. The seasonal distributions of acute "viral" CNS infections: data derived from the Walter Reed Army Institute of Research study from 1953 to 1963 showing the seasonal distributions of the commonest etiologic agents of viral meningitis, encephalitis, and poliomyelitis. (Data from Meyer et al., 1960; and Buescher et al., 1968.)

some viruses tend to cause more benign disease (e.g., the enteroviruses), whereas other viruses are only rarely associated with aseptic meningitis and tend to cause severe disease when the CNS is invaded (e.g., the arboviruses and herpes simplex virus). In contrast, the clinical syndrome of paralytic poliomyelitis was caused almost exclusively by polioviruses, although small numbers of cases were due to coxsackieviruses and echoviruses. With elimination of wild-type poliovirus infections in the Western Hemisphere, other enteroviruses have emerged as the commonest causes of the paralytic poliomyelitis syndrome (Figueroa et al., 1989; Dietz et al., 1995).

In retrospect, the study has defects: the laboratory methods and diagnostic criteria used probably underestimated infections with group A coxsackieviruses, echoviruses, Epstein–Barr virus, and *Mycoplasma*. On the other hand, some of the associations of herpes simplex virus infections with aseptic meningitis and nonfatal encephalitis are probably in error, because of our naiveté then regarding the capriciousness of serologic studies in confirming this diagnosis (Johnson et al., 1968b) (see Chapter 6).

The seasonal distribution of acute neurologic diseases caused by these viruses is shown in Fig. 5.1. Coxsackieviruses and echoviruses follow the same seasonal distribution historically recognized with polioviruses. Lymphocytic choriomeningitis virus causes more human infections during winter, and

TABLE 5.2. *Historical data and systemic physical findings that suggest the cause of acute encephalitis*

Variable	Virus(es)[a]
Historical data	
Season	Arboviruses in tick and mosquito season; mumps virus in spring; enteroviruses in late summer and fall; lymphocytic choriomeningitis virus in winter (*Borrelia burgdorferi* in summer)
Travel	Other arboviruses, exotic viruses (regional bacteria, fungi, and parasites)
Family illnesses	Enteroviruses cause family outbreaks of varied disease (*Mycobacterium tuberculosis*)
Recreational activity	California encephalitis virus in woodlands (*Leptospira* in farm ponds; *Naegleria* in quarry water)
Animal exposures	Lymphocytic choriomeningitis virus carried by mice or hamsters; rabies virus transmitted by bat, wild carnivore, dog, or cat bites
Immunization and drugs	
Systemic physical findings	
Rash	Viruses causing childhood exanthems, enteroviruses, human herpesvirus 6 (*Rickettsia rickettsii, B. burgdorferi*)
Herpangina	Coxsackieviruses
Adenopathy	HIV, Epstein–Barr virus, cytomegalovirus (*Bartonella henselae, Brucella*)
Parotitis and/or orchitis	Mumps virus, lymphocytic choriomeningitis virus
Pneumonitis	Adenoviruses, lymphocytic choriomeningitis virus (*Mycoplasma*)

[a]Nonviral agents are in parentheses.
Modified from Johnson (1996a).

mumps virus causes more during the spring. The arboviruses are restricted to seasons between the frosts, unless they are imported from other climes. Leptospiral infections, which may be clinically indistinguishable from viral CNS infections, show a preponderance of human infections during the summer. These patterns are helpful in formulating an educated guess as to the cause of aseptic meningitis or encephalitis in an individual patient (Table 5.2). On the basis of the nonneurologic signs and symptoms of these infections, and with knowledge of their epidemiologic behaviors, the physician can limit the differential diagnosis and, therefore, select optimal specimens to obtain a definite diagnosis from the virology laboratory.

ENTEROVIRUSES

Enteroviruses cause 40% to 60% of all cases of viral meningitis, most cases of paralytic poliomyelitis, and a small number of cases of encephalitis.

Enteroviruses compose a large genus of nonenveloped RNA viruses that together with the rhinoviruses and several other genuses constitute the giant family of picornaviruses. Although structurally similar to enteroviruses, the rhinoviruses are temperature sensitive and acid pH sensitive, which restricts their replication largely to the cool mucosa of the nasopharynx and sinuses, where they cause the common cold. They have not been implicated in neurologic diseases. The enteroviruses, which commonly infect the CNS, also replicate within the oropharyngeal tissues, but their lack of a lipid envelope, their stability at low pH, and their optimal replication at 37°C facilitate their growth in the intestinal tract and their potential to disseminate. Enteroviruses are known in many animal species, but each agent tends to be species specific in its replication. Over 70 human enteroviruses are known. Originally, enteroviruses were subcategorized by laboratory host ranges (Table 5.3), but time and knowledge have eroded clear-cut classifications (Hypiä et al., 1997). Some group A coxsackieviruses grow in

TABLE 5.3. *Differentiation of enteroviruses*

Subgroup	No. of serotypes	Host range	
		In vivo disease	*In vitro* in primate cells
Poliovirus	3	Primates (poliomyelitis)	+
Coxsackievirus			
Group A	23	Newborn mice (widespread myositis)	–
Group B	6	Newborn mice (focal myositis, pancreatitis, and encephalitis)	+
Echovirus	31	—	+
Enterovirus	10	Variable[a]	Variable

Cosackievirus A23 is now echovirus 9, echovirus 10 is now reovirus, and echovirus 28 is now rhinovirus 1A.

[a]Enterovirus 70 and 71 case "poliomyelitis" in monkeys.

tissue culture, and some echoviruses and polioviruses cause disease in mice. With the blurring of the original definitions, newly isolated enteroviruses are now simply assigned numbers as "enteroviruses," with no distinction between coxsackieviruses and echoviruses.

General Epidemiology

Under unusual circumstances, enteroviruses are spread by respiratory transmission, but they tend to be shed from the oropharynx in small amounts for only 1 to 7 days. In contrast, large amounts are shed from the gut, and fecal excretion continues for 1 to 3 weeks or longer. Epidemiologic data support transmission by fecal contamination, usually by hand-to-mouth human contact. Bacterial and viral cultures of human skin usually reflect the enteric flora, which has led to the epidemiologic euphemism of human "fecal veneer." As is evident to parents and physicians, this veneer is both more abundant on children and more effectively spread by children. Isolation of enteroviruses both in disease and in health is more frequent from children than from adults. Enteroviruses appear to spread horizontally between small children, with subsequent introduction into the family unit, where intimate contact leads to family outbreaks. Longitudinal family studies have shown that introduction of a coxsackievirus into a family unit results in infection of 76% of the nonimmune members of the household, and similar introduction of an echovirus leads to infection of 43% of the nonimmune members within a few days. This difference appears dependent on the longer fecal excretion of coxsackieviruses than echoviruses (Kogon et al., 1969).

Importance of close contact is also exemplified by several outbreaks of enteroviral meningitis among high-school football players. Although the viruses were spreading in the community, the football players had higher case–infection ratios and more hospitalizations than did other students; the explanation could be related to returning early for preseason practice, the close physical contact, and the sharing of water bottles (Moore et al., 1983).

Crowding and poor sanitation facilitate the hand-to-mouth spread of enteroviruses, but dissemination is also enhanced in suburban developments, modern urban-planning units, and communal child-care centers where small children share their daytime hours and their enteroviruses, with subsequent infection of their respective families (Johnson et al., 1960b). Flies or cockroaches may carry fecal contamination, and enteroviruses have been isolated from water sources and sewage. However, insects, water, and fomites are not major vehicles of dissemination. Those of us over 50 years of age recall the sad closings of swimming pools and the burgeoning sales of flypaper during the polio epidemics, but the perennial parental admonition to wash our hands undoubtedly was a better public health measure.

Enteroviruses are worldwide in their distribution, and they circulate throughout the year. In temperate climates, they cause epidemics during the late summer and early fall months. In tropical areas, infections occur at high prevalence through the year; one study found that over 50% of children in Pakistan were excreting one or more enteroviruses at any given time (Parks et al., 1967).

Epidemic Poliomyelitis

The appearance of epidemic poliomyelitis and, indeed, some aspects of its disappearance still remain unexplained (Nathanson and Martin, 1979; Nathanson et al., 1993). Epidemics were first seen among small children in Scandinavia in the late 19th century and in North America and the remainder of northern Europe in the early 20th century. Until the introduction of polio vaccines, the age of patients developing paralytic poliomyelitis increased from epidemic year to epidemic year. During the great epidemic of 1916, in New York City alone 9,000 cases of paralysis were reported, and 80% involved children under 5 years of age. During epidemics in the 1950s, the peak incidence of paralysis was in children from 5 to 9 years of age, and one-third of the cases and two-thirds of the deaths occurred in persons over 15 years of age. The peak poliomyelitis rate was reached in the United States in 1952, when over 21,000 cases of paralysis were reported. Some decline in rates was seen even before the introduction of killed poliovirus vaccine in 1955 and oral live poliovirus vaccine in 1961 (Strebel et al., 1992).

The popular hypothesis to explain this geographically localized appearance and subsequent age shift is based on several observations: (a) Paralysis is age dependent and is a more frequent complication of infection with increasing age (Weinstein, 1957). Adults and adolescents with primary infection are 10 times more likely to develop paralysis and, in virgin-population epidemics, a majority of all deaths are of patients over 40 years of age. (b) Prior to immunization programs, essentially all individuals experienced infections with all three strains of virus. This is documented by serologic surveys even in isolated populations. Therefore, it is assumed that as sanitation improved, virus dissemination among the very young declined, exposing a more susceptible population of older children and adults to primary infection (Nathanson and Martin, 1979). Quite possibly, during the period preceding epidemics of poliomyelitis, children were infected with all three strains during infancy when still protected from penetration beyond the gut by passive maternal antibody. Therefore, the accepted hypothesis is that changes in living patterns and sanitation delayed acquisition of infection, which led to the buildup of nonimmunes and the appearance of epidemic paralytic disease.

However, not all the aspects of poliomyelitis epidemics of the first half of the 20th century can be explained by this formulation. For example, strains of poliovirus recovered during epidemics usually showed greater neurovirulence in monkeys than strains recovered during endemic periods. This suggests that virus mutations may have contributed to the emerging epidemics. Also, climatic factors clearly played a role, with epidemics occurring in temperate zones, and infection remained largely endemic in the tropics. Facilitation of spread in high humidity or the prevalence of other enterovirus infections causing interference may be additional factors that inhibit epidemics.

A vigorous campaign to eradicate polio worldwide is under way, with a goal of global eradication by the year 2000 (Hull et al., 1997). The success of this campaign has already been seen in the Western Hemisphere, where the last case of poliomyelitis due to an indigenous wild poliovirus was found in 1991 in Peru [Centers for Disease Control (CDC), 1993c]. In 1993, wild-type virus was found to be circulating among members of a religious community in Canada that opposes vaccinations, but no cases of paralysis occurred. Members of this community had visited with an affiliated community in the Netherlands, where an outbreak of paralytic poliomyelitis was in progress (CDC, 1993b). The last outbreak of paralytic poliomyelitis in the United States occurred in an Amish community in Pennsylvania in 1979 (CDC, 1979).

Since 1980, no case of paralytic poliovirus due to indigenous wild-type virus has been reported in the United States. Between 1980 and 1994, however, there were 125 cases of vaccine-associated paralytic poliomyelitis and 6 cases of imported disease. Vaccine-associated cases have included, primarily, infants receiving their first dose of oral poliovirus vaccine; immunologically normal persons in contact with vaccinees, many of whom were inadequately vaccinated; and immunologically compromised individuals. This represents an incidence of one paralytic case per 1.2 million first doses, a remarkably low complication rate. Nevertheless, a return to killed vaccine followed by oral attenuated vaccine has been advocated (CDC, 1997a, 1997b). Arguments regarding optimum modes of immunization are discussed in Chapter 17.

Poliomyelitis remains a threat, but in many areas physicians fail to diagnose vaccine-associated disease because of their unfamiliarity with paralytic poliomyelitis or the atypical forms that the vaccine-associated disease may present (Arlazoroff et al., 1987; Querfurth and Swanson, 1990).

Varied Manifestations of Coxsackie and Echovirus Infections

Coxsackie and echoviruses remain major endemic and epidemic infections associated with varied diseases. A World Health Organization (WHO) surveillance program over a 4-year period recorded isolation of over 10,000 nonpolio enteroviruses from patients with clinical diseases. During the interval of that study, echovirus 9 was the most frequent cause of enteroviral disease and the most prominent cause of large epidemics; however, no regular pattern emerged of recurrence of different serotypes, and echovirus 30 has been the more prominent cause of viral meningitis epidemics in recent years (CDC, 1991a). The majority of infections and diseases in the WHO study occurred in children younger than age 14. The Northern Hemisphere enterovirus infections were concentrated from July to October, and the Southern Hemisphere infections were concentrated from October to February (Assaad and Cockburn, 1972). Superficially, this seasonal variation might appear explicable by the scant clothing and greater contact of children during the summer months. However, seasonal epidemics occur even in constant climates, such as that of Hawaii. Furthermore, undefined factors appear to facilitate enterovirus dissemination in general, because during major epidemics multiple enteroviruses are often involved. During a large epidemic of echovirus 9 in Milwaukee, Wisconsin, more than ten enteroviruses were recovered from the community (Sabin et al., 1958). In an epidemic of poliomyelitis in Hawaii, "nonparalytic poliomyelitis" proved to be associated not only with poliovirus but also with three different coxsackieviruses and three different echoviruses (Johnson et al., 1960a).

The majority of coxsackievirus and echovirus infections are not associated with significant clinical symptoms. Males and females are infected with equal frequencies, but clinical disease is more frequent in males. Although enteroviruses cause more cases of aseptic meningitis in children than in adults, the frequency of meningitis as a complication of an enterovirus infection is greater in adults than in children. CNS infections are the most important and prevalent diseases associated with enterovirus infections, but the varied manifestations of these infections also include undifferentiated fever, nonspecific respiratory disease, pleurodynia, carditis, diarrhea in small children, and a variety of rashes.

The coexistence of rash may be helpful in the diagnosis of the meningitis or encephalitis. Rashes have been associated with coxsackieviruses A5, A9, and A16 and with echoviruses 4, 6, 9, and 16. Rashes range from macular to papular to vesicular lesions, and one patient with echovirus 6 infection was reported with bulbous lesions over a localized area that resembled the lesions of shingles (Meade and Chang, 1979). In echovirus 9 epidemics, the rash has often been petechial, and this rash associated with meningitis may be confused with meningococcemia. Coxsackievirus A16 and, on rare occasions, A4, A5, A9, and A10 may be associated with vesicular lesions on the hands, feet, and oropharynx, so-called hand-foot-and-mouth disease. Group A coxsackieviruses also cause herpangina characterized by grayish vesicular lesions on the tonsillar fauces, soft palate, and uvula.

Respiratory symptoms with most enterovirus infections are mild, but pleurodynia, as well as pericarditis and myocarditis, can complicate group B coxsackievirus infections and, rarely, echovirus infections. Enterovirus 70 and coxsackievirus A24 have been associated with an acute hemorrhagic conjunctivitis.

Coxsackievirus and Echovirus CNS Infections

The single most common clinical manifestation of both the group B coxsackievirus and echovirus infections is meningitis (Grist et al., 1978). There is little to differentiate enterovirus meningitis from viral meningitis caused by other agents, except for the frequent coexistence of the more characteristic systemic signs of enteroviral infection in patients or their family members.

Typically, the onset of aseptic meningitis is abrupt and without prodrome, and disease lasts for several days or weeks. Cerebrospinal fluid examined early in the disease may contain polymorphonuclear cells, causing concern that a bacterial infection may be present, but usually the fever is below 40°C, and the patient does not appear gravely ill. A repeat lumbar puncture 12 to 24 hours later usually will show a conversion to lymphocytes. The electroencephalogram, even in very benign viral meningitis, may show disquieting amounts of slowing, and serial electroencephalograms may show persistence of slowing even after the patient is asymptomatic. The long-term prognosis of meningitis due to enteroviruses is excellent, although prolonged asthenia with muscle tenderness can extend for weeks or even months (Lepow et al., 1962). Concerns about intellectual development have been expressed for infants and toddlers with enteroviral meningitis who are under 24 months of age, but several recent follow-up studies have shown no cognitive deficits even in those children suffering seizures and severe obtundation during the acute disease (Bergman et al., 1987; Rorabaugh et al., 1993).

Signs of encephalitis, paralysis, or other localizing signs occur in less than 2% of clinically apparent coxsackievirus and echovirus CNS infections. Mild obtundation, seizures, or transient focal abnormalities have been reported with a variety of these infections, but permanent sequelae are rare. With the exception of the fatal encephalitis and myocarditis seen with fetal or neonatal infections with group B coxsackieviruses (see Chapter 13), severe encephalitis is very rare. Deaths do occur, however, particularly among children with acute encephalitis, and coxsackievirus B1 and echoviruses 9, 17, and 21 have been isolated from or identified in the brain after fatal encephalitis (Kibrick, 1964; Grist et al., 1978; Kamei et al., 1990). Fatal echovirus 11 infections in babies have been associated with disseminated intravascular coagulation and intracerebral hemorrhages (Berry and Nagington, 1982).

In some reports, however, the cause-and-effect relationship of virus to death or sequelae has not been entirely convincing. For example, during an epidemic of coxsackievirus B5 in Essex, England, two adults died (Heathfield et al., 1967). One had acute encephalitis, and a coxsackievirus was isolated from the cerebrospinal fluid early in the course of disease. However, the patient died after 4 months of coma and an "acute" encephalitis, with medial temporal lobe necrosis, was found at autopsy. Although this was accredited to the coxsackievirus infection, the localization of the encephalitis raises the possibility of activation of a herpesvirus during or subsequent to the original enterovirus infection. The other patient who died during the epidemic had an acute hemorrhagic leukoencephalitis. Coxsackievirus B5 was isolated from feces at autopsy; however, during an epidemic, many persons in a community will have the epidemic virus in their feces. Its relationship to the neurologic disease must remain doubtful. An even more dubious cause-and-effect relationship was drawn in the report of a middle-aged patient who had encephalitis, with coxsackievirus B2 found in stool, and who developed Parkinson's disease 3 months later (Walters, 1960). We all have multiple enterovirus infections during our lives, and therefore all of our illnesses either precede or follow these infections within weeks, months, or years.

Unusual neurologic complications of enterovirus infections are seen. Acute cerebellar ataxia has been reported in children infected with polioviruses, echoviruses 6 and 9, and coxsackieviruses A2 and A9, as well as all group B coxsackieviruses (Feldman and Larke, 1972). Acute hemiplegia with coxsackievirus A9 and opsoclonus–myoclonus with coxsackievirus B3 have been reported in children with viruses recovered from spinal fluid (Rodden et al., 1975; Kuban et al., 1983). Focal encephalitis with hemichorea was reported in a child with serologic evidence of an echovirus infection (Peters et al., 1979). Polyradiculitis has been reported with echovirus 9 recovered from cerebrospinal fluid, but the patient had a concomitant significant increase in herpes simplex virus antibody between acute-phase and convalescent-phase sera (Forbes et al., 1967).

Two enteroviruses have been associated with novel epidemics. In the summer of 1969 at the time of the Apollo landing on the moon, an explosive epidemic of hemorrhagic conjunctivitis erupted in Accra, Ghana. Locally, it was called Apollo disease, with the clear implication that it was nature's revenge for the lunar intrusion. The epidemic spread across Africa, to Eastern Europe, India, Taiwan, and Japan; in 1 per 10,000 infections, lower motor neuron paralysis was seen and, in some cases, severe paralytic sequelae were seen that resembled classic poliomyelitis (Hung and Kono, 1979; Wadia, 1989). Over the following year, the epidemic abated, only to recur in India in 1980, with spread to Asia and South America, Central America, and the Caribbean; a small number of cases were seen in southern Florida and North Carolina. Another decade passed, and the disease reappeared on Samoa but failed to spread (Bern et al., 1992). This unusual disease is caused by enterovirus 70, which spreads by hand-to-eye contact and is not isolated from stool specimens. This aberrant mode of spread probably explains the explosive nature of the epidemics, and the rapid spread probably explains the exhaustion of nonimmune hosts and the disappearance of the virus until sufficient mutations can accumulate to initiate another epidemic (Johnson, 1994a, 1996b).

In 1975, an epidemic of poliomyelitis-like disease associated with enterovirus 71, including fatal bulbar disease, occurred in Bulgaria (Chumakov et al., 1979). Similar epidemics occurred in Hungary in 1978 and in Brazil in 1989 and 1990 (da Silva et al., 1996). Two children developed transient paralytic disease during an enterovirus 71 outbreak in New York State (Chonmaitree et al., 1981). Both enteroviruses 70 and 71 produce paralytic disease in monkeys, and pathologic lesions resemble those of polioviruses (Kono et al., 1973; Hashimoto and Hagiwara, 1982).

Persistent infections of the CNS with enteroviruses are recognized only in patients with agammaglobulinemia. This chronic meningitis is related to echoviruses in 90% of these cases, with a disproportionate number being caused by echovirus 11 (McKinney et al., 1987). The use of intravenous immunoglobulin for the treatment of agammaglobulinemia has largely eliminated this chronic infection, but, occasionally, immunodeficient children still develop chronic enteroviral meningitis despite therapy (Misbah et al., 1992).

Other Enteric Viruses

In 1959, a group of respiratory and enteric orphan (REO) viruses previously classified as the echovirus 10 group were reclassified as reoviruses—viruses that subsequently proved to have little in common genomically or structurally with enteroviruses. Under the old classification, we had associated echovirus 10 with aseptic meningitis (Meyer et al., 1960) and, since reclassification, rare cases of reovirus-related meningitis and encephalitis have been reported (Johansson et al., 1996).

Encephalomyocarditis viruses are a group of rodent enteroviruses transmitted enterically or by ectoparasites. Their role in human disease remains in dispute. Original isolates were from rodents inoculated with specimens from poliomyelitis, and these recoveries probably represented activations of latent rodent viruses. However, accidental infection and encephalitis in a laboratory worker working with the Mengo strain did establish their potential pathogenicity in humans (Dick et al., 1948). Following that case report, several reports of encephalitis, poliomyelitis, myelitis, and polyradiculitis related to encephalomyocarditis viruses appeared from Europe (Gajdusek, 1955), and serologic surveys showed antibody to these viruses in human sera. Nevertheless, subsequent isolation and serologic studies of large numbers of patients with meningitis and encephalitis have failed to implicate these rodent enteroviruses in human disease (Meyer et al., 1960).

MUMPS VIRUS

Mumps virus had been the single commonest cause of aseptic meningitis and mild encephalitis in North America and Europe, but the routine inclusion of mumps vaccine with measles vaccine has resulted in a 90% decrease in the incidence of natural mumps in the United States. As with the enteroviruses, humans are the only known natural hosts, but mumps has a very different epidemiologic pattern.

Mumps virus is a large, pleomorphic paramyxovirus. Although different isolates of mumps virus show marked variability in the types of cytopathic effects in cell cultures and in neurovirulence in experimental animals, no antigenic difference has been demonstrated to form subtypes of mumps virus (McCarthy et al., 1980). Furthermore, no obvious differences in virulence, in terms of rates of parotitis, orchitis, or CNS complications are evident from outbreak to outbreak.

Epidemiology

Mumps is spread by the respiratory route and can readily be recovered from saliva or respiratory secretions. The virus can also be found in urine and in breast milk, but viruria and breast-feeding have not been incriminated as modes of transmission. As with many other viruses spread by the respiratory droplets, exposure is greater during the winter months. The incubation period is approximately 16 to 18 days.

Mumps virus has a worldwide distribution. Although sporadic infections maintain the virus throughout the year, attack rates increase in March and April in northern temperate climates. Major epidemics occur at intervals from 2 to 3 up to 7 years, depending on the development of a critical susceptible population. Prior to recent immunization programs, 80% to 90% of persons in urban populations had serologic evidence of prior infection by age 16, and 50% of infections occurred between the ages of 5 and 9. Slightly more than half of those infected show signs of clinical disease. In a virgin-population epidemic, 65% of those infected had clinical signs of disease, 11% had meningitis or encephalitis, and 35% had subclinical infections (Philip et al., 1959). Clinical signs associated with infection, however, are twice as frequent in males as in females, and the neurologic complications are three times more frequent in males (Johnstone et al., 1972).

Clinical manifestations include respiratory symptoms with swelling and tenderness of the parotid glands in approximately half of the cases. Orchitis, which is usually unilateral, develops in approximately one-third of postpubertal males, and minor enlargement and tenderness of mammary tissue occurs in approximately one-third of postpubertal females. More unusual manifestations include signs of pancreatitis, with acute abdominal pain; oophoritis, with lower abdominal tenderness; or thyroiditis, with tenderness and fullness of the thyroid.

CNS Infections

Involvement of the CNS is common, but the incidence of neurologic complications with mumps depends on one's threshold of suspicion. Headache is an almost universal feature of clinical mumps. Routine cerebrospinal fluid examinations on a large number of patients with mumps parotitis showed that over 50% had a pleocytosis, even though the majority had no nuchal rigidity (Bang and Bang, 1943). Conversely, only about 50% of patients with mumps meningitis and encephalitis have parotitis (Azimi et al., 1969). When both manifestations are present, the meningitis frequently develops several days after the onset of parotitis, but it may develop a week or more later. In rare cases, meningitis may precede the parotitis by a full week (Levitt et al., 1970). The spinal fluid pleocytosis may persist for months, and oligoclonal immunoglobulin G (IgG) proteins may persist for a year after mumps meningitis, despite complete clinical recovery (Vandvik et al., 1978).

More severe neurologic disease can occur. Mumps is a common cause of mild encephalitis (Meyer et al., 1960), but severe encephalitis is rare, and only four or five deaths were reported per year to the CDC prior to immunization programs. Strange neurologic complications of mumps encephalitis have included transient cortical blindness with ataxia (Davis et al., 1971), isolated cerebellar ataxia (Cohen et al., 1992), and myelitis with or without a sensory level (Scheid, 1961). These manifestations may represent postinfectious encephalomyelitis, and, indeed, pathologic studies of fatal mumps virus encephalitis have shown acute encephalitis in some cases and perivenular demyelination typical of postinfectious encephalomyelitis in others (see Chapter 8).

Like the coxsackieviruses and echoviruses, mumps virus infections occasionally cause signs of lower motor neuron disease simulating mild paralytic poliomyelitis. Paralysis is usually mild, but residua do occur: one study found sequelae in 4 of 11 patients with paralysis (Lennette et al., 1960). This rare lower motor neuron paralysis should not be confused with facial palsy that can occur with parotitis and is believed to represent a compression palsy or local peripheral neuritis. Permanent unilateral hearing loss is also a complication of mumps; this probably represents a peripheral lesion, with infection of the cochlea (see Chapter 16). Although one study reported permanent sequela in 25% of patients years after mumps encephalitis (Julkunen et al., 1985), most series report few sequelae and long-term total recovery in the vast majority (Johnstone et al., 1972).

The possibility of a chronic encephalomyelitis due to mumps virus has been suggested in several reports. Persistent intrathecal synthesis of antibodies to mumps virus has been found in patients with sequelae of mumps virus encephalitis (Julkunen et al., 1985), in a child with progressive mental deterioration with severe seizures following parotitis (Ito et al., 1991), and in an adult with multifocal inflammatory CNS disease (Vaheri et al., 1982). However, prolonged intrathecal synthesis of antibodies has been documented after uncomplicated mumps meningitis, and in some patients a specific intrathecal antibody response may result from a nonspecific activation of cells producing antibodies to an unrelated antigen (Vandvik et al., 1982). In view of these findings, virologic and immunocytopathologic studies of neural tissues are needed before concluding that mumps virus can cause chronic CNS disease.

Although attenuated live mumps virus vaccine has reduced neurologic complications, the Urabe vaccine strain of mumps virus has proved to cause occasional cases of meningitis in Europe, Japan, and Canada (Miller et al., 1993; Rebiere and Galy-Eyraud, 1995; Saito et al., 1996). The Jeryl Lynn strain used in the standard trivalent vaccine in the United States has not been associated with neurologic complications.

Other paramyxoviruses (parainfluenza viruses and respiratory syncytial viruses) are among the commonest causes of childhood respiratory infections. CNS complications are rare, but one—parainfluenza virus 3—has been associated with rare cases of encephalitis (McCarthy et al., 1990).

ADENOVIRUSES

Adenoviruses cause common infections with varied clinical manifestations, but neurologic complications are rare. Adenovirus infections do provide interesting epidemiologic comparisons with enterovirus and mumps virus infections, because adenoviruses are spread by both gastrointestinal and respiratory routes, and route of spread is an important disease determinant. Adenoviruses also differ from the other two virus groups in their propensity to persist.

Adenoviruses are nonenveloped, icosahedral viruses containing double-stranded DNA. Many serotypes are associated with human disease, but the features of disease depend on the strain of virus and host factors, as well as on the route of virus entry.

Epidemiology

Transmission in early life and among families is predominantly by fecal–oral spread similar to that of the enteroviruses. Epidemics of adenovirus respiratory disease are prominent in military and boarding-school populations. Furthermore, adenoviruses have physicochemical stability and can be transmitted in water and by fomites. Pharyngoconjunctival fever can be acquired in swimming pools (types 3 and 7), and epidemic keratoconjunctivitis can be spread by fingers and tools in offices of ophthalmologists (primarily type 8).

More adenovirus infections occur in the late winter and spring. In children, approximately 50% of the infections cause clinical disease, which may present as croup, pharyngitis, pneumonitis, and conjunctivitis, or as intussusception or hemorrhagic cystitis. Complications are more likely to occur if the virus is transmitted by the respiratory route than by the gastrointestinal route.

CNS Infections

Neurologic complications are seen almost exclusively in children and accompany severe respiratory disease. When the CNS is involved, encephalitis rather than aseptic meningitis tends to occur, and a number of deaths have been reported. However, the rarity of these complications is supported by our studies of over 1,000 cases of acute viral CNS disease in which virtually all patients without an established diagnosis were tested serologically for adenovirus infection, and none was found (Meyer et al., 1960). Other series have associated adenoviruses with about 1% of cases of encephalitis (Roos, 1989).

Lelong and colleagues (1956) first established an association of acute CNS disease with adenoviruses: in an epidemic of type 7 adenovirus, they reported five cases of encephalitis, including one fatal case in which adenovirus type 7 was recovered from brain. A similar epidemic with type 7 was described in Finland, with eight cases of encephalitis and two deaths (Simila et al., 1970). Although type 7 adenovirus has been the primary cause of encephalitis, types 1, 2, 3, 5, 6, and 12 have been isolated from cerebrospinal fluid or brain of children with meningitis or encephalitis (Roos, 1989). Other serotypes have been isolated from stool or respiratory tract in patients with aseptic meningitis and encephalitis, but these isolations must be interpreted with caution, because adenoviruses cause persistent infections and, indeed, can be isolated from half of all tonsils removed surgically. Adenoviruses have been recovered from stool for periods of more than 2 years. For diagnosis of concurrent infections, a significant rise in antibody must be demonstrated over the course of the disease; even then, sero-conversion during adenovirus epidemics may be so common that intercurrent inflammatory diseases may be unrelated (Johnson et al., 1961).

An unusual adenovirus encephalitis has been described in an adult with terminal lymphoma. This patient had a subacute encephalitis, and type 32 adenovirus was recovered (Roos et al., 1972). Histologically, intranuclear inclusion bodies showed adenovirus-like particles (Chou et al., 1973). Adenovirus encephalitis also has been described in patients with leukemia, a cerebellar astrocytoma, after bone marrow transplantation (Davis et al., 1988), and in AIDS (Hierholzer, 1992), but adenoviruses are not common opportunistic infections in AIDS.

PARVOVIRUS

Parvovirus B19 is a newly recognized human pathogen, and the only parvovirus known to cause human disease. It is a common respiratory infection at all ages, with seropositive rates reaching 50% in young adults and 90% in the elderly.

Parvoviruses are single-stranded DNA viruses that replicate via palindromic loops at either end of the DNA strand that serve as self-primers (Rotbart, 1990). Parvoviruses usually replicate in mitotic cells; parvovirus B19 infects hematopoietic cells and is associated with transient leukopenia and thrombocytopenia. Childhood parvovirus B19 infections cause erythema infectiosum or 5th disease, a spring and summer disease with major epidemics at 3- to 4-year intervals. Children with erythema infectiosum are usually not seriously ill, have "slapped cheek" facial erythema, and show a reticular, effervescent maculopapular rash over the trunk and proximal extremities. In older persons, arthralgias are common and, in adults, frank arthritis may occur. In patients with underlying hemolysis, such as sickle cell anemia, infection can precipitate serious aplastic crises; in pregnant women, infection can cause hydrops fetalis (see Chapter 13).

CNS complications are rare. Prior to detection of parvovirus B19, signs of meningitis and encephalopathy occasionally have been reported during erythema infectiosum, often with normal spinal fluid (Hall and Horner, 1977). Since 1990, a small number of children with aseptic meningitis have been reported with the typical clinical syndrome, a pleocytosis, and parvovirus B19 DNA detected in spinal fluid by polymerase chain reaction (PCR) (Koduri and Naides, 1995). In addition, a child with encephalopathy with seizures and drowsiness, and a 35-year-old healthy adult with headache, neck pain, and photophobia have been reported without a pleocytosis but with parvovirus B19 DNA in spinal fluid (Cassinotti et al., 1993; Watanabe et al., 1994). Further studies of neurologic illnesses during childhood erythema infectiosum, adults with acute arthritis, and patients with thrombocytopenia are needed to define the neurologic complications of parvovirus B19 infections better.

ARENAVIRUSES

Lymphocytic Choriomeningitis Virus

Lymphocytic choriomeningitis virus was the first virus isolated from aseptic meningitis, and the virus and the clinical syndrome were initially equated. In a review in 1937, Reimann stated that lymphocytic meningitis was "established as a specific infectious disease caused by *a* filterable virus." Even though lymphocytic choriomeningitis virus is recognized now as the cause of only 1% to 10% of the cases of aseptic meningitis and mild encephalitis, the clinical use of the term lymphocytic choriomeningitis (admittedly a superior descriptive term) for the aseptic meningitis syndrome continues to cause confusion.

Epidemiology

Lymphocytic choriomeningitis virus is of biologic interest as a zoonotic infection in which humans acquire the virus from mice or hamsters. It is a member of the arenavirus family, a group of enveloped, segmented, negative-stranded RNA viruses, several of which are transmitted from rodents to humans. Lymphocytic choriomeningitis virus is the only member of this family found in Europe and North America, but related agents are associated with diseases in Africa and South America (Table 5.4).

Lymphocytic choriomeningitis virus causes a common persistent infection in the house mouse, *Mus musculus*. In rodent populations carrying this virus, there

TABLE 5.4. *Arenaviruses causing CNS disease*

Virus	Animal reservoir	Geographic localization	Major human disease	Human-to-human spread
Old World				
Lymphocytic choriomeningitis virus	Common mouse (*Mus musculus*) and hamster (*Mesocricetus auratus*)	Europe and Americas	Aseptic meningitis, mild encephalitis	Not reported
Lassa virus	Wild rodents (*Mastomys natalensis*)	West Africa	Lassa fever	Frequent
New World				
Junin virus	Wild rodents (genus *Calomys*)	Northeast Argentina	Argentinian hemorrhagic fever	Occasional
Machupo virus	Wild rodents (genus *Calomys*)	Beni region of Bolivia	Bolivian hemorrhagic fever	Occasional
Guanarito virus	Wild rodents	Rural central Venezuela	Venezuelan hemorrhagic fever	?
Sabiá virus	Unknown	Brazil	Hemorrhagic fever	?

is apparent transovarian or early fetal infection. All or most of the cells of the carrier mouse are infected, including the ovarian germinal cells (Mims, 1966). The virus does not persist as a silent integrated nucleic acid; quite the contrary, infected cells in carrier mice produce large amounts of infectious virus, and viremia is maintained throughout life. Congenitally infected mice excrete virus in respiratory droplets, in feces, and in urine. This virus in mice represents the classic example of infection during fetal life that leads to a relative lack of immune response or tolerance (see Chapter 4). Infection of noncarrier adult mice or passive transfer of immune lymphocytes to carrier mice causes an acute fatal encephalitis, so the noncytopathic virus is capable of inciting murine disease mediated by cellular immune responses against virus-infected cells.

The geographic distribution of lymphocytic choriomeningitis virus infections is multifocal over much of Europe and North America. Scandinavia and Australia appear free of the infection. Human disease is found more frequently in the winter, because in temperate zones *M. musculus* leaves the fields and enters homes to seek warmth. Antibody surveys in both Germany and the United States have shown that 5% or less of human sera have antibody to the virus (Lehmann-Grube, 1971; Childs et al., 1992). Although human infection can occur from dust containing the excreta of these mice, many patients suffering clinical infections have a history of actually handling or killing mice. One of our patients with meningitis was a barn painter who made a habit of exterminating mice that ran across his painted sills by splattering them with the side of his brush, probably creating a potent infectious aerosol.

Clinical Disease

The incubation period after exposure is 6 to 13 days. Initial symptoms include fever, malaise, myalgia, and coryza. Leukopenia, thrombocytopenia, and radiologic evidence of pneumonitis may be present. In some cases, a diphasic course occurs, with defervescence and a clearing of symptoms before the acute onset of headache, recrudescence of fever, and stiff neck. No age or sex differentiation is evident in the development of clinical CNS disease. Whether or not the CNS disease in humans represents a cell-mediated immune response to a noncytopathic infection is unknown. Although this mechanism is suggested by the frequent diphasic course of the disease, no other data implicate an immune basis for the human CNS disease.

Occasionally, the meningitis is associated with parotitis. In one man, parotitis, orchitis, and meningitis were present, yet lymphocytic choriomeningitis virus was isolated from blood and spinal fluid, and no increase in antibodies to mumps virus was found (Lewis and Utz, 1961). Mild encephalitis with focal signs is common, but an extensive review by Lehmann-Grube (1971) found only eight fatal cases. Unlike the situation with most forms of aseptic meningitis, symptoms of headache and weakness, as well as the pleocytosis, may persist for a month or more; one child had an eosinophilia of 14% and 25% in spinal fluid 5 and 7 weeks after onset of symptoms (Chesney et al., 1979). Recovery usually is complete, and sequelae are rare, although a recent serologic study indicated that hydrocephalus may be more frequent in the progeny of women infected with this virus (see Chapter 13).

The hamster also has been a source for human infections. In 1974, tumor research workers in Rochester, New York, suffered an outbreak of respiratory disease, with some cases of meningitis and encephalitis. Lymphocytic choriomeningitis virus was implicated. The majority of affected workers handled hamsters, and all but 1 of 48 infected persons had entered the room where the hamsters were housed (Hinman et al., 1975). These research animals were epidemiologically linked to pet hamsters in New York State that were found to be infected. In 1974, 12 cases of meningitis and encephalitis, 34 cases of flulike illness, and 13 other paired sera showed evidence of lymphocytic choriomeningitis virus infections. Of these 60 persons, 55 had pet hamsters, and 4 others were employees of wholesalers or retailers of hamsters (Deibel et al., 1975). Other outbreaks have occurred in research facilities; the most recent involved nude mice (Dykewicz et al., 1992). Laboratory workers and pet owners clearly represent new populations at risk.

Hemorrhagic Fevers

Four other arenaviruses cause human disease with neurologic complications, but the primary illness in each of these infections is a hemorrhagic fever (Table 5.4). Lassa fever virus has an ecology similar to lymphocytic choriomeningitis virus but represents a more frightening public health problem. First recognized in Nigeria in 1969, the disease of Lassa fever in West Africa affects about 300,000 persons and kills 5,000 persons per year (Holmes et al., 1990). The Lassa fever virus causes a persistent infection of the *Masomys* genus of rats and presumably spreads to humans by aerosols of droppings, but this virus also has proven hazardous because of human-to-human spread from hospitalized patients to health workers and from human specimens to laboratory personnel. Hospital outbreaks have been associated with mortality rates of 30% to 66% among infected personnel. Clinically, there is pneumonitis, myocarditis, nephropathy, hemorrhage, and frequent signs and symptoms of encephalitis. In Africa, Lassa fever virus is a major cause of sensorineural deafness (Cummins et al., 1990). Clinicopathologic studies have been limited; indeed, the pathologist who performed the initial autopsies contracted Lassa fever and died. Experimentally infected rhesus monkeys show only scattered infiltrates of lymphocytes around cerebral vessels and in meninges but consistent infiltration of the choroid plexus with plasma cells and lymphocytes reminiscent of the pathologic findings in murine lymphocytic choriomeningitis (Callis et al., 1982). In human infections, pathologic changes in the CNS are nonspecific and less dramatic than those found in Argentinean and Bolivian hemorrhagic fevers (Walker et al., 1982).

In recent years, Argentinean hemorrhagic fever, due to the Junin virus, has been reported in more than 20,000 persons in agricultural areas of Buenos Aires province and adjacent areas. The virus is carried primarily in the corn rat, *Calomys* species. Mainly, field workers who handpick the corn have been infected, but with the introduction of modern harvesting equipment, the rat excrement and the rats themselves are aerosolized, causing some infections in neighboring communities and persons driving through the endemic areas. Human infection is characterized by high fever, headache, lymphadenopathy, and an erythematous exanthem over the face and thorax, with focal hemorrhages in skin and mucous membranes. Cerebellar signs and abnormalities of extraocular movements may be found, if sought, in very ill patients (*personal observation*). Death results from uremia or hypovolemic shock in 15% to 30% of patients. Perivascular inflammatory reactions and hemorrhages are found in the brain, and the virus has been recovered from brain (Elsner et al., 1973).

Administration of human immune plasma to patients within 8 days of the onset of illness has reduced the mortality to only 1%. This treatment, however, has resulted in a "late neurologic syndrome," consisting of isolated cerebellar ataxia and oculomotor abnormalities without systemic symptoms. This evolves 4 to 6 weeks after therapy in about 10% of treated patients (Maiztegui et al., 1979). This intriguing new syndrome suggests that immune plasma clears systemic virus but not virus in the CNS, and that after clearance of passively transferred immunoglobulins, an isolated, albeit self-limited, cerebellar and brainstem encephalitis recurs. A model of this sequela of immunotherapy has been developed in Junin virus-infected guinea pigs, so its pathogenesis can be studied (Kenyon et al., 1986).

Bolivian hemorrhagic fever is a similar clinical disease due to a related agent, Machupo virus. This virus is also found in *Calomys* species, but the disease occurs primarily in villages along the forest edge after heavy rains, when flooding drives rodents into the villages. Approximately one-fourth of the patients with Bolivian hemorrhagic fever have neurologic complications (Child et al., 1967).

In 1989, a similar hemorrhagic fever was recognized in central rural Venezuela, and the rodent-borne virus isolated from this disease has been named Guanarito virus (Salas et al., 1991). In 1994, an agricultural engineer in Brazil with no history of rodent exposure developed fatal hemorrhagic fever with tremor, convulsions, and coma. An arenavirus named Sabiá was recovered from her blood, and two nonfatal cases of hemorrhagic fever developed in laboratory workers studying the virus (Coimbra et al., 1994; Barry et al., 1995).

Other viral hemorrhagic fevers that are not arenavirus-related diseases are found in varied parts of the world. Korean hemorrhagic fever, although similarly spread by persistently infected rodents, is caused by hantavirus of the *Bunyavirus* family, and Congo–Crimean hemorrhagic fever virus is a tick-borne bunyavirus. Dengue, Omsk hemorrhagic fever, and Kyasanur Forest disease are all caused by flaviviruses spread by arthropods.

FILOVIRUSES

The filovirus family includes Marburg and Ebola viruses, which have been related to outbreaks of hemorrhagic fever in humans and subhuman primates. These are almost certainly zoonotic infections that can spread from primate to primate, but the natural history and reservoirs harboring these agents between outbreaks remain a mystery. These strange agents have elongated enveloped virions containing a single strand of negative-strand RNA.

In 1967, in Yugoslavia and Germany, outbreaks of hemorrhagic fever occurred in laboratory workers handling African green monkey organs and subsequently occurred among the medical personnel who cared for them (Kissling et al., 1968). The Marburg agent was recovered from the monkey cells and the patients. Subsequent Marburg virus outbreaks have occurred in East and South Africa, with fatality rates in excess of 30%. Ebola virus was the cause of major hemorrhagic fever epidemics in Zaire and Sudan in 1976 and 1979 and more recently in Zaire in 1995 and Gabon in 1996. Again, person-to-person transmission has occurred in family and hospital settings. Fatality rates in these epidemics have been 70% to 90% (Sanchez et al., 1995). Exposure to contaminated blood and reused needles, and close direct contact, such as preparing bodies for burials and sexual spread, have all been implicated in transmission (Feldmann et al., 1996). The concerns of international spread with jet travel mirror those regarding Lassa fever (see Chapter 18).

With both virus infections, disease begins abruptly with fever, chills, headache, vomiting and diarrhea, and widespread hemorrhage. Stupor, abnormal behavior, coma, and hemiparesis are common, although the cerebrospinal fluid is usually acellular. A multifocal nodular encephalitis is found, with lymphocytes, perivascular infiltrates, and perivascular extravasations of red cells (Jacob, 1971). The clinical and pathologic features are similar to those of rickettsial diseases, which suggests that the target of CNS infection may be cerebrovascular endothelial cells.

ARBOVIRUSES

Arthropod-borne viruses (arboviruses) are important causes of encephalitis in many areas of the world. Since these agents are restricted to specific species of mosquitoes or ticks and to specific ecologic systems, the arboviral encephalitides show marked geographic restriction. They also are seasonal diseases, dependent on the breeding and feeding seasons of the arthropod host.

Arboviruses are agents of several virus families that can replicate in both invertebrate and vertebrate cells. Arbovirus is no longer an official taxonomic term, but the term remains useful biologically, epidemiologically, and clinically for viruses that undergo biologic transmission by arthropods; that is, replication and infection of the hematophagous host must occur prior to injection of the vertebrate host. This is in contrast to mechanical transmission in which virus may be spread by contaminated mouthparts, as in the spread of equine infectious anemia virus by biting flies, or the contaminated feet of flies or cockroaches as postulated for enteroviruses.

TABLE 5.5. *Arboviruses that cause encephalitis*

Family / Genus / Complex / Virus Species	Vector	Animal Resevoir	Geographical location	Importance in encephalitis[a]
Togaviridae				
Alphavirus[b]				
Eastern encephalitis	Mosquitoes (*Culiseta Aedes*)	Birds	Eastern and gulf coasts of US, Caribbean, and South America	++
Western encephalitis	Mosquitoes (*Culex*)	Birds	Widespread; but disease in western U.S. and Canada	++
Venezuelan equine encephalitis	Mosquitoes (*Aedes, Culex, Mansonia*, etc.)	Horses and small mammals	South and Central America, Florida, and southwest U.S.	+
Flaviviridae[c]				
St. Louis complex				
St. Louis	Mosquitos (*Culex*)	Birds	Widespread in U.S.	+++
Japanese	Mosquitoes (*Culex*)	Birds	Japan, China, southeast Asia, and India	++++
Murray Valley	Mosquitoes (*Culex*)	Birds	Australia and New Guinea	++
West Nile	Mosquitoes (*Culex*)	Birds	Africa, Middle East, and southern Europe	++
Ilheus	Mosquitoes (*Psorphora*)	Birds	South and Central America	+
Rocio	Mosquitoes (?)	Birds	Brazil	++
Tickborne complex				
Far Eastern tickborne encephalitis[d]	Ticks (*Ixodes*)	Small mammals and birds	Siberia	+++
Central European tickborne encephalitis	Ticks (*Ixodes*)	Small mammals and birds	Central Europe	+++
Kyasanur Forest	Ticks (*Haemophysalis*)	Small Mammals and Birds	India	++

Louping ill	Ticks (Ixodes)	Small mammals and birds	North England, Scotland, and Ireland	+
Powassan	Ticks (Ixodes)	Small mammals and birds	Canada and northern U.S.	+
Negishi	Ticks(?)	Small mammals and birds	Japan	+
Bunyaviridae[e]				
Bunyavirus				
California group				
California encephalitis	Mosquitoes (Aedes)	Small Mammals	Western U.S.	+
La Crosse	Mosquitoes (Aedes)	Squirrels, chipmunks	Midwestern and eastern U.S.	++
Jamestown Canyon	Mosquitoes (Culiseta)	Whitetailed deer	U.S. and Alaska	+
Cache Valley	Mosquitoes (Culiseta)	Livestock and large mammals	North and South America	+
Snowshoe hare	Mosquitoes (Culiseta)	Snowshoe hare	Canada, Alaska, northern U.S., and Russia	+
Tahnya	Mosquitoes (Aedes, Culiseta)	Small mammals	Central Europe	+
Inkoo	Mosquitoes (?)	Reindeer, moose	Finland and Russia	+
Phlebovirus				
Rift Valley	Mosquitoes (Culex, Aedes)	Sheep, cattle, camels	East Africa	+
Reoviridae				
Coltivirus				
Colorado tick fever	Ticks (Dermacentor)	Small mammals	Rocky Mountain area	+

[a]++++, over 10,000 cases/year; –, common outbreaks of >100 cases/year; ++, irregular outbreaks +, rare occurrences.
[b]Formerly group A arboviruses.
[c]Formerly group B arboviruses.
[d]Formerly Russian spring–summer encephalitis
[e]Several other Bunyaviridae (Arbia and Toseana viruses of genus Phlebotovirus; Erve virus of genus Nairovirus), and Reoviridae (Lipovnik and Tribec viruses of genus Orbivirus; Eyach of genus Coltivirus) and single tick-borne members of Bunyaviridae (Bhyanjavirus) and Orthomyxoviridae (Thogotobirus) have been tentatively associated with CNS disease in Europe, Asia, and Africa (Dobler, 1996).
Modified from Johnson, 1990.

There are over 400 arboviruses, including the alphavirus group of Togaviridae, the *Flavivirus* genus of Flaviviridae, most Bunyaviridae, and the coltivirus genus of Reoviridae. Four major clinical syndromes have been associated with human arbovirus infections: (a) encephalitis, caused by over 20 agents (Table 5.5); (b) yellow fever caused by a single flavivirus that has both jungle and urban cycles that cause endemic and epidemic disease, respectively; (c) hemorrhagic fevers; and (d) undifferentiated tropical fevers. The arboviral encephalitides show different epidemiologic patterns, disease incidences, ratios of inapparent to clinical infections, age effects, and severity (Table 5.6). Following a discussion of the infection in arthropods, the major arboviral encephalitides of humans are reviewed, beginning with those in North America.

Arthropod Infection

A susceptible female arthropod is infected by ingestion of blood with a critical concentration of virus; the virus must penetrate the gut and eventually infect

TABLE 5.6. *Examples of Arboviral encephalitis with different epidemiological patterns and varying severity of human disease.*

Epidemiological pattern Virus	Number of cases per year	Inapparent/ Apparent infection	Mortality rates	Sequelae
Annual epidemic disease				
Japanese encephalitis	>20,000	1,000:1 As high as 50:1 (adults)	20%–30% 50% >50 years	30%
Annual endemic disease				
Tickborne encephalitis	>2,000	>30:1	Russia 20% Europe <5%	30%–60%
California	±100	26:1 under age 15	<1%	Mild
Annual endemic/ intermittent epidemic disease				
St. Louis encephalitis	Interepidemic years <50 Epidemic years up to 2,000	19:1–470:1	8% Young 2% Elderly >20%	30%–50% mild <10% severe
Western	Interepidemic years <50 Epidemic years up to 1,000	1,000:1	10%–20% <1 year < 3% adults	55% age <1month 5% adults
Eastern	Interepidemic < 5 Outbreaks 6–40	20:1	50%–80%	70% of young
Intermittent epidemic disease				
Murray Valley	Interepidemic 0 Outbreaks 12–60	800:1	20%	40%

Modified from Johnson, 1990.

the arthropod's salivary glands. The time from the blood meal to the salivary gland is called the extrinsic incubation period, and its duration is highly dependent on virus and host species and on ambient temperature. An increase in environmental temperature shortens the extrinsic incubation period, so high temperatures promote epidemics. Infection is noncytopathic in the arthropod, and it remains infected for life. Mosquitoes can be maintained in the laboratory for many months, but in its natural habitat life is perilous, with about a 10% mortality per day. This short survival of mosquitoes makes the extrinsic incubation period very critical in nature; in contrast, ticks have long survivals.

Studies of an alphavirus, eastern encephalitis virus in its natural host vector, *Culista melanura*, showed initial infection of the gut, with rapid dissemination via the hemolymph to all organs examined, except the ovarioles. The muscles showed the largest amount of virus antigen. All mosquitoes had disseminated infections by 3 days, and maximum amounts of virus were found on day 7 (Scott et al., 1984).

In contrast, studies of a flavivirus, Japanese encephalitis virus, inoculated into its natural host vector, *Culex tritaeniorhynchus*, showed a prolonged and highly temperature-dependent extrinsic incubation period. Virus infected the phagocytic hemolymph cells within 2 days, but intervening muscle fibers never showed antigen. By days 3 to 5, cells of the nervous system were infected, with consistent infection of all retinula cells in the compound eyes and patchy involvement of neural cells in the cephalic, thoracic, and abdominal ganglia. This neural infection preceded involvement of salivary gland by several days, and when temperature was lowered from 32° to 26°C, the nervous system infection preceded the salivary gland infection by 2 weeks. Whether nervous system infection is a prerequisite for salivary gland infection, as in rabies virus infections, remains unknown (Leake and Johnson, 1987).

Japanese encephalitis virus proved to be not only neurotropic in the mosquito, but also highly selective in which neurons it infected. The neurons of the compound eyes were consistently infected, and no neurons were infected in Johnston's organs, which lie at the base of the antennae and form the auditory organs and probable synaptic sites of the chemoreceptors on the antennae (Leake and Johnson, 1987). Despite the noncytopathic nature of this infection, this selectivity may have functional significance, because mosquito-trapping studies in Thailand yielded a higher ratio of infected mosquitoes in light traps baited with CO_2 than in traps without CO_2. This raises the intriguing possibility that noncytopathic infection of specific neuronal populations may modify behavior, enhancing transmission to CO_2-emitting targets such as humans. Increased probing behavior of biting mosquitoes infected with La Crosse virus suggests a similar viral effect to facilitate transmission to vertebrate hosts (Grimstad et al., 1980).

In tropical areas, virus transmission may occur throughout the year, but how arboviruses persist after the first frost in temperate zones has been a mystery. Persistence in ticks or mites that overwinter has been suggested. Overwintering of the occasional female mosquito after a blood meal has been postulated, but normally only nulliparous mosquitoes hibernate. Transovarian transmission occurs with bunyaviruses and may occur in flaviviruses (Rosen, 1987) and alphaviruses (Fulhorst et al., 1994).

Eastern Encephalitis Virus

Eastern encephalitis virus is found in the eastern half of the United States primarily along the freshwater marshes of the Atlantic and Gulf coasts, on Caribbean islands, and on the Atlantic Coast of Central and South America to Argentina (Scott and Weaver, 1989). Human infections are rare, particularly with South American strains of virus. This rarity of human disease is explained, in large part, by the epornitic cycle of the virus (Fig. 5.2). In most areas, the virus

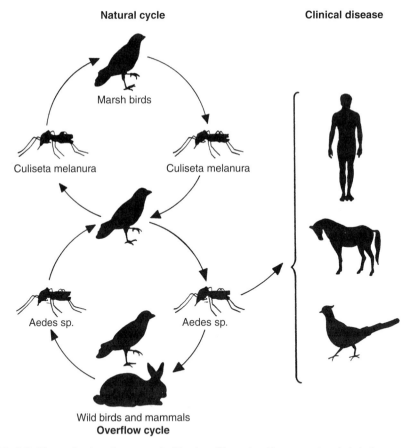

FIG. 5.2. The cycle of eastern encephalitis virus. The natural inapparent cycle is between small birds and *Culiseta melanura*, a swamp-marsh mosquito that does not bite large birds or mammals. Overflow of the cycle into various species of *Aedes* mosquitoes can amplify the virus into other wild birds and mammals, and *Aedes* species may bite humans, horses, and pheasants that can develop clinical encephalitis.

is transmitted between marsh birds and *Culiseta melanura* mosquitoes, which do not feed on large vertebrates. With alterations in the conditions of the marshes, changes in rainfall, different bird populations, and variations in mosquito breeding, the virus can spill over into other mosquito vectors that feed on mammals. Human outbreaks usually are heralded by deaths among pheasants and horses. Penned exotic birds, such as pheasants, can spread virus directly by pecking and cannibalism, shortcutting the arthropod cycle. Horses, which are particularly important sentinel animals in warning of impending human outbreaks, are, like humans, dead-end hosts for the virus. Therefore, the traditional term eastern equine encephalitis is a misnomer unfairly implying an equine guilt for human disease and leading to ill-conceived public health decisions, such as the proposed closure of pari-mutuel racing in New Jersey during the 1957 epidemic.

When human infection occurs, the ratio of inapparent infections to apparent infections is remarkably low. In children, the ratio is estimated to be from 2:1 to 8:1; in adults, from 4:1 to 50:1. The disease tends to be fulminant, characterized by the usual signs of encephalitis, but often with death during the first 2 to 5 days of disease. Periorbital edema has been described during the acute disease. Of patients with clinical encephalitis, 36% die and 35% of survivors are moderately or severely disabled (Deresiewicz et al., 1997). Age is not a major factor in mortality, but severe sequelae are more pronounced in children younger than 10 years of age (Feemster, 1957). Five of nine patients died in the 1989 outbreak, and only one of the four survivors was free of serious neurologic sequelae (Letson et al., 1993). Neuropathologic changes include meningeal and perivascular inflammatory reactions, neuronophagia, and microglial clusters in the parenchyma of brain and spinal cord. The neuropathologic findings are the same in fatal infections with western and St. Louis encephalitis viruses.

Eastern encephalitis virus has the highest rates of clinical infections and the highest mortality rates of the major arboviruses, but, fortunately, because of its natural cycle, it has been a rare infection of humans (Table 5.5). Therefore, the recovery of eastern encephalitis virus from *Aedes albopictus* mosquitoes in Florida in 1991 has raised major concerns (Mitchell et al., 1992). This mosquito, also known as the Asian Tiger mosquito, was imported into Houston, Texas, in 1985 in a shipment of used tires (Francy et al., 1990) and has since become established in wide areas of the United States, extending as far north as Chicago. The mosquito is an aggressive biter of humans, thrives in suburban as well as forest habitats, and could become a treacherous host for the eastern encephalitis virus.

Western Encephalitis Virus

Western encephalitis virus has been found over most of the United States, but human infections are limited to the western two-thirds of the country, where the natural cycle is between *Culex tarsalis* mosquitoes and small birds, such as finches and sparrows (Fig. 5.3). In California, an additional transmission cycle involves the blacktail jackrabbit and *Aedes melanimon* (Hardy, 1987). Both of

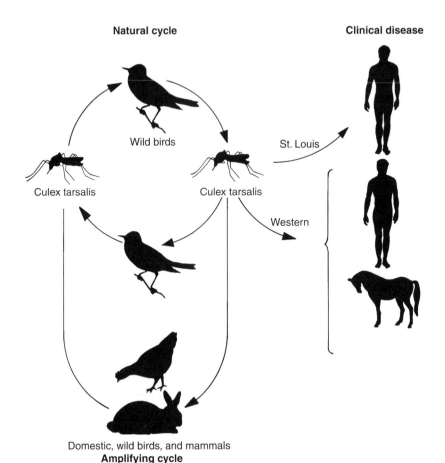

FIG. 5.3. The sylvatic cycles of western and St. Louis encephalitis viruses. The natural inap-parent cycle is between *Culex tarsalis* and nestling and juvenile birds, but this cycle may be amplified by infection of domestic birds and wild and domestic mammals. Western encephalitis virus can replicate in mosquitoes at cooler temperatures, so epidemic disease in horses and humans may occur earlier in the summer and farther north into Canada. St. Louis encephalitis virus in the eastern Untied States involves *Culex pipiens* and other urban mosquitoes and causes urban epidemics.

these mosquitoes readily feed on large vertebrates, so human or equine cases occur. The number of cases depends on rainfall, because mosquito breeding is largely in ground pools. In the San Joaquin Valley of California, disease inci-dence has been correlated with irrigation practices. Since 1987, there has been a dramatic decrease in the number of reported human cases, and this decline remains unexplained (CDC, 1994). The virus is found also in mosquitoes and birds on the East Coast and in Florida, but primarily in Culiseta mosquitoes that do not feed on humans.

The ratio of inapparent to apparent clinical infections is estimated at 50:1 to 8:1 in children and over 1,000:1 in adults. The encephalitis can be clinically severe but is rarely fatal. Sequelae are seen primarily in children younger than 2 years of age (Earnest et al., 1971) and include retardation, seizures, and spasticity. These children may appear to have progressive encephalitis, but longitudinal clinical studies clearly indicate that the apparent progression represents the failure of the maturing impaired child to meet developmental milestones (Finley et al., 1967).

St. Louis Encephalitis Virus

Geographically, St. Louis encephalitis virus is the most widespread arbovirus in the United States and the commonest cause of epidemic viral encephalitis. The virus is transmitted in three distinct cycles, all involving passerine birds, such as the house sparrow. In the western areas of the United States, its cycle is the same as that for western encephalitis virus and involves *C. tarsalis* mosquitoes (Fig. 5.3). In the Mississippi Valley, the urban Midwest, and rarely extending to the Mid-Atlantic area, the virus is found in other culicine mosquitoes that breed in urban environments where there is stagnant water with high organic content, particularly poorly draining sewage. Paradoxically, urban St. Louis encephalitis epidemics occur in drought years because of poor drainage, whereas rural St. Louis encephalitis outbreaks occur in years with high rainfall (Shope, 1980). In Florida, a rural cycle involves *Culex nigripalpus*, and cases of human encephalitis occur into early December.

In 1975, a record epidemic of St. Louis encephalitis spread up through the Midwest, extending over 31 states from Arizona to New York, Maryland, North Carolina, and Georgia and into Canada. Almost 2,000 laboratory-documented cases were reported, with 171 deaths, including over 500 cases with 47 deaths in Illinois, the hardest hit state (Creech, 1977). Since then, increased state and local surveillance has monitored viral transmission in enzootic cycles; these measures anticipated subsequent outbreaks in Houston and Florida but failed in more focal outbreaks (CDC, 1991c).

The ratio of inapparent to apparent infections is in the range of 60:1, but in striking contrast to the situation with eastern and western encephalitis viruses, the attack rate and the case fatality rate are greater among the elderly (Monath and Tsai, 1987; Tsai et al., 1988). Furthermore, in most urban epidemics, infection and disease are more frequent in the lower socioeconomic groups, presumably because of proximity to stagnant water, inadequate screening, absence of air conditioning, and crowding. The Chicago epidemic of 1975, however, was most intense in middle-class suburban areas.

Some patients with the St. Louis encephalitis virus develop benign aseptic meningitis, but when clinical disease occurs, encephalitis is three times more common. Several clinical features of St. Louis encephalitis are unusual. A prodrome of urinary symptoms, with pyuria and dysuria occurs in some patients, and the encephalitis is sometimes associated with opsoclonus and myoclonus.

Inappropriate secretion of antidiuretic hormone is found in as many as 25% of the patients (Southern et al., 1969), and unusual brainstem findings, with oculomotor paralysis, have been described (Kaplan and Koveleski, 1968).

The fatality rate is approximately 5% to 10%, but most of the survivors recover completely. However, prolonged neurasthenia, emotional instability, and resting and intention tremors are observed in elderly survivors (Lawton et al., 1966).

California Encephalitis Viruses

The California serogroup of bunyaviruses represent a large family of viruses, several of which have been related to human encephalitis (Table 5.5). The original California virus was isolated and first associated with mild encephalitis in California; the La Crosse strain of the California serogroup, which causes more severe disease in the Midwest, now represents the commonest endemic arboviral encephalitis in the United States (Fig. 5.4).

In 1960, the La Crosse virus was recovered from a child with fatal encephalitis in Wisconsin (Thompson et al., 1965). This virus has subsequently been related to many cases of mild to severe encephalitis in children in 23 states, with 90% of cases in six Midwestern states: Ohio, Wisconsin, Minnesota, Illinois, Indiana, and Iowa (Fig. 5.4). In recent years, about 80 cases per year have been reported, but because of the sporadic and widespread nature of infections, underreporting certainly occurs. The La Crosse virus appears more neurovirulent than the virus originally isolated in California or those found in other areas of the world.

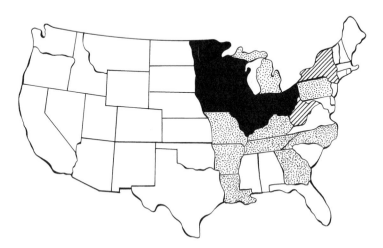

FIG. 5.4. The geographic distribution of California encephalitis due to the La Crosse strain of virus. The states that reported more than 100 cases between 1964 and 1991 are *heavily shaded*, the *lined* states reported 50 to 99 cases, the *stippled* states reported 5 to 49 cases, and the *clear* states reported 4 or fewer cases. (Data from Centers for Disease Control and Prevention reports.)

Unlike eastern, western, and St. Louis encephalitis, the transmission cycles of the California viruses do not involve avian reservoirs. Even experimentally, birds cannot be infected. The natural mosquito host of the La Crosse virus is *Aedes triseriatus*, a tree-hole mosquito of woodlands, and the natural cycle involves small woodland mammals, including chipmunks, squirrels, and rabbits (Fig. 5.5). The infection is apparently amplified by a venereal cycle: following transovarian infection, the infected male can infect the hematophagous female, which can then transmit to vertebrates and transmit virus to male and female progeny (Thompson and Beaty, 1977). The mosquito has a limited flight range, and humans are

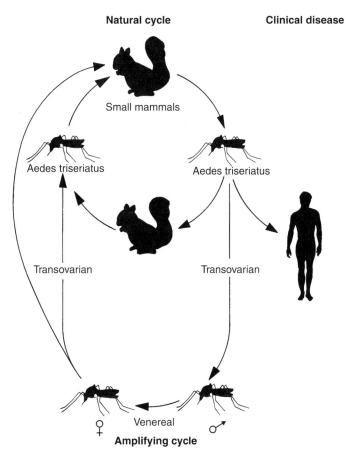

FIG. 5.5. The cycle of La Crosse encephalitis virus. The inapparent cycle of the La Crosse virus is between *Aedes triseriatus*, a woodland mosquito, and chipmunks and tree squirrels. The virus is maintained over winters by transovarian transmission and is amplified by venereal transmission between the infected male nonbiting mosquito and the uninfected female, which can in turn transmit either by biting or by transovarian transmission to the next generation. Humans are the only known hosts to develop clinical disease and are dead-end hosts for the virus.

bitten when they go into the woods or when old tires are left in yards providing "synthetic tree holes." Forestry workers have a high frequency of antibody, and children with the disease often have a history of outings in the woods.

The acute CNS infection in children can range from a benign aseptic meningitis to severe forms of encephalitis (Johnson et al., 1968a); fatalities occur in fewer than 1% of these children. Boys are affected twice as frequently as girls. Sequelae, consisting primarily of behavioral changes, irritability, inattentiveness, and associated abnormalities on electroencephalogram, have been found in approximately 15% of the patients. Severity of sequelae correlates directly with the severity of the initial encephalitis (Balfour et al., 1973).

Several other California serogroup viruses have been related to encephalitis. In 1980, a child with severe encephalitis in Michigan had evidence of infection with the Jamestown Canyon virus, a virus whose major vertebrate host is deer (Grimstad et al., 1982). Subsequent cases of Jamestown Canyon virus encephalitis have been reported in the Midwest, New York State, and Canada, and, interestingly, the mean age of patients has been 35 years, a striking contrast to La Crosse virus encephalitis, where the mean age is 7 to 8 years (LeDuc, 1987). Snowshoe hare virus in the northern United States, Canada, and Eastern Russia; Tahyna virus in Eastern Europe; and Inkoo virus in Finland and Russia have also been associated with mild encephalitis. A single case of life-threatening Cache Valley virus encephalitis has occurred in a young adult in North Carolina (Sexton et al., 1997).

Venezuelan Equine Encephalitis Virus

Venezuelan equine encephalitis occurs in both endemic and epidemic forms, and mosquitoes of both the *Aedes* and *Culex* genera are involved. For many years, the endemic form has been recognized in Central America and in Florida. In the Florida Everglades, the virus is cycled between swamp mosquitoes and small rodents, and humans can be infected when entering these swamps. Indeed, 50% of Indians in these areas of southern Florida have antibodies. Clinical cases of encephalitis are rare, and all patients in Florida have recovered without sequelae (Ehrenkranz and Ventura, 1974).

The epidemic form of disease was first recognized in South America, where major epidemics periodically recur (Weaver et al., 1996). Over the 1950s and 1960s, epidemics spread northward through Central America and Mexico. The first incursion across the Rio Grande occurred in 1971, when an epidemic led to the death of over 100 horses and to over 100 nonfatal human cases in the southwestern United States. The epidemic disease involves a cycle between a variety of mosquitoes and horses; in this instance, the horse is culpable, and immunization of horses can control epidemics.

The clinical disease in humans resembles influenza, with fever lasting for only 1 to 4 days. Occasionally, shock and coma are associated with widespread destruction of lymphoid tissues. Encephalitis develops in 3% of clinical cases, it is more severe in children, and 75% of all fatal cases have involved children under 5 years of age. During the Texas epidemic in 1971, two cases of children with encephalitis were reported. Both children survived, but one had severe sequelae (Ehrenkranz and Ventura, 1974).

Tick-borne Encephalitis Viruses

The tick-borne encephalitis viruses of the flavivirus family represent a number of antigenically related agents that infest tick populations throughout the northern-latitude woodlands of the world. The distribution of those viruses is from Siberia across to Scandinavia, through the Vienna Woods and Black Forest of Europe into Belgium, to Scotland and Northern Ireland, across forested Canada, dipping into some northern areas of the United States, and into Japan. Most of these tick-borne viruses have been associated with human disease, but there is a gradation of virulence. The Far Eastern (Siberian) strains (formerly called Russian spring–summer encephalitis virus) cause severe encephalitis, often with bulbar and cervical cord involvement, a high fatality rate, and frequent sequelae. In Scandinavia and Central Europe, the disease is frequently biphasic, with an influenza-like illness followed by defervescence and then recrudescence of fever and signs of encephalitis (Holmgren and Forsgren, 1990; Günther et al., 1997). The strains of virus found in Scotland and Northern England cause a sheep disease called louping-ill, so named because of a characteristic cerebellar ataxia. Human infections with louping-ill virus are rare and have primarily involved laboratory workers, shepherds, or abattoir workers. Infection has been associated with mild encephalitis and occasionally flaccid paralysis (Brewis et al., 1949; Davidson et al., 1991). Paralytic disease resembling paralytic poliomyelitis (Likar and Dane, 1958) and an ascending myelitis (Grinschgl, 1955) has also been associated with Western European strains. A virus of the tick-borne complex was isolated in Japan from the brains of two patients dying of acute encephalitis in 1948, but antibody to this virus, Negishi virus, has not been found in humans or birds, and the virus has not been related to subsequent cases of encephalitis (Okuno et al., 1961).

A virus of the tick-borne encephalitis complex was first discovered in North America in 1959 (McLean and Donohue, 1959). The virus was recovered from the brain of a 7-year-old boy who died of encephalitis after a tick bite while vacationing near Powassan, Ontario. Subsequently, Powassan virus has been found in mammals and birds across Canada and the northern parts of the United States; 24 human cases have been recorded in North America since 1959, and 11 have been in the United States (CDC, 1995a). Infections are usually not fatal (Shope, 1980).

A remarkable twist occurred in the geographic distribution of tick-borne encephalitis viruses in 1957, when monkey deaths were noted in the Kyasanur Forest in Mysore State in India. Initially, there was fear that yellow fever virus had invaded the Indian subcontinent, but the virus recovered was identified as a variant of Russian spring–summer encephalitis virus. The vector was shown to be a tick, but the lack of prior monkey deaths suggested that the virus was a newly introduced agent, possibly carried by ticks on birds crossing the Himalayas into the Indian subcontinent. Human infections with the Kyasanur Forest disease virus usually result in an influenza-like illness with fever, headache, severe myalgia, and often hemorrhagic complications. As in tick-borne encephalitis in Europe, disease may be biphasic and, as long as 3 to 4 weeks after the initial illness, there is a recrudescence of fever with confusion, headache, tremor, abnormal reflexes, and a spinal fluid pleocytosis (Webb and Rao, 1961).

Colorado Tick Fever Virus

Colorado tick fever virus, which is an orbivirus transmitted by *Dermacentor andersoni*, is confined to the geographic distribution of the tick in the Rocky Mountains and causes a common infection in hikers and foresters during May and June. A febrile illness develops, with headache and myalgias, 3 to 6 days after the tick bite. A macular papular rash is seen in about 50% of patients.

In general, Colorado tick fever is a benign disease, but in very rare cases a bleeding diathesis may develop, and fatalities have been reported. About 18% of patients develop nuchal rigidity, and a pleocytosis may be found. Stupor, coma, delirium, and convulsions are rare, and only one patient with a long-term sequela has been reported (Spruance and Bailey, 1973; Goodpasture et al., 1978).

Japanese Encephalitis Virus

Japanese encephalitis virus has the widest geographic distribution of any single arbovirus serotype and causes more neurologic morbidity and mortality than all of the other arboviruses combined (Table 5.6). It is a flavivirus closely related to St. Louis encephalitis virus. Major epidemics of encephalitis have been recorded in Japan since the 1870s, and the virus was isolated there in 1934 (Okuno, 1978). The original designation as Japanese B encephalitis virus was intended to distinguish it from the cause of encephalitis A or von Economo disease, an encephalitis whose causative agent has never been recovered. The virus was associated with epidemic disease in Japan, Korea, Taiwan, and other temperate areas of Asia. In recent years, the disease in Japan has been controlled by immunization and changed agricultural practices, but over the past two decades, epidemic disease has spread into new areas. The disease is prevalent in all but three provinces of China, with more than 10,000 cases annually, the epidemics in Thailand appear to be spreading further south, endemic disease in Sri Lanka has become epidemic, and the disease has appeared for the first time in many areas of India and onto the Nepalese plateau (CDC, 1984). The virus habitat extends from maritime Siberia, to Indonesia, and west to Pakistan.

The natural cycle of virus is between herons and other water birds and culicine mosquitoes that breed in rice fields, particularly *C. tritaeniorhynchus*. Pigs and young water buffalo are important amplifying hosts, whereas mature immune buffalo provide a blocking host (Fig. 5.6).

In epidemic areas, encephalitis is primarily a childhood disease, because almost all adults have antibody. Movement or travel of adults into epidemic areas shows that adults are fully susceptible to disease (Johnson et al., 1986). Viral meningitis is rare; in 1 of 1,000 persons, when virus does invade the nervous system, severe encephalitis is the rule. The course is fulminant, with rapid depression of consciousness. More intense involvement of the basal ganglia, thalamus, brainstem, and cervical spinal cord often leads to coarse tremors, sudden cardiorespiratory failure, and flaccid paralysis in the upper extremities (Johnson et al., 1985). Death occurs in 20% to 35%, usually within the first week of disease

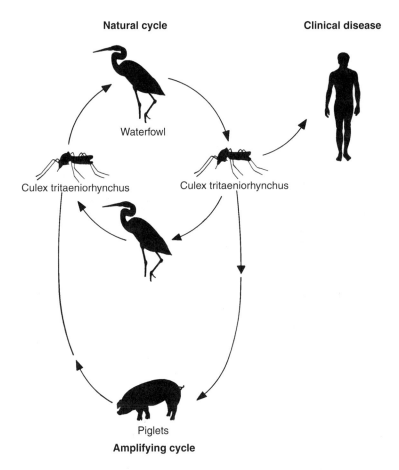

FIG. 5.6. The cycle of Japanese encephalitis virus. The natural cycle is between water birds and mosquitoes, predominantly *Culex tritaeniorhynchus*. Amplification occurs in piglets and juvenile water buffalo, but older buffalo are blocking hosts. Humans are dead-end hosts.

(Burke et al., 1985; Hoke et al., 1992); sequelae, including mental defects, paralysis and dystonia, and movement disorders, occur in about 30%.

Recently, rare recurrences of disease have been reported months after recovery, and virus has been recovered from blood (Sharma et al., 1991) and spinal fluid months after the acute illness (Ravi et al., 1993). This suggests that Japanese encephalitis virus, similar to tick-borne viruses, may have the potential to persist in the CNS.

Effective vaccine is available for Asian children and for travelers to rural Asia during the epidemic season (Hoke et al., 1988; CDC, 1993a).

Other Mosquito-borne Arboviral Encephalitides

Murray Valley encephalitis posed an intriguing mystery for many years, with long periods of disappearance and then reappearance in Southern Australia. In 1917 and 1918, an epidemic of severe encephalitis with a case fatality rate of 70% occurred in New South Wales; the disease was called Australian X disease. In 1922 and 1925, small numbers of encephalitis patients were seen in Queensland and New South Wales, but not until 1951 did another major epidemic of encephalitis occur along the Murray–Darling River Basin of New South Wales. During this epidemic, the Murray Valley encephalitis virus was recovered. This virus is now recognized as an endemic agent in the tropical but relatively unpopulated northern areas of Australia. During some years when the dry riverbeds and bilibongs of the Australian outback contain sufficient water to facilitate bird movement and to allow mosquitoes to breed, the virus can spread into the more heavily inhabited southeastern area of the country (Mackenzie et al., 1994). Encephalitis is seen more commonly in children but does not present features that differentiate it from other forms of encephalitis (Bennett, 1976).

Rocio virus caused an abrupt epidemic along the south coast of Brazil in 1975, with 400 cases of encephalitis and 61 deaths. Inexplicably, the virus has been quiescent since.

In the Middle East, West Nile virus infections have been associated with meningitis (Marberg et al., 1956), and in the 1950 outbreaks of West Nile virus infections in Israel, more severe encephalitis was seen. Among elderly patients with clinical infections, 25% to 50% suffered severe morbidity and some mortality. One young patient with rising antibody titers to West Nile virus had flaccid motor weakness resembling poliomyelitis (Gadoth et al., 1979). Rift Valley fever virus in Africa and Ilheus virus of northern South America also have been associated with encephalitis on rare occasions.

Dengue viruses are flaviviruses that cause widespread morbidity and mortality in the Americas, Africa, and Asia. The fever, rash, arthritis, and the hemorrhagic shock syndrome of dengue notably exclude the nervous system. Neurologic signs occasionally accompany dengue hemorrhagic fever, but they have been assumed to be due to hemorrhage. The spinal fluid is acellular and lacks virus specific IgM found in infections with neurotropic flaviviruses, and neuropathologic studies even in fatal cases show no neuronophagia, perivascular infiltrates, or gliosis

(Bhamarapravati et al., 1967). Nevertheless, in rare cases, children have been reported with clinical signs and laboratory findings suggesting CNS invasion (Lum et al., 1996), so, under unusual and inexplicable circumstances, dengue virus may show neuroinvasive, neurotropic, or neurovirulent properties.

DIFFERENTIAL DIAGNOSIS

The first obligation of a physician dealing with a suspected acute viral infection of the nervous system is to differentiate herpes simplex encephalitis, because of the necessity to institute specific therapy (see Chapter 6), and to rule out nonviral causes that may require other therapies. Although a definitive etiologic diagnosis in viral meningitis or encephalitis must rest on the laboratory, in most patients clues can be obtained from community epidemiologic data, clinical history of immunization, exposures to animals, travel, and family health or physical findings to enable an educated guess that can guide laboratory studies (Table 5.2).

Traditionally, laboratory diagnosis depends on isolation of virus from clinical specimens and demonstration of a significant increase in antibody in serum specimens obtained in the acute and convalescent phases of disease (Table 5.7).

TABLE 5.7. *Specimens for conventional diagnosis of acute CNS infections*

Virus	Specimens for virus isolation					Sera acute and convalescent
	Throat washings	Stool	Spinal fluid	Blood	Other	
Enteroviruses						
Polioviruses	+	+++	–	–		+
Coxsackie viruses and echoviruses	+	+++	+++	–		+
Mumps virus	+++	–	++	–	Saliva, urine	+
Adenovirus	+++[a]	+	+	–		+
Lymphocytic choriomeningitis virus	–	–	+++	+		+ and 2–3 month convalescent
Arthropod-borne viruses	–	–	+	++		+
Herpesviruses						
Herpes simplex virus						
type 1	+[a]	–	–	–	Brain	+[a]
type 2	–	–	+	+	Vesicular fluid	+[a]
Herpes zoster virus	–	–	+	–	Vesicular fluid	+[a]
Epstein–Barr virus	+[a]	–	–	+[a]		+[a]
Cytomegalovirus	–	–	–	+[a]	Urine[a]	+[a]
Rabies virus	–	–	+	–	Saliva, brain	+

[a]Isolations or antibody responses may represent nonspecific activation.
From Jackson and Johnson, 1989.

Alternatively, diagnosis is possible by recovery of virus from biopsy or autopsy tissues. Recovery of virus from brain or spinal fluid provides greater assurance that the virus is directly related to disease. Although polioviruses, herpes simplex virus (type 1), and arboviruses are usually not recoverable from spinal fluid, coxsackieviruses and echoviruses may be more readily isolated from spinal fluid obtained early in disease than from throat washings or stool specimens (Johnson et al., 1960a).

Recognition of viral DNA or RNA by PCR in serum, spinal fluid, or brain has been used in many infections (Darnell, 1993), but these tests are not readily available, except for herpesviruses. Detection of virus-specific IgM by antibody-capture enzyme-linked immunosorbent assay in serum has been used for rapid diagnosis of enterovirus and arbovirus infections (Monath et al., 1984; Calisher et al., 1986; Day et al., 1989); in Japanese encephalitis, over 90% of patients are positive for virus-specific IgM in spinal fluid on arrival at the hospital (Burke et al., 1982).

Many nonviral infectious diseases can present with fever, headache, nuchal rigidity, and a predominantly mononuclear cell pleocytosis (Table 5.8). Particu-

TABLE 5.8. *Infectious diseases that can masquerade as viral CNS infections.*

Rickettsia	Rocky Mountain spotted fever
	Typhus
	Q fever
Bacteria	Spirochetes
	Syphilis (secondary of meningovascular)
	Leptospirosis
	Borrelia burgdorferi (Lyme disease)
	Mycoplasma pneumoniae infection
	Cat scratch fever
	Listeriosis
	Brucellosis (particularly *B. melitensis*)
	Tuberculosis
	Typhoid fever
	Whipple disease
	Parameningeal infections (epidural, petrositis)
	Partially treated bacterial meningitis
	Subacute bacterial endocarditis
	Brain abscess
Fungi	Cryptococcosis
	Coccidiodomycosis
	Histoplasmosis
	North American blastomycosis
	Candidiasis
Parasites	Toxoplasmosis
	Cysticercosis
	Echinococcosis
	Trichinosis
	Trypanosomiasis
	Plasmodium falciparum infection
	Amoebiasis (*Nagleria* and *Acanthamoeba*)

lar vigilance must be maintained in immunocompromised patients predisposed to unusual bacterial, fungal, and parasitic infections of the CNS. In infections such as tuberculosis and brucellosis, and in fungal infections, the disease process is chronic, and the subsequent progressive rise in protein and decline in sugar in the spinal fluid may clarify initial confusion with acute viral disease. Some fulminant infections, such as those produced by free-swimming amoeba, may resemble acute viral encephalitis, but polymorphonuclear cells usually predominate in the spinal fluid. *Brucella melitensis* infection can present as acute viral meningitis, encephalitis, transverse myelitis, or radiculitis mimicking viral disease (Al-Deeb et al., 1988).

A variety of noninfectious diseases must also be considered in patients with signs of meningitis and encephalitis and a pleocytosis. Carcinomatous meningitis, gliomatosis cerebri, granulomatous angiitis, sarcoidosis, systemic lupus erythematosus, rheumatoid meningitis, rupture of cysts into the subarachnoid space, drug-induced meningitis, Behçet's disease, and oculocephalic syndromes must be considered (see Chapter 10).

Several infectious diseases clinically masquerade so successfully as viral meningitis and encephalitis that they are often differentiated only by serologic studies. As shown in the studies discussed earlier in this chapter (Table 5.1), this is true of rickettsia, such as Rocky Mountain spotted fever, several spirochetes, *Mycoplasma pneumoniae*, and cat-scratch fever. Indeed, Lyme disease and cat-scratch fever were both discussed as putative viral illness in the prior edition of this book.

Rickettsial Infections

Like viruses, rickettsiae are obligatory intracellular parasites, but they contain some intrinsic energy systems and maintain cellular integrity during reproduction. The rickettsia that infect humans selectively infect the vascular endothelium of small vessels, and through this common pathogenesis cause rashes, hemorrhagic disorders, and neurologic disease. Nervous system complications are most severe in Rocky Mountain spotted fever, epidemic typhus, and scrub typhus, and findings are similar in each disease.

Rocky Mountain spotted fever is caused by *Rickettsia rickettsii*, which has a natural reservoir in wild animals and is spread to humans by ticks. Unlike Colorado tick fever, which is limited to the Rocky Mountain area, this rickettsia infects not only *Dermacentor andersoni*, the wood tick of the Rockies, but also *Dermacentor variabilis*, the common dog tick prevalent in the eastern half of the United States. Thus, despite its geographic name the disease is most frequent in the South-Atlantic and South-Central states, where the majority of human cases are now recognized. In some Mid-Atlantic areas, over 5% of ticks are infected. After increasing incidence in the early 1980s, the number of cases declined and has now plateaued with about 600 reported cases a year (CDC, 1993d). Almost all cases occur between April and September, when the ticks are feeding. The majority of cases occur in children, with a slightly higher incidence in males than females, presumably related to contact with household pets and outdoor activities.

The disease starts with fever, headache, and frequently gastrointestinal symptoms. The rash, the hallmark of the disease, develops 2 to 4 days after the fever, usually beginning on the wrists and ankles, spreading to the palms and soles and then centripetally. The rash is initially macular but often becomes purpuric (Kirk et al., 1990).

Neurologic complications occur in 60% of patients with Rocky Mountain spotted fever. In addition to intense headache, depression of the state of consciousness is common, although there may be delirium with hallucinations. Varied focal neurologic signs are seen, but fewer than 5% of patients have convulsions. Coma is an ominous sign, because it is almost invariably present in the fatal cases and, in surviving patients, coma correlates with sequelae. Behavioral and learning disorders are the major sequelae, and seizures and motor deficits are rare (Gorman et al., 1981). During the acute neurologic disease, the spinal fluid shows a paucity of abnormalities. Only about 20% to 50% of patients have a pleocytosis, and the protein is often normal. This is consistent with the neuropathologic findings of minimal meningeal inflammation. However, small vessels throughout the brain have swollen endothelia and are cuffed by lymphocytes. Vascular occlusions and microinfarcts are found primarily in white matter.

Diagnosis depends on the recognition of the characteristic rash and confirmation by serologic studies. Historically, up to 40% of patients with Rocky Mountain spotted fever died, but increasingly early recognition and the institution of therapy with tetracycline or chloramphenicol have produced a tenfold reduction in the fatality rate. Diagnosis has also been facilitated by the virtual eradication of measles, because confusion with measles or measles encephalitis commonly delayed appropriate therapy in the past. In rare instances of fulminant disease, coma and even death occur before the development of rash, and a late onset of rash frequently is associated with fatality. Therefore, in endemic areas such as ours, a low threshold of suspicion must be maintained during the spring and summer months.

A variety of other tick-borne typhuses occur throughout the world. All of these produce similar but less severe disease, with fewer neurologic complications and very few deaths (Shaked, 1991). Q fever is caused by *Coxiella burnetti*, a rickettsia common in animals worldwide, and spreads to humans by respiratory droplets. Symptomatic infection is usually a pneumonitis, but meningitis, meningoencephalitis, and myelitis have been reported on rare occasions (Ferrante and Dolon, 1993; Hwang et al., 1993; Sempere et al., 1993).

Spirochetal Infections

All three genera of spirochetal bacteria that infect humans can cause infections of the nervous system that resemble viral infections. Secondary syphilis can present as an acute aseptic meningitis with initial spirochetal invasion of the nervous system, and early tertiary syphilis—meningovascular syphilis—can simulate acute encephalitis with focal neurologic signs (Reik, 1987).

Leptospira

Leptospira are major causes of "viral" meningitis and mild encephalitis. Leptospiral infections are zoonoses, and many species infect rats, dogs, field mice, pigs, and cattle throughout the world. Leptospira are threadlike spirochetes with a thin external membrane that cannot tolerate either drying or salt water. They persist in animals only in the kidney, brain, and eye, and the chronic infection of the brush border of the proximal tubules of the kidney seeds the spirochetes into urine. Leptospiras can remain viable in fresh water for several months.

Human exposure can be either occupational or recreational. Sewer and abattoir workers, veterinarians, and farmers are exposed at their work, and rural residents are exposed by swimming and wading in ponds and creeks contaminated by the urine of dogs or livestock. With these modes of exposure, it is not surprising that over three-fourths of those with leptospirosis are males, predominantly teenagers and young adults. The disease occurs year round, with an increase during summer because of the greater recreational exposure (Heath et al., 1965; Martone and Kaufmann, 1979).

The three serotypes most frequently associated with neurologic disease in the United States are *L. icterohaemorrhagiae*, the species most often carried by rats and the cause of Weil's disease; *L. canicola*, carried primarily by dogs; and *L. pomona*, commonly found in pigs and cattle and the agent of swineherd's disease. The former two are cosmopolitan diseases because of the urban concentrations of sewer rats and dogs. The latter is localized to rural areas where pigs and cows may share bathing or drinking water with humans. Leptospiral infections account for nearly 10% of cases of "viral" aseptic meningitis and a small percentage of cases of mild encephalitis. In our study at Walter Reed Army Institute of Research, *L. pomona*, the species least likely to produce overt liver and kidney disease, was the strain most frequently implicated in CNS infections (Meyer et al., 1960).

The clinical disease is typically biphasic, with initial high fever, severe muscle pain, and frequent conjunctivitis. Five to 6 days later, specific organ involvement may present as jaundice, nephritis, or meningitis, any of which may be complicated by a hemorrhagic diathesis. The commonest of these is meningitis, which complicates 60% of cases and is twice as common as overt jaundice or renal disease. In patients with benign meningitis, the presence of mild abnormalities in liver function tests, proteinuria or pyuria, and neutrophilia may suggest the diagnosis to alert clinicians. The cerebrospinal fluid is typical of viral meningitis, although polymorphonuclear cells may predominate, and rarely a low sugar content is seen. Neurologic sequelae and fatalities are rare. A limited study of the pathologic findings in these infections has shown an inflammatory encephalitis similar to viral infections (Gsell, 1978).

In most cases, the meningitis is a benign self-limited disease, and specific diagnosis and treatment are not imperative. Penicillin therapy has not been proved to alter the course of the meningitis. However, meningitis may become indolent and may persist for several weeks, and possibly this can be aborted by antibiotic therapy.

Borrelia

In the summer of 1975, Lyme, Connecticut, suffered an outbreak of arthritis. Epidemiologic analysis implicated *Ixodes dammini* ticks, and clinical data showed a large percentage of patients had had an antecedent annular rash. In Europe, this tick-bite-related rash, erythema chronicum migrans, had been associated with neurologic disease known as lymphocytic meningoradiculitis or Bannwarth's syndrome (Reik, 1987). Lyme disease has spread and increased in incidence, so that Lyme now accounts for the majority of arthropod-borne diseases in the United States and over 12,000 cases per year (Barbour and Fish, 1993). It has now been reported in all 48 contiguous states, with major foci in the Northeast and Central Atlantic coastal area, California, and Wisconsin and neighboring states. Although initially assumed to be a viral disease (Johnson, 1982), a spirochete, *Borrelia burgdorferi*, has been shown to be the causative agent (Burgdorfer et al., 1982; Steere et al., 1983).

At the site of the tick bite, a red macule develops after 2 to 20 days. Low-grade fever, malaise, headache, and gastrointestinal symptoms are common at this time. As the erythematous lesion enlarges, central clearing gives an annular appearance. Approximately half of the patients have more than one skin lesion. At the time of the rash or 1 to 6 weeks after its resolution, neurologic symptoms and signs appear in 10% of patients; 80% of these present with meningitis resembling viral meningitis (Reik, 1987). After intervals of up to 10 months, recurrent monoarthritis or polyarthritis develops in about 50% of patients, and 8% develop cardiac conduction abnormalities.

Subacute and chronic central and peripheral nervous system complications are common. Severe meningoencephalitis with multifocal signs, chorea, cerebellar ataxia, and myelitis are seen. Cranial nerve palsies are very frequent, particularly facial diplegia. Peripheral neuropathies may involve roots, plexuses, or individual peripheral nerves. The spinal fluid shows a mononuclear pleocytosis and moderate protein elevation. Chronic encephalopathy and an axonal polyneuropathy have been reported years after Lyme disease infection, with intrathecal antibody synthesis against the spirochete and, in some cases, improvement after antibiotic treatment (Logigian et al., 1990).

Mycoplasma Infections

Mycoplasma pneumoniae, the major cause of "viral" pneumonia, was long regarded as a virus, because it is a filterable agent that was originally propagated only in laboratory animals and embryonated eggs. It ultimately proved to be a bacteria lacking a cell wall. *Mycoplasma pneumoniae* has no known host other than humans and is spread by the respiratory route. The incubation period is approximately 2 weeks, but the agent can be harbored in the upper respiratory tract and transmitted for prolonged periods. Infections occur throughout the year, but are most frequent in winter and more frequent among schoolchildren and other closed populations. When the atypical pneumonia is associated with bullous myringitis, the etiologic diagnosis is relatively certain. Patients may develop cold agglutinins in blood, hemolytic anemia, myopericarditis, arthralgias, and a variety of rashes (Murray et al., 1975).

The commonest extrapulmonary complications of *M. pneumoniae* infections are neurologic. They occur more frequently in males than in females, in the young more than in the old, and in 1% to 5% of patients with clinical pneumonitis. Neurologic complications typically develop a week after the onset of respiratory disease, but they may occur concurrently or even precede respiratory symptoms. A remarkable variety of neurologic syndromes have been described, including meningitis, encephalitis, polyradiculitis (Guillain–Barré syndrome), cranial nerve palsies, acute cerebellar ataxia, and transverse myelitis (Koskiniemi, 1993; Thomas et al., 1993). Thus, this curious bacteria can cause almost the full gamut of neurologic complications associated with viruses.

The spinal fluid usually shows a pleocytosis, predominantly of lymphocytes, an elevation in protein, and a normal sugar—mimicking viral infection. The clinical course in most instances is benign, but among those patients with severe encephalitis the death rate approaches 15%, and sequelae, including mental retardation, seizures, cerebellar ataxia, and optic atrophy, are frequent (Ponka, 1980). The organism is sensitive to antibiotics, but their benefit in the neurologic diseases is uncertain.

The pathologic changes are varied. In most cases, cerebral edema is found, with perivascular inflammation. Changes in vessels are inconstant, but in some cases vascular occlusion leads to infarcts (Visudhiphan et al., 1992). There has been no recovery of the organism from brain, although there are seven reported recoveries from cerebrospinal fluid. Both the pathologic findings and the usual failure to isolate *Mycoplasma* from CNS tissue raise questions about the pathogenesis of the neurologic diseases.

Mycoplasma cause neurologic disease in two natural animal hosts: *M. gallisepticum* causes fatal cerebral arteritis in turkeys, and an exotoxin elaborated by *M. neurolyticum* causes "rolling disease" in mice and rats. In both diseases, capillary endothelial swelling with occlusion is prominent (Manuelides and Thomas, 1973).

Mycoplasma infections not only mimic many virus-associated neurologic illnesses but also pose many of the same questions of pathogenesis. Disease may represent direct invasion of the brain by the agent; a vascular infection may cause vasculitis similar to that seen in rickettsial infections and some viral infections; a bacterial toxin or protein may be important, as suggested by animal

Mycoplasma infections; or disease may be immune mediated, as suggested by the associated arthritis, autoimmune hemolytic anemia, and rashes.

Cat-Scratch Disease

Although long suspected of having a viral etiology, cat-scratch disease is a benign febrile adenitis that commonly develops after scratches or bites from apparently healthy, but usually immature, cats. *Bartonella henselae* has been shown to cause most cases (Bergmans et al., 1995); some have been associated with *B. quintana*, the cause of trench fever usually transmitted by lice. Transmission of *B. henselae* or *B. quintana* to humans by fleas has been suspected.

Over 22,000 cases occur each year in the United States. More than 50% of patients are under 18 years of age, and 90% have a history of cat exposure (Marra, 1995). Three to 14 days after the scratch, a red, raised papule develops at the site. A low-grade fever may develop with painful regional adenopathy that may be fluctuant and even appear to suppurate. The adenopathy may persist for several months, and complications include Parinaud's oculoglandular syndrome, erythema nodosum, thrombocytopenic purpura, and osteolytic lesions.

About 2% of the patients with cat-scratch fever develop a mild meningitis or encephalopathy days to weeks after the initial skin lesion. Neurologic complications begin abruptly with depressed consciousness or combative behavior, headaches, and occasionally seizures, paralysis, and ataxia (Carithers and Margileth, 1991). An acute hemiplegia with angiographic evidence of arteritis in the internal carotid artery has been described in one child (Selby and Walker, 1979). Neurologic signs and symptoms may persist for days or weeks, followed by full recovery, although one adult was reported with persistent dementia after infection (Revol et al., 1992). The spinal fluid may be acellular or show a mild pleocytosis, and the protein content is usually elevated.

Diagnosis traditionally has been dependent on the patient's history of cat exposure, the typical clinical course, and a positive skin test using antigen of sterilized pus from pooled lymph nodes. Lymph node biopsy can demonstrate typical histology. Serologic methods and PCR of serum and spinal fluid now are becoming available in the diagnosis of this disease transmitted by mankind's second-best friend.

SUPPLEMENTARY BIBLIOGRAPHY

Calisher CH, Thompson WH, eds. *California serogroup viruses.* New York: Alan R Liss, 1983.

Evans AR, Kaslow RA, eds. *Viral infections of humans,* 4th ed. New York: Plenum Publishing, 1997.

Monath, TP, ed. *St. Louis encephalitis.* Washington, DC: American Public Health Association, 1980.

Scott TW, Weaver SC. Eastern equine encephalomyelitis virus: epidemiology and evolution of mosquito transmission. *Adv Virus Res* 1989;37:277–328.

6

Herpesvirus Infections

In the not so remote biologic past, some thousands of years ago, neolithic man was living in small family groups of 30–60 persons upon the watersheds, prevented from frequent intercourse with his neighbours on the other watersheds by the forest and bogs of the intervening valleys. In such communities an outbreak of varicella would have used up all available susceptibles in a few weeks, and the causal viruses would have disappeared forever. Bartlett (1957) has shown that an aggregation of some 200,000 people is needed for continuous support of such a virus, and yet varicella shows all the marks of an ancient parasitism of man; we know of no alternative host, and it does not seem, like measles or variola, to be a recent mutant of an animal epizootic virus.

R. Edgar Hope-Simpson,
The Nature of Herpes Zoster: A Long-term Study and a New Hypothesis, Wander lecture to the Royal Society of Medicine, 1965

This riddle of virus survival in Neolithic man is solved by the phenomenon of latency. After the acute exanthem of varicella, 20 or 30 years may elapse before the reactivation of virus in the form of shingles. This reactivation can inaugurate a new epidemic of varicella within a new generation. Latency occurs with other DNA viruses and with retroviruses, but the latency and reactivation of herpesviruses are of particular relevance because they are related to an array of human diseases.

Most herpesviruses are restricted to their natural hosts. Of nearly 100 known herpesviruses of subhuman species, only B virus (herpes simiae or Cercopithecine herpesvirus 1) of macaque monkeys causes significant human disease. The eight human herpesviruses (herpes simplex viruses, types 1 and 2; varicella–zoster virus; Epstein–Barr virus; cytomegalovirus; and human herpesviruses 6, 7, and 8) are prevalent in all human populations. Initial infection may or may not be associated with disease. Seven of these viruses are capable of persisting for life, and primary or reactivated infection may cause significant acute neurologic diseases (Table 6.1). Type 1 herpes simplex virus, the cause of cold sores, is the commonest cause of nonepidemic fatal encephalitis. Type 2 herpes simplex virus, a common venereal disease agent, causes fatal encephalitis in newborns and recurrent meningitis in adults. Varicella–zoster virus causes both chickenpox with varied acute neurologic complications and shingles, an

133

TABLE 6.1. Diseases associated with human herpesviruses

Virus	Primary infection		Latency	Reactivated infection	
	Systemic	Neurologic		Systemic	Neurologic
Herpes simplex, type 1	Gingivostomatitis or pharyngitis	Childhood and adult encephalitis	0	Herpes labialis	Encephalitis
Herpes simplex, type 2	Herpes genitalis	Neonatal encephalitis,[a] adult meningitis	Cervical cancer (?)	Herpes genitalis	Recurrent meningitis and radiculitis
Varicella–zoster	Varicella	Parainfectious encephalomyelitis, Guillain–Barré syndrome, Reye's syndrome[b]	0	Herpes zoster	Radiculitis, myelitis, encephalitis
Epstein–Barr	Infectious mononucleosis	Encephalitis, Guillain–Barré syndrome[b]	Burkitt lymphoma, nasopharyngeal carcinoma(?), and B-cell lymphomas (?)	Recurrence only with immunodeficiency	?
Cytomegalovirus	Infectious mononucleosis	Fatal encephalitis,[a] Guillain–Barré syndrome[b]	0	Pneumonia, hepatitis, thrombocytopenia (immunosuppressed)	Encephalitis, Guillain–Barré syndrome (?)
Human herpesvirus 6	Exanthem subitum	Encephalitis	0	?	Encephalitis (?)
Human herpesvirus 7	Exanthem subitum	Meningitis or encephalitis	0	?	?

[a]Discussed in Chapter 13.
[b]Discussed in Chapter 8.

increasing problem with the aging population, with the increasing use of immunosuppressive drugs and with the emergence of AIDS. Epstein–Barr virus causes infectious mononucleosis and its neurologic complications, and it is the herpesvirus most convincingly linked to human neoplasms. Cytomegalovirus in the fetus is a major cause of mental retardation and sensorineural deficits; activation of this virus in immunosuppressed patients can cause fatal systemic disease with CNS involvement. Newly discovered human herpesvirus 6 causes exanthem subitum in children, occasionally with encephalitis, and has already been targeted as a possible cause of chronic fatigue syndrome (see Chapter 9) and multiple sclerosis (see Chapter 10). Human herpesvirus 7 probably holds a similar future.

Herpesviruses are large, highly complex viruses. The size of the herpesvirus DNA varies from 150 to 230 kb; herpes simplex virus DNA, one of the smallest, encodes for at least 77 genes. In the virion, the two strands of linear DNA are encased by a capsid of about 11-nm diameter comprising 162 capsomeres characteristic of all herpesviruses. Additional proteins form a variably sized tegmentum, which is enclosed by an envelope containing an array of viral glycoproteins, at least 11 in the case of herpes simplex viruses. Virions range in size from 120 to 300 nm.

After attachment to a host cell surface, the envelope fuses with the cytoplasmic membrane, and the nucleocapsid is transported to the nucleus, where the DNA is released and immediately circularized. DNA is replicated in the nucleus.

The first group of herpes simplex genes to be expressed are the "immediate early" or α genes, which are expressed prior to viral protein production, and several are essential to virus replication. The α genes activate the early or β genes, many of which encode enzymes involved in nucleotide metabolism; they then activate late or γ genes, which code for viral structural proteins. Capsid proteins are translated in the cytoplasm and transported to the nucleus, where the core or nucleocapsid is assembled. The envelope is added as the nucleocapsid moves through a modified portion of the nuclear membrane. Between the core and the envelope, matrix proteins are added, forming the tegmentum, but the amount of this tegmentum is variable between species of herpesviruses and even between virions of the same species. Virions are transported to the extracellular space through the Golgi. Thus, in electron-microscopic studies of infected cells, cores are found in the nucleus with or without tegmental coating, and mature virions in the cytoplasm are often of variable diameter. Productive infection is accompanied by host cell destruction (Fawl and Roizman, 1994).

Herpesvirus replication is inefficient: less than 10% of viral DNA is integrated into virions, and large excesses of proteins are produced, including nonstructural proteins. The excess of viral protein accounts for the characteristic inclusion bodies of herpesvirus infections. During the early phase of infection with herpes simplex virus, the bluish ground-glass nuclear inclusion contains many virus core particles. However, the classic Cowdry type A inclusion body, with marginated chromatin forming a halo, contains few, if any, particles.

An additional important property of herpesviruses is their ability to move from cell to cell by the fusion of cell membranes. This enables spread into cells that lack receptors for the virus and enables virus spread in the presence of antibody, a phenomenon of probable importance in the localization of herpes simplex virus encephalitis or the dermatomal restriction of zoster vesicles.

LATENCY

The term *latency* has been used in two ways. Virus persistence with continuous shedding of small amounts of virus has been referred to as dynamic latency (Roizman, 1965). However, latency usually implies persistence of the virus genome, without production of infectious particles, but from which reactivation can lead to a recrudescence of virus replication and disease. The viral or proviral DNA is sequestered in nonreplicating form. In this volume, the term *latency* is used to refer to this static form of latency.

The human herpesviruses establish latency in either neural cells (herpes simplex viruses and varicella–zoster virus) or hematopoietic cells (Epstein–Barr virus, cytomegalovirus, and herpesviruses 6 and 7). Unlike some DNA viruses and retroviruses that integrate viral DNA into the host cell genome, herpesvirus DNA is latent episomally in the nucleus in circular or concatemeric form. Multiple copies are usually present within the latently infected cell, and there is limited transcription from these latent viral genomes. Latent herpes simplex transcribes a limited region, varicella–zoster transcribes several separate regions of its genome, and Epstein–Barr not only transcribes long transcripts but translates multiple proteins in latently infected cells (Stevens, 1989). One nuclear protein in Epstein–Barr virus-infected lymphocytes appears essential to the maintenance of latency.

Induction of latency is largely host cell dependent rather than virus dependent. Herpes simplex virus type 1 latency can be established in dorsal root ganglion cells of mice without virus replication (Speck and Simmons, 1991); in mice, one cell population of ganglion cells is productively infected and destroyed, while another produces latency-associated transcripts and no detectable viral proteins (Margolis et al., 1992). These latency-associated transcripts do not belong to any of the three sets of viral gene classes expressed during virus replication in cell culture and they are, in part, antisense messages (Stevens et al., 1987). Their demonstration in human trigeminal ganglia (Croen et al., 1987) caused great interest, because they were thought to be critical to establishment or maintenance of latency. However, mutant virus lacking the appropriate coding areas can establish and maintain latency (Sedarati et al., 1989; Leib et al., 1989), but reactivation is delayed or inhibited (Steiner and Kennedy, 1993). Latency-associated transcripts may play other roles in reactivation, possibly by activating a neuronal inhibitory factor that prevents lytic infection or by being involved in transfer of the virus nucleic acid down the axon to the periphery, where replication can resume without irreparable damage of the neuron (Steiner and Kennedy, 1995).

A role for host immune responses in maintaining latency has long been suspected because of the clinical activation of herpesviruses in immunodeficient patients. Antibody responses as well as cytokines may be involved in maintaining latency as well as activation.

Reactivation is poorly understood but depends on the virus type and the site of infection. For example, genital infection with type 2 herpes simplex virus has a reactivation rate of 85% within 1 year of primary infection, whereas genital infection with type 1 virus has an activation rate of 55% within 1 year. Furthermore, oral infection with both types shows lower reactivation rates, but type 1 activates more frequently than type 2 (Lafferty et al., 1987). The comparative patterns of reactivation of herpes simplex and varicella–zoster viruses are even more striking. Herpes simplex virus reactivations are frequent, usually are localized to the cutaneous distribution of a single sensory root, do not cause great pain, and often decrease in frequency with age. Conversely, varicella–zoster virus activations rarely occur more than once, involve an entire dermatome, cause severe pain, and increase in frequency with age (Kennedy and Steiner, 1994).

HERPES SIMPLEX VIRUSES

Herpes simplex viruses include two closely related human viruses: types 1 and 2. These viruses are morphologically identical, have about 50% sequence identity, and share common antigens, making them difficult to differentiate serologically. Nevertheless, these two viruses have different modes of spread, present different epidemiologic patterns, and cause different neurologic diseases. B virus (Cercopithecine herpesvirus 1) is related to herpes simplex viruses and is a rare cause of human encephalitis and myelitis.

Although herpes simplex virus types 1 and 2 are natural infections only in humans, the viruses grow readily in a wide range of cultured cells from many species, in embryonated eggs, and in a variety of laboratory animals. Thus, of all the human herpesviruses, they have been most amenable to experimental studies.

Type 1 Herpes Simplex Virus

Epidemiology

Type 1 herpes simplex virus is a ubiquitous agent: half the population has antibody by age 15, and approximately 90% of adults show serologic evidence of infection. Despite its usual benign manifestations, the rare involvement of the CNS represents the commonest cause of nonepidemic fatal viral encephalitis. Approximately 2,000 cases occur each year in the United States: over half of those who are untreated die and many of the treated or untreated survivors suffer severe sequelae.

Type 1 virus is spread by salivary or respiratory contact. Primary infection usually is asymptomatic but can cause gingivostomatitis, pharyngitis, or respiratory disease. In some primary infections, fever, adenopathy, parotitis, and constitutional symptoms are present. In children with malnutrition or immunodeficiencies, the virus may disseminate with widespread cutaneous lesions. Primary infection usually occurs in the oropharynx, but epithelial surfaces may be involved, as in whitlow or paronychia, a disease seen primarily in medical and dental personnel whose fingers probe the mouths of patients, and in herpes gladiatorum, seen in wrestlers who suffer abrasions at their shoulders, which are then "inoculated" with the saliva of the adversary. Whitlow and herpes gladiatorum support the concept of viral spread by saliva. Exogenous reinfection may occur, so childhood infection may not provide total protection to the dentists, wrestlers, and others who have unusual salivary exposure.

Latency and Activation

During the primary infection, virus is transported up the local sensory nerve fibers by a fast retrograde transport system and establishes latency in the sensory ganglia (Fig. 6.1). This sequence is well established in animals experimentally infected with herpes simplex viruses, and it is presumed to occur in humans, because type 1 virus can be isolated from explants of one or both trigeminal ganglia in the majority of routine autopsies (Baringer and Swoveland, 1973). In some instances, virus can be recovered from geniculate, superior cervical, and vagus ganglia as well (Warren et al., 1978; Furuta et al., 1992b). This latency persists for life.

Activation of herpes simplex virus infection in the human trigeminal ganglion was first suggested by Cushing (1904), who devised the operation of extirpation of the ganglia for the treatment of trigeminal neuralgia. He found that herpetic eruptions frequently developed adjacent to the area of anesthesia. Carton (1953), after sectioning of the proximal root of the ganglia, found that herpetic lesions occurred in 90% of patients; however, if a peripheral nerve segment had previously been sectioned, the area of prior hypesthesia was spared. Two interpretations of Carton's data are possible: (a) that herpes simplex virus is present and remains latent in 90% of trigeminal ganglia, or (b) that virus in the trigeminal ganglia may be related to the pathogenesis of trigeminal neuralgia. Studies of nonselected autopsies have not achieved recovery rates to match the surgical reactivation rates, but they support the first alternative (Baringer, 1975).

Between 20% and 40% of the population suffer spontaneous reactivation in the form of labial herpes or cold sores. These recurrences occur at a frequency of one per month for 5% of these persons and at a frequency of less than once a year in 60%. Attacks may be precipitated by emotional stress, febrile illness, ultraviolet light, and a variety of other nonspecific events, but individuals often accredit some very specific event to their personal reactivations. Reactivation also occurs without the development of mucocutaneous lesions; in 1% to 3% of normal individuals, herpes simplex virus can be isolated from the oropharynx at any point in time, suggesting that infection of oropharyngeal cells occurs asymptomatically with great frequency (Douglas et al., 1970). Such isolations are more frequent

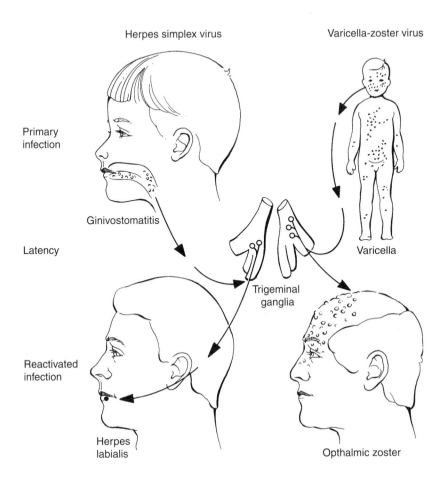

FIG. 6.1. Diagram of primary childhood infection, trigeminal ganglia latency, and later-life activation of herpes simplex and varicella–zoster viruses. Primary infection with herpes simplex is most often a gingivostomatitis or pharyngitis during which virus ascends along local sensory nerves and becomes latent in the third division of the trigeminal ganglia. Later activation can cause lesions in the oropharynx or the mucocutaneous junction. Primary infection of varicella causes a viremia and widespread lesions over the trunk and face, and latency can develop in any sensory ganglia. The first division of the trigeminal ganglia is the single most frequent involved, and later activation causes ophthalmic zoster, with characteristic dermatomal distribution of lesions over the first division of the trigeminal nerve.

when patients are in stressful situations or have unrelated acute diseases. There-fore, the isolation of the herpes simplex virus from the oropharynx cannot be accepted as significant evidence of an etiologic relationship with a coexistent dis-ease, because many diseases, particularly febrile illnesses, reactivate the virus.

Similar latency in sensory ganglia can be established in animals, and in mice the virus can be reactivated in explants. In mice, a tegument structural protein (Vmw 65), which activates immediate early genes, may influence whether pro-ductive infection or latency occurs in ganglion neurons; and neurons may express factors, such as nerve growth factor, that may inhibit expression of herpes sim-plex virus immediate early genes (Steiner and Kennedy, 1995). In animals and subsequently in humans, it was shown that the neurons of the sensory ganglia har-bored the viral DNA either in a circularized molecular or in concatemeric form. A minority of neurons maintain latency with estimates of 10 to 100 copies of viral DNA in their nuclei. In mice, neural cells of the adrenal medulla, retina, and brain can be latently infected (Stevens, 1994), and recent studies using polymerase chain reaction (PCR) indicate that some humans harbor herpes simplex viral sequences in their brains as well (Baringer and Pisani, 1994).

Neurons lack thymidine kinase, but herpes simplex virus has its own thymi-dine kinase. Viral mutants lacking the enzyme can replicate in systemic cells but not in nonreplicating neurons. Nevertheless, they establish latency in neurons in mice, again demonstrating that latency is host cell directed, and produce latency-associated transcripts in 95% to 100% of ganglia, even though these mutants cannot be reactivated (Tenser et al., 1989; Tenser, 1991).

The mechanisms of reactivation remain poorly understood. In mice, reactiva-tion can be induced by skin or nerve trauma, by treatment with immunosuppres-sive agents, or with x-ray irradiation. Reactivation normally occurs in the pres-ence of antiviral antibody, implicating a central role of cell-mediated immune responses (Shimeld et al., 1996). On the other hand, cytotoxic agents and x-ray irradiation may damage ganglion cell DNA directly, and their immunosuppres-sive effects may be of secondary importance in reactivation.

The mechanisms of the reactivation in ganglion cells pose an additional bio-logic dilemma. Herpes simplex virus is a highly lytic virus and "activation" that leads to productive infection should destroy the host cell. Therefore, recurrent herpes labialis in humans should eventually lead to an area of anesthesia in the area of the recurrent cold sores. This does not occur. Therefore, virus may be activated in a subunit form without lysis of the host cell. This subunit would be transported down the axon to the mucosal or cutaneous cells where lytic infec-tion occurs (Stevens, 1978). It is even possible that viral DNA is transported with transfection of susceptible peripheral cells.

Pathogenesis of Encephalitis

The acute, severe encephalitis due to herpes simplex type 1 in humans may rep-resent primary infection, reinfection, or reactivation of latent infection. The disease presents with distinctive clinical features because of a remarkable localization of the encephalitis to the orbital–frontal and temporal lobes (Fig. 6.2). Pathologic studies have shown localized inflammation, necrosis, and inclusion bodies, and this frontal–temporal localization is often strikingly unilateral. This is in contrast to the diffuse encephalitis in neonates caused by either type 1 or type 2 herpes simplex virus (see Chapter 13). The localization of disease in adults and children cannot be explained solely by selective vulnerability of specific cell populations, because inclusions and virions are found in both neurons and glia over a contiguous anatomic area. This pathologic finding gives the impression that virus is spread from cell to cell along the base of the brain within the middle and anterior fossae. In immunodeficient or anergic patients, the same localization and necrosis have been reported, although the histopathologic changes show an abundance of inclusion bodies and a paucity of inflammation (Tan et al., 1993).

This unique localization might be explained by the route of virus entry into the CNS and subsequent limitation of spread by antibody, such as entry of virus by the olfactory route, with subsequent spread along the base of the brain (Johnson and Mims, 1968). Immunofluorescence and electron-microscopic studies have localized virus to the olfactory nerve ipsilateral to major temporal lobe involvement (Ojeda, 1980), but infection of the olfactory bulbs is not uniformly

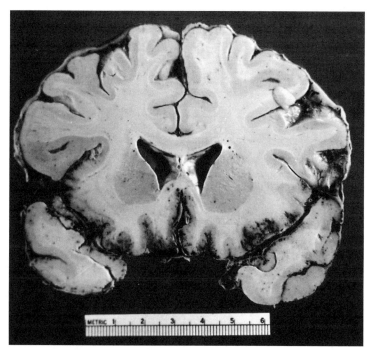

FIG. 6.2. Herpes simplex virus encephalitis. Coronal section of brain shows hemorrhagic necrosis localized primarily to the orbital frontal and medical temporal cortex.

found in patients dying of herpetic encephalitis (*personal observations*). Furthermore, herpetic encephalitis in adults is not usually a primary encounter with the virus, as previous believed, and latency of virus in the trigeminal ganglia is now recognized as almost universal.

These findings have led to the alternative hypothesis that encephalitis may result from reactivation and spread of virus from the trigeminal ganglia (Davis and Johnson, 1979). Anatomic studies in both primates and humans have shown that the meninges in the middle and anterior fossae are innervated by nerve fibers derived from the trigeminal nerve. A recurrent branch, the nervous tentorii, originates from the upper border of the ophthalmic division within the lateral wall of the cavernous sinus 1 cm distal to the ganglion. This nerve travels within the trochlear nerve sheath and fans out over the floor of the middle fossae. Fibers clearly innervate the dura of the middle and anterior fossae, form perivascular plexuses about the meningeal arteries, and contribute to the nerve fibers seen in the pia. The nervus meningeus medius and nervus spinosus derived from the second and third divisions of the trigeminal nerve may also contribute to dural innervation of the middle and anterior fossae (Fig. 6.3), whereas meningeal nerves

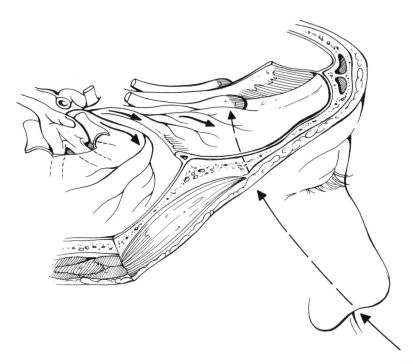

FIG. 6.3. Possible anatomic explanations for the orbital–frontal and temporal localization of herpes simplex virus encephalitis. Direct invasion of the olfactory bulb **(right)** could produce orbital–frontal infection, with spread to the temporal lobes. Small sensory fibers from the trigeminal ganglia **(left)** send fibers to the basilar meninges of the anterior and middle fossae.

derived from upper cervical branches and traveling with vagus and hypoglossal nerves innervate the dura of the posterior fossa. Thus, fibers from the trigeminal ganglia are concentrated in basilar structures corresponding to the anatomic localization of herpetic encephalitis. Therefore, we postulated that virus activated in the trigeminal ganglia that usually travels down the fibers of the trigeminal ganglia to the face or lip might rarely transverse back along the tentorial nerves, causing encephalitis in which dissemination of virus in spinal fluid or brain is inhibited by preexisting antibody. This proposed route of spread is supported by a murine model in which selective retrograde spread along the mandibular branch of the trigeminal after distal pulp inoculation leads to ipsilateral temporal lobe infection (Barnett et al., 1994a).

Another option is that encephalitis follows activation of latent virus within the brain. Latent infection in brain has been found in experimental animals, and a recent study using PCR in humans to amplify herpes simplex virus sequences detected viral sequences in 14 of 40 brains. Furthermore, topographic analysis showed localization to medulla, olfactory bulbs, pons, gyrus rectus, amygdala, and hippocampus (Baringer and Pisani, 1994). The same anatomic issues of nasal and olfactory spread are raised by these localizations.

Analysis of viral DNAs isolated from the brain and from trigeminal ganglia of patients suggests that encephalitis may result from trigeminal activation in some instances and from primary infection or reinfection in others. Using restriction endonucleases to cleave the herpesvirus DNAs, minor differences in the complex genome can be detected, and these vary from one isolate to another. Thus, common-source infections show viruses with the same restriction pattern as do isolates from two ganglia of a given patient. Trigeminal ganglia isolates from unrelated patients each show different patterns. If virus in the brain originated from the trigeminal ganglia, the same endonuclease cleavage pattern should be present in viruses from both brain and trigeminal ganglia; if virus in the brain was acquired from a different source, possibly by olfactory spread, different patterns should be found. Studies of a small number of patients with fatal encephalitis from whom virus has been isolated from both brain and trigeminal ganglia have shown that approximately half of the viruses are identical, which suggests that virus in brain originated from the trigeminal ganglia, and half are different, which suggests that the virus causing encephalitis and the virus infecting the ganglia originated from separate infections (Whitley et al., 1982).

Studies of virus mutants in mice have identified genes that modulate both neuroinvasiveness and neurovirulence. In the former case, the mutant virus replicates equally well in peripheral tissue and in brain when inoculated intracerebrally, but fails to enter the CNS after peripheral inoculation. The altered viral membrane glycoprotein coded by the mutant gene sequences is important in stimulating protective immune responses that may alter neuroinvasiveness, but this membrane protein also may be involved in gaining access to nerve terminals or the axonal transport system (Izumi and Stevens, 1990; Stevens, 1993). Deletion of a different gene that is not essential for viral growth in cell culture results in failure of virus replication of CNS even after intracerebral inoculation (Chou et al., 1990). Thus, viruses of variable neuroinvasiveness or neurovirulence exist, but the lack of familial or geographic clustering of cases of herpes simplex encephalitis provides no evidence for the importance of strain variations in human disease.

Clinical Presentation of Encephalitis

Epidemiologic studies show that herpes encephalitis has no seasonal distribution and no gender preference. Although primarily an adult disease, a diphasic age distribution is evident, with persons under 20 years and over 40 years of age being affected more frequently than persons in the third and fourth decades of life. Herpes encephalitis can occur in patients with immunodeficiencies or other diseases, but most individuals are in good health. Approximately one-fourth of the patients with herpes encephalitis have a past history of cold sores, an incidence similar to that for the general population (Whitley et al., 1977).

Herpes encephalitis may have an insidious or a fulminant onset. Fever is almost always present and may be in the range of 40° to 41°C. Headache is a prominent early symptom, and 90% of patients develop symptoms or signs that suggest local involvement of one or both temporal lobes. These symptoms may take the form of personality changes, which can dominate the clinical picture for a few days or even a week before other signs evolve. Patients may have acute episodes of terror, may experience hallucinations, or may show bizarre behavior (Drachman and Adams, 1962). One teenage girl's first sign was to awaken in the middle of the night, pack her bag, and tell her family that she was leaving to visit her grandmother, who had recently died. A dentist on route to work one morning entered his garage, came out with an ax, and chopped down his neighbor's picket fence. Such bizarre behavior may lead to an initial admission to psychiatric services. These early behavioral changes, however, are followed by other signs such as seizures, that are often focal and occur early in the disease in about 40% of patients (Olson et al., 1967). Hemiparesis is seen in one-third of patients and frequently shows greater involvement of face and arm, corresponding to the inferior frontal and temporal origin of the disease. Aphasia, superior-quadrant visual-field defects, and paresthesias may suggest the same localization. The anterior opercular syndrome with paralysis of masticatory, facial, pharyngeal and tongue muscles has been described (McGrath et al., 1997). Some patients progress rapidly from stupor to coma, with few if any clinical clues to suggest localization (Irani and Johnson, 1996; Sköldenberg, 1996).

Cerebrospinal fluid often shows an increased pressure. A mononuclear cell pleocytosis ranging from 10 to 1,000 cells/mm³ is present, but early in the disease no cells or significant numbers of neutrophils may be found. Red blood cells frequently are found, but their presence does not clearly indicate herpetic encephalitis, nor does their absence exclude it. Protein content is invariably elevated, and the sugar content usually is normal. The electroencephalogram may show only diffuse slowing, but often a unilateral or bilateral periodic discharge in temporal leads suggests a localized process. In some patients, characteristic slow wave complexes are seen at regular intervals of 2 to 3 per second, similar to the pattern in subacute sclerosing panencephalitis (Lai and Gragasin, 1988).

The abnormalities revealed by computerized tomography tend to appear late in the disease, and the major finding is a low-density abnormality in one or both temporal lobes. Magnetic resonance imaging with enhancement demonstrates lesions earlier and is superior in localizing lesions to temporal lobes (Schroth et al., 1987).

Diagnosis of Herpetic Encephalitis

Virus isolation from autopsy or brain biopsy tissue has been the gold standard for the diagnosis of herpes encephalitis with 100% specificity. The commonest cause of a false-negative biopsy is failure to obtain the specimen from the area with clinical or laboratory evidence of involvement. For example, if a patient has aphasia or left hemiparesis, and scans or electroencephalograms show abnormalities primarily in the left temporal lobe, the biopsy specimen should be taken from that lobe, despite the temptation to sample the nondominant temporal or frontal lobe. The disease can be remarkably localized, and virus may be recovered from one area when not recoverable from the contralateral temporal or frontal lobes. Although needle biopsy through a burr hole seems a conservative approach, this procedure is more hazardous than open biopsy. In view of the increase in intracerebral pressure, craniotomy with decompression of the affected temporal lobe may have a therapeutic effect and allows direct visualization of the brain for selection of an optimal biopsy specimen (Hanley et al., 1987).

Tissue specimens should be fixed for routine histology, immunocytochemical staining and possibly *in situ* hybridization, and electron microscopy, and unfixed portions should be inoculated into cell cultures for virus isolation. Isolation studies yield the most definitive positive results. Histologic studies alone give a low positive yield, because inclusion bodies are recognized in only half of virus-positive biopsy specimens, but they quickly confirm an inflammatory encephalitis and effectively rule out many other diseases. Both electron-microscopic examination and immunohistochemical staining can be rapid and useful if experienced microscopists are available. However, electron microscopy and immunocytochemical studies yield a number of false negatives and a small number of false positives (Whitley et al., 1981).

Although spinal fluid cultures are typically negative, detection of viral DNA in spinal fluid with PCR is rapidly replacing biopsy as a sensitive and specific method of diagnosis. The sensitivity is 75% to 98% in varied studies of child and adult patients with definitive biopsy or late serologic diagnoses. In biopsy-positive cases from the collaborative studies, 53 of 54 cases were positive by PCR, and all 18 spinal fluid specimens obtained prior to biopsies were positive (Lakeman and Whitley, 1995). The specificity is 100% if done with optimal techniques in a laboratory with experienced personnel (Sköldenberg, 1991; Troen-dle-Atkins et al., 1993; Lakeman and Whitley, 1995). With the proper PCR primers, the method can also differentiate type 1 and 2 herpes simplex viruses (Aurelius et al., 1993). False positives still pose a problem in some hospital diag-nostic laboratories. Unlike any other method, PCR also can be used to study autopsy specimens of patients dying with "burnt out" encephalitis for retrospec-tive diagnoses (Nicoll et al., 1991).

Detection of viral antigens in spinal fluid by a variety of methods has not proved more sensitive and has lacked specificity above 90% (Lakeman et al., 1987). A technique for detecting antigen by measuring antigen–antibody com-plex-activated complement-stimulated chemiluminescence has been reported (Kamei et al., 1994). Sensitivity and specificity appear excellent in the initial report, but these results need confirmation.

The diagnosis of herpetic encephalitis by serologic studies poses too great a time delay to affect decisions on antiviral therapy. Patients with herpetic encephalitis generally develop fourfold or greater increases in antibody to the virus, but antibody can be nonspecifically boosted during reactivation of the virus during the course of other intercurrent infections such as pneumonia or hepatitis (Johnson et al., 1968b). Increases in antibodies in spinal fluid 2 to 3 weeks after the onset of disease are more specific but may reflect leakage of antibody with increasing disruption of the blood–brain barrier. Unless markers for other viral antibodies are included, sensitivity and specificity are only about 80% (Whitley and Lakeman, 1995). Interestingly, intrathecal antibody synthesis may persist for many months, and in one individual it was recorded after 8 years (Taskinen et al., 1984; Vandvik et al., 1985).

Treatment of Encephalitis

Treatment of herpes simplex virus encephalitis has had an interesting and instructive history. In 1966, there was a report of a single patient who survived after treatment with 5-iodo-2′-deoxyuridine (idoxuridine), a thymidine analogue (Breeden et al., 1966); the same patient, however, was cited in another article that described the therapeutic benefits of surgical subtemporal decompression in herpetic encephalitis (Page et al., 1967). Nevertheless, this case report was fol-lowed by many anecdotal case reports and small uncontrolled series claiming efficacy for idoxuridine, even though the natural history and prognosis of the untreated disease were unclear (Johnson, 1972b). Subsequently, other drugs were tried, and finally in 1972 collaborative controlled trials of idoxuridine and adenine arabinoside (vidarabine), a purine nucleoside, were undertaken in com-parison with placebo. Early in the course of that study, idoxuridine demonstrated clear-cut toxicity without efficacy and was withdrawn (Boston Interhospital Virus Study Group, 1975). Thus, for 9 years, idoxuridine had been widely used as a therapeutic agent, and it probably did more harm than good; yet at the out-set of the collaborative study, critics believed that the "proven" efficacy of idoxuridine made it unethical to include a placebo in the trials. In view of the results, the ethical basis of permitting the use of a toxic drug without a controlled study appears more germane.

In 1977, the Collaborative Antiviral Study Group reported the efficacy of vidarabine versus placebo in biopsy-proven cases of herpes simplex encephalitis. The mortality was 70% for those receiving placebo and 28% for those receiving vidarabine, and the subsequent open study of 75 patients with biopsy-proven herpes simplex encephalitis treated with vidarabine showed a similar acute mortality of 32% (Whitley et al., 1977). Concurrently, a British study compared nontreatment and treatment with cytosine arabinoside. The mortality in both groups was between 70% and 80%, which confirmed the fatality rate without treatment or with ineffective treatment. In the open study, two important determinants of outcome were evident: age and level of consciousness at time of initiating treatment. Treated patients under 30 years of age showed a mortality of 24% compared with 52% in those over age 30. Patients who were lethargic at the initiation of treatment had a long-term mortality of 26% versus 53% for the semicomatose or comatose patient population.

Between 1981 and 1985, the collaborative group tested acyclovir, an acyclic purine nucleoside analogue, versus vidarabine, again using brain biopsy as the standard for diagnosis. Acyclovir reduced the mortality rate to 19% by 6 months after therapy compared with 54% treated with vidarabine (Whitley et al., 1986). Almost the same mortality rates had been reported in a Swedish study where diagnosis was supported by brain biopsy or antibody responses in serum and spinal fluid (Sköldenberg et al., 1984). Again, age and level of consciousness at institution of therapy were important determinants of outcome. For example, patients under 30 years of age with a Glasgow Coma score greater than 6 all survived, and 8 of 13 had only mild or no long-term morbidity; all 3 patients over 30 years of age and with a Glasgow Coma score less than 6 died or had severe sequela. Acyclovir has been used successfully during pregnancy without damage to the offspring (Hankey et al., 1987).

Of the 208 patients who were admitted to the study on the basis of having suspected herpes simplex encephalitis with evidence of disease localization, herpes simplex virus was recovered from tissue in only 33%. This rate was below the 40% and 50% positive diagnosis by virus isolation in the controlled and open vidarabine studies. There is no evidence that the participating physicians had deteriorated in clinical acumen, but based on the earlier studies greater effort was made to establish diagnoses earlier and thus biopsies were done earlier. Even with extensive clinical experience, one cannot anticipate greater than 50% accuracy in diagnosis of herpes simplex virus encephalitis early in the course of disease. It is true that this encephalitis is unique in being the only viral encephalitis that *characteristically* presents with signs and symptoms indicating a temporal lobe localization. On the other hand, herpes simplex virus causes only about 10% of the cases of viral encephalitis (see Chapter 5), and enteroviruses, arboviruses, and other agents that cause diffuse infection, by chance, may cause signs pointing to the temporal lobes. Nonviral illnesses, many of which are treatable, also may localize to temporal lobes, mimicking herpes simplex encephalitis. A by-product of the long-term studies of herpes simplex encephalitis by the Collaborative Antiviral Study Group requiring diagnosis by brain biopsy has been an extensive list of the diseases that may mimic herpes simplex encephalitis, often as very atypical presentations of these varied diseases (Table 6.2). Over the years, 45% of patients suspected of having herpes simplex virus encephalitis who underwent brain biopsy have had herpes simplex virus isolated from brain, 22% have had other diagnoses established by biopsy, and 33% remained without a diagnosis (Whitley et al., 1989).

Patients who survive herpes simplex encephalitis may have severe debilitating sequelae, including major motor and sensory deficits, aphasia, and often an amnestic syndrome (Korsakoff's psychosis). Even after early acyclovir treatment and good recovery with normal performance on a standard clinical mental status test, more detailed cognitive testing may show dysnomia and impaired new learning (Gordon et al., 1990).

Patients who survive acute encephalitis maintain high cerebrospinal fluid levels of antibody against herpesvirus for several years (Sköldenberg et al., 1981), and several patients who have died after a full course of antiviral therapy have had virus isolated from brain. In a number of patients, further clinical deterioration has appeared 1 week to 3 months after initial stabilization or partial recovery after vidarabine or acyclovir therapy (Wolinsky, 1980; Barthez et

TABLE 6.2. *Diseases diagnosed by brain biopsy or autopsy from patients with suspected herpes simplex encephalitis*

Other viruses	Other infections	Other diseases
Arboviruses	Abscess or empyema	Tumor
St. Louis encephalitis		Subdural hematoma
Western encephalitis	Bacterial	Systemic lupus erythematosus
California encephalitis	Meningococcal meningitis	Adrenal leukodystrophy
Eastern encephalitis	Mycoplasma	Vascular disease
	Tuberculosis	Toxic encephalopathy
Other herpesviruses		Reye's syndrome
Epstein–Barr virus	Fungal	
Cytomegalovirus	Cryptococcosis	
Herpesvirus 6	Mucormycosis	
Echovirus	Rickettsia	
Influenza A	Toxoplasmosis	
Mumps		
Adenovirus		
Lymphocytic choriomeningitis		
Progressive multifocal		
leukoencephalopathy		
Subacute sclerosing		
panencephalitis		

Modified from Whitley et al. (1989).

al., 1987; Kimura et al., 1992). In some cases, this recurrence has a smoldering course or multiple relapses (Brochet et al., 1990). Virus isolated from brain during relapses after a full course of therapy have been acyclovir sensitive (Van Landingham et al., 1988), but concern persists that drug-resistant strains may develop in the CNS (Gateley et al., 1990). Therefore, retreatment with additional courses of acyclovir with or without vidarabine usually has been instituted.

Other Neurologic Diseases

Atypical forms of herpes simplex encephalitis do occur. In experimental herpes simplex virus infections in rabbits, virus is transported centripetally along the trigeminal nerve proximal to the ganglia and causes an initial encephalitis in the pons. Some human cases of brainstem encephalitis may be due to herpesvirus infections. Herpes simplex virus has been implicated in brainstem encephalitis by immunofluorescence (Ellison and Hanson, 1977), by morphological localization of inclusion bodies and viruslike particles (Roman-Campos and Toro, 1980), by *in situ* hybridization for viral DNA (Schmidbauer et al., 1989; Rose et al., 1992), and by demonstration of DNA in spinal fluid of patients with brainstem encephalitis (Mertens et al., 1993), including one patient with recurrent signs of brainstem encephalitis (Tyler et al., 1995). Myelitis in immunocompetent patients has been seen with evidence of type 1 herpes simplex virus infections (Folpe et al., 1994; Petereit et al., 1996), including one patient with recurrent ascending myelitis (Shyu et al., 1993).

Since herpes simplex virus involves nerves and establishes latency in the geniculate ganglion, it has also been proposed as a potential cause of idiopathic facial paralysis (Bell's palsy). This hypothesis is supported by anecdotal reports, such as that of an 8-year-old who developed Bell's palsy during recovery from herpes simplex virus stomatitis (Smith et al., 1987), by several series demonstrating antibody increases in a small percentage of patients with Bell's palsy (Morgan and Nathwani, 1992), and by a higher incidence of anti–herpes simplex virus antibody in patients with facial palsy than in age-matched controls (Adour et al., 1975). Recently, herpes simplex virus DNA was demonstrated by PCR in endoneurial fluid or posterior auricular muscle specimens obtained during surgical decompression of facial nerves in 11 of 14 patients; the specificity of these results is strengthened by negative findings and positive PCR findings for varicella–zoster virus in patients with facial palsy in Ramsay Hunt syndrome (Murakami et al., 1996). Bell's palsy also occurs during the course of mumps and *Borrelia* infection and rarely during herpes zoster virus, Epstein–Barr virus, rubella virus, and HIV infections.

Type 1 herpes simplex virus has been detected on several occasions in spinal fluid from patients with cervical and lumbar radicular pain (Morrison et al., 1979) and with Mollaret's meningitis (Steel et al., 1982; Yamamoto et al., 1991). These syndromes, however, are more often associated with type 2 virus.

Type 2 Herpes Simplex Virus

Type 2 herpes simplex virus is spread primarily by venereal contact and accounts for most herpetic lesions below the waist. Primary infection can occur *in utero* or during parturition through an infected birth canal (see Chapter 13), but the majority of infections occur between the ages of 14 and 35 years, when up to 30% of people develop antibody. The incidence of infection is higher in women than men and has increased markedly in the past two decades. Because the rate of infection varies with numbers of sexual partners, antibodies are found in over 75% of prostitutes and are virtually absent among nuns. Symptoms of primary infection are usually more severe in women. Local pain and itching, dysuria, and adenopathy are common. Aseptic meningitis accompanies 8% of primary infections, and sacral nerve root dysfunction with saddle anesthesia and urinary retention occur in a small number (Corey et al., 1983).

Similar to type 1 virus, type 2 herpes simplex virus spreads to corresponding sensory ganglia and is recoverable from the second through fourth sacral ganglia at routine autopsies (Baringer, 1974). In about 60% of those infected, virus is intermittently activated, producing recurrent herpes genitalis.

The neurologic infections of greatest severity are seen in infants infected at the time of birth, who develop disseminated herpetic infections with hepatic and adrenal necrosis and a diffuse encephalitis (see Chapter 13). Unlike type 1 virus, this virus can be recovered from both cerebrospinal fluid and blood (Craig and Nahmias, 1973). Prior to the differentiation of type 1 and 2 virus, most older reports in the literature of herpes simplex virus isolation from cerebrospinal fluid probably represented type 2 viruses.

The infected sacral ganglia receive sensory fibers from the external genitalia, the medial side of the thigh, and the back of the thigh. Recurrences are most frequent over the genitalia and frequently are associated with local dysesthesias. With exacerbation of genital lesions, meningitis or radiculitis may recur (Bergström et al., 1990; Cohen et al., 1994). Pain may be a lancinating or burning dysesthesia, and when the S-2 dermatome is affected, virus activation may simulate sciatica produced by disc disease. Recurrent lymphocytic meningitis can also occur in the absence of genital lesions (Schlesinger et al., 1995), and recently has been associated with Mollaret's meningitis, a long-recognized syndrome of suspected viral etiology. A PCR study of 13 cases of recurrent lymphocytic meningitis detected herpes simplex virus DNA in the cerebrospinal fluid of 11: ten were type 2 virus and one was type 1 (Tedder et al., 1994).

Type 2 herpes simplex virus has recently been found in the temporal lobe of a 40-year-old man with chronic genital lesions and a 3-year history of escalating temporal lobe seizures. This smoldering encephalitis in an immunocompetent adult is unique (Cornford and McCormick, 1997). Severe cerebral herpes simplex virus type 2 infections in adults are usually limited to severely immunocompromised patients. Fatal disseminated herpesvirus infections, including encephalitis, have been seen in patients with thymic dysplasia and other severe immunodeficiency states (Sutton et al., 1974). Severe, often fatal, meningoen-cephalitis has been associated with herpesvirus type 2, as well as type 1, in patients undergoing intensive immunosuppressive therapy or with AIDS (Dix et al., 1985; Chrétien et al., 1996).

B Virus (Cercopithecine Herpesvirus 1)

This simian virus is related to herpes simplex virus and produces an analo-gous latent infection, with recurrent oral lesions, in rhesus monkeys and other *Macaca*. Severe myelitis and encephalitis have occurred in at least 25 laboratory workers after contact with macaques or their cells, resulting in 16 fatalities (Wei-gler, 1992). The first fatality was that of a 29-year-old research physician (Dr. B.) who was bitten by an apparently normal rhesus monkey (Sabin and Wright, 1934). Three days after the bite, pain and swelling developed at the site of the wound, followed by a local lymphangitis and vesicles at the site of the original bite. He subsequently suffered limb paralysis, urinary retention, and a rapidly progressive myelitis and died. In the late 1950s, cases occurred during the devel-opment of polio vaccines, primarily among laboratory workers and animal atten-dants with histories of monkey bites. However, one technician developed fatal myelitis after he broke a glass culture tube containing monkey renal cells into his hand, causing minor lacerations (Davidson and Hummeler, 1960).

The myelitis and encephalitis usually are rapidly fatal, and severe residua have persisted in most survivors. One was an eminent virologist with no history of contact with monkeys for 10 years. His disease began with a zosterlike lesion in the trigeminal nerve distribution, followed by severe encephalomyelitis. B virus was isolated later from a vesicular rash that developed over his thorax. The dis-ease was ascribed to B virus, but alternatively could have represented reactiva-tion of latent B virus in a severely ill patient with herpes zoster who was treated with steroids (Fierer et al., 1973). In 1987, three workers in a Florida laboratory were infected, and one spouse became infected presumably when she applied ointment to her husband's lesions and used the same cream to treat her own der-matitis. She and her husband were treated with acyclovir prior to neurologic involvement, and both survived [Centers for Disease Control (CDC), 1987]. The current clinical examination and serologic screening of rhesus monkeys used in medical research have reduced the risk of this infection in laboratory workers.

VARICELLA–ZOSTER VIRUS

Varicella–zoster virus causes two distinct clinical diseases: varicella (chicken-pox), a generalized exanthem that affects almost all children; and herpes zoster (shingles), an exanthem restricted to one or more adjacent sensory dermatomes that represents a reactivation of the same virus in the immune host. Varicella and herpes zoster were long suspected of being caused by the same agent. von Bokay

(1909) observed that children could acquire varicella after contact with elders with shingles. This clinical relationship was observed by others, as were the histopathologic similarities of the cutaneous lesions with giant cells and intranuclear inclusions. The serologic and tissue culture studies of Weller and Witton in 1958 firmly established that the two diseases are due to a single agent.

Epidemiology

The virus probably has no natural nonhuman host, although varicella has been observed in anthropoid apes in zoos. In the laboratory, the virus is similarly restricted to growth in primate cells, with some experimental evidence of transmission to monkeys (Wenner et al., 1977). This virus is avidly cell associated and usually can be experimentally transmitted only by the inoculation of infected cells, even though the virus is remarkably stable in cell-free form in vesicular fluid. Morphologically, the virus resembles herpes simplex virus, and, indeed, they share several common antigens, despite their striking differences in experimental host range and the infectivity of cell-free virus.

Varicella is spread by the respiratory route. Most children are infected during early school years, with outbreaks every 2 to 4 years predominantly in the winter and spring. The majority of infections are clinically obvious, and fewer than 4% escape recognition. The rash begins with small, rose-colored vacuoles on an erythematous base that then develop a central vesicle. Successive crops of vesicles develop every 2 to 4 days, corresponding to several waves of viremia, and the rash spreads centripetally from the face and trunk toward the extremities. It is usually a benign illness, although there are rare fatal pulmonary infections in adults and fatal disseminated disease in immunodeficient children, particularly children with leukemia. In the fatal cases, infection is concentrated in vascular endothelial cells. Severe neurologic complications are rare but varied (Table 6.3). In large part, these appear to be postinfectious complications and are discussed in Chapters 8 and 9.

Herpes zoster shows a completely different epidemiologic pattern. Zoster does not occur in epidemics, either by year or season, and no increase in the incidence of zoster is found during the years of varicella epidemics; indeed, the incidence may decrease slightly during the years of varicella epidemics (Hope-Simpson, 1965). Herpes zoster occurs at a rate of 125 to 350 per 100,000 population per year; 75% of these cases involve patients over 45 years of age, and less than 10% involve children under age 15. Contrary to folklore, an attack of zoster does not confer immunity to zoster; indeed, the immunocompetent patient is at about equal risk of future eruption as the person who has not had the disease. It is estimated that half of the people who reach age 85 will have suffered at least one attack of shingles. Severity correlates with age, because zoster is more benign in the young and more painful and protracted in the elderly, with a higher rate of postherpetic neuralgia (Portenoy et al., 1986). Rates are higher in persons with malignancies or diabetes and in those immunosuppressed by

TABLE 6.3. *Varied neurological complications of varicella–zoster virus infections*

Varicella	Acute ataxia[a]
	Postinfectious encephalomyelitis[a]
	Myelitis[a]
	Guillain–Barré syndrome[a]
	Reye's syndrome[b]
	Vasculitis with stroke
	Limb deformities after maternal infection[c]
Zoster	Postherpetic neuralgia
	Cranial nerve palsies
	Segmental motor paralysis
	Aseptic meningitis
	Meningoencephalitis
	Transverse myelitis
	Ascending myelitis
	Delayed contralateral hemiplegia
	Small vessel disease with demyelinative lesions (immunocompromised patients)
	Ventriculitis (immunocompromised patients)
	Guillain–Barré syndrome[a]

[a]See Chapter 8.
[b]See Chapter 9.
[c]See Chapter 13.

drugs, radiation, or HIV infection. These groups are also predisposed to dissemination of zoster, usually defined as the spreading of lesions over more than three dermatomes. The role of trauma in the precipitation of exacerbations remains controversial. A history of antecedent trauma in about 1% or 2% or patients with zoster has been found, but this may be no more than expected by chance (Hope-Simpson, 1965; Ragozzino et al., 1982). Juel-Jensen (1970) reported a rate of 3.8%, however, and he suggested that the higher rate of ophthalmic to mandibular shingles might be explained by the greater likelihood of bumping one's forehead than one's chin. This logic falters, though, considering that lesions are more common over the thorax than over the extremities, although trauma to the chest is certainly less frequent than trauma to fingers and toes.

Pathogenesis of Herpes Zoster

Details of the pathogenesis of herpes zoster are uncertain, but the following scenario can be formulated from analogies to herpes simplex and from clinical, pathologic, and virologic data: A mononuclear cell-associated viremia occurs in susceptible children, and skin infection originates from the blood, with infection of capillary endothelium. Vesicles develop primarily over the face and trunk. The virus is assumed to be transported centripetally along sensory nerves to the sensory ganglia, where it becomes latent within the neurons. By PCR, virus DNA has been found in trigeminal ganglia in 87% and in thoracic ganglia in 53% of adults who had not recently had chickenpox or shingles (Mahalingam et al., 1990), and 69% of geniculate ganglia were positive in another study (Furuta et al., 1992a). Subsequent studies showed the same ganglia can be latently infected with both herpes simplex and varicella–zoster viruses (Mahalingam et al., 1992), but whether the same cell can harbor both viruses is unknown.

Identification of the precise cells containing latent varicella–zoster virus has been contentious: initial reports of *in situ* hybridization showed viral DNA limited to neurons (Hyman et al., 1983; Gilden et al., 1987), whereas other studies have found RNA latency transcripts restricted to satellite cells (Croen et al., 1988; Meier et al., 1993). Recent studies convincingly show latent varicella–zoster virus primarily localized to neurons (D.H. Gilden, *personal communication*). The nature of the cell–virus relation is clearly different from that of herpes simplex in ganglia because varicella–zoster virus cannot be recovered by *in vitro* explantation of ganglia. Furthermore, despite its presence in many sensory ganglia throughout the neuraxis, varicella–zoster virus reactivates with far lower frequency.

Reactivation in some patients is associated with local malignancy, local irradiation, trauma, or tumor entrapment of the dorsal root ganglia or nerve root. In most patients, however, no obvious inciting cause is evident, and because the frequency of reactivation increases with age, a decline in immunity and lack of reexposure to chickenpox have been postulated as factors (Hope-Simpson, 1965). Indeed, a decline in cell-mediated immunity to the virus has been correlated with age (Miller, 1980). When virus replication is reactivated, a ganglionitis develops that causes pain along the corresponding sensory distribution. Virus or virus subunits may then pass down the nerve, multiply again in the skin, and cause characteristic clusters of vesicles along the dermatome (Fig. 6.1). The more frequent involvement of thoracic and trigeminal dermatomes corresponds to the major areas of eruptions during the antecedent varicella. The immune response may limit the infection and prevent dissemination, although the clearance of the rash in zoster correlates better with the collection of inflammatory cells and interferon in vesicular fluid than it does with antibody development (Stevens et al., 1975). Waning immunity could explain the occurrence of the disease with increasing age and the lack of seasonal association with chickenpox.

Pathologic studies have documented an acute ganglionitis, with an intense inflammatory response, cell necrosis, and occasional hemorrhages in the ganglia (Ghatak and Zimmerman, 1973). Inflammation is also found in adjacent segments of the cord or brainstem, and this inflammation tends to be more intense ipsilateral to the cutaneous lesions and most prominent in the dorsal root entry zone. Inflammation is also found in roots distal to the ganglia; thus, a true peripheral mononeuritis exists.

In considering the dermatomal distribution of the lesions, it is natural to recall the standard diagram of the sensory dermatomes, which usually is footnoted as being "modified from Head and Campbell (1900)." Contrary to popular assumption, this was not an anatomic paper on the sensory dermatomes but the classic early paper on shingles. The sensory dermatomes were defined by the virus—a contribution of virology to neuroanatomy that is not generally appreciated.

Disease Description

The eruption of shingles usually is preceded by several days of malaise and fever, and segmental dysesthesia usually precedes the rash for 4 to 5 days. This dysesthesia may be a superficial tingling or burning, a severe deep pain, or only a mild itching, and the dysesthesia may be intermittent or constant. Tenderness and hypesthesia often can be detected along the dermatome during the preeruption stage. The cutaneous lesions begin, like the varicella lesions, as reddish papules that later develop central vesiculation. On about day 3, the vesicular fluid becomes turbid as inflammatory cells collect and, in 5 to 10 days, the vesicle usually is dry and a crust has formed. In severe cases, vesicles may become confluent, giving a gangrenous appearance, and the lesions may fail to heal for several weeks. Spread to adjacent dermatomes is usual, although usually not to the other side of the body. A significant number of patients over the age of 40 develop pain that persists for months to years, and this occurs in half of the patients who develop the disease after age 80.

Zoster can occur over any sensory dermatome, but thoracic dermatomes are the sites in over half of the patients. Cranial nerve involvement is next in frequency, and this involvement tends to cause greater pain, more meningeal inflammation, and a higher rate of neurologic complications (Table 6.3). The commonest cranial nerve involvement is the ophthalmic division of the trigeminal nerve, accounting for 10% to 15% of all cases of zoster. Lesions over the nasociliary branch are harbingers of ocular involvement (uveitis, keratitis, and corneal ulceration) (Harding et al., 1987). The maxillary or mandibular branches may also be involved. During varicella, vesicles develop on the buccal mucosa, palate, and anterior pillars, and this can lead to latent infection not only of the trigeminal ganglia but also of the petrosal ganglia, which receive sensory fibers via the glossopharyngeal nerve from the posterior tongue, tonsils, posterior fossa, uvula, and posterior wall of the pharynx. Later activation may lead to zoster of the oropharyngeal mucosa. Similarly, the somatic sensory fibers of the facial nerve from the external auditory meatus may carry virus to the geniculate ganglia, and later activation may lead to vesicles and pain in the external auditory meatus, loss of taste in the anterior two-thirds of the tongue, and an ipsilateral facial palsy—the so-called Ramsey Hunt syndrome. The facial palsy presumably is due to inflammation and compression of the motor fibers of the facial nerve as they pass through the ganglion (Aleksic et al., 1973). However, with zoster of the face, oropharynx, or ear, there often are other associated neurologic signs. In ophthalmic zoster, involvement of ocular motor function, ptosis, and paralytic mydriasis are common. In otitic zoster with facial palsy, hearing loss, vertigo, and other signs are common, indicating involvement of multiple cranial nerves or ganglia or localized involvement of the brainstem (Denny-Brown and Adams, 1944).

Motor function may be affected not only with cranial nerve localization but with zoster in the cervical, thoracic, and lumbar segments. Segmental motor paralysis occurs in about 5% of episodes of shingles and takes an array of forms (Kennedy, 1987). Paralysis usually corresponds to the dermatome involved by the rash, but dissociated paresis is seen, such as rash over the deltoid with a contralateral weakness of intrinsic muscles of the hand (Christie, 1969). This presumably results from a localized myelitis. Diaphragmatic paralysis often accompanies cervical zoster, but paralysis usually is unilateral and unrecognized (Weiss et al., 1975b). Horner's syndrome has been described with zoster of second and third thoracic dermatomes (Wimalaratna et al., 1987). Asymptomatic paralysis of individual intercostal muscles may be found, if carefully sought. On rare occasions, thoracic lesions are associated with constipation and hypomotility (Juel-Jensen and MacCallum, 1972) or even paralytic ileus (*personal observation*). Urinary retention or urinary and fecal incontinence may occur with zoster of sacral dermatomes (Jellinek and Tulloch, 1976). Since the primary lesions are in the ganglia, spinal fluid frequently shows pleocytosis and protein elevation, even when clinical signs of meningeal irritation are absent.

Zoster sine herpete is typical radicular pain over a localized dermatomal distribution, without the development of vesicles. This has long been suspected to be an activation of the virus without cutaneous spread, and two physicians with transient radicular pain and no vesicles documented increases in antibody to varicella between their own acute and convalescent sera (Easton, 1970; Juel-Jensen and MacCallum, 1972). Varicella–zoster DNA has been demonstrated in the spinal fluid of several patients who had experienced years of radicular pain without zoster rash (Gilden et al., 1994; Amlie-Lefond et al., 1996). Whether activation without rash is a common cause of the many transient minor radicular pains in the face and chest remains a matter of speculation. Attempts to associate trigeminal neuralgia and facial palsy (Bell's palsy) with zoster sine herpete have been unsuccessful or inconclusive. Occasionally, zosterlike lesions both of the face and trunk in otherwise healthy people have been associated with herpes simplex viruses (Kalman and Laskin, 1986).

Unusual Neurologic Complications

Since episodes of herpes zoster often are associated with meningitis, the question had naturally followed whether meningitis can occur without the exanthem. Varicella–zoster virus DNA has been identified in spinal fluid by PCR in several cases of aseptic meningitis and encephalitis without the skin lesions (Shoji et al., 1992; Echevarría et al., 1994; Bergström, 1996). Further studies are needed to determine whether clinically unsuspected varicella–zoster virus reactivation is a substantial cause of aseptic meningitis.

Life-threatening encephalitis and myelitis have also been described with zoster, and most, but not all, have been in immunocompromised patients (Peterslund, 1988). Fourteen cases of herpes zoster encephalitis were found in the archives of New York City between 1932 and 1960; none of the patients died acutely, and only three patients had sequelae (Appelbaum et al., 1962). More recently, a number of cases have been reported, including two patients who had relapsing courses (Norris et al., 1970). Both of these patients were being treated with corticosteroids, and one was also receiving an antimetabolite for treatment of Hodgkin's disease. Another report described two fatal cases of varicella–zoster virus encephalitis in patients receiving immunosuppressant drugs; virus was cultivated from brain of one, and viruslike particles were demonstrated electron microscopically in glial cells in both (McCormick et al., 1969). A patient with T-cell lymphoma has been reported who had fatal varicella–zoster virus meningoradiculitis without skin involvement (Dueland et al., 1991). In a single patient with fatal nodular brainstem encephalitis and no cutaneous rash, varicella–zoster antigens and DNA were detected in lesions (Schmidbauer et al., 1992).

Acute transverse myelitis and fatal ascending myelitis have also been reported (Hogan and Krigman, 1973; Chapman and Beaven, 1979; Aizawa et al., 1996). With increased use of immunosuppressant drugs and the emergence of AIDS, more cases of zoster myelitis are being reported. Viral infection of neuroecto-dermal cells, particularly oligodendrocytes, have been shown by immunocyto-chemistry and by the presence of typical intranuclear inclusions (Devinsky et al., 1991). Two patients with relapsing–remitting courses have also been reported (Gilden et al., 1995).

Delayed contralateral hemiplegia after ophthalmic zoster is a unique vasculitic complication of herpes opthalmicus that has been recognized in over 50 patients (Kleinschmidt-DeMasters et al., 1996). Two to 10 weeks after the onset of the facial lesions, usually with involvement of the eye, the patient suddenly devel-ops a contralateral hemiplegia. The spinal fluid may or may not show pleocyto-sis and protein elevation. Angiography usually shows a segmental narrowing of the proximal middle and anterior cerebral arteries on the side of the antecedent herpetic lesions, but widespread segmental narrowings or aneurysms also have been found. The fatality rate is about 20%.

In several fatal cases, a granulomatous arteritis with giant cells has been found in the occluded vessels and in cerebral vessels over a wider area (Rosen-blum and Hadfield, 1972; Hilt et al., 1983). The assumption is that vasculitis may develop locally near the ganglion and then spread more diffusely. Her-pesvirus-like particles were found by electron microscopy in outer layers of cerebral vessel walls in one patient (Linneman and Alvira, 1980) and in smooth muscle cells of the middle cerebral artery in another (Doyle et al., 1983). Vari-cella–zoster virus antigen was reported in the media of affected vessels in another case (Eidelberg et al., 1986). In one patient, varicella–zoster DNA was detected by PCR of arteries dissected from the affected side of the brain, but from the contralateral arteries (Melanson et al., 1996). Variations on this clas-sic pattern have included central retinal artery occlusion 2 weeks after ipsilat-eral facial zoster (Hall et al., 1983), thalamic infarction 8 days after zoster oti-cus (Joy et al., 1989) and 10 days after lingual zoster (Geny et al., 1991b), and brainstem infarctions after cervical zoster (Ross et al., 1991). Sudden death 10 weeks after C2 zoster was found associated with a ruptured basilar aneurysm. The basilar artery showed granulomatous angiitis with herpesvirus-like particles and varicella–zoster antigen in infiltrating inflammatory cells (Fukumoto et al., 1986). A waxing and waning CNS vasculitis has been reported with antecedent zoster in which a patchy distribution of viral DNA and antigen was found in cerebral arteries (Gilden et al., 1996).

Several children have developed hemiplegia 6 weeks to 3 months after varicella, and a similar pathology has been postulated (Caekebeke et al., 1990; Ichiyama et al., 1990; Liu and Holmes, 1990). The most unusual childhood case was a 17-month-old whose mother had chickenpox at 8 months' gestation; the infant developed left trigeminal zoster at 16 months of age and a right hemiplegia 4 weeks later, with angiographic evidence of occlusion of left lenticulostriate arteries (Leis and Butler, 1987).

In most of the instances of vasculitis, the late evolution and the morphology of the angiitis suggest an immune pathogenesis; on the other hand, the findings of viruslike particles and antigen in vessel walls suggest a direct viral effect. Because of this ambiguity, a number of patients have been treated with antiviral drugs and steroids but without convincing therapeutic efficacy.

Another unusual zoster-associated lesion that has been reported in cancer patients involves multifocal demyelinating lesions of the brain that resemble progressive multifocal leukoencephalopathy. These patients had cutaneous zoster over thoracic or cervical dermatomes many months before the onset of progressive multifocal neurologic signs and symptoms. At autopsy, Cowdry type A intranuclear inclusions were found in oligodendrocytes, astrocytes, and neurons bordering the demyelinating foci. Electron microscopy showed herpesvirus-like particles, and immunoperoxidase staining detected varicella–zoster virus antigens in these cells (Horten et al., 1981). A vasculopathy has been found in subsequent studies involving smaller vessels than seen in the acute contralateral hemiplegia; inclusions are seen in oligodendrocytes surrounding small areas of infarction causing small ovoid demyelinative lesions (Amlie-Lefond et al., 1995; Kleinschmidt-DeMasters et al., 1996). Thus, varicella–zoster virus, like herpes simplex virus, cytomegalovirus, measles virus, and adenoviruses, appears capable of causing a smoldering subacute infection in the brain of immunocompromised patients, and, as with papovaviruses, this opportunistic infection may cause a demyelinating disease (see Chapter 10).

Unusual and varied varicella–zoster infections of the CNS have been described in patients with AIDS. These have been reported months after the dermatomal rash and without the characteristic skin eruption. Progressive encephalitis (Ryder et al., 1986; Gilden et al., 1988), brainstem encephalitis (Moulignier et al., 1995), and necrotizing myelitis (Gomez-Tortosa et al., 1994; Manian et al., 1995; Lionnet et al., 1996) have been described. Pathologic studies in some cases have shown a necrotizing vasculitis with ventriculitis, meningomyeloradiculitis, and involvement of leptomeningeal vessels with cerebral infarcts (Gray et al., 1994b).

Postherpetic Neuralgia

Postherpetic neuralgia is a common complication of zoster that carries an enormous morbidity. Postherpetic neuralgia is usually defined as pain persisting for more than 30 days in the area of the eruption.

Pain usually precedes the dermatomal eruption of zoster by several days and, on rare occasions, pain can precede the rash by more than a week (Gilden et al., 1991). Acute pain is assumed to be caused by the acute inflammation of the ganglia and nerve roots, where there is often intraneural hemorrhage. Once the cutaneous eruption has occurred, there is also a burning sensation of the skin presumed to arise from excitation of nociceptors in the skin (Bennett, 1994). The precise mechanism for continued pain after clearing of the rash is not known. A decrease in inhibitory, large, myelinated fibers leaves a predominance of small, unmyelinated, afferent pain fibers, increasing pain transmission to the spinal cord. Abnormal gating of sensory input may also occur at the level of the ganglion. A central mechanism of abnormal processing has also been postulated, because section of the nerve root proximal to the ganglia does not necessarily interrupt pain. Suggestions have also been made that small microfibromas may occur with regeneration. The recent finding of varicella–zoster virus DNA in peripheral mononuclear cells of patients with postherpetic neuralgia and not in convalescent persons without neuralgia suggests an ongoing productive infection in the ganglia, with spillover being detected in the blood (Vafai et al., 1988; Mahalingam et al., 1995). Nevertheless, the pain has not been shown to be responsive to acyclovir treatment.

Postherpetic neuralgia occurs in 9% to 15% of patients after zoster; half of these abate within the second month and less than one-fourth or approximately 2% of the total persist for longer than 1 year. These numbers, however, are highly dependent on several risk factors, including age, the dermatomes involved, and the severity of pain with the initial attack. Postherpetic neuralgia is extremely rare in patients with herpes zoster who are younger than 20 years of age but occurs in nearly 50% of those older than age 60. Several independent, population-based studies have shown that about 50% of patients over age 60 continue to have pain 1 month after onset of zoster, approximately 25% still have pain at 3 months, and as many as 10% continue to have pain 6 months after the rash (Wood, 1991). Postherpetic neuralgia is also more frequent after trigeminal zoster than after involvement of thoracic dermatomes. The postherpetic pain may take a variety of forms, from a deep aching pain to ticlike lancinating sensations as well as varied dysesthesias. Particularly in the elderly, it may cause severe disability.

Treatment

Varicella vaccine is now recommended for all children, but nonimmunized children with leukemia and other immunodeficiency states, as well as immunocompromised adults without a history of varicella, should be treated with zoster-immune globulin after exposure to chickenpox or zoster (CDC, 1996b). Immunoglobulin does not protect against zoster in children or adults with a past history of chickenpox. Varicella in normal children usually requires no specific treatment, except that aspirin should be avoided because of the association with Reye's syndrome (see Chapter 9). Immunocompromised patients who develop zoster or adults who show evidence of dissemination of zoster for than more three contiguous dermatomes are usually treated with intravenous acyclovir. Acyclovir has been shown to halt the progression and to accelerate the rate of clearance of virus from vesicles (Balfour et al., 1983). Comparative trials of acyclovir and vidarabine show that both are effective (Whitley et al., 1992). Myelitis in AIDS has also been reported to resolve with acyclovir treatment (Lionnet et al., 1996).

The major undecided issue is the treatment of normal adults who have uncomplicated zoster. For many years, steroids have been used: they reduce pain, impose some risk of causing spread, and do not prevent postherpetic neuralgia (Esmann et al., 1987). Initially, acyclovir was seldom used in immunocompetent patients with zoster because of the need to use intravenous therapy, and equivalent oral dosages were not effective. With larger oral doses, however, it has been established that acyclovir shortens the healing time of lesions and decreases the duration and severity of acute pain. Therefore, it has been widely used particularly in patients over 60 years of age. A number of studies agree on this efficacy, but opinion is divided as to whether there is any effect on the frequency of postherpetic neuralgia (Huff et al., 1993; Wood, 1994).

The drug that has proved in many studies to be the most effective for treatment of established postherpetic neuralgia is amitriptyline, a blocker of both norepinephrine and serotonin reuptake. The lack of efficacy of drugs that more specifically block serotonin reuptake suggests that its primary effect on the treatment of postherpetic neuralgia is the effect on norepinephrine reuptake (Max, 1994). Anesthetic and surgical therapeutic approaches to postherpetic neuralgia have been of limited value (Portenoy et al., 1986).

EPSTEIN–BARR VIRUS

Epstein–Barr virus is the major cause of infectious mononucleosis, as well as an occasional cause of respiratory disease in children and the probable cause of Burkitt's lymphoma and nasopharyngeal carcinoma and possibly CNS T-cell lymphomas (see Chapter 15). The virus was originally isolated from cells grown from a Burkitt's lymphoma (Epstein et al., 1964). Several years later, a technician working with the virus in a virology laboratory developed infectious mononucleosis, and her convalescent serum showed a rise in antibody titer against the agent. Subsequent serologic and virologic isolation studies conclusively established the virus as the cause of heterophil-positive infectious mononucleosis and of about 10% of heterophil-negative cases (Henle et al.,

1968). Cytomegalovirus, human herpesvirus 6, HIV, and adenoviruses, as well as *Toxoplasma gondii*, may cause heterophil-negative infectious mononucleosis.

Epstein–Barr virus is structurally similar to herpes simplex virus. Laboratory propagation is difficult because only primate lymphocytes can be infected, and very little extracellular virus is released. To culture the virus, lymphocytes are grown from cord blood that is free of antibody; after exposure to inoculum containing the virus, cells show accelerated growth. Only the B lymphocytes have virus receptors, and they are the major sites for replication. The virus produces a number of antigens, and the immune responses to various antigens does, in part, differentiate acute from chronic from reactivated infection, in contrast to the situation with other herpesviruses.

Epidemiology

Serologic surveys have shown that Epstein–Barr virus has a worldwide distribution and appears to be spread solely from human to human. In underdeveloped countries, nearly all children are infected in the first year of life. In the United States, approximately 50% of college students are still free of antibody. This is important, because childhood infections usually are asymptomatic, and infectious mononucleosis is primarily the result of adolescent or adult infection.

Epidemiologic studies have suggested that the virus is spread in saliva. Although potentially it can be acquired from shared drinking containers, intimate oral contact ("kissing of more than filial intensity") often is incriminated in its transmission (Hoagland, 1969). This explains the low contact rate among roommates of the same sex and a low contact rate in families, where only about 10% of susceptibles acquire infection. In contrast, a history of intimate kissing with a seropositive partner is common. Seasonal variation is not seen except under special circumstances, such as those at the U.S. Military Academy, where a sudden increased incidence was observed 1 to 2 months after Christmas and summer leaves. Infectious mononucleosis affects the sexes equally, but it occurs earlier in girls (mean age, 16) than in boys (mean age, 18). It is more common in higher socioeconomic groups, such as college students and white-collar workers, who were sheltered from early asymptomatic childhood infection.

Disease Description

The incubation period of infectious mononucleosis is 4 to 7 weeks. The virus can be isolated from the pharynx in approximately 80% of symptomatic patients, and it may be persistently shed for many months, with recurrent shedding over years. About 20% of seropositive persons are shedding at one time point, and over 50% of persons immunosuppressed for organ transplants are shedding. Virus is also present in the lymph nodes.

The classic clinical triad of infectious mononucleosis is fever, pharyngitis, and lymphadenopathy. Petechial hemorrhages are sometimes seen on the hard palate. Approximately 50% of patients have splenomegaly; only 10% have hepatomegaly, but a majority have abnormalities on liver function tests. Atypical lymphocytes are frequently found on blood smears; however, these lymphocytes do not represent the infected B cells that proliferate during the first week of infection but rather natural killer and T cells that are activated between weeks 2 and 4. Some patients are anergic during the T-cell proliferation; abnormalities of B-cell function are less common, but acquired hypogammaglobulinemia has followed infectious mononucleosis (Provisor et al., 1975). An X-linked proliferative disorder in some boys leads to fulminant mononucleosis after Epstein–Barr virus infection. Other complications of infectious mononucleosis include pneumonia, myocarditis, nephritis, autoimmune hemolysis or thrombocytopenic purpura, and varied neurologic disorders (Khanna et al., 1995).

In patients with typical clinical signs, an absolute lymphocytosis with more than 10% atypical cells, and a high heterophile antibody titer, the likelihood of primary Epstein–Barr virus infection is over 90%. Heterophile antibody is not directed against viral components and can develop in other inflammatory diseases and therefore is not specific for Epstein–Barr virus infections. Furthermore, approximately 10% of cases of Epstein–Barr virus infectious mononucleosis in adolescents and adults are heterophile negative, and this rate is even higher in childhood infections. Virus is difficult to recover and only very rarely has been recovered from the spinal fluid or CNS tissue (Schiff et al., 1982). Recovery of virus from the throat is of dubious significance, because the virus may persist for many months after an initial infection. Because virus is latent in B cells and can be activated during the course of other diseases, isolation from blood or even demonstration of some antibody responses may only reflect activation.

Viral antibody responses are complex. IgM against the virus capsid antigen (anti-VCA) develops promptly, persists for weeks, and usually does not appear with reactivation, so its presence is presumptive evidence of recent primary infection. IgG anti-VCA rises and falls during acute infection but persists for life. Antibody against early antigens (anti-EA) develops in most primary infections and wanes with time. Antibody against Epstein–Barr nuclear antigen (anti-EBNA) develops late, so its absence may suggest ongoing infection. Interpretations of serologic results, however, are fraught with problems. Persistence of anti-EA, unusually high titers of IgG anti-VCA, and absence of anti-EBNA are found in the lymphoproliferative disease that can follow Epstein–Barr virus infections, but these same findings can be seen in other patients with impaired cellular immunity (Straus et al., 1993). Furthermore, most of these tests are performed with immunofluorescence, leading to subjective differences among technicians and between test cells on different days. Comparing results done on different days or by different laboratories is not valid.

Even detection of Epstein–Barr virus DNA by PCR requires careful interpretation. If techniques are sufficiently sensitive, the normal latent DNA in B lymphocytes may give a meaningless positive result; in immunocompromised seropositive individuals, more Epstein–Barr virus-infected cells are found in blood. What is needed, particularly in evaluating neurologic diseases that are not temporally associated with typical infectious mononucleosis, is some *in situ* assay to determine specific cell infection (Pedneault et al., 1992).

Neurologic Complications

Neurologic complications occur during Epstein–Barr virus infections. Headache is almost universal during symptomatic infections. Stiff neck is fairly common but may be symptomatic of the marked cervical adenopathy rather than meningeal irritation. Routine spinal fluid examination frequently shows a pleocytosis and protein elevation (Gautier-Smith, 1965). The frequency of clinical neurologic complications in mononucleosis is difficult to determine: over 5% of hospitalized patients have been reported to have abnormal neurologic findings (Silverstein et al., 1972), but in nonhospitalized patients the incidence of such findings is probably less than 1%. On the other hand, neurologic complications are the commonest causes of the rare deaths during infectious mononucleosis, being more frequent than splenic rupture (Penman, 1970).

The reported neurologic complications include aseptic meningitis, encephalitis, optic neuritis, cranial nerve palsies, cerebellar ataxia, transverse myelitis, Guillain–Barré syndrome, and acute autonomic neuropathy (Connelly and DeWitt, 1994; Bennett et al., 1996). When these complications occur during heterophile-positive infectious mononucleosis, it is reasonable to assume an association. The onset of Mollaret's recurrent meningitis during classic infectious mononucleosis also has been reported (Graman, 1987). Many neurologic abnormalities have been described in the absence of the typical disease, and in these cases serologic analysis must be scrutinized carefully. In primary infection, early acute-phase serum should show high levels of antibody to VCA, the presence of the anti-EA or virus-specific IgM antibody (or both), and the absence of antibody to EBNA, but it is important to show a fourfold or greater decrement in anti-VCA or anti-EA antibodies or both or a late decline in anti-VCA or loss of anti-EA antibodies to EBNA in subsequent serum specimens. Furthermore, comparisons of early and late sera must be in the same test because of the aforementioned variables. Using these criteria, Grose and colleagues (1975) documented primary Epstein–Barr virus infections in 7 of 24 patients with Guillain–Barré syndrome, 3 of 16 patients with Bell's palsy, several patients with meningoencephalitis, and 2 patients with transverse myelitis.

The pathogenesis of the diverse neurologic complications is unknown. Some autopsies have shown perivascular mononuclear cells in the brain and inflammatory infiltrates in peripheral nerves (Ricker et al., 1947). Others have shown only cerebral congestion or edema, or have shown inflammatory demyelinating lesions that suggest an autoimmune encephalitis (Ambler et al., 1971). The occasional demonstration of exceedingly high levels of antibody to Epstein–Barr virus in cerebrospinal fluid of patients with cerebellar ataxia or transverse myelitis favors direct viral invasion of the CNS (Lascelles et al., 1973; Feinberg et al., 1984), as does the presence of Epstein–Barr DNA in brain tissue and spinal fluid in patients with encephalitis and myelitis complicating infectious mononucleosis (Pedneault et al., 1992; Landgren et al., 1994; Tselis et al., 1997). The data suggest that some complications are due to direct Epstein–Barr virus infection of CNS and others are postinfectious autoimmune demyelinating diseases of CNS and peripheral nerves (see Chapter 8).

In summary, varied neurologic complications occur during the course of primary Epstein–Barr virus infections, and these clearly can take the diverse forms of aseptic meningitis, encephalitis, acute cerebellar ataxia, cranial nerve palsies, and Guillain–Barré syndrome (DeSimone and Snyder, 1978). However, the problems of serologic diagnosis and the uncertain significance of virus recovery or viral DNA detection make it impossible to determine the frequency of such complications. Activation of the virus during intercurrent infections or disease obscures the possible role of Epstein–Barr virus in chronic or recurrent neurologic disease.

CYTOMEGALOVIRUS

Cytomegaloviruses are species-specific herpesviruses that cause a distinctive cytopathologic enlargement of host cells, with intranuclear and cytoplasmic inclusion bodies. Human cytomegalovirus is a ubiquitous agent that is a major cause of serious diseases in infected fetuses and immunosuppressed patients. As with Epstein–Barr virus, latency is established in hematogenous cells, but the nature of latency is less well defined and may primarily involve monocytes (Taylor-Wiedeman et al., 1991). Also, like Epstein–Barr virus, this agent is activated nonspecifically, with frequent presence in saliva, breast milk, semen, vaginal secretions, and blood. Relating the virus to disease causes similar dilemmas, except in tissue sections where the distinctive cytopathologic findings are found.

Antibody to human cytomegalovirus is found in 50% to 90% of adults. About 1% are infected *in utero*; in an urban American population, 25% are infected by age 2, with higher rates in infants who were breast-fed, and 33% are seropositive by 10 years of age (Yow et al., 1986). Serologic surveys show a rather steady rate of antibody acquisition throughout life, and respiratory or salivary spread is probably of primary importance. In late adolescence and young adult life, however, seroconversion increases, and this is more striking in venereal disease clinic patients and absent in celibates, suggesting venereal transmission. About 40% to 50% of women of childbearing age are still seronegative, and approximately 2% to 2.5% have primary infections during pregnancy, with high rates of transmission to the fetus. Reactivation also is common in pregnancy, and 10% of pregnant women have virus in cervical secretions and 3% to 6% in urine (Stagno et al., 1975). The most dramatic and important clinical diseases caused by cytomegalovirus result from fetal infections and are discussed in Chapter 13.

In healthy adolescents and adults, primary infection can cause an infectious-mononucleosis-like syndrome, with fever, atypical lymphocytes, and abnormal liver function test results. Pharyngitis and lymphadenopathy are usually less prominent. Thrombocytopenia and anemia can occur. Cytomegalovirus is a common cause of these signs after blood transfusions and in the "postperfusion syndrome." In immunosuppressed patients, cytomegalovirus infections cause fever, leukopenia, pneumonitis, and hepatitis and are major causes of death. This is assumed to represent an activation of latent virus, but it could represent primary infection or exogenous reinfection.

Cytomegalovirus has been implicated in several acute neurologic syndromes in immunocompetent adolescents and adults. During cytomegalovirus mononucleosis, 5% of patients have been reported to have meningitis, encephalitis, or Guillain–Barré syndrome (Cohen and Corey, 1985); this is a similar frequency and spectrum of diseases reported in Epstein–Barr virus infectious mononucleosis. These illnesses have been documented by isolations of cytomegalovirus from spinal fluid of patients with meningitis and encephalitis (Studahl et al., 1994) and from brain biopsy of one patient with encephalitis (Phillips et al., 1977). We reported the case of a patient with recurrent focal signs and a pleocytosis who had recurrent increases in anticytomegalovirus antibodies (Richert et al., 1987). The problem of causation, as in other herpesvirus infections, is confounded by the nonspecific activation of cytomegalovirus. For example, two patients with acute meningitis have been described with significant increases in antibody to cytomegalovirus and coxsackievirus B5, which raises the possibility that an enterovirus meningitis can activate cytomegalovirus (Klemola et al., 1967). The same explanation is applicable to other reports in which increases in antibody to cytomegalovirus have been documented. Similarly, isolation of virus from the throat or the urine of a patient with meningitis, encephalitis, or neuritis (Chin et al., 1973; Duchowny et al., 1979) fails to establish a causal role, because this could represent nonspecific reactivation or simply chronic secretion of virus.

Many attempts have been made to incriminate cytomegalovirus in the Guillain–Barré syndrome. In a number of patients, the virus has been isolated from throat or urine (Leonard and Tobin, 1971), and IgM antibody against cytomegalovirus has been found in sera of 10 of 94 patients with Guillain–Barré syndrome (Schmitz and Enders, 1977). Although virus isolation or IgM antibody is evidence for active infection, IgM antibodies may reappear in reactivated infections (Schmitz et al., 1977), and in one study 27% of healthy seropositive individuals were found to have anticytomegalovirus IgM (McVoy and Adler, 1989), so neither finding establishes primary infection. During the course of the Guillain–Barré syndrome, activated lymphocytes are found in blood that incorporate radiolabeled thymidine, presumably in preparation for mitotic activity. In mice, cytomegalovirus harbored in B cells can be activated nonspecifically with B-cell mitogens (Olding et al., 1975). Since activated mononuclear cells are present in the blood of patients with the Guillain–Barré syndrome, similar activation by other agents or mitogens could account for the serologic results seen in these patients (see Chapter 8).

In immunocompromised patients, CNS infection with cytomegalovirus is more obvious and intense. Invasion of the CNS by cytomegalovirus is frequent during immunosuppression for the maintenance of organ allografts. Characteristic cytomegalic cells are found in the brains of many patients who die after renal or cardiac transplantation, but neurologic findings may not be noted ante-mortem (Schneck, 1965; Schober and Herman, 1973). In a series examined retrospectively, however, confusion, acute psychotic reaction, disturbance of consciousness, tremor of the limbs, and spastic quadriparesis appeared to correlate with neuropathologic evidence of cytomegalovirus infection (Dorfman, 1973). The pathologic changes in these patients were not dramatic: numerous scattered glial nodules were found, particularly in the gray matter, and infrequently cytomegalic cells were found within these glial aggregates. Inflammation usually was minimal.

All human herpesviruses exhibit activation during HIV infections, but none as dramatically or frequently as cytomegalovirus. These complications include two syndromes with distinct clinical and pathologic features: cytomegalovirus ventriculoencephalitis and polyradiculomyelopathy. Cytomegalovirus retinitis is the most frequent neurologic complication, occurring in nearly 20% of patients with AIDS. Evidence of cytomegalovirus infection in brain has been found in 11% of 347 consecutive autopsies in our studies and in up to 50% in other studies (Wiley et al., 1986). Most of these patients have diffuse micronodular encephalitis, with scattered microglial nodules containing cytomegalic cells or viral antigen. The uncertainty of clinical correlates and the paucity of inflammation are similar to the issues in transplant patients. A recent comparison of patients with cytomegalovirus micronodular encephalitis with patients with HIV-associated dementia without opportunistic infections suggested that those with cytomegalovirus disease were more severely immunodeficient, had more rapid onset of dementing disease, and were more likely to have delirium and focal neurologic signs (Holland et al., 1994). Cytomegalovirus retinitis and viremia are also more common in patients with cytomegalovirus encephalitis.

Ventriculoencephalitis is clinically and pathologically distinct from the micronodular encephalitis (McCutchan, 1995). In advanced stages of immunodeficiency, this acute illness is characterized by lethargy, cranial nerve palsies, ventriculomegaly with subependymal enhancement on imaging studies, and striking inflammation in the spinal fluid, often with polymorphonuclear cells and a depressed glucose concentration (Kalayjian et al., 1993; Salazar et al., 1995). Periventricular enhancement is common, but ring-enhancing space-occupying lesions on magnetic resonance imaging may mimic tumors (Moulignier et al., 1996). Pathologically, necrosis of ependyma and subependymal regions suggests a fulminant centrifugal infection from ventricles rather than the diffuse, presumably hematogenous, spread of virus seen in nodular encephalitis (Wiley et al.,

1986). Vasculitis with hemorrhagic lesions and infarction has also been found (Golden et al., 1994).

Direct cytomegalovirus infection of peripheral nerves occurs in AIDS, causing mononeuritis multiplex with necrotizing vasculitis of epineural arteries (Said et al., 1991). A unique lumbosacral root and cord involvement is called cytomegalovirus polyradiculomyelopathy. Patients develop ascending motor weakness, lower extremity areflexia, loss of sphincter control, painful saddle paresthesias, and variable sensory loss. Polymorphonuclear cell pleocytosis and hypoglyorrhachia are seen (Cohen et al., 1993). Imaging of cord may show swelling of the conus medullaris. The localization has suggested that this infection may result from an ascending neuritis originating from cytomegalovirus proctitis.

Detection of cytomegalovirus DNA by PCR in cerebrospinal fluid has proved helpful in the diagnosis of encephalitis and polyradiolmyelitis. The response of cytomegalovirus encephalitis, myelitis, and neuritis to ganciclovir or foscasnet has been variable. Some have improved, some have developed while the patient was on antivirals for treatment of retinitis, and others have progressed while on treatment (Cinque et al., 1995; Cohen, 1996). With the exception of retinitis, guidelines for treatment of cytomegalovirus infections in AIDS are not resolved (McCutchan, 1995).

HUMAN HERPESVIRUSES 6 AND 7

Human herpesviruses 6 and 7 are newly recovered agents. Human herpesvirus 6 was initially recovered from peripheral blood cells of patients with immunodeficiencies. The agent has a genetic organization and sequence similar to cytomegalovirus. Infection usually occurs in infancy and has been associated with childhood exanthem subitum (rosiola infantum) (Yamanishi et al., 1988). Up to one-third of first febrile seizures in children under 2 years of age have been related to herpesvirus 6 infections (Hall et al., 1994). Virus remains latent in mononuclear cells, predominantly T cells, and possibly in the brain (Luppi et al., 1994). A number of infants with exanthem subitum develop meningitis and encephalitis, including several fatal cases (Asano et al., 1992; Suga et al., 1993). Viral sequences have been shown in spinal fluid of these infants by PCR. One HIV-infected infant developed fulminant fatal encephalitis, and herpesvirus 6 was shown to be widespread in all cell types by immunocytochemistry (Knox et al., 1995).

Subsequently, human herpesvirus 6 has been associated with disease in older children and adults. Of patients with non-Epstein Barr–noncytomegalovirus heterophile-negative mononucleosis-like illnesses, 30% showed serologic evidence of active herpesvirus 6 infection (Steeper et al., 1990). In a retrospective study of 138 patients with focal encephalitis in which herpes simplex virus had been suspected but unverified, 9 had herpesvirus 6 DNA detected by PCR in spinal fluid (McCullers et al., 1995). Since the virus has been alleged to persist in the

CNS and the mononuclear cells, the specificity of this test in encephalitis needs verification. Immunocytochemical staining has demonstrated herpesvirus 6 antigen in tissues of an elderly woman with a 2-year history of myelopathy and a 27-year-old woman with a subacute leukoencephalitis of 13 months' duration (Mackenzie et al., 1995; Carrigan et al., 1996). Fatal encephalitis also has been reported in an adult following bone marrow transplantation, with viral antigen predominantly in glial cells of white matter (Drobyski et al., 1994).

Human herpesvirus 7 has also been recovered from T lymphocytes and also may cause exanthem subitum and possibly similar neurologic complications (Torigoe et al., 1995). Human herpesvirus 8 (Kaposi's sarcoma-associated herpesvirus) has not yet been associated with neurologic disease.

A Cautionary Note

In the preceding chapter, the acute meningitides and encephalitides of humans were more straightforward. Acute CNS infections with human, zoonotic, and arthropod-borne RNA viruses are rather two-dimensional: characteristic clinical presentations; helpful ancillary data on season, exposure, or immunization; ease of serologic or virologic diagnosis; and straightforward outcomes of recovery with or without sequelae or death.

The latency and nonspecific reactivations of all herpesviruses pose knotty problems in relating these viruses to diseases, because shedding of virus or renewed antigenic stimulation may only reflect the stress induced by other illnesses. The repeatedly documented presence of virus in appropriate cells convincingly links herpes simplex viruses with neonatal and adult encephalitis, zoster with ganglionitis and encephalomyelitis, and cytomegaloviruses with disease in the neonate and rare cases of encephalitis in healthy adults as well as immunosuppressed patients. The more discriminating serologic methods sometimes can tie primary Epstein–Barr virus infections to various neurologic diseases.

Of the alleged associations of human herpesviruses with Guillain–Barré syndrome, cancer, chronic fatigue syndrome, multiple sclerosis, atherosclerosis, and schizophrenia, one or more may be true. However, the ubiquitous presence of these agents, common contamination from the oropharynx of medical and laboratory personnel, the capricious serologic responses, and the interactions with other agents all contribute to ambiguous findings. True to their propensity to reactivate, herpesviruses will keep reappearing in subsequent chapters.

SUPPLEMENTARY BIBLIOGRAPHY

Roizman B, Whitley RJ, Lopez, C. *The human herpesviruses.* New York: Raven Press, 1993.

7

Rabies

Finally there appears a symptom practically constant in established rabies in man, the horror of water. The sight of this liquid often suffices to bring on a general tremor; but it is, above all, when the patient wishes to bring water to his lips that this special horror comes on, those convulsions of the face and of the entire body which make such a vivid impression on those who witness an attack. The rabid man completely preserves his reason; he is thirsty; he wishes to drink, he bids his hand carried to his lips the vessel filled with liquid, but no sooner does it touch him that the unhappy creature withdraws terrified, sometimes he cries out that he cannot drink; his face shows agony, his eyes are fixed, his features contracted; then his limbs shake and his body quivers. The crisis lasts several seconds, gradually calm seems to return, at the least contact, even a breath of air, suffices to start a new crisis, such is the hypersensitivity of the skin. He cannot wash hands or face or comb his hair without being menaced by convulsions ...

A. Trouseau,
Clinique Medical de l'Hôtel-Dieu de Paris, 1865
(translated by Bloomfield, 1958)

He walked erratically, as if his right legs were shorter than his left legs. He reminded me of a car stuck in a sandbed ... I thought mad dogs foamed at the mouth, galloped, leaped and lunged at throats, and I thought they did it in August. Had Tim Johnson [the dog] behaved thus, I would have been less frightened. Nothing is more deadly than a deserted, waiting street. The trees were still, the mockingbirds were silent.

Harper Lee,
To Kill a Mockingbird, 1960

The images of rabies in humans or animals evoke a unique horror—whether they are the 18th-century tales of mad dogs running through the streets of London or the more recent descriptions of wolf attacks on entire villages in the Middle East, the stealthful feeding of vampire bats on sleeping Trinidadians, or my own memories of a quiet afternoon in Cleveland, Ohio, several years ago when a rabid fox ran amuck from yard to yard, attacking suburbanites. Rabies is unique in its mode of transmission by biting, its spread to the CNS along nerves, its long incubation period, its bizarre clinical manifestations, and its almost universally fatal outcome.

Rabies virus is a rhabdovirus, a group of negative-strand RNA viruses with a distinctive bullet shape. Antigenically, rabies virus differs from the other major rhabdoviruses, such as vesicular stomatitis virus of cattle, but several viruses that are antigenically related to rabies have been found in bats, shrews, midges, and arthropods in Africa and in bats in Europe and fruit bats in Australia. These rabieslike viruses have more limited host ranges, but several have been related to human disease (Familusi et al., 1972; Rupprecht et al., 1995; Hemachudha and Phuapradit, 1997). Rabies virus can grow in a wide variety of cell cultures, but it is generally noncytopathic, a curious feature in view of the fatal outcome of infection in virtually all warm-blooded animals. Susceptibility is variable between species, in terms of their ability to be infected, the periods of virus latency and infectivity, and in their efficiency in transmission because of variable salivary excretion, degrees of aggressive behavior with infection, and propensity to bite.

ECOLOGY

Rabies virus continues to be endemic in all continents of the world except Antarctica, although it has been excluded or eliminated by rigid quarantine from some island populations, such as those of New Zealand, Japan, Hawaii, and Great Britain. Over 35,000 persons die of rabies each year, and in India alone there are over 25,000 cases. In most countries of Asia, Africa, and South America, dogs are the major reservoir of rabies; dog and cat bites account for over 90% of the world's cases of human rabies. In specific areas, other species also play a significant role in epizootic transmission, such as the mongooses and meerkats of South Africa, the pariah dogs and jackals of Southeast Asia, and the cattle and vampire bats of South America. During the 19th and early 20th centuries, dogs and cats were the major carriers of rabies in the United States; the peak year of reported human cases was 1890, with 143 fatal human cases, and number of reported canine cases peaked in 1944 at over 9,000.

Since World War II, programs to eliminate stray dogs and immunize pets in North America and Europe have led to a near eradication of urban rabies, but rabies cannot be totally eliminated, because the virus is sustained in wild carnivores and bats. Thus, with the control of dog rabies in North America and Europe, the primary reservoirs and sources of human infection have shifted to wild animals. From 1980 to 1997, only 34 cases of fatal human rabies have been reported in the United States, and 14 of these were acquired from exposures outside the country or along the Texas–Mexico border [Centers for Disease Control (CDC), 1995c and 1996a].

Historically, foxes and wolves have represented the major sylvatic reservoirs of rabies virus, and they are efficient transmitters of the disease. Foxes are affected throughout Northern Europe (with the exception of Great Britain and the Scandinavian Peninsula) and in several areas of the United States and all of Canada and Alaska. Epizootics of rabies in arctic foxes remain a problem with attacks on sled dogs. In the continental United States, fox rabies poses a problem in upstate New York, bordering on the Canadian epizootic area, and in central Texas, where coyotes are also involved. For unknown reasons, fox rabies in Europe is spreading and in the United States it is declining. Indeed, fox rabies now accounts for less than 15% of the wildlife rabies in the United States and accounts for fewer isolates than those from skunks, raccoons, or bats (Fig. 7.1).

During the 1980s, skunks became the predominant reservoir of wildlife rabies in the United States, and skunk bites resulted in a number of human deaths. Rabies has been found in pet skunks, including some allegedly bred in captivity.

Since 1990, the raccoon has been the most frequent sylvatic host, and the movement of this epizootic has been dramatic. A focus of raccoon rabies in Georgia and Florida had been recognized for many years. From 1971 to 1977, raccoons from this area were transported to Virginia to replenish hunting stocks (Rupprecht et al., 1995). The newly established focus in Virginia crossed the Potomac into Maryland in 1981 and spread north, crossing the Hudson River into Connecticut in 1991. New York and New Jersey now represent the centers of raccoon rabies (CDC, 1994a). In 1997, it crossed the Appalachian Mountains into Ohio. Although the epizootic has moved south into the Carolinas, the predominant northern movement of the epizootic is puzzling.

The semidomesticated behavior of raccoons that thrive on urban garbage puts them in frequent contact with humans and their domestic pets. Although no

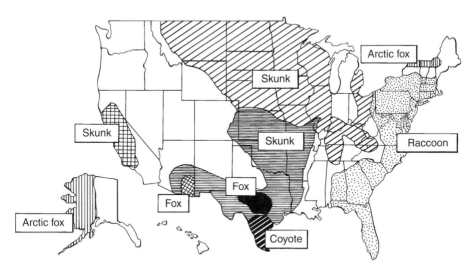

FIG. 7.1. Distribution of major terrestrial mammal reservoirs of rabies in the United States. The Florida–Georgia focus of raccoon rabies has recently converged in the Carolinas with the Northeast focus, but the sequence and antigenic similarities confirm the common origin of these variants. The same arctic fox rabies variant is present in both Alaska and northern New England and across Canada. Three distinct variants are present in skunks involving large regions, and two different fox variants are found in small regions in the southwestern gray foxes. The coyote focus in southern Texas is a spillover of dog rabies. Hawaii remains rabies free. (Modified from Krebs et al., 1995.)

human case of rabies as yet has been attributed to a raccoon bite, the greatest threat of the spreading raccoon epizootic is the reintroduction of rabies into dogs and cats.

The foolishness of translocation of raccoon rabies to the Northeast apparently did not deter hunters, since coyote rabies from Texas recently was transported into Florida fox-hunting pens, with a resultant canine rabies outbreak (CDC, 1995d). Other urban animals, such as squirrels and rats, remain a concern, because they are susceptible. In Europe, rare isolates of rabies from squirrels and brown rats have been reported, but the rats and squirrels of North America have not, as yet, been involved, and bites from these animals do not warrant postexposure therapy.

The insectivorous bat is a relatively new or newly recognized reservoir of rabies virus. Derriengue, the limping illness of cattle, has plagued Latin America since colonial times. Early in this century, this disease was recognized to be paralytic rabies transmitted by vampire bats, but human disease from bat bites was unobserved or unappreciated. In 1929 and 1930, over 100 cases of ascending flaccid paralysis occurred in Trinidad. Initially, poliomyelitis was suspected, but pathologic examinations revealed Negri bodies. The vampire bat was implicated as the vector by epidemiologic studies (Hurst and Pawan, 1932). Apparently, the hematophagous bats slipped through the open eaves of houses at night and drank blood from the feet or toes of sleeping victims, often without even arousing them. Vampire bats do not exist north of the Mexican border. In 1953, a 7-year-old boy in Florida was looking for a baseball in shrubs when a bat attacked and clung to his chest. This insectivorous bat was examined for rabies and found to be positive; the boy, after postexposure treatment, remained well. Since that dramatic incident, many species of bats throughout North America and, indeed, in other areas of the world have been found to harbor rabies virus, and human cases of rabies in North America, Europe, Africa, and India have been associated with bites of insectivorous bats. Bat-associated variants of rabies virus have been found in 17 of the 34 cases of human rabies in the United States since 1980, yet a history of bat contact was obtained in only 7 of the 17 cases and a definite history of a bat bite in only one (CDC, 1996a).

Using monoclonal antibodies and, more recently, sequence data, rabies virus variants can be defined that are specific to geographic locations and species. In the United States, eight variants are found in terrestrial mammals with restricted species and geographic distributions (Krebs et al., 1995) (Fig. 7.1). Eight variants are found in bats, and bat rabies is distributed across the contiguous 48 states. The silver-hair bat variant has been identified in a number of recent fatal human cases even though a history of bat bites was missing. Even more puzzling is the relative rarity of this bat species, the uncommon documentations of rabies in this species, and this bat's solitary lifestyle where transmission would be less likely than among communal cave bats that bite one another as they back into the bat horde (Morimoto et al., 1996).

Rabies is a zoonotic disease, and transmission from human to human has not been well documented. There are old anecdotal tales of a Victorian gentleman who allegedly developed rabies after being bitten while kissing the scullery maid, and of a nursing rabid mother who allegedly transmitted disease to her infant. Recently in Ethiopia, parallel anecdotes have been reported of rabies in a mother bitten by her rabid 5-year-old son and rabies in a 5-year-old child after repeatedly being kissed by a rabid dying mother (Fekadu et al., 1996). Indeed, human transmission is a potential threat, because virus is present in saliva of patients with clinical rabies.

Rare transmission of rabies by routes other than animal inoculation has occurred. Airborne transmission among humans was first suspected when two men developed rabies after exploring Frio Cave in Texas, and both denied being bitten by bats. Subsequently, animals placed in caves in bat-proof cages contracted rabies by the respiratory route presumably from the atmosphere heavily contaminated with bat excreta (Constantine, 1971). Further cases of presumed respiratory transmission of rabies virus have occurred among laboratory workers exposed to aerosols of the virus. Both of these men had received preexposure immunization against rabies; in the one fatal case, no demonstrable serum antibody had developed (Winkler et al., 1973), whereas, in the investigator who survived with severe sequelae, postimmunization antibodies had been documented (CDC, 1977).

Even more bizarre are recent reports of rabies in recipients of corneal transplants. The donor for the first case was a patient in Idaho who had no known exposure to rabies. The donor died of presumed Guillain–Barré syndrome, which in retrospect proved to be rabies (Houff et al., 1979). Five subsequent cases have been reported, including an instance in which two corneas from a single rabid donor transmitted disease to two recipients (CDC, 1980a).

PATHOGENESIS

After experimental inoculation analogous to the bite, rabies virus has been shown to infect individual muscle cells near the site of inoculation, including the muscle spindle, giving virus access to endings of both the sensory and the motor nerve fibers (Murphy, 1977). The acetylcholine receptor may serve as a rabies virus receptor in muscle (Lentz et al., 1982), but movement along noncholinergic pathways indicates that it is not the sole receptor (Kucera et al., 1985). The long or variable incubation period of rabies appears to be determined, in large part, by persistent infection of muscle fibers before ascending in the nerves (Baer and Cleary, 1972).

Invasion of the CNS via nerves is well documented (Johnson, 1970a; Murphy, 1977) and appears to occur by rapid axonal transport to the soma of sensory or motor neurons where virus can be replicated (see Chapter 3). In electron-microscopic studies of infected mice, replication is seen in perikaryon and dendritic processes of neurons (Johnson and Mercer, 1964). Presumably, the early involvement of the dorsal root ganglia correlates with the dysesthesias at the site of the bite often seen during the prodrome of clinical rabies. After invasion of the CNS, virus is rapidly disseminated along axonal pathways utilizing the neuronal microtubulin network, and spread is inhibited by colchicine (Ceccaldi et al., 1989).

In some virus host systems, early selective infection of specific neuronal populations is seen, with localization to neurons of the limbic system and relative sparing of neocortex (Johnson, 1965a); this or specific functional effects on infected neurons provide a fascinating clinical–pathologic correlate. The alertness, loss of natural timidity, abnormal sexual behavior, and aggressiveness that typify furious rabies represent a diabolical adaptation of virus to selected neuronal populations—neurons capable of driving the host in a fury to transmit the virus to another host animal. By natural selection, strains that cause paralytic or dumb rabies are not maintained in nature. Eventually, widespread infection of neurons leads to terminal coma.

After involvement of the CNS, virus is transmitted centrifugally along nerves to the neural cells of the gut, retina, pancreas, adrenals, muscle spindles, urinary bladder, papilla of the tongue, the cornea, and hair follicles (Fischman and Schaeffer, 1971). The latter localizations permit corneal smears, buccal mucosal biopsies, or hair follicle biopsies as methods for premortem diagnosis. Biopsy of the skin on the neck, with immunohistochemical staining for rabies antigens in the hair follicles, has proved to be a reliable rapid diagnostic test during the late clinical stage (Warrell et al., 1988). The biologically important centrifugal spread, of course, is to salivary glands. This spread is along nerves, and denervation of one salivary gland in the dog will selectively prevent its infection (Dean et al., 1963). In the salivary glands, virus replicates primarily in acinar cells, with budding of virions directly into the salivary ducts.

In some species, including laboratory rodents, rabies virus may cause paralytic disease and neuronal infection with recovery. Long-term infection with prolonged salivary excretion of virus can occur in bats. These variations in pathogenesis clearly depend on host genetics, route of exposure, and immune responses (Lodmell and Ewalt, 1985), but neurovirulence of the laboratory-attenuated virus strains has been localized to a single amino acid site on the envelope glycoprotein. A single mutation at position 333 can attenuate pathogenicity (Dietzchold et al., 1983; Seif et al., 1985). Viruses with this single amino acid substitution still infect neurons, but they show less efficiency in spread rather than altered topographical distribution of infection (Jackson, 1991).

HUMAN DISEASE

Development of human rabies after an animal bite necessitates that the animal be actively secreting virus in saliva at the time of biting. Nearly 50% of dogs with documented rabies do not have virus in their saliva. Thus, even severe bites about the face lead to rabies in only 60% of untreated persons, and the overall rate of rabies in persons bitten by rabid dogs is only 15%. The likelihood of developing rabies after a bite of a rabid animal depends on the species of animal, location and severity of the bite, and whether the bite is through clothing that mechanically can remove saliva from the teeth. The dog does not excrete virus in saliva longer than 5 to 7 days before the onset of clinical rabies, so quarantine after a bite can determine whether the dog had the potential for salivary infection at the time of the bite. This interval of salivary secretion is not the same for other carnivores, and therefore quarantine and observation of wild animals after a bite is of no use. Indeed, bats may excrete virus for long periods without clinical evidence of rabies.

The incubation period of rabies in humans generally is between 15 days and 1 year. Longer incubation periods have been proposed in the literature but regarded with skepticism; recently, however, three cases of rabies in the United States have occurred in immigrants from Laos, the Philippines, and Mexico, and studies with monoclonal antibodies and amplified viral sequences identified antigenic and genetic characteristics of viruses in their countries of origin and not known strains in the United States. In these three patients, these findings suggest incubation periods of 4 years, 6 years, and 11 months (Smith et al., 1991). The incubation period tends to be shorter after bites on the head than after bites on extremities, and the incubation period is also shorter in children, who represent a large percentage of the cases of rabies. During the last two decades in the United States, almost half of patients with rabies have had no history of a bite.

Clinical rabies begins with a prodromal period of malaise and anorexia, headache, and fever. Over half of the patients have pain or paresthesias at the site of the bite for 1 to 14 days before the onset of other clinical signs. The encephalitic form (furious rabies) often begins with anxiety and nervousness and a paucity of objective findings. Within hours or days, periods of confusion, with bizarre behavior and autonomic signs, such as dilated pupils and piloerection, alternate with lucid periods. As symptoms become more extreme, periods of intense agitation and aggressiveness may alternate with drowsiness. Aerophobia and hydrophobia with pharyngeal and inspiratory diaphragmatic spasms occur in almost all the patients but abate with the onset of terminal coma (Hemachudha, 1989). The paralytic form (dumb rabies) occurs in about 20% of patients, particularly those with bat-transmitted disease. Progressive flaccid paralysis with areflexia and respiratory failure resembles the Guillain–Barré syndrome, except that fever is a constant finding in rabies (Hemachudha, 1994). Signs of classic rabies may be minimal or absent. The regional distribution of virus or intensity of inflammation in the CNS does not appear to account for these different forms of clinical disease (Tirawatnpong et al., 1989), but studies in both humans and mice suggest that host immune responses differ in the encephalitic and paralytic forms of disease (Hemachudha et al., 1988c, 1993; Sugamata et al., 1992; Weiland et al., 1992). The spinal fluid shows mild pleocytosis in only about half of patients, but protein is modestly elevated in most patients.

Anecdotal reports suggest occasional survival following clinical rabies. In addition to the survival of the aforementioned preimmunized laboratory worker, three patients, who developed probable rabies despite postexposure treatment after bites, have reportedly survived. A 7-year-old boy in Ohio (Hattwick et al., 1972), a middle-aged woman in Argentina (Porras et al., 1976), and a 9-year-old boy in Mexico (Alvarez et al., 1994) developed unusual clinical signs of rabies but recovered, with sequelae. The two children survived only after prolonged intensive care. The diagnosis in all patients was based on development of antibody levels to rabies virus in serum and spinal fluid not recorded after injection of vaccine. In the most recent case, intrathecal antirabies antibody synthesis was documented. However, definitive diagnosis was not made by virus recovery or demonstration of antigen on biopsy specimens.

The bland pathologic findings in rabies are in stark contrast to the dramatic clinical disease. The brain appears grossly normal or shows only mild congestion. Histologically, perivascular inflammation can usually be found, but inflammatory cells may be scarce and quite localized. Unlike other encephalitides, tissue necrosis is absent, and neuronophagia is uncommon (Dupont and Earle, 1965). The neuropathology is so minimal that prior to description of the Negri body and the introduction of immunofluorescent staining, the tentative diagnosis in dogs was made by examining their stomachs rather than their brains, looking for sticks and stones as stigmata of their deranged behavior. The Negri body, a neuronal cytoplasmic inclusion of 1 to 7 μ with a dark central inner body, is pathognomonic for rabies virus infection. These inclusions are most readily identified in the neurons of Ammon's horn and in the Purkinje cells of the cerebellum. An additional pathologic finding is a striking proliferation of capsular cells of the dorsal root ganglia. The paucity of cellular pathology has provided hope that intensive care might sustain patients through the formidable clinical illness with minimal sequelae similar to the three patients just described. Unfortunately, heroic measures of intensive care and even intraventricular interferon and intrathecal antirabies immunoglobulin have not led to further reports of survival (Warrell et al., 1976; Merigan et al., 1984; Hemachudha, 1994).

PREVENTION

The most effective prevention of rabies depends on quarantine and immunization of pet dogs and cats and control of strays. Control of the wild animal species is highly problematic. In some European countries, bait laced with an attenuated live virus has been successfully used to control fox rabies by immunization. This specific vaccine strategy would be of little use in the United States, because that attenuated virus has been shown to cause rabies in skunks and to be ineffective in immunization of raccoons. A more promising strategy utilizes recombinant DNA, expressing the surface glycoprotein, G protein, in the vaccinia virus. A large-scale campaign to eradicate fox rabies in southern Belgium employed this vaccine: helicopter drops of this bait over a 2,200-km^2 area achieved remarkable success (Brochier et al., 1991). Control of bat populations is not feasible, but some reduction of contact of humans and domestic animals with bats can be achieved by physically excluding bats from human dwellings and discouraging the capturing or handling of bats.

When a patient reports a bite, first the risk of rabies must be assessed before initiation of postexposure immunization (Table 7.1). Bites of carnivorous animals, such as dogs, cats, foxes, coyotes, raccoons, and skunks, as well as bites of bats, woodchucks, and beavers, may be infective in North America, whereas bites of squirrels, rabbits, mice, hamsters, gerbils, and rats require only local treatment. The behavior of the animal, circumstances of the bite, and the nature of the wound all influence decisions regarding therapy. In countries with widespread canine rabies, provocation of a dog bite probably should not be a factor in the treatment decision (Siwasontiwat et al., 1992).

Local treatment of the bite wound with either soap and water or quaternary ammonium compounds is an effective means of decreasing the risk of rabies. If

TABLE 7.1. *Postexposure prophylaxis for rabies exposure*

Animal	Condition of animal at time of attack	Treatment
Dog and cat	Healthy and available for 10-day observation	None,[a] unless animal develops rabies
	Rabid or suspected rabid	Rabies immune globulin[b] and diploid cell vaccine[c,d]
	Unknown or escaped	Consult public health officials in local area regarding risk
Skunk, bat, fox, raccoon, coyote, bobcat, woodchucks, and other carnivores	Regard as rabid until proved negative by laboratory tests	Rabies immune globulin and diploid cell vaccine
Livestock, rodents, and lagomorphs	—	Consult local public health officials; livestock may be rabid; rodents and lagomorphs are almost never involved

[a]The World Health Organization recommends administration of vaccine immediately for minor bites on uncovered skin, licks over broken skin, or minor scratches or abrasions with no bleeding an administration of rabies immunoglobulin *and* vaccine immediately for single or multiple transdermal bites or scratches or licks over mucosa. Treatment can be stopped if the dog or cat remains healthy through the observation period or if the animal is killed and found to be free of rabies by fluorescent antibody test.

[b]Human rabies immune globulin (HRIG), 20 IU/kg. As much as possible should be infiltrated around the wound(s) as soon as it is cleaned with soap and water; the remaining is given intramuscularly in the gluteal area; if HRIG is unavailable, equine antirabies (40 IU/kg) serum can be used, but serum sickness will develop in some recipients.

[c]Five 1-mL intramuscular injections of human diploid cell vaccine or rabies vaccine, adsorbed (a fetal rhesus lung diploid cell culture vaccine) *not* at the site of HRIG injection and *not* with the same syringe given on days 0, 3, 7, 14, and 28.

[d]In previously vaccinated individuals, HRIG is not given but vaccine 1.0 mL intramuscularly is given on days 0 and 3.

From CDC (1991b).

further postexposure treatment is needed, a combination of active and passive immunization is used. Vaccines induce active immune responses that take 7 to 10 days to develop, but persist for a year or more; immunoglobulins provide immediate passive immunity over the initial few weeks after the exposure. Vaccines have had a long and colorful history, beginning with Pasteur's vaccine, which consisted of mildly attenuated live virus in desiccated rabbit spinal cord. Viruses grown in neural tissue and inactivated with phenol or β-propriolactone have been used for many years but are complicated by allergic reactions to neural antigens. To reduce immune reactions to the CNS proteins, viruses grown in suckling rodent brains or in duck embryo were subsequently used—the former in Latin America and the latter in North America. The former proved to cause severe and often fatal demyelinating polyneuritis, and the latter showed poor antigenicity; therefore, many countries with high rates of rabies continued to use inactivated virus grown in sheep brain or other neural tissue. However, no carefully controlled study of the efficacy of any of these vaccines had been done; it is estimated that the overall rate of 15% of rabies after bites by rabid dogs is reduced by approximately one-half by a complete series of injections.

The development of high-titered inactivated virus vaccine grown in cell cultures has been a major advance, because these vaccines are free of neural antigens and induce excellent immune responses with small numbers of injections. No cases of rabies developed in 45 patients in Iran who received human diploid cell vaccine after being bitten by rabid wolves or dogs, even though one patient was not immunized until 14 days after the bite (Bahmanyar et al., 1976). Only a single patient has been described who developed rabies despite timely and appropriate treatment with human diploid cell vaccine and rabies immune globulin (Shill et al., 1987), although vaccine was administrated into the gluteal rather than the deltoid muscle as recommended. Some minor allergic reactions occur with these vaccines, but they have been free of major neurologic complications, except for three reports of subsequent Guillain–Barré syndrome that may have been fortuitous occurrences (CDC, 1991b).

The use of hyperimmune serum as an adjunct has undergone controlled trials. The most dramatic of these tests occurred in 1954, when a rabid wolf entered an Iranian village and bit 29 persons in succession. The patients were transported immediately to Teheran and given the inactivated nervous tissue vaccine; 17 were also treated with immune serum. In the group receiving serum, there was only one death (6% of the total number or 8% of those with severe wounds), whereas, in the group not receiving immune serum, there were three deaths (25% of the total or 75% of those with severe wounds) (Baltazard and Bahmanyar, 1955). However, the use of hyperimmune horse serum leads to serum sickness in many patients, a problem that can be circumvented by use of human immune rabies globulin obtained primarily from veterinarians who have been given preexposure immunization.

Prior to the introduction of the human diploid cell vaccine, postexposure immunization was attended by significant complications. With the nervous tissue vaccines, approximately 1 in 1,000 developed neurologic complications and 1 in 35,000 died. With the duck embryo vaccine, 1 in 25,000 was reported to have neurologic complications and 1 in 200,000 died (Rubin et al., 1969). Even though only 34 cases of human rabies have occurred in the United States between 1980 and 1997, over 10,000 persons receive postexposure therapy annually. The problems of public panic and cost are not trivial; recently, a single rabid kitten in a New Hampshire pet store led to postexposure treatment of 665 persons at a cost of over 1 million dollars for biologics alone (Noah et al., 1996). In South America over 300,000 persons are treated annually, and in India over 3 million treatments for rabies exposure are reported annually.

The complications of the neural tissue vaccines have taken the form both of an acute perivenular demyelinating encephalomyelitis and an acute Guillain–Barré syndrome with demyelination of the nerve roots and peripheral nerves. With the new vaccines, these complications should become of only historical importance, but these complications of rabies vaccines have given insights into the pathogenesis of other neurologic diseases—the subject of the next chapter.

SUPPLEMENTARY BIBLIOGRAPHY

Baer GM, ed. *The natural history of rabies,* 2nd ed. Boca Raton, FL: CRC Press, 1991.
Hemachudha T. Human rabies: clinical aspects, pathogenesis and potential therapy. *Curr Top Microbiol Immunol* 1994;187:121–143.
Tsiang H. Pathophysiology of rabies virus infection of the nervous system. *Adv Virus Res* 1993;42:375–412.

8

Postinfectious Demyelinating Diseases

> To me, it is a profound biological phenomenon to learn that the tissues of a person or animal can create antibodies that will result in disease or in the death of that person or animal . . . The work I did on demyelinating encephalitis is probably the nicest piece of work I ever did, and it wasn't in virology. To be sure, I was trying to get an answer to what might follow an infection of viruses but it turned out to be a whole new field. Today a lot of people talk a great deal about allergic encephalitis and the ironic part is they don't connect me with it at all.
>
> Tom Rivers,
> *Reflections on a Life in Medicine and Science,* 1967

Experimental allergic (autoimmune) encephalomyelitis was indeed discovered in the 1930s by the patriarch of American virology. Rivers worked extensively with vaccinia virus, and his interest was piqued by the demyelinating encephalomyelitis that occasionally complicated vaccination against smallpox. He noted the similarity to the perivenular demyelination found in fatal "neuroparalytic accidents" complicating rabies vaccines. On the basis of these histologic comparisons, he prepared homogenates of normal rabbit brains that he injected repeatedly into monkeys. After 6 months, several monkeys developed an inflammatory, demyelinating encephalitis simulating postvaccinal encephalomyelitis and the reactions to rabies vaccines (Rivers and Schwentker, 1935). This first induction of experimental autoimmune encephalomyelitis launched the studies from which present concepts of autoimmunity are derived and focused attention on alternative pathways by which viruses can produce disease.

In this chapter, demyelinating diseases of the central and peripheral nervous system are discussed in which there is a clear temporal relationship to infections. These diseases differ from acute meningitis and encephalitis by virtue of the presentation of neurologic signs late in the course of the clinical infection or weeks after recovery. They differ pathologically by the presence of inflammation and demyelination. They differ virologically by the usual failure to isolate viruses from neural tissues. Nevertheless, sundry viruses are sporadically recovered, and clinical or serologic data have implicated antecedent infection with a host of common viruses. Although these postinfectious demyelinating syndromes are associated with viruslike illnesses, the diseases are not specific to viruses. Postinfectious encephalomyelitis can follow immunization and bacterial infections, and the Guillain–Barré syndrome can follow immunization, bacterial infections, surgery, or fever therapy. Despite new information on the pathogenesis of postinfectious demyelinating disease of the central and peripheral nervous systems, gaps still persist in our knowledge of how viral infections trigger these illnesses.

CONSIDERATIONS OF MECHANISMS

Autoimmune Encephalomyelitis and Neuritis

Experimental autoimmune encephalomyelitis became a practical and reproducible experimental disease for investigation after Kabat and associates (1947) found that the encephalomyelitis can be precipitated by a single injection, if the brain tissue is emulsified in Freund's complete adjuvant. In addition, they showed that the acute inflammatory demyelinating disease could be produced with homologous tissue; that is, brain removed from an animal and injected back into the same animal after recovery can cause the disease. Subsequent studies have established experimental autoimmune encephalomyelitis as the prototype autoimmune disease. Several myelin antigens can induce the disease, including specific amino acid sequences of the basic protein and the proteolipid protein of CNS myelin. Both have many common sequences across species. Cellular and humoral immune response to myelin proteins occurs, but the disease can be passively transferred only with sensitized lymphocytes (Paterson, 1960). In transgenic mice with no mature lymphocytes except CD4 T cells expressing a T-cell receptor specific for myelin basic protein, experimental autoimmune encephalomyelitis develops spontaneously, indicating that CD8, B cells, and antibodies are not critical in disease induction (Lafaille et al., 1994). The fine specificity, major histocompatibility complex restriction, lymphocyte secretion, activation requirements, and T-cell receptor usage of the encephalitogenic T cells have been studied extensively (Martin and McFarland, 1995). Antibodies against myelin basic protein do not passively transfer the disease in animals, but in organotypic cultures these antibodies inhibit myelination and induce demyelination, and passive antibody administration in experimental animals after cell transfer enhances the demyelination.

Experimental autoimmune encephalomyelitis has a latency of 7 to 21 days, similar to classic delayed hypersensitivity responses. Clinically, animals show weakness and paralysis. Histologically, changes in vascular permeability are found first, followed by a mononuclear cell infiltrate consisting of small lymphocytes and macrophages. This is most prominent in a perivenular distribution in the white matter. Demyelination then occurs, with a separation of myelin lamellae and focal vesicular disintegration and with the stripping of myelin by the cytoplasmic projections of macrophages (Lampert, 1978). Experimental autoimmune encephalomyelitis is more readily induced in specific species and in selected inbred strains; the severity and course of disease can be modified not only by changing the species but also by the nature of the inoculum and the age of the inoculated animals. For example, inclusion of pertussis vaccine as adjuvant in the inoculum causes a hyperacute disease in rats that is characterized by acute polymorphonuclear cell infiltrates and hemorrhages (Levine and Wenk, 1965). Use of whole brain as antigen, modification of adjuvant, and selection of specific host ages and strains can lead to a relapsing–remitting form of the disease (Wisniewski and Keith, 1977).

In 1955, Waksman and Adams reported that emulsions of peripheral nerve and adjuvant injected into rabbits led to an acute demyelinating neuropathy, which they termed experimental allergic neuritis. In this experimental disease, the major antigen has proved to be a basic protein (the P2 protein) generated by Schwann cells, and the demyelination again is initiated by cell-mediated immune responses (Arnason and Chelmicka-Szorc, 1972). After a latency period of approximately 2 weeks, the rabbits develop a severe flaccid paralysis, with elevated spinal fluid protein, but few, if any, inflammatory cells in the fluid. Histologic studies have shown that mononuclear cells initially infiltrate around the endoneural venules and that segmental demyelination follows, characterized by vacuolization of myelin and by the stripping of myelin by phagocytic cells. This segmental demyelination, when severe, can be accompanied by wallerian degeneration. A variable degree of accompanying CNS demyelination is seen with the acute neuritis in some species but not in others.

Rabies Vaccine-induced Demyelination

Neurologic complications of postexposure rabies immunization represent the human counterparts of these two experimental diseases. In the 1890s, neuroparalytic accidents were recognized after immunization with Pasteur's attenuated virus vaccine and with initial phenol-inactivated vaccines. It was thought that these neuroparalytic accidents resulted from virus that escaped inactivation or from activation of a second agent latent in the brain. Rivers's demonstrations that the lesions could be reproduced by repeated injection of nervous system tissue alone, coupled with the observation that the neurologic complications in 1 of 300 to 1 of 1,000 vaccinees developed 1 to 3 weeks after the initiation of multiple injections of nervous tissue, provided compelling evidence that the neuroparalytic accidents represented autoimmune encephalomyelitis (Fig. 8.1).

In many countries, rabies vaccines still are prepared from infected adult rabbit, sheep, and goat brain or spinal cord. Our studies of Thai patients with neurologic complications of Semple vaccine showed that their lymphocytes proliferated in the presence of purified myelin (Hemachudha et al., 1987b) and their antibody responses indicated that myelin basic protein was the encephalitogenic antigen in post–rabies vaccine encephalitis and polyneuritis (Hemachuda et al.,

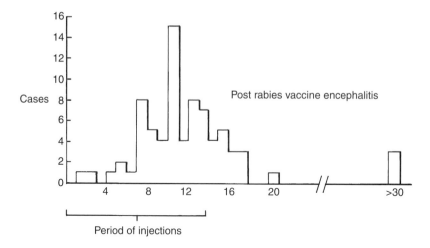

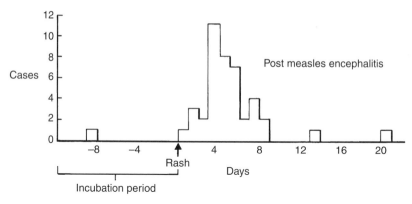

FIG. 8.1. Time of onset of rabies vaccine-induced encephalomyelitis **(top)** and postmeasles encephalomyelitis **(bottom)** measured from the initiation of vaccine injections and the beginning of the inoculation period, respectively. (Modified from Griffin et al., 1989a.)

1987a). As in experimental autoimmune encephalomyelitis, recurrent–relapsing disease is occasionally seen (Hemachuda et al., 1988b).

In an effort to reduce or eliminate the risk of sensitization by myelin proteins, antirabies vaccines have been developed in embryonated eggs and cell cultures. An alternative strategy was employed in South America. Virus was grown in newborn mouse brains, where large quantities of virus can be prepared in a tissue relatively free of myelin. Neurologic complications continued to occur: 1 of 8,000 vaccinees developed disease, with a fatality rate of approximately 22%. Of these vaccine complications, 80% are acute polyradicular neuropathies that resemble Guillain–Barré syndrome, but in our experience those patients had more extensive cranial nerve involvement (Cabrera et al., 1987). Various explanations have been proposed for the altered complications of this vaccine (Held and Adaros, 1972), but the simple explanation is that the vaccine probably contains peripheral nerve myelin. During rapid removal of suckling mouse brains, cranial nerves usually are included, and it would be surprising if these fully myelinated peripheral nerves were not present in the vaccine. Nevertheless, in patients with Guillain–Barré following vaccine made from either suckling mouse brain or mature sheep brain, we were unable to detect antibody to the P2 protein and assumed that some alternative antigen induced the human autoimmune neuritis (Hemachudha et al., 1988a). Inactivated Japanese encephalitis virus vaccine is also prepared in mouse brain, and rare cases of disseminated encephalomyelitis have followed its use (Plesner et al., 1996; Fukuda et al., 1997).

The histologic similarities are remarkable between experimental autoimmune encephalomyelitis and post–rabies vaccine encephalomyelitis and postinfectious encephalomyelitis, as are those between experimental autoimmune neuritis and post–mouse brain vaccine polyneuritis and the Guillain–Barré syndromes. Immunologic studies have strengthened these parallels (Tables 8.1 and 8.2).

TABLE 8.1. *Comparisons of experimental autoimmune encephalomyelitis with encephalomyelitis after rabies vaccine and viral infections*

	Experimental autoimmune encephalomyelitis	Postrabies vaccine encephalomyelitis	Postinfectious encephalomyelitis
Inducing event	Inoculation with CNS tissue or myelin basic protein	Inoculation with CNS tissue	Infection with enveloped viruses
Latent period (days)	10–21	7–42	10–40[a]
Clinical forms			
Acute onset	+	+	+
Monophasic disease	+	+	+
Occasional chronic or relapsing forms	+	+	+
Pathologic findings			
Perivenular lymphocytes	+	+	+
Perivenular demyelination	+	+	+
Immunologic studies			
Lymphocytes stimulated *in vitro* by myelin basic protein	+	+	+
In vitro demyelination by lymphocytes	+	?	+
Antimyelin protein antibodies	+	+	-

[a]From the beginning of the incubation periods.

TABLE 8.2. *Comparisons of experimental autoimmune neuritis with neuritis after rabies vaccine and Guillain–Barré syndrome*

	Experimental autoimmune neuritis	Postrabies vaccine polyneuritis	Guillain-Barré syndrome
Inducing event	Inoculation with nerve or P2 protein	Inoculation with nervous system tissue	Infection immunization, surgery, or fever therapy
Latent period (days)	10–21	10–42	10–30
Clinical forms			
Subacute onset	+	+	+
Monophasic disease	+	+	+
Rare chronic or relapsing forms	+	+	+
Cerebrospinal fluid			
Lymphocytes	Few	Few	Few
Increased protein	+	+	+
Electrophysiology studies			
Conduction block	+	+	+
Slow nerve conduction	+	+	+
Polyphasic responses	+	+	+
Pathologic findings			
Lymphocytic infiltrates	+	+	+
Activated macrophages	+	+	+
Segmental demyelination	+	+	+
Wallerian degeneration in severe cases	+	+	+
Immunologic studies			
Lymphocytes stimulated *in vitro* by peripheral nerve protein	+	+	+
In vitro demyelination by lymphocytes	+	?	+
Antinerve antibodies	+	+	+

Adapted from Arnason and Soliven (1993) and Server and Johnson (1982).

Virus-induced Demyelination

The obvious, but often disregarded, missing link in the parallels between autoimmune encephalomyelitis and neuritis and postinfectious encephalomyelitis and Guillain–Barré syndrome is that patients with the latter diseases have not been injected with myelin proteins. The majority are recovering from various viral infections, and the role of these antecedent infections needs to be addressed.

A number of laboratory models of acute and chronic virus-induced demyelination have been reported (Table 8.3). Many invoke a direct cytotoxic or indirect cytokine role of the immune response. Virus replication within glial cells can produce demyelinating disease without invoking an immunopathologic mechanism. This is best demonstrated in the chronic demyelinating disease of immunocompromised monkeys caused by simian virus 40, which selectively infects oligodendrocytes (see Chapter 10).

TABLE 8.3. *Animal models of demyelinating diseases*

Virus family	Virus	Host animal	Proposed mechanism
Papovavirus	SV40	Monkeys	Opportunistic infection of oligodendrocytes in immunodeficient animals
Coronavirus	Mouse hepatitis virus	Mice Rats	Persistent oligodendrocyte infection and probable humoral immune responses
Picornaviruses	Theiler's virus	Mice	Persistent infection of oligodendrocytes and macrophages and immune responses
	Encephalomyocarditis virus	Mice	?
Rhabdovirus	Chandipura virus	Mice	Cell-mediated immune responses
	Vesicular stomatitis virus	Mice	
Togavirus	Semliki Forest virus	Mike	Neuronal infection and
	Venezuelan equine encephalitis virus	Mice	immune-mediated demyelination
	Ross River virus	Mice	Direct lysis of oligodendrocytes
Paramyxovirus	Canine distemper virus	Dogs	Predominantly astrocytic infection with probable indirect demyelination
Lentivirus	Visna virus	Sheep	Macrophage and monocyte infection with cytokine-mediated demyelination
	Caprine arthritis–encephalitis virus	Goats	

Modified from Johnson (1994b).

Murine Coronaviruses

The JHM strain of mouse hepatitis virus, originally isolated from the brain of a mouse with spontaneous paralytic disease, produces acute lesions of the brain and spinal cord characterized by loss of myelin, with relative sparing of axons. Murine hepatitis virus infects various neural cells in rodent hosts, but, with manipulation of host age and inoculation, reproducible multifocal demyelination can be found 5 to 7 days after infection (Weiner, 1973). Immunocytochemistry shows patchy infection of glial cells in white matter, and electron microscopy shows virions within oligodendrocytes (Lampert et al., 1973). Mouse hepatitis viruses are known to persist in tissue, and examination of mice surviving for over a year after the initial infection shows small foci of active demyelination, with virus particles in these late lesions (Herndon et al., 1975a).

Despite initial impressions that JHM virus simply infected and lysed oligo-dendrocytes, extensive pathogenesis studies have shown the disease to be far more complex. Acuteness of disease, relative greater infection of neurons and astrocytes, relapses of the disease, and the resultant pathology have proved to be dependent on strain and age of mice, strain of mouse hepatitis virus, mutations in the surface glycoprotein of the virus, and antibody against specific epitopes of virus proteins (Buchmeier et al., 1984; Fleming et al., 1986; Yokomori et al.,

1995; Stohlman et al., 1997). Furthermore, immunosuppression with irradiation prevents demyelination (Wang et al., 1990); and congenitally immunodeficient mice (that is, mice with severe combined immunodeficiency) fail to show demyelination, although athymic mice and mice lacking major histocompatibility complex class I or II expression show robust demyelination but fail to clear virus (Houtman and Fleming, 1996a). The humoral immune response and cytokines appear to play a key role in the demyelination.

Rats infected with JHM virus develop a demyelinating encephalomyelitis after several weeks to months. Lymphocytes from these rats can be stimulated *in vitro* with myelin basic protein, and subsequent adoptive transfer to inbred rats leads to lesions resembling experimental autoimmune encephalomyelitis (Watanabe et al., 1983). This demonstrates the potential for infection of oligodendrocytes to sensitize the host to myelin antigens, but this may be an epiphenomenon and does not necessarily clarify the mechanism of demyelination in the infected host.

Theiler's Virus

Theiler's murine encephalomyelitis virus strains are divided into two subgroups based on the different diseases that they induce. The GDVII-like strains infect predominantly neurons and cause an acute fatal polioencephalomyelitis. In contrast, the TO strains cause a less widespread infection of neurons, glia, and macrophages (Hubert and Brahic, 1995; Simas et al., 1995). Mice surviving the acute phase of flaccid paralytic infection have later paralysis that was initially assumed to represent an immune-mediated postinfectious demyelination (Lipton, 1975).

The relative roles of immune response and virus lysis of oligodendrocytes again are complex. In surviving mice, virus persists for years to a limited extent in oligodendrocytes but predominantly in macrophages, demyelinating lesions correspond to sites where viral RNA is expressed, and demyelination occurs in nude mice (Roos and Wollmann, 1984). Apoptosis of oligodendrocytes has been demonstrated in spinal cord in chronic infection (Tsunoda et al., 1997). Unlike JHM virus infections, demyelination depends on ongoing Theiler virus infection. Nevertheless, immunosuppression treatment with antibodies to class 2 MHC decreased cellular immune responses to viral epitopes, and macrophage depletion all decrease demyelination, even though demyelination can occur in the absence of either CD4 or CD8 cells (Rodriquez et al., 1987 and 1997; Pena Rossi et al., 1997).

Since GDVII and TO strains have 95% identity at the amino acid level, molecular determinants of neurovirulence and demyelination have been studied with recombinants and mutants (Jakob and Roos, 1996). Determinants of neurovirulence of GDVII are multigenic and located in the virus protein (VP1) region and in the 5' region, the latter being reminiscent of the neurovirulence studies of human polioviruses (see Chapter 2) (Pritchard et al., 1993). Susceptibility to demyelination also is multigenic, with linkage to the major histocompatibility complex class I locus, H-2D (Lipton et al., 1995), possibly related to the immune response in demyelination, and a region of viral protein (VP1) believed to lie adjacent to the putative receptor-binding site (Senkowski et al., 1995), which might be related to specific glial cell infection. Mutations in the gene coding for a protein L* dramatically decrease demyelinating activity; this protein is associated with cell membrane and its presence suggests that it may interact with the immune system in mediating demyelination (Chen et al., 1995).

Other Viruses

Experimental infections of mice with temperature-sensitive mutants of two rhabdoviruses—Chandipura and vesicular stomatitis viruses—show initial neuronal infection with later demyelination similar to murine hepatitis virus, JHM strain. These mutants in nude mice cause only acute neuronal necrosis, without the later demyelination, which suggests a pathogenetic role of mature T cells in the demyelination (Dal Canto et al., 1979; Dal Canto and Rabinowitz, 1981).

Demyelination has also been described in three alphavirus infections of mice. Avirulent strains of Semliki Forest virus cause primarily neuronal infection, but foci of demyelination are found without ultrastructural evidence of oligodendrocyte infection (Chew-Lim et al., 1978). Studies in nude mice and prevention of demyelination with CD8 cell depletion suggest an immune-mediated pathogenesis (Jagelman et al., 1978; Fazakerley and Webb, 1987; Subak-Sharpe et al., 1993). Venezuelan equine encephalitis virus in mice causes similar neuronal infection and demyelination in spinal cord, and the latter lesions fail to develop in nude mice (Dal Canto and Rabinowitz, 1981). In contrast, similar demyelinating lesions develop with Ross River virus infections of young mice, but virus particles have been identified in oligodendrocytes, and immunosuppressive drugs did not diminish demyelination (Seay and Wolinsky, 1982 and 1983).

Canine distemper virus can cause both acute and chronic demyelination in dogs. The acute demyelination is noninflammatory and is related to active virus replication in astrocytes, with possible restricted infection of oligodendrocytes (Blakemore et al., 1989). In the persistent infection, demyelination is associated with inflammatory infiltrates and may be related to immune responses or the so-called bystander effect (Miller et al., 1995). The possible role of cytokines in demyelination as well as neuronal death is dealt with in Chapters 11 and 12.

Theoretical Mechanisms

A number of mechanisms have been proposed to explain the potential role of immune responses in viral demyelination (Weiner et al., 1973a) (Table 8.4). Virus or viral products theoretically could cause demyelination by damaging myelin membranes directly, without infecting the myelin-supporting cells. Fusion proteins of virus envelopes can dramatically alter membranes, even of cells insusceptible to infection or after virus has been inactivated by ultraviolet

TABLE 8.4. *Possible mechanisms of virus-induced demyelination*

Direct viral effects
    Virus infection of oligodendrocytes or Schwann cells causing demyelination through cell
      lysis or an alteration in cell metabolism
    Myelin membrane destruction by virus or viral products

Virus-induced immune-mediated reactions
    Antibody and/or cell-mediated reactions to viral antigens on cell membranes
    Sensitization of host to myelin antigens
      Breakdown of myelin by infection with introduction into the circulation (epitope spreading)
      Incorporation of myelin antigens into virus envelope
      Modification of antigenicity of myelin membranes
    Cross-reacting antigens between virus and myelin proteins (molecular mimicry)
    Cytokine and/or protease-mediated demyelination (innocent-bystander effect)

Viral disruption of regulatory mechanisms of the immune system

Adapted from Johnson and Weiner (1972).

light (Harter and Choppin, 1971). Many, but not all, of the viruses that have been associated with postinfectious encephalomyelitis and the Guillain–Barré syndrome, including measles, mumps, influenza, and varicella viruses, contain a fusion protein in their envelope. Another mechanism for potential myelin destruction is suggested by the finding that purified myelin basic protein is an excellent substrate for the protein kinase in the vaccinia virus core. The release of this viral enzyme by a neighboring cell could have a profound effect on myelin structure and function (Steck et al., 1976).

In some viral infections, virus-specified polypeptides are inserted into the plasma membrane of the host cell. If myelin-supporting cells are infected, an antibody or cell-mediated immune reaction against the viral antigen in the cell membrane could lead to myelin destruction. Alternatively, a viral infection of myelin-supporting cells could introduce sequestered myelin antigens into the circulation by direct release or by incorporation of these antigens into the virus envelopes, with the released virion acting as the vehicle to incite autoimmunity. During experimental autoimmune encephalomyelitis and JHM and Theiler virus infections, immune responses develop against noninoculated endogenous epitopes, which are presumably released into the circulation during the CNS inflammation. This evolution of expanding responses to different myelin protein epitopes over a period of weeks to months has been called epitope spreading, and, once established, it has been shown to be self-perpetuating after viral clearance (Miller et al., 1995; Vanderlugt and Miller, 1996). This is an attractive hypothesis to explain relapsing experimental autoimmune encephalomyelitis and to consider in the pathogenesis of multiple sclerosis (see Chapter 10).

An alternate mechanism for virus-induced immune-mediated demyelination in the absence of direct infection of myelin-supporting cells is molecular mimicry. If virus polypeptides shared common antigenic determinants with central or peripheral nerve myelin, an anatomically distant infection could cause an autoimmune reaction. Molecular mimicry has been sought in the gene bank by looking for the viral protein sequence most resembling the encephalitogenic sequence in myelin basic protein. The nonstructural polymerase protein of hepatitis B virus showed the best match, and a polypeptide was synthesized and injected into rabbits. Mild CNS inflammatory lesions resembling experimental autoimmune encephalomyelitis developed (Fujinami and Oldstone, 1985). Some have tried to cash in on this finding by claiming demyelination may result from the vaccine, ignoring the fact that the P protein is not in the recombinant hepatitis B vaccine. Another twist on molecular mimicry is seen in transgenic mice expressing the nucleoprotein or glycoprotein of lymphocytic choriomeningitis virus as self in oligodendrocytes. A self-limited peripheral infection with the virus in an adult was followed by a bout of CNS inflammation and demyelination (Evans et al., 1996). To date, the best example of molecular mimicry in human neurologic disease is the infection with strains of *Campylobacter* bacteria leading to an axonal form of the Guillain–Barré syndrome discussed later (Ho et al., 1995; Oomes et al., 1995).

Tertiary structure as well as sequence alignment may lead to mimicry. For example, a single T-cell receptor can recognize distinct, but structurally related, peptides from different pathogens (Wucherpfenning and Strominger, 1995). Therefore, an encephalitogenic sequence of a myelin protein might be mimicked by peptides of a variety of viruses, a phenomenon that might explain how diverse agents can induce demyelinating encephalomyelitis or polyneuritis.

Demyelination induced by soluble substances released by inflammatory cells was originally termed the innocent-bystander effect (Cammer et al., 1978). During the inflammatory response evoked by a delayed hypersensitivity reaction, activated lymphocytes or macrophages release factors (probably proteases or cytokines) that can disrupt myelin. For example, guinea pigs previously sensitized to tuberculin and later inoculated intracerebrally with tuberculin purified protein develop demyelination associated with the inflammatory reaction around the inoculation site (Wisniewski and Bloom, 1975). Thus, an immune reaction against a viral antigen in the vicinity of central or peripheral nerve myelin can result in demyelination without concomitant infection of the myelin-supporting cell.

Finally, infections may precipitate autoimmune disease by pertubating immunoregulatory mechanisms. Paterson (1979) said these mechanisms "effectively restrain our ever-present capacity to react immunologically against our own nervous tissues." Originally, the phenomenon of self-tolerance was thought to result from deletion, at an early age, of the potential "self" reactive clones of lymphocytes. Tolerance, however, is an active process in which autoimmune reactions are suppressed by regulatory mechanisms of the immune system (Cunningham, 1976).

Within this context, several mechanisms can be envisioned by which viral infections could trigger a reaction against myelin proteins. An antecedent viral infection could increase the vulnerability of nervous tissue to attack from a persisting, previously subclinical, autoimmune process. Alternatively, viral infection affecting myelin-supporting cells or myelin sheaths could alter the pattern of myelin breakdown, thereby upsetting a balance by which circulating endogenous myelin might regulate autoimmune reactivity. Finally, the most attractive hypothesis for diverse viral infections leading to central or peripheral demyelination is that virus acts directly on T-cell subsets or receptors, disturbing the balance that normally prevents a symptomatic autoimmune reaction. Both measles virus, the commonest agent related to postinfectious encephalomyelitis, and Epstein–Barr virus, the virus most convincingly associated with Guillain–Barré syndrome, alter T-cell activity during primary infections (Griffin et al., 1994a; Karp et al., 1996).

In summary, the demyelinating abnormalities of postinfectious encephalomyelitis and Guillain–Barré syndrome can be mimicked by immune responses to the basic proteins of central and peripheral nervous system myelin, respectively. Virus infections can cause demyelination without intervention of immune responses, by virus-induced immune response, by nonspecific mechanisms that can cause myelin dissolution, or by disrupting immune regulation. To differentiate these mechanisms in acute human demyelinating disease, we need to know whether virus is present within the neural cells, the antigenic determinants of the virus, whether systemic immune responses to myelin components as well as viral components can be detected, and the effect of the infection on subsets of lymphocytes. However gratifying it might be to find a single mechanism to explain these complications, we know that a given pathologic response may derive from different pathogenic mechanisms, and we have no reason to assume that a unitary mechanism will explain all cases of postinfectious demyelination.

POSTINFECTIOUS ENCEPHALOMYELITIS

Postinfectious encephalomyelitis is known under a surfeit of names. Parainfectious, postexanthematous, postvaccinal, and postinfluenzal encephalomyelitis have been used to describe the clinical setting. Acute disseminated encephalomyelitis describes the common pathology, as do the terms perivascular myelinoclasis, perivenous encephalitis, and acute demyelinating encephalomyelitis. Other names that have been proposed to imply knowledge of pathogenetic mechanisms include allergic encephalomyelitis, immune-mediated encephalomyelitis, hyperergic encephalomyelitis, and disseminated vasculomyelinopathy (Johnson and Griffin, 1987).

Historically, postinfectious encephalomyelitis was of major importance as a complication of vaccinia and measles virus infections (Table 8.5). However, the discontinuation of vaccination against smallpox has eliminated the former, and immunization against measles virus has greatly reduced the latter. The last patient with natural smallpox was reported in 1977, and the complications of smallpox and its vaccination are now only of historical interest. Encephalomyelitis complicating measles has almost disappeared in North America and Europe with the widespread use of measles virus vaccine, but measles remains

TABLE 8.5. *Postinfectious encephalomyelitis with perivenular demyelination associated with exanthematous viral infections*

	Case rate	Fatality rate	Sequelae rate
Vaccinia	1:63 to 1:200,000	10%	Rare
Measles	1:1000	25%	Frequent
Varicella[a]	1:10,000	5%	10%
Rubella[a]	1:20,000	20%	Very rare

[a]Estimates are difficult to determine because of the frequency of toxic encephalopathy or Reye's syndrome (different pathology) and acute cerebellar ataxia (unknown pathology) and the rare documentation of perivenular demyelinating disease.

a major epidemic disease in many areas of the world and, because of high incidence of demyelinating complications and clinical ease of diagnosis, measles encephalomyelitis has been the focus of clinical pathogenesis studies. Postinfectious complications of mumps and rubella also have declined in many countries where vaccines strains have been routinely included with measles vaccine. With these dramatic advances in disease control, postinfectious encephalomyelitis is now most frequently seen after nonspecific upper respiratory infections, where the specific etiologic agents usually are unknown (Johnson et al., 1985b).

These changes in immunization practices and precipitating infections have made the differential diagnosis of viral encephalitis and postinfectious encephalitis difficult. The history of preceding respiratory or gastrointestinal symptoms may be fortuitous or may not be recalled. Both encephalitis and postinfectious encephalomyelitis can present with abrupt signs of fever, nuchal rigidity, multifocal neurologic abnormalities, and depression of consciousness. Cerebrospinal fluid cells and protein in postinfectious encephalomyelitis may be normal, but the same may be true early in the course of encephalitis. Magnetic resonance imaging has proved an effective method of differentiation in some cases; multifocal white matter lesions, which may or may not enhance, are characteristic of postinfectious encephalomyelitis (Kesselring et al., 1990; Caldemeyer et al., 1994). These imaging abnormalities resolve over many months, so lesions may be obvious even after complete clinical recovery.

As with experimental autoimmune encephalitis and rabies vaccine complications, a lag usually occurs between encounter with the antigen and the onset of an acute monophasic disease. In each instance, the pathologic hallmarks are perivenular inflammation and demyelination.

Vaccinia

In retrospect, acute perivenular demyelination was found in brains of patients dying of smallpox, but this complication was overlooked during early epidemics—immersed under the devastating systemic disease (Marsden and Hurst, 1932). The encephalomyelitis surfaced with the introduction of immunization using the related virus of cowpox (vaccinia virus). Use of vaccination was widespread by the end of the 18th century, but moral as well as scientific controversy continued to impede its use: under the close scrutiny of the religious and medical detractors, complications of vaccination were unlikely to have gone unnoticed. Nevertheless, reports of postvaccinal encephalomyelitis did not appear until the late 1920s. This conundrum about the emergence of the postvaccinal encephalomyelitis is compounded by its variable incidence in different vaccinated populations in different years, varying from a high of 1 in 63 in one Dutch experience (DeVries, 1960) to 1 in 4 million in other programs. The basis for these astonishing differences in attack rates never has been clarified but could reflect differences in the genetic susceptibility in different populations, variations in the batches of vaccinia virus, or other factors.

Acute postvaccinal encephalomyelitis was more frequent after primary immunization but did occur after revaccination. Fever, nuchal rigidity, and obtundation were the usual first signs. Movement disorders, tremor, ataxia, and signs of pyramidal tract disease were all seen (Spillane and Wells, 1964). Trismus and myoclonus were frequent findings in this particular encephalomyelitis (Miller, 1953). The cerebrospinal fluid usually showed a pleocytosis and an elevation of protein content. The reported fatality rates ranged from 10% to 40%. Recovery of survivors was generally complete.

Although virus replication usually was limited to the dermis, a viremia was documented in some patients. In vaccinees who developed encephalomyelitis, virus was found in blood for longer intervals, and virus occasionally was recovered from brains and cerebrospinal fluid of patients with encephalomyelitis (Angulo et al., 1964; Gurvich et al., 1975; Brooks, 1979). Studies to determine which CNS cells are infected and to evaluate immune responses to myelin proteins in these patients were not reported.

Measles

Globally, measles is a major epidemic disease causing about 1.5 million childhood deaths per year (Assaad, 1983). Measles remains one of the three commonest infectious causes of childhood mortality and a major cause of neurologic deficits in many areas of the world. The most frequent fatal complications of epidemic measles are disseminated infections with pneumonitis, gastroenteritis, and secondary bacterial infection. These result from the depression of cell-mediated immune responses for 1 to 4 weeks after acute measles virus infections; prior to the emergence of HIV infections, measles was the most profound cause of virus-induced acquired immunodeficiency. A second important complication and a major cause of sequelae is postinfectious encephalomyelitis, which because of analogies to experimental autoimmune encephalomyelitis and post–rabies vaccination reactions, is presumed to be an autoimmune reaction. Thus, we have a paradox, with some complications believed to be due to depression and others to augmentation of immune responses.

In contrast to the situation with vaccinia virus infection, the incidence of postinfectious encephalomyelitis after measles is relatively constant at about 1 per 1,000 infections, although this incidence is lower in children younger than 2 years of age. Acute encephalomyelitis accounts for 95% of the neurologic complications of measles virus infections, although myelitis, polyneuritis, toxic encephalopathy, and acute hemiplegia are reported (Miller et al., 1956).

Measles is a highly contagious disease with an incubation period of 10 to 14 days. After a prodrome of coryza, conjunctivitis, dry cough, and Koplik spots on the buccal mucosa, a maculopapular rash develops on the face and trunk and then spreads to the extremities. Virus is recoverable from blood during the prodrome and from the maculopapular skin lesions. In children who have died within 5 days after rash, viral antigen or RNA has been found in epithelial cells of lung, gut, bile duct, bladder, skin, and lymphoid organs, as well as brain endothelial cells (Moench et al., 1988; Esolen et al., 1995). Even though no neural cells are infected, a large percentage of children with rash have subclinical CNS dysfunction, since half have abnormal electroencephalograms (Gibbs et al., 1959) and 30% have pleocytoses, occasionally with more than 50 cells (Ojala, 1947; Hanninen et al., 1980).

Characteristically, the encephalomyelitis occurs 4 to 5 days after the onset of the rash, but it can predate the rash or evolve 3 weeks after the rash (Griffin et al., 1989a) (Fig. 8.1). Typically, the patient has defervesced, and the rash is fading, when suddenly fever returns and headache develops. Some patients become rapidly obtunded, whereas others show gradual depression of consciousness. Half of the patients have generalized or focal convulsions. Focal neurologic signs of involvement of cerebral hemispheres, basal ganglia, spinal cord, cerebellum, brainstem, or optic nerves may be evident. The cerebrospinal fluid may be normal, but the majority of patients have mild pleocytosis of mononuclear cells and moderate to dramatic elevations of protein content. Myelin basic protein can be found in the majority, with highest levels earlier in disease (Johnson et al., 1984). The electroencephalogram shows diffuse slowing.

Mortality is high, ranging from 10% to 40% in different series. A majority of the survivors have neurologic sequelae, including mental retardation, hemiparesis, paraplegia, and ataxia (Johnson and Griffin, 1987). The prognosis has been related to length of coma or stupor (Miller et al., 1956; Tyler, 1957), but we found remarkable exceptions. One of our patients showed progressive deterioration for 3 weeks and remained semicomatose for an additional 3 weeks, responding to pain only with decorticate posturing. Nevertheless, over the subsequent 2 months, she made an almost total recovery, achieving normal levels of intellectual function and physical activity, with only minor residual spasticity in her legs (Johnson et al., 1984). Neuropathologic examinations show perivenular infiltration of mononuclear cells with demyelination. The pattern of loss of myelin proteins is the same as that in experimental autoimmune encephalomyelitis (Gendelman et al., 1985b).

Since the vaccine for measles is a live attenuated virus, the question arose as to whether encephalomyelitis could follow vaccination. In 40 children inoculated during the vaccine development, electroencephalograms showed no alterations (Gibbs et al., 1961). After introduction of widespread immunization, only one case of encephalitis per million children was reported following immunization. This figure is actually lower than the estimated background of two cases of encephalitis per million children per month, but some clustering of the cases was noted during the 6 to 15 days after immunization (Landrigan and Witte, 1973). Because no encephalitis deaths have been reported after immunization, the pathologic abnormalities in these patients are unknown.

In contrast to the situation with postvaccinal encephalomyelitis, virus has seldom been recovered from nervous system specimens of patients with measles encephalomyelitis. Virus was recovered from spinal fluid from one child with measles encephalitis (Shaffer et al., 1942) and by cocultivation of spinal fluid cells of another (Purdham and Batty, 1974). In contrast to the acute viral encephalitis, we found a lack of intrathecal synthesis of antibody against measles (Johnson et al., 1984), found no increase of interferon in cerebrospinal fluid despite high plasmid levels (Griffin et al., 1990), and by both immunocytochemistry and *in situ* hybridization failed to show measles virus infection of brain in patients who died with encephalomyelitis (Gendelman et al., 1984; Moench et al., 1988).

In our studies of measles virus infections in Peru from 1980 to 1991, we addressed the apparent paradox posed by the complications related to immunosuppression and the encephalomyelitis with a possible autoimmune basis. Conversion of tuberculin reactions during measles and for weeks thereafter had been described by von Pirquet in 1908, and this anergy was confirmed in children immunized with Calmette–Guérin bacillus (Tamashiro et al., 1987). The severe inhibition of lymphocyte responses to mitogens (Whittle et al., 1978) also was confirmed, but it did not appear to differ in patients with uncomplicated measles, pneumonia, or encephalomyelitis (Hirsch et al., 1984). In all three groups, antibody responses to major viral proteins were distinguishable (Graves et al., 1984), and similar leukopenias developed with maintenance of normal CD4/CD8 ratios (Griffin et al., 1986). It became clear, however, that there was parallel evidence of immune activation, with spontaneous proliferation of CD4, CD8, and B lymphocytes (Griffin et al., 1989b; Ward et al., 1990); spontaneous suppressor cell activity (Hirsch et al., 1984); increased lymphocyte activation markers (Griffin et al., 1986); monocyte activation (Ward et al., 1991; Griffin et al., 1992b); elevated levels of soluble interleukin 2 and CD8 (Griffin et al., 1989b); elevated C-reactive proteins and plasma immunoglobulin E (IgE) levels (Griffin et al., 1983 and 1985); and elevated plasma levels of interferon α and neopterin (Griffin et al., 1990). Measles virus produces activation of cells, and lymphoproliferation of lymphocytes in presence of myelin basic protein was found in 15% of cases of uncomplicated measles and in 47% of those with encephalomyelitis (Johnson et al., 1984).

These data, compared with parallel data in viral encephalitis, strongly argue for a very different pathogenesis, with primary measles virus infection of lymphoid cells, disruption of immune regulation, and cellular immune responses directed inappropriately against host myelin (Johnson, 1987).

Varicella

Significant neurologic complications occur in about 1 in 10,000 patients with chickenpox. Acute cerebellar ataxia accounts for about half of these complications, with an incidence of 1:4,000 varicella cases among children (Guess et al., 1986). This ataxia has an excellent prognosis (Connolly et al., 1994), and the underlying pathologic changes are unknown. The most frequent life-threatening neurologic complication of varicella is acute toxic encephalopathy or Reye's syndrome, in which the acute cerebral edema is not accompanied by inflammation or demyelination.

True postinfectious encephalomyelitis as a complication of varicella is rare (Griffith et al., 1970; Johnson and Milbourn, 1970; Takashima and Becker, 1979). Encephalomyelitis tends to occur 4 to 14 days after the onset of rash, but it can, on occasion, precede the rash. The clinical presentation is similar to that seen after measles and vaccinia, with sudden fever, obtundation, and meningeal signs. Seizures, focal neurologic signs, and movement disorders can develop (Gollomp and Fahn, 1987). Computed tomography and magnetic resonance images have shown nonenhancing bilateral hypodense basal ganglion lesions as well as diffuse hypodense lesions (Darling et al., 1995). The spinal fluid usually shows a mild lymphocytosis and mild elevation of protein. Perivenular demyelination has been documented postmortem (Fig. 8.2).

On rare occasions, acute transverse myelitis has been reported (McCarthy and Amer, 1978; Magliulo et al., 1979; Rosenfeld et al., 1993), bilateral optic neuritis has been seen following chickenpox (Selbst et al., 1983), and, on one occasion, myelitis was accompanied by optic neuritis (Chusid et al., 1979). Whether these represent demyelinating diseases is unknown. One child has been described with fatal intracerebral hemorrhage secondary to thrombocytopenia with varicella (Tobin and ten Bensel, 1972). Transient protein S deficiency, lupus anticoagulant, and antiplatelet antibodies have all been reported in children with varicella (Manco-Johnson et al., 1996; Mayer and Beardsley, 1996).

There is a paucity of virologic data on any of these complications. Virus has not been isolated from cerebrospinal fluid or brain tissue. Spinal fluid cells containing virus antigen have been reported in two children with cerebellar ataxia complicating chickenpox, which suggests direct virus invasion of the CNS (Peters et al., 1978), but fluorescent antibody staining of spinal fluid sediment is a capricious procedure. Inclusion bodies have been demonstrated in brain in several children with varicella, but these patients had been receiving steroids or suf-

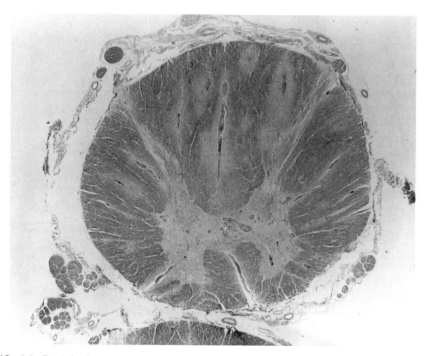

FIG. 8.2. Postinfectious encephalomyelitis showing extensive perivenular demyelination in spinal cord. This 12-year-old girl developed dysesthesias in legs and paraparesis abruptly 2 weeks after uncomplicated varicella. Three days later, she developed upper arm weakness and abrupt blindness, respiratory distress, and seizures and then died. (Courtesy of Dr. Carlos Pardo.)

fered from immunodeficiency disorders and had unusual forms of disseminated disease (Takashima and Becker, 1979). Several children with acute cerebellar ataxia have had lymphoproliferative responses to myelin basic protein, which suggests a pathogenesis similar to postmeasles encephalomyelitis and experimental autoimmune encephalomyelitis (Lisak et al., 1977; Johnson et al., 1984).

Rubella

Rubella is the fourth viral exanthem associated with postinfectious encephalomyelitis. However, the neurologic complications with postnatal rubella are even less well defined than with varicella. Approximately 1 in 20,000 cases of rubella involves some neurologic complication. During the week following the onset of rash, fever, depression of consciousness, and headache often develop in conjunction with seizures but generally without focal neurologic signs. Transverse myelopathy and polyradiculitis have been reported (Bechar et al., 1982; Bitzan, 1987). Spinal fluid usually shows a pleocytosis. The fatality rate is high, with approximately 20% of the children with encephalitis dying acutely during the first days, but those who recover are almost invariably free of sequelae.

In the majority of fatalities, perivenular demyelination is not found. Many show only congestion or multiple petechial hemorrhages in the brain. Others have vascular changes or occlusions, and in one child with acute hemiplegia leading to death, rubella virus antigen and particles resembling rubella virus were found in brain even though virus was not recovered (Connolly et al., 1975). Inflammatory cells may be present in a perivenular distribution, and this inflammation may be more prominent in white matter, but clear-cut perivenular demyelination is rare (Hart and Earle, 1975). The paucity of demyelination has been accredited to the brevity of illness (Miller et al., 1956). Clearly, less is known of these rare neurologic complications of acute rubella than is known about the congenital rubella encephalitis (see Chapter 13) or even the very rare adolescent progressive rubella panencephalitis (see Chapter 10).

Rubella virus vaccine has not been implicated in encephalitis, although transient paresthesias and objective evidence of peripheral neuropathies have been reported in a number of vaccine recipients. Two teenage women were reported with transverse myelitis 4 and 14 days after receiving rubella virus vaccine (Holt et al., 1976), but similar patients have not been reported to corroborate a causal relationship.

Other Viral Infections

Perivenular demyelination has been described with a variety of nonexanthematous diseases, including mumps, influenza, and Epstein–Barr virus infections. The fatal cases of mumps virus encephalitis provide the greatest challenge to a clear-cut distinction between viral encephalitis and postinfectious encephalomyelitis. As discussed in Chapter 5, prior to vaccine programs mumps was the virus that most frequently invaded the CNS. The virus causes both aseptic meningitis and mild encephalitis and is readily recoverable from spinal fluid. Fatalities from acute mumps encephalitis are rare. Nevertheless, in nearly half of these patients, perivenular inflammation with demyelination has been found (Schwarz et al., 1964; Hart and Earle, 1975).

How often demyelination is associated with the frequent invasion of the CNS by mumps virus is unknown. In our studies of ultrastructure of cerebrospinal fluid sediment from patients with mumps meningitis, ependymal cells containing virus nucleocapsid were evident, but myelin fragments were not seen (Herndon et al., 1974). In two patients with mumps meningitis, we have not detected myelin basic protein in spinal fluid by radioimmunoassay, and in further contrast to the situation with measles encephalomyelitis, peripheral blood lymphocytes showed no proliferative response after exposure to myelin basic protein (*unpublished data*). Demyelination in mumps encephalitis may simply reflect severity of the disease, or two different neurologic complications of mumps virus infection may occur that defy clinical differentiation.

With declining frequency of childhood exanthems, postinfectious encephalo-myelitis is now most frequent after flulike illnesses. The precise role of the influenza viruses, however, is not clear, because in contrast to the characteristic clinical features of measles, varicella, rubella, and mumps, differentiation of influenza virus from other respiratory virus infections requires laboratory confirmation. A large number of reports of encephalitis complicating the Asian influenza epidemics in the late 1950s appeared (Horner, 1958), and subsequently smaller numbers of patients have been noted with encephalitis during epidemics of influenza B and more recent strains of influenza A (Hawkins et al., 1987). In a number of these patients, the influenza virus infection has been established serologically (Sulkava et al., 1981). However, the course of these diseases has in general been benign, so whether they represent perivenular demyelinating disease or other pathologic forms of encephalitis is undetermined. Rarely, perivenular demyelination has been convincingly linked epidemiologically and serologically with influenza virus infection (Hoult and Flewett, 1960), but no definitive isolations of influenza virus have been reported from the nervous system of patients with perivenular demyelinating encephalitis. The evidence relating the influenza viruses with toxic encephalopathy, Reye's syndrome, acute transverse myelitis, and the Guillain–Barré syndrome is more convincing; postinfectious encephalomyelitis appears to be a rare complication of influenza virus infections (Wells, 1971; Davis and Kornfeld, 1980).

Epstein–Barr virus has also been related to pathologically documented postinfectious encephalomyelitis (Paskavitz et al., 1995) and postinfectious cerebellar ataxia (Ito et al., 1994). Hepatitis A virus has also been implicated in postinfectious encephalomyelitis (Davis et al., 1993). In addition, the syndrome is not specific for viral infections, because it has been seen after *Mycoplasma* infections, after immunizations and serum treatment, and as an adverse reaction to drugs (Miller and Stanton, 1954; Behan and Currie, 1978; Fenichel, 1982; Nishimura et al., 1996; Pellegrini et al., 1996).

Localized Postinfectious Syndromes

Several localized postinfectious illnesses have been described similar to the localized cerebellar ataxia complicating varicella.

Transverse myelitis is an acute deficit in sensory and motor function below a demarcated level due to an intramedullary disease of the spinal cord. Causes include multiple sclerosis, paraneoplastic myelopathy, and vascular insufficiency, but 30% to 45% of patients have a history of preceding or concurrent "viral" infection (Jeffrey et al., 1993a). Myelitis may be the sentinel sign of diffuse postinfectious encephalomyelitis, but magnetic resonance imaging has aided in this distinction. Rather than the diffuse enhancing white matter lesions in patients with postinfectious encephalomyelitis, patients with acute transverse myelitis have normal imaging or show areas of T2 density or enhancement stretching through several adjacent segments of the spinal cord.

Acute transverse myelitis has been associated with measles, mumps, rubella, varicella, Epstein–Barr, cytomegalovirus, hepatitis A, adenovirus, and influenza A viruses, and recurrent transverse myelitis has been associated in one patient with a high-titered hepatitis B antigemia (Tyler et al., 1986a; Linssen et al., 1991; Breningstall and Belani, 1995; Matsui et al., 1996; Salonen et al., 1997). Nonspecific respiratory or gastrointestinal illnesses 1 to 3 weeks prior to the onset of weakness are the most common antecedent infections. Myelitis caused by rabies and B viruses in immunocompetent patients and caused by vari-cella–zoster and herpes simplex in immunodeficient patients represents a direct infection of spinal cord and usually presents as an ascending necrotizing myelitis rather than as a transverse myelitis.

The opsoclonus–myoclonus syndrome (dancing eyes–dancing feet) is charac-terized by chaotic, rapid, randomly directed eye movements associated with myoclonic jerking and often cerebellar ataxia. This syndrome occurs as a remote effect of cancer (particularly neuroblastomas in children) and as a postinfectious disorder of unknown pathology. There are individual case reports associating the disease with a number of specific viruses, but most postinfectious instances of this dramatic disease follow nonspecific upper respiratory or gastrointestinal febrile illnesses (Pranzatelli, 1992).

Acute Hemorrhagic Leukoencephalitis

Acute hemorrhagic leukoencephalitis is a rare disorder that may or may not represent a distinct syndrome. Some regard it as a severe form of postinfectious encephalomyelitis, whereas others maintain that its clinical features, pathologic changes, and association with different etiologic agents set it apart (Behan and Currie, 1978).

Like postinfectious encephalomyelitis, acute hemorrhagic leukoencephalitis usually appears 1 to 20 days following a "viruslike" infection. Similarly, the onset is abrupt, with recrudescence of fever, rapid deterioration of mentation, and development of seizures and focal neurologic signs. The disease is more ful-minant, and clinical findings often suggest an expanding cerebral mass, with progressive focal signs and elevated intracranial pressure. Rarely, the disease may be localized to the posterior fossa (Michaud and Helle, 1982). The major-ity of patients die within 5 days of onset, and most survivors have severe neuro-logic deficits. The cerebrospinal fluid shows pleocytosis, but with polymor-phonuclear cells and red blood cells. In addition, peripheral leukocytosis, markedly elevated sedimentation rate, and proteinuria usually are present.

Pathologically, postinfectious encephalomyelitis and acute hemorrhagic leukoencephalitis appear to represent a gradient of severity. In the latter disease, fibrinoid necrosis of vessels involves not only veins but also arterioles. This vascular necrosis is accompanied by transudates of fibrinous exudate into the perivascular area, extravasation of red blood cells, and large areas of tissue necrosis, with intense polymorphonuclear cell infiltration. Changes are most intense in the white matter, with myelin loss and relative preservation of axons.

Acute hemorrhagic leukoencephalitis has been clinically associated in rare cases with varicella and measles (Pearl et al., 1990) and, in several patients, with serologic evidence of influenza A virus infections (Sabin, 1959; Hoult and Flewett, 1960). Even before immunization practices changed, the majority of cases followed nonspecific upper respiratory tract infections. This difference from postinfectious encephalomyelitis is illustrated in an earlier autopsy series in which 38 cases of perivenular demyelinating disease were collected. Of the 30 cases fulfilling histopathologic criteria of postinfectious encephalomyelitis, 17 followed measles, 4 rubella, 6 mumps, 2 varicella, and 1 vaccinia. In contrast, of the 8 cases of acute hemorrhagic leukoencephalitis, 5 followed nonspecific upper respiratory disease, and in 3 there was no history of antecedent illness. Thus, the spectra of viruses precipitating the two diseases appear to differ (Hart and Earle, 1975).

The argument that acute hemorrhagic leukoencephalitis is a more intense form of postinfectious encephalomyelitis is supported by a continuum of human pathologic findings. In addition, modification of the adjuvant in the induction of experimental autoimmune encephalitis causes hyperacute encephalomyelitis that mimics the histopathologic findings of acute hemorrhagic leukoencephalitis, and lymphocytes from one patient with this disease demonstrated a proliferative response when cultured in the presence of myelin basic protein (Behan et al., 1968). These data support the concept that acute hemorrhagic leukoencephalitis is an intense form of postinfectious encephalomyelitis mediated by similar immune mechanisms but triggered by different agents.

GUILLAIN–BARRÉ SYNDROME

Guillain–Barré syndrome is an acute inflammatory demyelinating polyradiculoneuropathy that in the majority of cases follows a "viruslike" illness. The clinical delineation and nosology of the syndrome have been subjects of controversy for over a century. The syndrome was described as acute ascending paralysis by Landry (1859) and by many others in the late 19th century, including Osler (1892), who introduced the name acute febrile polyneuritis for patients with ascending motor paralysis who presented with fever. Following the introduction of spinal fluid examination as a clinical test, Guillain, Barré, and Strohl (1916) described a benign acute polyneuritis in two French soldiers and described the typical spinal fluid changes of elevated protein and no pleocytosis (the albuminocytologic dissociation). Numerous eponyms have been attached to the syndrome, with admonitions that Landry be included on the basis of precedent, Osler on the basis of chauvinism, or Strohl on the basis of fundamental fairness. The name Guillain–Barré syndrome seems established by usage, however, and at least it is preferable to "French polio," which was popularized by the news media during the outbreak of cases associated with swine influenza vaccine.

Guillain–Barré syndrome is a common disease, with an annual incidence of 1.5 to 2.0 cases per 100,000 population. Although often regarded as a winter disease, population-based studies have shown no significant annual or seasonal variation. All age groups are affected, although the disease is more common among individuals over 40 years of age. No HLA linkage has been found, although relapses of disease may be HLA dependent (Arnason and Soliven, 1993).

The literature abounds with anecdotal reports relating Guillain–Barré syndrome to antecedent events, including nonspecific and specific infections, vaccinations, surgery, fever therapy, trauma, pregnancy, alcoholic liver disease, collagen vascular disease, and malignancy (Leneman, 1966). However, case-controlled studies have documented a significant association with antecedent viruslike respiratory or gastrointestinal illnesses (Melnick and Flewett, 1964; Kennedy et al., 1978). In 1976, the disease clearly was related to injection with an inactivated vaccine against swine influenza virus.

Disease Description

The Guillain–Barré syndrome has a subacute onset; over half of the patients evolve their maximum deficit within 2 weeks and over 90% within 4 weeks. Progressive motor weakness commonly ascends from legs to arms, but weakness may begin in the face and descend. Half of the patients eventually develop facial weakness, but fewer than 5% develop weakness of the extraocular muscles. Sensory symptoms are frequent at the outset, but sensory findings rarely predominate. A symmetric pattern of weakness is usual but not absolute. Areflexia is usual in areas of weakness, but areflexia may be universal even in areas of minimal weakness. Dysesthesias and pain are common, but objective evidence of sensory deficits is usually less extensive than subjective dysesthesias suggest. Fever usually is absent at the outset. Autonomic dysfunctions, such as tachycardia, bradycardia, arrhythmias, and postural hypotension, are found in over half of the patients, and include anhidrosis and inappropriate secretion of antidiuretic hormone. Bowel and bladder functions transiently may be abnormal, but abnormalities seldom persist. Variants of the syndrome show cerebellar ataxia, severe sensory loss, or a relapsing clinical course.

Cerebrospinal fluid and electrodiagnostic studies confirm the clinical diagnosis. Cerebrospinal fluid protein is almost invariably elevated but often not until after the first week of symptoms. Several weeks into disease, this protein may exceed 2 g/dL and may be associated with increased intracranial pressure and papilledema. In contrast, cellular content usually is normal, although up to 50 mononuclear cells per cubic millimeter sometimes are found early in the disease and in cases associated with HIV infections (Cornblath et al., 1987). Electrophysiologic studies usually show multifocal conduction block, reduced nerve conduction velocities, prolonged distal latencies, and absent F waves or prolonged minimal F-wave latencies (Cornblath, 1990).

Although recovery may not be maximal for 4 to 6 months, 85% of patients have a good recovery. Approximately 5% of patients are permanently disabled, and some abnormal findings have been found in as many as 43% of patients after convalescence (Loffel et al., 1977). A poor prognosis correlates with the delay from the time of maximal involvement until the time when recovery begins, with evidence of axonal damage, and with advanced age. Mortality previously ranged from 10% to 20%, but intensive care, early respiratory support, and cardiorespiratory monitoring have reduced the mortality to 2% to 6%. Of these fatalities, more than 80% involve patients who die suddenly with cardiovascular complications that result from autonomic nervous system impairment (Keenlyside et al., 1980).

Corticosteroids and adrenocorticotropic hormone were advocated to alter the course of the disease, but several controlled studies have failed to show efficacy, and in a British study delayed recovery and a higher relapse rate were observed in steroid-treated patients (Hughes et al., 1978). Two methods have been shown in large controlled studies to shorten the course of disease: plasmapheresis and intravenous IgG treatment. The success of plasmapheresis has been a potent argument for a role of antibodies, immune complexes, or cytokines in the pathogenesis of the disease.

Pathologic studies have shown perivenous accumulation of mononuclear cells in patches throughout the length of peripheral nerves. In early lesions, CD4 cells dominate the infiltrates, but macrophages soon are predominant. Segmental demyelination is found in areas of the infiltrates (Asbury et al., 1969), with both vesicular myelin degeneration and stripping of myelin sheaths by macrophage processes. Later, Schwann cells proliferate. Similar abnormalities are found in the autonomic nervous system. At the light-microscopic and electron-microscopic levels, the pathologic changes are remarkably similar to those in experimental autoimmune neuritis. In some cases, axonal degeneration predominates, and these are discussed later.

Immunologic Studies

Studies of patients with Guillain–Barré syndrome further support the analogies to experimental autoimmune neuritis. In both diseases, activated lymphocytes are found in peripheral blood, and their number may correlate with disease severity (Cook et al., 1970). Furthermore, lymphocytes cultured in the presence of peripheral nerve extracts are activated, as shown by increased DNA synthesis (Abramsky et al., 1975) and by release of cytokines (Rocklin et al., 1971). However, the specific antigen may be different, because animals with experimental autoimmune neuritis show evidence of cell-mediated immunity to the P2 protein of peripheral nerve myelin, whereas patients fail to show antibody or cell-mediated immune responses to this protein (Iqbal et al., 1981). Finally, lymphocytes from both patients and experimental animals will demyelinate peripheral nerve in cultures of rat trigeminal ganglia (Arnason et al., 1969).

Soluble factors clearly are involved in paralysis, because plasmapheresis abbreviates the course. Serum from patients can cause demyelination in cultures (Cook and Dowling, 1981) and when injected directly into sciatic nerves of normal rats (Feasby et al., 1980; Saida et al., 1982). IgM antibodies that bind to carbohydrates of peripheral nerve have been found in 90% of patients (Koski et al., 1989). In early stages of disease, high-resolution immunocytochemistry shows complement activation marker C3d and the terminal complement complex neoantigen C5b-9 along the outer surface of the Schwann cells. Vesicular changes in the outermost myelin lamellae are seen on the complement-positive fibers, and this was seen prior to invasion of macrophages (Hafer-Macko et al., 1996a). This suggests that antibodies cross-reacting with epitopes on the Schwann cell cytoplasmic membrane may be critical in initiating the disease.

Viral Infections

The majority of patients with Guillain–Barré syndrome have prodromal "viruslike" illnesses involving the respiratory and gastrointestinal tracts. The

TABLE 8.6. *Viruses associated with Guillain–Barré syndrome*

Clinical association	Serologic evidence of recent infection[a]	Isolation from nervous tissue or cerebrospinal fluid
Strong association		
Infectious mononucleosis	Epstein–Barr virus	Hepatitis B virus
Chickenpox/herpes zoster	Cytomegalovirus	HIV
Hepatitis (A ,B and	HIV	
non-A–non-B)	Hepatitis B virus	
HIV		
Vaccinia		
Case reports		
Mumps	Adenovirus	Adenovirus 2
Measles	BK virus	Coxsackie viruses A2, 4,
Rubella	Coxsackie virus B5	and 6
	Delta hepatitis virus	Echoviruses 6, 7, 9
	Echovirus 7	Influenza A virus
	Hepatitis A and C viruses	Parainfluenza 3 virus
	Herpes simplex virus	
	Influenza A and C viruses	
	Mumps virus	
	Measles virus	
	Parainfluenza 2 and 3 viruses	
	Poliovirus 3	
	Respiratory syncytial virus	

[a]Fourfold or greater rise or fall in antibody titer, or, in the case of hepatitis, conversion from antigen positive to antibody positive.
Modified from Server and Johnson (1982).

latent period between these illnesses and neuropathic symptoms is usually 1 to 4 weeks, comparable to the latent period for experimental autoimmune neuritis. Although no specific etiologic agent is implicated in the majority of patients, a diverse selection of viruses have been sporadically incriminated by clinical diagnosis, antibody responses, or virus isolations (Table 8.6). Assuming a final common pathway involving sensitization to peripheral nerve myelin protein, it is difficult to envision how diverse viruses with no common antigenic characteristics and that grow in different sites could trigger a common response.

The viruses most consistently related to the Guillain–Barré syndrome have been Epstein–Barr virus, cytomegalovirus, HIV, and hepatitis viruses. Enteroviruses have been the viruses most often isolated from nervous system or spinal fluid, including the recovery of coxsackievirus A4 from brain, spinal ganglia, and spinal cord in three patients dying of Guillain–Barré syndrome (Estrada et al., 1975). Clearly, Guillain–Barré syndrome has been seen in patients with clinical infectious mononucleosis, with definitive serologic studies establishing a primary infection with Epstein–Barr virus (Grose et al., 1975). However, other serologic data must be interpreted cautiously (see Chapter 6). Data implicating cytomegalovirus are based on higher antibody levels in a case-controlled study and on increases in convalescent antibody levels (Dowling et al., 1977); yet these, like the antibody to herpes simplex virus (and human herpesvirus 6), might result from nonspecific virus activation (Merelli et al., 1992) (see Chapter 6). Both Epstein–Barr virus and cytomegalovirus remain latent in leukocytes, and, as noted earlier, lymphocytes are activated during the course of the Guillain–Barré syndrome. Lymphocyte activation alone can arouse these latent viruses. With herpesvirus infections, we are confronted again with the chicken-or-the-egg question: Is virus activation an epiphenomenon during the course of disease, or is virus infection or activation crucial in the pathogenesis of the disease?

Guillain–Barré syndrome has been associated with HIV infections at time of seroconversion, during the long asymptomatic period, and after onset of AIDS. The clinical course and response to plasmapheresis resemble the classic disease, but a pleocytosis of up to 100 mononuclear cells per cubic millimeter may be found (Cornblath et al., 1987).

Guillain–Barré syndrome has been clinically associated with hepatitis, and serologic studies have incriminated hepatitis A, B, and C, and delta viruses (Marés-Segura et al., 1986; Lin et al., 1989; De Klippel et al., 1993). In one report, hepatitis B immune complexes were found in spinal fluid of four patients, and serum levels of complexes correlated with clinical status. Hepatitis B antigen has been identified around endoneural small blood vessels and in endoneurium (Tsukada et al., 1987). In one case of chronic relapsing polyneuropathy, deposits of hepatitis B antigen, immunoglobulin, and C3 component were found in vasa nervorum (Inoue et al., 1987). Temporal association with Rocky Mountain spotted fever has also been reported (Toerner et al., 1996). *Mycoplasma* infections have been associated with some cases.

Guillain thought that the disease represented a direct viral infection of nerves. Although some viruses invade the nervous system by ascending or descending within nerve and, at times, infect Schwann cells, the only virus that has been associated with the infectious polyneuritis is Marek's disease virus, a herpesvirus that causes a demyelinating polyneuritis in poultry. Marek's disease is an economically important disease of domestic chickens, usually occurring in epidemic form in 3- to 5-day-old chicks. Paralysis with signs of spasticity or flaccidity, myoclonic spasms, abnormal postures of the legs, wings, and neck, and blindness secondary to iridocyclitis occur, as well as muscle atrophy. The disease runs a protracted course, although periods of transient improvement or even complete recovery are seen (Biggs, 1968). Both peripheral and CNS lesions are found in the natural disease. When transmitted experimentally, the disease is more acute, and visceral lymphomatosis is also seen. The peripheral nerves often are enlarged, showing marked infiltration of lymphoid cells; in some lesions these cells appear to be malignant cells of the lymphomatosis, but in others they cannot be differentiated from mononuclear cells seen in the Guillain–Barré syndrome (Lampert, 1978). Demyelination occurs in the infiltrated nerves.

In one study, explants of sciatic nerves and spinal ganglia from diseased birds were maintained in cultures with permissive primary chicken kidney cells, and replication of latent herpesvirus was induced. Ultrastructural and immunohistochemical studies of these tissues showed viral products in isolated Schwann cells, satellite cells, lymphocytes, fibroblasts, and macrophages, but not in neurons or in myelinating Schwann cells. Early in the course of the disease, cell-mediated and humoral immune responses to peripheral nerve and peripheral nerve myelin were detected. These investigators proposed the hypothesis that a persistent cell-associated viremia results in a latent infection of nonmyelinating Schwann cells and satellite cells, that viral antigens in the latently infected cells trigger a cell-mediated immune reaction that nonspecifically damages nearby myelin sheaths (bystander demyelination), and that myelin fragments from the damaged sheaths may also enter the circulation and stimulate an autoimmune reaction against peripheral nerve myelin (Pepose et al., 1981). This scenario is provocative in that it incorporates a number of the mechanisms of virus-induced demyelination.

Vaccine-associated Disease

Guillain–Barré syndrome has long been blamed on injected vaccines, including vaccinia, killed poliovirus, and influenza, but these reports have been anecdotal. In 1976, the National Influenza Immunization Program was established to provide a New Jersey (swine) influenza vaccine to most of the adult population of the United States, as well as to children at risk for serious complications from influenza virus infection. A nationwide surveillance system was organized to monitor complications. The vaccination program, which began on October 1, 1976, was suspended on December 16, 1976, when numerous reports of Guillain–Barré syndrome appeared among vaccinees.

Subsequent epidemiologic data confirmed that the incidence among vaccinees was significantly greater than that among nonvaccinated individuals over the same period of observation (Schonberger et al., 1979). Moreover, there was a striking nonrandom distribution of time intervals between the influenza vaccine and the onset of disease, with the period of increased risk concentrated within the 6-week period after vaccination. Some argued that this clustering of cases may have represented poor case definition and lack of follow-up, particularly since no increase in incidence of Guillain–Barré syndrome following swine flu immunization was observed in the U.S. military (Kurland et al., 1985). A reassessment analyzing individual cases in several states, however, confirmed the increase in risk (Safranek et al., 1991). The nature of the relationship between the vaccine and the syndrome has yet to be determined. Significantly, surveillance of subsequent influenza vaccines did not demonstrate their association with a significant excess risk of Guillain–Barré syndrome; this was particularly striking in the military, where over 5 million dosages of influenza vaccine were administered in October between 1980 and 1988, with no increase in November rates of the Guillain–Barré syndrome (Roscelli et al., 1991).

Somewhere in the swine flu vaccine program, a clue to the pathogenesis of the Guillain–Barré syndrome has eluded us. Nevertheless, an important lesson has been learned that in the risk/benefit analysis of an injectable foreign antigen or serum, into adults in particular, a possible heightened risk of this disease must be weighed in the analysis.

Axonal Neuropathies

Over the past two decades, large numbers of children in rural Northern China have developed acute flaccid paralysis, primarily in summer months. This is a Guillain–Barré syndrome in that it is an afebrile illness with ascending symmetric paralysis, with areflexia and the lack of a pleocytosis. The age of onset, geographic distribution, and seasonality all suggested a singular etiology. Reevaluation of this disease by a combined team of American and Chinese collaborators has shown by electrophysiologic and pathologic studies that this is an acute motor *axonal* neuropathy (McKhann et al., 1993; Griffin et al., 1995). This disorder is not restricted to China; in other patients with Guillain–Barré syndrome, about 10% to 20% have evidence of the axonal form of the disease, without sensory loss, and a more fulminant course, with poorer recovery (Rees et al., 1993). Antecedent disease in these patients is more often diarrheal. Electromyographic data reveal little or no evidence of demyelination (Visser et al., 1995). The pathology shows predominantly wallerian-like degeneration of nerve fibers, with only minimal demyelination and inflammation. Immunocytochemistry shows IgG and the complement activation product C3d bound to the axolemma of motor fibers, concentrated at the nodal axolemma, a striking contrast to the findings in the acute inflammatory demyelinating form of the Guillain–Barré syndrome (Hafer-Macko et al., 1996b).

Some patients with Guillain–Barré syndrome, especially the motor axonal form, have IgM antibodies against gangliosides, particularly GM-1. Lipopolysaccharides of *Campylobacter* have been found to react with monoclonal antibodies to GQIb ganglioside. Some Guillain–Barré syndrome patients, particularly those with the Miller–Fisher variant (ophthalmoplegia, ataxia, and areflexia) have this antiganglioside antibody, suggesting molecular mimicry between a bacterial component and neuronal antigen (Yuki et al., 1994). Attempts to use ganglioside preparations as therapeutic agents have led to Guillain–Barré syndrome with axonal degeneration (Illa et al., 1995).

Epidemiologic and serologic studies have implicated *Campylobacter jejuni* as the major cause of the diarrheal illness preceding the axonal form of the Guillain–Barré syndrome both in seasonal outbreaks in China and in sporadic cases worldwide (Ho et al., 1995; Rees et al., 1995; Jacobs et al., 1996). The circumstantial evidence is now supported by more direct proof: lipopolysaccharide of a Chinese strain of *C. jejuni* has produced flaccid paralysis and axonal degeneration after injection into chickens (Li, CY, *unpublished data*). If confirmed, this would represent the most convincing data to date of molecular mimicry as a pathogenic mechanism in a neurologic disease.

Brachial Neuritis

Acute brachial neuritis (also know as brachial plexus neuropathy or Parsonage–Turner syndrome) represents another acute axonal neuropathy related to antecedent infections. This acute painful localized paralysis involving one or both arms is characterized by the acute onset of intense shoulder–girdle pain that may persist for hours or weeks, followed by the development of weakness of muscles of the shoulder girdle that progresses for several weeks. Cerebrospinal fluid often shows a mild increase in protein and occasionally a mild mononuclear cell pleocytosis. Electrophysiology studies indicate an axonal disorder. Biopsies have shown striking multifocal mononuclear cell infiltrates in nerves (Suarez et al., 1996).

Clinically, about half the patients describe a viruslike illness or immunization during the 1 to 3 weeks prior to onset. It was a frequent complication of the postexposure treatment of rabies and tetanus when horse serum routinely was used. This led to the conclusion that brachial neuritis was a manifestation of serum sickness and was an immune-complex disease. Clinically, infectious mononucleosis, hepatitis, and herpes zoster infections have been implicated. Recently, several young adults have developed brachial neuritis following a febrile illness accompanied by arthralgias and rash shown serologically to be associated with parvovirus B19 infection (Denning et al., 1987; Walsh et al., 1988; Maas et al., 1996).

A similar acute lumbosacral radiculoplexopathy has been described with evidence of recent Epstein–Barr virus infection (Sharma et al., 1993). This appears to be an acute monophasic disease with good recovery and, therefore, in contrast to the severe progressive lumbosacral radiculoneuritis caused by cytomegalo-virus in patients with AIDS (see Chapter 6).

In both generalized demyelinating and axonal neuropathies and in focal neu-ropathies, no evidence implicates direct infections of the peripheral nervous sys-tem in humans, but increasing evidence implicates antibodies with complement-mediated injury or immune-complex diseases.

SUPPLEMENTARY BIBLIOGRAPHY

Asbury AK, Thomas PK, eds. *Peripheral nerve disorders 2.* Oxford: Butterworth, 1995.

Gilden DH, Lipton HL, eds. *Clinical and molecular aspects of neurotropic virus infections.* Boston: Kluwer Academic Publishers, 1988.

Hartung H-P, ed. *Baillière's clinical neurology,* vol 5: *Peripheral neuropathies.* London: Ballière Tindall, 1996.

9

Other Postviral Syndromes

Science seeks generally only the most useful systems of classification; these it regards
for the time being, until more useful classifications are invented, as "true."
S.I. Hayakawa,
Language and Thought in Action, 1939

Syndromes represent aggregates of symptoms and signs that "run together" and
therefore imply a common process. The three syndromes in this chapter are basically noninflammatory clinical complexes that have been repeatedly observed to
follow viral infections. All have been described during the past 35 years, and all
have been widely publicized in the lay media and, in some cases, politicized at
the national level.

Reye's syndrome was described in 1963 by Douglas Reye, an Australian
pathologist, who regarded it as a new disease. It became a clearly defined syndrome, sometimes clustering after outbreaks of varicella or influenza virus
infections. There was a dramatic increase in incidence through the 1960s and
1970s. In the early 1980s, contentious public hearings linked aspirin to the disease and demands of action led to warning labels and a public campaign against
the use of aspirin in children with respiratory infections or chickenpox. Subsequently, the syndrome has virtually disappeared, a phenomenon for which the
aspirin adversaries have enjoyed credit and about which critical observers are
perplexed.

Postpolio syndrome was first suggested by case reports in the 19th century. It
was formalized as the survivors of severe paralysis during the final epidemics of
the early 1950s reached maturity. Early in the 1980s, patient advocate groups
popularized the name and received extensive press coverage, yet recent studies
have questioned its very existence.

Chronic fatigue syndrome raises a question of what justifies labeling of a syndrome. In 1988, in response to public pressure, the Centers for Disease Control
and Prevention published a formal definition of chronic fatigue syndrome, an
ancient clustering of symptoms now marketed under a new label, the most recent
of many that this symptom complex has had through history. As Hayakawa has
suggested, "until more useful classifications are invented" we will accept these
three syndromes as "true."

VIRUS-INDUCED ENCEPHALOPATHY

Viral infection leading to a postinfectious, noninflammatory, metabolic encephalopathy presumably involves very different mechanisms than those in postinfectious, inflammatory, demyelinating diseases. Indeed, the pathogenesis may necessitate noncytopathic infection and exclusion of the immune responses. A number of viruses cause noncytopathic infections with acute cerebral disease. These can occur in immunocompetent hosts that fail to mount an inflammatory response, presumably because of a lack of some signal to initiate the inflammatory reaction (Johnson et al., 1979).

In experimental infections with some strains of rabies virus, and even in some cases of fatal human rabies, light-microscopic alterations are sparse, cytopathic effects on infected neurons are not seen, and inflammation is absent. Nevertheless, virus can readily be recovered, immunocytochemical staining shows copious virus antigen in neurons, and electron-microscopic studies show that virus particles abound (Johnson and Mercer, 1964).

Acute fatal encephalopathy can also occur with defective or nonpermissive infections of brain. Newcastle disease virus and neuroadapted strains of measles virus, which cause acute inflammatory encephalitis in infant mice, cause an acute fatal neurologic disease in adult mice, without obvious pathologic changes in the CNS. Minimal, if any, virus can be recovered. In Newcastle disease virus infections, virus antigen is found in very few cells, and the mechanism for fatal illness in this defective infection is uncertain (Burks et al., 1976). In the measles virus defective infection in adult mice, abundant antigen is formed in neurons (Griffin et al., 1974). Ultrastructural studies of these affected neurons show by immunoperoxidase staining that nucleocapsid and envelope viral proteins are diffusely distributed through the cytoplasm, but no viral structures are present in either nucleocapsid or virion form. Apparently, the mature mouse neuron restricts replication at a level before nucleocapsid assemblage, and the only structural correlate to the infection is depolymerization of neuronal polyribosomes (Herndon et al., 1975b). Nevertheless, the viral proteins or changes induced by the proteins apparently cause acute fatal neurologic disease.

Comparable types of virus-induced encephalopathy can readily be envisioned in toxic encephalopathy and in Reye's syndrome, where the primary alterations appear to be in mitochondria. A noncytopathic infection of the cells, a toxic effect of a viral protein, or some other indirect effect of virus replication not yet defined might disrupt hepatic and cerebral mitochondrial function.

REYE'S SYNDROME

Acute cerebral edema without inflammation is a long-recognized complication of viral and bacterial infections and immunizations (Lyon et al., 1961). This "toxic encephalopathy" is seen almost exclusively in young children. In rare instances before the 1960s, fatty changes in the liver had been seen accompanying toxic encephalopathy complicating varicella and other viruslike illnesses.

In 1963, Reye and his colleagues in Australia described the cases of 21 children between 5 months and 8.5 years of age who had acute cerebral edema and associated fatty changes of the viscera. The disease appeared to be postinfectious, and, indeed, subsequent data show that 75% of patients have respiratory symptoms as part of their antecedent illness, 15% have diarrhea, and 15% have varicella [Centers for Disease Control (CDC), 1980b].

Epidemiology

Reye considered the syndrome to be a new disease, which it clearly was not, because reports date back to the 1920s. It was a new disease, however, in the sense of an abrupt increase in incidence (Komori et al., 1992). The pathologic findings are sufficiently dramatic that its rarity in former years would be difficult to accredit to oversight. Furthermore, retrospective pathologic studies documented a genuine increase in the disease, rather than simply growing awareness (Chaves-Carballo, 1978). After 1963, Reye's syndrome was recognized as a worldwide disease, affecting primarily children up to 16 years of age, although occasional adults are affected. Only slight differences in attack rates between sexes and races are noted, but rural children have a three to four times greater risk than urban children (Hattwick and Sayetta, 1979). The disease occurs throughout the year, but with epidemic peaks in winter and a marked year-to-year variation. Outbreaks were associated with epidemics of influenza B and, to a less extent, with epidemics of influenza A. The numbers of reported cases increased through the 1970s. In 1980, a total of 555 cases were reported to the CDC. Then, coincident with warnings about the use of salicylates in children during viral illness or other factors, the incidence began to decline. Only 20 cases were reported in 1988 (CDC, 1989b).

Disease Description

The clinical disease parallels postinfectious encephalomyelitis in that the clinical "viral" illness may be abating when an abrupt recrudescence of illness occurs. In contrast to the situation with postinfectious encephalomyelitis, fever often is absent at the outset. Instead, severe vomiting is the cardinal feature. Lethargy may progress to agitated delirium, stupor, or coma within a few hours. Focal neurologic signs are absent, but a generalized increase in tone often develops, followed by decorticate or decerebrate posturing. Sympathetic hyperactivity and hyperpnea are prominent in severe disease. Engorgement of retinal veins occur, but papilledema seldom develops. Hepatomegaly is evident in about 50% of these patients, but jaundice is rare. Death results from increased intracranial pressure.

Laboratory studies show serum transaminase elevations at the outset of the disease and later elevations of plasma ammonia. Over half of the patients have prolonged prothrombin times. In early reports, hypoglycemia was considered a hallmark of the disease of pathogenetic importance, but hypoglycemia is now recognized to occur predominantly in children younger than age 2. The serum bilirubin level usually is normal. The spinal fluid shows elevated pressure without pleocytosis or an increase in protein content, and the electroencephalographic abnormalities are nonspecific (DeVivo and Keating, 1976).

In Reye's initial report, 17 of 21 children died and, during the 1960s, fatality rates in excess of 80% were reported. Although exchange transfusion, peritoneal dialysis, and varied metabolites and chemicals have been advocated for treatment, no treatment has proved superior to optimal intensive care, with strenuous efforts to reduce increased intracranial pressure (Corey et al., 1977). Recent mortality figures are quoted at 20%, but the denominator now often includes children with vomiting and laboratory evidence of liver dysfunction without neurologic signs. In those patients admitted with signs of increased intracranial pressure, the mortality is probably between 30% and 40%. Of the survivors, 10% have severe brain damage, and a much larger percentage have subtle disturbance of higher cognitive function (Brunner et al., 1979).

The brain in Reye's syndrome is swollen, and microscopy shows pyknotic neurons and swollen glia, but inflammation and demyelination are singularly absent. The liver shows a panlobar microvesicular steatosis with triglycerides in droplets and with depletion of glycogen. Inflammation and hepatocyte necrosis usually are absent, and this fatty metamorphosis is entirely reversible in children who survive. Fatty changes in the heart and kidney are frequent, with variable changes in lung, pancreas, muscle, spleen, and gastrointestinal tract (Partin et al., 1975). Electron-microscopic studies of both brain and liver obtained early in the disease show abnormalities in the mitochondria of neurons and hepatocytes, consisting of matrix disruption, moderate but not massive matrix swelling, and pleomorphism. These changes appear characteristic, if not specific, for the disease. An acute encephalopathy with hemorrhagic pancreatitis following virus infections has also been observed in children; this may represent a similar or related disease (Stover et al., 1968).

The ultrastructural changes have their counterpart in biochemical findings in which carbamyl phosphate synthetase, ornithine transcarbamylase, and other mitochondrial enzymes are reduced, whereas cytosolic enzyme activities remain normal (Woodfin and Davis, 1991). It is thought that β-oxidation is blocked, short-chain and medium-chain Acyl-Co A esters accumulate within mitochondria, and reduction of energy production and ATP within mitochondria prevent proper processing of imported protoenzymes and assembly of holoenzyme complexes (Glasgow and Moore, 1993).

Viral Infections

Epidemiologic associations with influenza and varicella virus infections are indisputable, yet isolations of these viruses from brain or liver have been rare or unknown. Serologic and virus isolation studies have implicated a plethora of different agents in individual cases or small numbers of cases (Davis, 1989a) (Table 9.1). The epidemiologic, pathologic, and biochemical investigations make it difficult to formulate a hypothesis of pathogenesis relating this spectrum of viral infections to hepatic and cerebral mitochondrial disease. Direct viral injury, virus precipitation of genetically determined metabolic defects, and virus in concert with some cofactor have been proposed.

The lack of inflammation, neuronophagia, or other histologic signs of encephalitis do not exclude a direct infection. A viral infection that invades neurons and hepatocytes and causes a selective mitochondrial injury is conceivable, as discussed earlier. The remarkable increase in incidence of Reye's syndrome during the 1970s and the plummeting incidence since 1980 could be related to mutational changes in the virus. Although influenza A viruses show annual mutations and periodic reassortments, this is much less true for influenza B, the more common precipitant of Reye's syndrome.

Intravenous inoculation of influenza B virus in mice can cause an acute encephalopathy, with seizures, coma, and death. The brain is swollen, with no inflammation but swelling of the astrocytic processes, and there is microvesicular fatty metamorphosis of the liver. Although no virus replication is found, viral antigen is found in cerebrovascular endothelial cells and hepatocytes, but the infection fails to spread to adjacent cells, indicating a defective infection (Davis, 1987; Davis et al., 1990). This appears to be a valid animal model for the disease, but other host factors or cofactors need to be evaluated to explain the epidemiologic patterns of the illness.

Some cases of acute metabolic encephalopathy diagnosed as Reye's syndrome result from infection of a patient with an inborn error in metabolism, such as an

TABLE 9.1. *Viruses associated with Reye's syndrome*

Epidemiologic and clinical	Serologic or extraneural isolation	Rare isolates from nervous tissue or spinal fluid
Strong association		
Influenza B virus	Influenza B virus	Influenza B virus
Varicella virus	Varicella virus	—
Influenza A virus	Influenza A virus	Influenza A virus
Case reports		
	Reoviruses 1–3	Reoviruses 1–3
	Coxsackie virus A10	Poliovirus 1
	Coxsackie viruses B1, B4, and B5	Coxsackie virus A9
	Echoviruses 3,8,11	Coxsackie viruses B2, B4, and B5
	Herpes simplex virus	Echovirus 8
	Epstein-Barr virus	Herpes simplex virus
	Measles virus	Cytomegalovirus
	Parainfluenza viruses 1–4	
	Respiratory syncytial virus	
	Adenoviruses 1, 2, 3, and 7	
	Rubella virus	

inherited abnormality of the urea cycle (Thaler, 1975). Indeed, the most striking decrease in cases since 1980 has been among 5- to 10-year-olds; those under 5 years of age continue to be affected, and alternative metabolic diagnoses are being made with increasing frequency in this younger age group (Hurwitz, 1989; Newton and Hall, 1993).

A number of medications, pesticides, and food additives were considered as possible cofactors with infections to explain the abrupt increase in incidence of Reye's syndrome during the 1960s and 1970s. Between 1980 and 1982, four case-controlled studies showed an association of Reye's syndrome with ingestion of aspirin during the prior viral illnesses. Aspirin companies and their champions attacked these studies on the basis of inherent biases. They delayed the mandate of a package label warning until 1986, after a prospective study not only confirmed the risk of aspirin but showed a dose response (Hurwitz et al., 1987).

Since the first warning of the dangers of aspirin, there has been a 50% to 70% reduction in use of aspirin in children under age 10 who have respiratory disease; yet, during the past decade, the incidence of Reye's syndrome has decreased more than tenfold despite several epidemics of influenza B and of chickenpox. Furthermore, a study in the children's hospital where Reye worked has shown that aspirin use in Australian children has been low for many years, yet the rise and virtual disappearance of the disease parallel the trends in the United States (Orlowski et al., 1987). The upsurge and subsequent fall in the incidence of Reye's syndrome are not adequately explained.

POSTPOLIO SYNDROME

Since the 19th century, reports have appeared of progressive motor neuron disease, often diagnosed as amyotrophic lateral sclerosis, occurring in patients bearing the stigmata of old paralytic poliomyelitis. Analysis of a series of these patients collected at the Mayo Clinic established criteria to differentiate new weakness years after paralysis, often with pain, atrophy, and fasciculations, from classic progressive amyotrophic lateral sclerosis. The weakness years after poliomyelitis differed from amyotrophic lateral sclerosis by the lesser severity and the lack of relentless progression of the motor neuron deficit and usually by the lack of upper motor neuron signs (Mulder et al., 1972; Jubelt and Cashman, 1987).

Over the past decade, the postpolio syndrome has received great attention in the medical literature and in the popular press. The term has come to encompass degenerative joint disease, marginal joint stability, mechanical respiratory problems associated with scoliosis, and late orthopedic complications of shortened limbs and tendon transfers. Postpolio syndrome discussed here is limited to "the development of new muscle weakness and fatigue in skeletal or bulbar muscles, unrelated to known cause, that begins 25 to 30 years after an acute attack of paralytic poliomyelitis" (Dalakas, 1995a).

Epidemiology

The frequency and prevalence of the postpolio syndrome largely depend on how the syndrome is defined and on how the study population is selected and queried. For example, in a follow-up of 283 patients with old paralytic poliomyelitis, 239 (84%) developed late dysfunctional worsening at a mean of 35 years after the paralytic illness. However, 170 had primarily orthopedic problems, only 35 had purely neurologic problems, and the remainder had combinations of difficulties (Kidd et al., 1997). Population-based studies give diverse incidences and prevalences. Of patients with prior paralytic poliomyelitis in Allegheny County, Pennsylvania, 28% were reported to suffer late progressive weakness with peak onsets 30 to 34 years after the acute paralytic episode. Weakness was more frequent in those who had more serious sequelae of their poliomyelitis and in females. Frequency was not related to the age at acquisition of poliomyelitis or to the severity of the original disease (Ramlow et al., 1992), although several prior studies correlated older age and severity of paralytic disease with the postpolio syndrome (Jubelt and Drucker, 1993). In a prevalence population-based study in a Swedish county, prevalence of postpolio syndrome was estimated at 92 per 100,000, which interestingly made the syndrome more prevalent than all other neuromuscular diseases combined; 80% of patients with sequelae of paralytic poliomyelitis reported late-onset symptoms of one type or another (Ahlström et al., 1993). A more widely accepted figure is that from the studies of Olmsted County, Minnesota, which determined that approximately 20% of patients have late progressive muscle weakening. The results of a recent study there, however, that selected 50 individuals who had had paralytic poliomyelitis between 1935 and 1960, and that performed detailed quantitative clinical and electrophysiologic studies at entry and 5 years later, showed remarkably stable neuromuscular function, even though 60% of patients were symptomatic from their sequelae; 20% did have unexplained muscle pain, fatigue, and a perception of weakness, but mechanical disorders were thought to explain these symptoms (Windebank et al., 1996). This does not contradict the observation that late muscular atrophy can occur years after paralytic poliomyelitis, but indicates only that it is probably not as frequent as has been assumed and that reliance on patient reporting of progressive weakness may give falsely high incidence and prevalence rates.

Disease Description

At the onset of the typical neurologic postpolio syndrome, strength and function have been relatively stable since the convalescence from acute paralytic poliomyelitis years before. Patients then have the insidious onset of increased weakness. This is most frequent in the previously weakest muscles and is often associated with pain and muscle atrophy. In patients who suffered from bulbar paralysis with respiratory compromise, new weakness may be noted in bulbar and respiratory muscles. Fasciculations are less frequent than in amyotrophic lateral sclerosis, but they tend to be coarser, indicating that larger fascicles are involved. Fatigue and pain are common symptoms of the disease, but they are difficult to differentiate from the fatigue and pain due to deteriorating orthopedic or respiratory problems that may complicate old but stable muscle weakness. Initially, electromyographic evidence of denervation and increased "jitter" on single-fiber electromyography were thought to characterize the postpolio syndrome, but these signs of denervation have not proved to distinguish between stable patients with prior paralytic poliomyelitis and those with new weakness. Immunocytochemical studies have shown that myofibrils expressing the neural cell adhesion molecule are also found in both stable patients and in those with progressive weakness (Cashman et al., 1987).

The progression of disease is highly variable from patient to patient. Often after an initial period of progressive weakness, there are periods of up to 10 years of stability. Over a 10-year period, the average progression has been estimated at 1% loss of strength in the involved muscle per year (Dalakas, 1995a).

Disease Mechanisms

The delayed onset and progression of paralysis and muscle wasting years after acute infectious poliomyelitis have raised this question: Does this represent a late sequelae resulting solely from attrition of overloaded, damaged, and aging neurons or does it represent ongoing infection (Table 9.2)?

Following loss of anterior horn cells during acute poliomyelitis, axonal sprouting of remaining neurons occurs. The slow recovery of function seen in the acute disease results from this reinnervation, and consequently larger fascicles are observed in muscles previously paralyzed. This overloading of residual motor neurons might lead to their premature demise, causing further denervation, more stress of wider reinnervation, and more demands on additional neuronal cell bodies. In addition, normal aging may be a factor. Morphological studies quantitating motor neurons at different ages and physiologic studies estimating the size of motor units with aging both indicate that attrition of ante-

TABLE 9.2. *Proposed mechanisms of postpolio syndrome*

Attrition of overloaded motor neurons
Normal aging loss with lack of reserve neurons
Immunopathologic reaction
    Persistent inflammation in spinal cord and muscle
    Abnormal antibodies or cytokines in spinal fluid
Persistent poliovirus infection
    Poliovirus IgM in serum
    Intrathecal poliovirus antibody synthesis
    Poliovirus RNA in spinal fluid by PCR

Ig, immunoglobulin; PCR, polymerase chain reaction.
Modified from Dalakas (1995b).

rior horn cells begins in humans after the sixth decade of life (McComas et al., 1973; Tomlinson and Irving, 1977). Although this may have little significance in normal patients, in patients with depleted motor neuron populations and no reserves this natural attrition might lead to progressive weakness (Johnson, 1984). The argument against normal cell aging being the sole factor in the onset of postpolio syndrome is that normal motor neuron loss is not evident before age 60, yet postpolio syndrome often begins at younger ages.

An autoimmune process or autoimmune dysregulation has been proposed based on the finding of inflammatory cells in sections of spinal cords from patients with prior poliomyelitis (but this occurs with and without postpolio syndrome), as well as some endomysial inflammation. In some reports, there has been high GM_1 antiganglioside antibodies or higher levels of interleukin 2 and its receptors, suggesting some ongoing abnormal immune response. These, however, have not been consistent findings (Dalakas, 1995b).

Persistence of virus seems highly unlikely in view of the rapid cytolytic nature of poliovirus infection. Nevertheless, enteroviruses can persist in animals. Theiler's encephalomyelitis virus persists in both the gut and the nervous system of mice and can produce chronic neurologic disease (see Chapter 8). The mouse-adapted Lansing strain of type 2 poliovirus causes classic acute poliomyelitis in mice, but persistence for over 2 months has been found in the brains of asymptomatic infected mice (Miller, 1981). Mouse-adapted poliovirus type 1 and Lansing type 2 RNAs have been found in mouse spinal cord by polymerase chain reaction (PCR) 12 months after paralysis (Destombes et al., 1997). Persistence of polioviruses in human nervous system has been demonstrated in children with hypogammaglobulinemia attended by chronic neurologic disease (Davis et al., 1977b). The presence of antipoliovirus immunoglobulin M (IgM) has been reported in occasional sera of patients with postpolio syndrome (Leon-Monzon and Dalakas, 1995). A very dramatic paper reported oligoclonal IgM bands specific for poliovirus in the spinal fluid in 21 of 36 patients with postpolio syndrome and in none of the controls. The investigators found no increased synthesis of IgM to measles, herpes simplex, or varicella–zoster viruses, and the report concluded that recurrence of muscle weakness may be caused by persistence or recurrent infection with polioviruses (Sharief et al., 1991). Nevertheless, a number of studies, some that predated and some subsequent to that report, have not supported these abnormalities despite the use of the same techniques (Salazar-Grueso et al., 1989; Jubelt et al., 1995).

Several laboratories have reported detection of poliovirus or enterovirus RNA in spinal fluid by using PCR. In one using primers from the $5'$ noncoding region and from the replicase gene of poliovirus, sequences were found in 4 of 40 spinal fluids of patients with postpolio syndrome but in none of the controls (Leon-Monzon and Dalakas, 1995). In another study, primers for a sequence common to many enteroviruses detected enteroviral RNA in the spinal fluid in 3 of 24 patients with postpolio syndrome but in none of 36 patients with stable poliomyelitis or 36 patients with other neurologic diseases. The study also reported positive reaction in spinal cord tissue from three of seven patients with a history of paralytic poliomyelitis (Muir et al., 1995). The third study using primers for a viral protein region amplified RNA segments in the spinal fluid of five of eight postpolio syndrome patients but also of two patients with amyotrophic lateral sclerosis and of one normal control (Leparc et al., 1995). Other studies conclusively have shown no poliovirus in the spinal fluid, muscle, or serum of patients with postpolio syndrome (Melchers et al., 1992) or have found enterovirus sequences of a nonpolio type in patients with and without neurologic disease (Muir et al., 1996).

Attempts to implicate persistent or recurrent viral infection by serologic and PCR studies of virus remain contradictory. The early demise of overloaded motor neurons in an already damaged spinal cord compounded by the normal aging process probably explains the late muscle weakness after paralytic poliomyelitis, but our changing concepts of RNA virus persistence in neurons make it necessary that we not glibly discard the possible role of polioviruses. The availability of new molecular tools, transgenic mice, and fresh viewpoints on how cells die or harbor RNA viruses make this a fitting time to reevaluate the possibility of persistent infection (Johnson, 1995a).

CHRONIC FATIGUE SYNDROME

Prolonged periods of lassitude often follow viral meningitis and encephalitis as well as many systemic infections, such as hepatitis, infectious mononucleosis, Lyme disease, and *Mycoplasma* pneumonia. Debilitating fatigue can be the chief complaint in a number of noninfectious diseases, such as multiple sclerosis, collagen vascular disease, and sleep apnea. Also, chronic fatigue may be the presenting symptom of somatization disorders and depression. The recent introduction of the all-encompassing term chronic fatigue syndrome has muddied clinical distinctions between the many illnesses in which fatigue may be a symptom and has given the dubious impression that this represents a new disease.

The terms used to describe an illness characterized by prolonged fatigue often accompanied by headaches, myalgia, low-grade fevers, sleep disorders, impaired concentration, postexertional malaise, and an array of other symptoms have mirrored the biases of the times. In the early 19th century, the terms nervous exhaustion and neurasthenia were coined. Da Costa's effort syndrome was proposed during the Civil War, shell shock during World War I, and battle fatigue after World War II. Chronic brucellosis and functional hypoglycemia became popular but overused explanations of these symptoms during the first half of this century. Total allergy syndrome, chronic candidiasis ("the yeast connection"), sick building syndrome, and mercury poisoning from dental fillings still have their proponents to explain chronic unexplained fatigue (Straus, 1991). Two features give credence to an infectious cause in some patients: the outbreaks of epidemic neuromyasthenia and the history in a majority of sporadic patients that their chronic fatigue began following a flulike illness.

Epidemic Neuromyasthenia

Over the past 60 years, over 50 outbreaks have been recorded of this curious disease, also known as Iceland disease, benign myalgic encephalomyelitis, and the Royal Free disease. Most outbreaks have occurred within closed institutional settings or rural communities; the majority of patients have been young adults, with women outnumbering men in most outbreaks. Early outbreaks were described during summer months when poliomyelitis was epidemic, and some epidemics were described as atypical poliomyelitis, but the attack rates were far higher than ever seen in paralytic poliomyelitis. For example, nearly 400 were affected at Los Angeles County Hospital in 1934 and over 300 at the Royal Free Hospital in London in 1955.

The epidemic disease typically begins abruptly with headaches and severe muscle pains; cervical lymphadenopathy and fever are variable findings. During the epidemics prior to 1960, motor and sensory neurologic symptoms and signs, including hyperreflexia, myoclonus, involuntary movements, diplopia, and facial paralysis, were occasionally seen. Despite these findings, the spinal fluid was normal in 95% of cases. Recent outbreaks have tended to be less stereotyped and have fewer objective neurologic findings (Briggs and Levine, 1994). The disease tends to have a protracted course; most patients recover completely within 3 months, but relapses of weakness and myalgia are frequent, and emotional disturbances, particularly complaints of memory loss, depression, and emotional lability, may be prolonged (Henderson and Shelokov, 1959).

Several of the early epidemics occurred during epidemics of poliomyelitis, and the high rates among young female hospital workers and the paucity of objective clinical or laboratory findings led some to assume a psychological causation; on the other hand, the stereotyped features of geographically and temporally dispersed outbreaks, the presence of objective findings in a significant number of patients, and the occurrence in closed communities, where spread of an infectious agent would be optimized, give credence to a viral cause (Acheson, 1959).

Sporadic Cases

The failure to recognize sporadic interepidemic cases was not surprising, because the spectrum of symptoms and variable findings would make sporadic cases difficult if not impossible to diagnose. The interest in sporadic cases of chronic fatigue was kindled in the 1980s with studies implicating coxsackieviruses in the United Kingdom and the Epstein–Barr virus in the United States.

Investigators in Glasgow initially reported a greater frequency of high levels of antibodies to coxsackie B viruses in patients with chronic "myalgic encephalomyelitis" than in controls or patients recently admitted to psychiatric hospitals (Bell and McCartney, 1984; Bell et al., 1988). Subsequently, using the diagnostic term postviral fatigue syndrome, groups in Glasgow and London reported a higher frequency of detection of coxsackie B viral RNA in muscle biopsy specimens from patients with chronic fatigue than in specimens from patients undergoing surgery for other reasons (Cunningham et al., 1990; Gow et al., 1991). A larger extended study comparing muscle biopsies of patients with chronic fatigue syndrome to biopsies of other neuromuscular diseases has failed to confirm a difference in the frequency of detection of coxsackievirus sequences in muscle (Gow et al., 1994). The issue is not settled, however, because the results of PCR studies of serum and throat swabs of patients with chronic fatigue syndrome using primers for a highly conserved region were positive more frequently in patients with chronic fatigue syndrome than in healthy controls, and sequence data indicated distinct sequences, suggesting the presence of a previously unknown (or unsequenced) enterovirus (Galbraith et al., 1995).

In 1985, two American groups reported patterns of antibody responses to Epstein–Barr virus that suggested active infection in patients with persisting fatigue; many but not all of these patients had symptoms or signs of infectious mononucleosis at the onset of their chronic illness (Jones et al., 1985; Straus et al., 1985). The cute tag of "yuppie flu" heightened popular press interest. Commercial laboratories responded with batteries of "chronic EB tests," and many patients shopped from doctor to doctor, seeking confirmation of what seemed to be a fashionable diagnosis. The criteria for diagnosis included high titers of antibody against viral capsid, persistent antibody to early antigen, and lack of antibody to nuclear antigen. Many asymptomatic people may show these variations years after primary infection, many patients with chronic fatigue had no antibodies to the virus, and a large overlap of results was found between fatigued and asymptomatic individuals. Most of the tests were done by indirect immunofluorescence involving subjective readings with major differences between cell cultures and observers. The lack of correlation of antibody levels with clinical status (Straus, 1988), the failure of acyclovir treatment (Straus et al., 1988), and the failure to find increased virus load in blood even in those patients with variant antibody levels (Swanink et al., 1995) dampened enthusiasm for the Epstein–Barr virus as a major cause of chronic fatigue.

Other herpesviruses, particularly human herpesviruses 6 and 7 (Buchwald et al., 1992), have been implicated with epidemic and sporadic cases of chronic fatigue, but increased amounts of antibody may represent nonspecific reactivation of virus at a time of stress (Table 9.3). In 1986, an outbreak of epidemic neuromyasthenia occurred around Lake Tahoe, Nevada, and was concentrated among high school students and casino workers. High frequencies of minor cerebral dysfunction, anosmia, lack of concentration, and emotional lability and lymphadenopathy were described. Of those affected, 60% had antibodies to human herpesvirus 6 compared with only 30% prevalence of antibodies in healthy controls. Human herpesvirus 6 has been reported to be five times more frequent in lymphocytes among sporadic cases of chronic fatigue syndrome, than in healthy controls (Di Luca et al., 1995).

TABLE 9.3. *Virus implicated in chronic fatigue syndrome*

Virus family Specific agent	Means of implication
Enteroviruses Coxsackie, group B viruses	Higher prevalence of antibodies Demonstration of viral RNA in muscle biopsies

Herpesviruses
  Epstein–Barr virus
  Human herpesvirus 6
 	
  Human herpesvirus 7
	
	Antibody patterns suggesting active infection
	Elevated titers of IgA; presence of IgM
	Antigen and DNA in lymphocytes
	Isolation from blood monocytes of a single patient

Retroviruses
  Human T-lymphotropic virus II
 	
  Human spumavirus (foamy)
	
	Virus antibody in serum
	Virus sequences in peripheral blood lymphocytes
	Virus isolation

Ig, immunoglobulin.

A possible relationship of retroviruses with chronic fatigue syndrome was raised by the report of human T-lymphotropic virus, type II, gag sequences in blood cells and antibodies in sera of both adults and children with symptoms, as well as in their close contacts but not in noncontact controls (DeFreitas et al., 1991). This and other retroviruses have not been implicated by subsequent studies (Gow et al., 1992; Khan et al., 1993; Heneine et al., 1994). A recent case-controlled study at the CDC found no serologic evidence to incriminate enteroviruses, herpesviruses, or retroviruses (Mawle et al., 1995).

Other studies have emphasized immunologic abnormalities presumably induced by the viral infection precipitating the fatigue and leading to the activation of herpesviruses. Low levels of immunoglobulins, circulating immune complexes, T-lymphocyte dysfunction, monocyte dysfunction, elevated cytokines, and a high rate of skin test reactivity to common antigens have been variably reported. Decreased natural killer cell activity or marginal differences in cytokine responses has been the most consistent finding (Swanink et al., 1996; Mawle et al., 1997). None of these abnormalities correlate with severity of symptoms, are found in all patients, or are of sufficient severity to lead to opportunistic infections (Shafran, 1991; Barker et al., 1994).

Attempts to Define a Syndrome

In 1988, the CDC convened a consensus meeting to define the chronic fatigue syndrome, and British and Australian groups have proposed similar working definitions. All propose the new onset of disabling fatigue of at least 6 months' duration and the exclusion of other clinical conditions that may cause fatigue. Both British and Australian definitions include cognitive dysfunction; the American definition includes neuropsychiatric symptoms among 14 minor criteria, 11 based on symptoms (fever, sore throat, lymphadenopathy, weakness, myalgias, prolonged postexertional fatigue, headaches, arthralgias, neuropsychiatric complaints, sleep disturbances, and description of onset over a few hours or days) and three based on findings confirmed at least 1 month apart (low-grade fever, nonexudative pharyngitis, and palpable or tender cervical or axillary nodes). Case definition requires the two primary criteria and six or more minor symptoms plus two or more physical criteria or eight or more minor symptoms (Holmes et al., 1988). Some working definition may seem necessary for studies, but nearly half of the cases followed in chronic fatigue clinics fail to meet these criteria (Bates et al., 1994). In clinical practice, about 20% of men and 25% of women state that they "always feel tired," so unexplained fatigue is a major health problem (Wessely and Powell, 1989). In a community-based prevalence study, chronic fatigue alone ranged from 1,775 to 6,321 cases per 100,000 persons, but chronic fatigue syndrome fulfilling defined criteria ranged from 75 to 267 cases per 100,000 (Buchwald et al., 1995). The sufferers are dominantly female (60% to 85%) and are a mean of 30 to 40 years of age. A four-site CDC study estimated a prevalence of 4.0 to 8.7 per 100,000 population (Reyes et al., 1997).

The prognosis is good in children (54% to 94% definite improvement or complete recovery) but poor in adults (fewer than 10% improve, and 10% to 20% worsen). In addition to age, a comorbid psychiatric disorder, a firm belief that the illness is due to a physical cause, abstinence from alcohol, and membership in a self-help organization have all been associated with a poor outcome (Sharpe et al., 1992; Joyce et al., 1997).

The contrary view is that chronic fatigue syndrome is not a syndrome. It is vaguely defined. Official labeling may satisfy distressed patients but may cut short the pursuit of causes of distress in the individual—whether it is a somatization disorder needing psychiatric treatment, chronic brucellosis or giardiasis needing antimicrobials, sleep apnea needing surgery, or postviral meningitis fatigue needing reassurance.

SUPPLEMENTARY BIBLIOGRAPHY

Dalakas MC, Bartfeld H, Kurland LT, eds. The post-polio syndrome: advances in the pathogenesis and treatment. *Ann NY Acad Sci* 1995;753:1–412.
Levine PH, ed. Chronic fatigue syndrome: current concepts. *Clin Infect Dis* 1994;18[Suppl 1]:S1–S167.

PART III

Chronic Neurologic Diseases

Traditionally, viral infections of the nervous system were associated only with acute inflammatory diseases. Over the past three decades, studies of human diseases and of natural and experimental animal diseases have shown that viruses can cause chronic and relapsing demyelinating diseases, degenerative diseases, malformations, tumors, and vascular diseases of the nervous system. The mechanisms of pathogenesis of these chronic diseases are as varied as their clinical and pathologic expressions.

In considering the array of actual and potential diseases associated with viral infections, we must differentiate between chronic infection and chronic disease. The static sequelae of acute infection, such as the paralytic residua of poliomyelitis or the amnestic state following herpes simplex encephalitis, are chronic diseases but are not thought to be related to chronic infection. In later life, the patients with the residua of paralytic poliomyelitis may develop further diminution of motor strength; this progressive disease may be independent of chronic infection. Ongoing demyelinating episodes can be due to epitope spreading or other mechanisms that can cause chronic or relapsing disease initiated by an acute viral infection but that do not require persistent infection to propagate the disease. Fetal and neonatal acute self-limited infections may appear to be progressive when failure to achieve developmental milestones with maturation may erroneously suggest progressive deterioration.

Conversely, persistent active or latent infections of the nervous system can occur without clinical signs, as seen in human immunodeficiency virus infections or latent herpesvirus infections. This persistence can be punctuated by acute relapses, as in recurrent herpetic infections, or by evolution of disease in the face of static or mounting quantities of virus.

The next five chapters address chronic infections and the evolution of acute and chronic diseases. They also address an array of diseases of unknown cause in which viruses have been implicated in inconclusive ways.

10

Chronic Inflammatory and Demyelinating Diseases

If the word chronic is taken to mean not only protracted, but also something which lingers on, has an irregular and unpredictable course and may end in any one of several different ways, then the expression should not be used about the diseases I have discussed here; these infections should perhaps rather be called slow infections . . .

In my opinion a number of such infections exist and the following criteria could be tentatively suggested for the group:

1. A very long initial period of latency lasting for several months to several years.
2. A rather regular protracted course after clinical signs have appeared usually ending in serious disease or death.
3. Limitation of the infection to a single host species and anatomical lesions in only a single organ or tissue system.

Björn Sigurdsson,
Rida; a Chronic Encephalitis of Sheep with General Remarks on Infections which Develop Slowly and Some of Their Special Characteristics, lecture at the University of London, 1954

In a series of lectures, Sigurdsson, an Icelandic pathologist who worked for many years with chronic sheep diseases, described the characteristics of maedi (an interstitial pneumonitis), paratuberculosis (a chronic bacterial infection), and rida (a degenerative disease of the brain, also known as scrapie). In the final lecture, he first coined the term "slow infections" and set forth his definition, stating that the final criterion might need future modification, as it has. Three years later, Sigurdsson described an inflammatory and demyelinating CNS disease of sheep related to maedi that was called "visna," the Icelandic word for wasting (Sigurdsson et al., 1957). Visna and scrapie of sheep have become the prototypes of slow infections (Table 10.1). They have in common long incubation periods after either natural or experimental transmission. The onset of both clinical diseases is insidious, followed by an afebrile progressive neurologic disease that leads to death. However, the two diseases differ sharply in pathologic and virologic features. Visna is an intensely inflammatory disease localized primarily to white matter, with attendant leukomalacia and demyelination; the causative

TABLE 10.1. *The prototype slow infections of sheep*

	Visna	Scrapie
Distribution	Classic disease limited to Iceland; other forms probably worldwide	Worldwide; Australia and some islands are exempt
Clinical features		
Incubation period		
Natural	2–7 years	2–7 years
Experimental	2–5 years	1–7 years
Onset	Insidious, afebrile onset of neurologic signs	Insidious, afebrile onset of neurologic signs
Prominent signs	Paralysis	Ataxia
Course	Progressive or intermittent course of many months	Relentless progression over 1–6 months
Cerebrospinal fluid findings	Chronic, pleocytosis, elevated protein and IgG	Normal
Pathology		
Neuropathology	Localized to white matter, with inflammation and demyelination	Localized to gray matter, with spongiform changes and no inflammation
Extraneural	Often interstitial pneumonia	None
Causal agent	RNA retrovirus	Prion
Host range		
Animal	Only sheep	Sheep, goat, mice, hamster, primates, and many others
Cell cultures	Sheep, goat, bovine, and other cells	None[a]
Immune response	Humoral and cell-mediated immune responses	None

Ig, immunoglobulin.
[a]Replication but not cytopathologic effects in neural cell line (PC 12 cells).

agent is a conventional virus. Scrapie, which is a noninflammatory disease of gray matter, is characterized by neuronal vacuolar degeneration and astrocytosis; the causative agent lacks most properties of viruses and has become the prototype of the so-called subacute spongiform encephalopathy agents or prions.

This and the subsequent two chapters deal with chronic diseases caused by persistent infections with conventional viruses. The spongiform encephalopathies caused by prions is addressed in Chapter 14.

MECHANISM OF VIRUS PERSISTENCE IN THE CNS

A remarkable variety of viruses can persist in the CNS. In addition to the herpesviruses, enteroviruses, arenaviruses, rhabdoviruses, and coronaviruses, which have been discussed in previous chapters, there is evidence of neural persistence of adenoviruses, papovaviruses, parvoviruses, paramyxoviruses, rubella virus, retroviruses, togaviruses, and flaviviruses—virtually the full gamut of animal viruses. Furthermore, the CNS appears to be the favored site for persistence; the majority of the slow infections of humans cause chronic neurologic diseases.

Both anatomic and immunologic factors foster virus persistence in the CNS. The unique lack of vascular permeability and the tightly packed parenchymal structure of the CNS, discussed in Chapter 3 as barriers against virus invasion, also form deterrents to clearance once virus has penetrated the CNS. Under normal circumstances, the CNS appears to be devoid of lymphatics or immunocompetent cells, and phagocytic cells are sparse. The levels of immunoglobulins and complement within the CNS are small fractions of serum levels, and these low levels may have more implications than solely the failure to neutralize or lyse viruses. Antibody and complement in high levels will cause antibody-dependent destruction of infected cells, whereas at low levels the same antibody may attach to viral antigens on the cell surface and cause capping, with extrusion or endopinocytosis of the antibody–antigen complexes. Thus, a cell infected with a budding virus may be lysed by extraneural levels of antibody and complement, but a comparable infected cell in the CNS may simply have surface antigens removed, which may allow the preservation of the nucleic acid and internal proteins within the cell. An infection cleared from extraneural tissues may be "modulated" in the CNS.

The absence of major histocompatibility-complex antigens on functional neurons eliminates the major mechanisms of clearance of intracellular virus by cytotoxic T cells. The relative protection of mature neurons from apoptosis is an additional factor in preserving their integrity (see Chapters 2 and 4).

The static nature of CNS cells also encourages persistence. In the congenital rubella syndrome, for example, chronic noncytopathic infection of cells in most organs is rapidly overgrown by the normal replacement populations, but virus persists in the static cell populations of the CNS. Similarly, the DNA of a herpesvirus sequestered in the nucleus of a hepatic cell might soon be lost, but the DNA in a ganglion cell of the nervous system secures its preservation for life.

Both DNA viruses, as discussed in Chapter 6, and retroviruses, such as visna, are capable of establishing static latency by sequestration of viral or proviral DNA. The mechanisms by which other RNA viruses persist in the CNS are more complex and depend on factors within the viral genome, the machinery of the host cell, and modifications of infection by immune responses. Several decades ago, there was a flurry of excitement about the possible persistence of nonretrovirus RNA viruses via DNA intermediates (Zhdanov, 1975; National Institutes of Health, 1976). It was speculated that these viruses might acquire or utilize a reverse transcriptase of an endogenous retrovirus already residing in the animal host or cell culture system. However, investigations have failed to uncover DNA intermediates in persistent animal infections with RNA viruses other than retroviruses. Instead, interactions of virus, host, and immune mechanisms appear to channel many of these infections into persistent form (Table 10.2).

Noncytopathic infections can persist if immune responses do not lyse host cells with viral antigens on their surfaces. Cell-associated fetal rubella virus

TABLE 10.2. *Mechanisms of virus persistence in CNS*

Standard virus and no immunologic determinant
    Sequestration of viral DNA (herpesviruses) or proviral DNA (retroviruses)
    Noncytopathic infection (rubella and lymphocytic choriomeningitis viruses)
    Lytic infection of population of replicating cells
Defect in virus gene or its expression
    Modulation by defective interfering particles
    Slow expression of conditional mutants
Defective maturation (measles in subacute sclerosing panencephalitis)
    Virus gene defect
    Host expression defect
    Immune modulation
Immune determinants
    Immune deficits (papovavirus in progressive multifocal leukoencephalopathy)
    Blocking factors
    Suppressor T cells
    Interferon

infections can persist for long periods in cells with low turnover rates (see Chapter 13). Noncytopathic productive infections of mice with lymphocytic choriomeningitis virus can persist for life, if infection occurs at the time of conception, *in utero*, or in the neonatal period, and leads to relative immunologic tolerance. Persistence of picornaviruses is difficult to explain, because they are not enveloped and therefore do not have known defects of maturation. Furthermore, an early function of their genome usually mandates host cell destruction. Nevertheless, picornaviruses such as Theiler's virus or type 2 human poliovirus in mice can be recovered from tissues, including the CNS, for months or years at low levels of infectivity (Miller, 1981; Destombes et al., 1997). Either an unrecognized mechanism to moderate infection exists in the animal host or the infection may be limited to a small population of cells capable of repopulation. This might occur in ependymal or arachnoid cells or in the subventricular zone, where even after maturation a vestigial group of cells continue to undergo mitosis but fail to migrate, degenerating *in situ*. These cells might provide an ideal host cell population for a smoldering lytic virus infection. Alternatively, virus might be sequestered in mature neurons that fail to express major histocompatibility antigens and that resist apoptosis.

Mutant or defective viruses can also modulate infection (see Chapter 2). Conditional mutants and defective interfering particles have been studied extensively in cell cultures and to a limited extent in animals. With temperature-sensitive mutants in animals, the incubation period may be prolonged and the clinical disease more protracted, presumably because of "leakiness" of the mutant at body temperature. Inoculation of mixtures of standard and defective interfering particles can dampen the tempo of infection by inhibition of the standard virus replication. Other mutations or impairment of gene reexpression dependent either on virus or host cell also could be important in persistent infections, but the recovery of defective or mutant viruses in persistently infected animals does not establish their role in the initial infection. The mutation rate is high in RNA viruses because they are not subjected to proofreading of DNA. During acute infections, there is a natural selection against avirulent or less infectious mutants, and their production, even at high rates, is irrelevant. In chronic infections, however, natural selection favors retention of these mutants, which are too enfeebled to kill the host cell. Orgel (1963) postulated that the accuracy of protein synthesis would deteriorate in the absence of cellular selection and lead to an "error catastrophe." He devised this hypothesis to explain cellular senescence, but such a phenomenon may be more relevant in persistent infections with RNA viruses, in which a cascade of mutations would occur. In turn, these mutant viruses might favor further persistence of infection, even though not crucial in its initiation. Thus, the recovery of temperature-sensitive mutants, defective particles, and other mutants in chronic infections, where survival of the meek is fostered, leaves their role in the initiation and even the maintenance of such infections ambiguous (Johnson et al., 1981).

Immune mechanisms may also promote persistence. An immune deficit may lead to failure of viral clearance, and this deficit may either be preexistent in the host or be induced by the viral infection itself. Epstein–Barr virus, measles virus, and HIV infect lymphoid cells and alter immune responses. Blocking factors, suppressor T cells, and interferon induced by the virus may, in turn, modulate the infection to promote persistence.

The roles of defective virus maturation, host cell factors in gene expression, and immune modulation have been extensively studied with measles virus in subacute sclerosing panencephalitis. Therefore, these factors are best discussed within the content of that human disease.

SUBACUTE SCLEROSING PANENCEPHALITIS

Descriptions of the pathologic findings in subacute sclerosing panencephalitis exist in the older German literature, but the current clinical and pathologic characteristics were defined by Dawson in the 1930s. As the epidemic of encephalitis lethargica abated in the United States, Dawson (1933) described what he regarded as an atypical form of that disease in which he found intranuclear inclusion bodies. Later he described the clinical and pathologic features under the title "subacute inclusion encephalitis" (Dawson, 1934). In subsequent years, nosologic confusion arose with the descriptions by European neuropathologists under the appellations of nodular panencephalitis of Pette and Doring (1939) and subacute sclerosing leukoencephalitis of Van Bogaert (1945). Dawson, a general pathologist, relied primarily on hematoxylin–eosin stains, which maximize inflammatory response and the presence of inclusion bodies; Van Bogaert, a neuropathologist, used myelin stains, which emphasize the demyelination and fail to show the inclusion bodies. Finally, Greenfield (1950) obtained their blocks, restained them, and showed the unity of the diseases; in the spirit of international compromise, the epithets of the three classic descriptions were combined into the cumbersome name subacute sclerosing panencephalitis.

Although Dawson postulated a viral cause, 35 years intervened before the disease was conclusively related to measles virus. Even now, questions about pathogenesis are unresolved.

Disease Description

Subacute sclerosing panencephalitis is a worldwide disease with an incidence of about one case per million children per year in nonimmunized populations. The disease has been reported in patients who are between 1 and 35 years of age, with average age of onset between 8 and 10 years of age. Males are affected three times more often than females, and there is a curious high preponderance among males of rural origin (Detels et al., 1973; Modlin et al., 1977). The most important risk factor for the disease is measles infection early in life (prior to age 2 in 50% or prior to age 4 in 80%). The disease is not contagious; no horizontal or vertical transmission is seen.

Although the tempo of the disease is highly variable, it progresses through rather stereotyped stages. The onset usually is insidious, with behavioral problems and decline in school performance. The counsel of a school psychologist or a psychiatrist often is sought because of lethargy, slovenliness, temper tantrums, aggressive outbursts and other unusual behavior. The second stage of the disease begins weeks or months later, with obvious intellectual decline and episodic disturbance of motor function, particularly with the development of myoclonic jerks. Seizures occur in some patients, and chorioretinitis, optic atrophy, cerebellar ataxia, and dyskinesias may develop. In the third stage, the child lapses into a stuporous state, with increased choreoathetosis, dystonia, and rigidity. Autonomic instability may lead to temperature fluctuations, diaphoresis, and tachycardia. A fourth stage is characterized by loss of cortical function, mutism, and flexed posture. In a typical patient, the course is ingravescent, progressing to death in 1 to 3 years. In approximately 10%, however, fulminating disease leads to death within 3 months, and in as many as 20% the disease may be protracted, with survival from 4 to 14 years (Cobb et al., 1984). Particularly in this latter group, prolonged periods of stabilization are seen, and in about 10% of patients transient periods of objective improvement are documented.

Clinical symptoms and signs and laboratory tests do not suggest an infection. Fever and headache are not present, and laboratory studies show no abnormality of peripheral leukocytes or sedimentation rate. The electroencephalogram, particularly during the second stage of the disease, often shows a very characteristic pattern of repeated discharges of high-amplitude slow waves followed by a relatively flat pattern. This "suppression burst" pattern is characteristic but not pathognomonic of the disease. The spinal fluid typically shows no pleocytosis and normal protein and sugar content. Despite the normal total protein, a first-zone colloidal gold curve was recognized in early cases, a finding now known to represent a relative increase in gammaglobulin in relation to albumin. In addition to the elevation of immunoglobulin G (IgG), agarose gel electrophoresis shows oligoclonal bands of IgG. The spinal fluid antibody titers against measles virus are high, as they are in serum, and a distorted serum–spinal fluid ratio relative to other antibody titers indicates local antimeasles antibody synthesis in the CNS. Indeed, 50% to 80% of the IgG in the spinal fluid may represent specific antibody against measles virus proteins. The findings on computerized tomography of brain remain normal during early stages, and late in disease show only ventricular enlargement and some attenuation of white matter. Periventricular and subcortical white matter abnormalities are more evident by magnetic resonance imaging. Both imaging methods may show generalized cortical atrophy and usually fail to show areas of enhancement (Anlar et al., 1996).

Pathologic abnormalities are limited to the CNS. Both gray and white matter are involved, but changes often are more prominent in the posterior cerebral hemispheres and less prominent in the rostral hemispheres, brainstem, cerebellum, and spinal cord. There is a mild leptomeningitis, and small cuffs of lymphocytes and plasma cells are found around cerebral vessels. Gliosis and the microglial reaction often are striking, and variable degrees of demyelination are found. Eosinophilic intranuclear inclusion bodies are characteristic, and although they are seen in all cell types, they are most frequent in oligodendrocytes. Immunocytochemical staining and *in situ* hybridization show measles virus antigen and RNA in the nuclei and cytoplasm and in processes of neurons and glia, including many cells that fail to show inclusion bodies (Allen et al., 1996).

Recovery of Measles Virus

The frequency of intranuclear inclusion bodies and the rarity of cytoplasmic inclusion bodies initially suggested a herpesvirus, and many of us made unsuccessful attempts to isolate a herpesvirus from this disease. The possible relationship with measles virus was not entertained until ultrastructural studies of the inclusions showed tubular structures with measurements corresponding to the nucleocapsid of morbilliviruses (Bouteille et al., 1965) (Fig. 10.1). Following this lead, high levels of measles antibody in serum and spinal fluid were promptly demonstrated, and immunofluorescent staining of brain tissue documented the presence of measles virus antigen (Connolly et al., 1967). Despite this convincing evidence for the presence of measles virus, no budding virus could be found in brain by electron microscopy, and the virus could not be recovered by standard methods. This could not be ascribed to neutralization by the high levels of antibody, because trypsinized cultures of brain cells subcultured multiple times in the laboratory failed to yield virus. After removal of antibody, the cells continued to contain nucleocapsid and antigen but released no infectious virus. Finally, cocultivation of these cultures of human brain tissue with cells of nonneural origin yielded cell-free measles virus (Horta-Barbosa et al.,

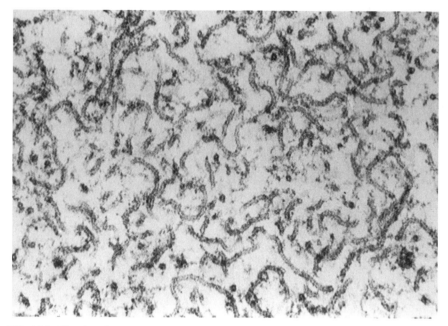

FIG. 10.1. Measles virus nucleocapsids in subacute sclerosing panencephalitis. This electron micrograph of a brain biopsy shows the ultrastructure of an intranuclear inclusion body in a child with subacute sclerosing panencephalitis. The 18-nm nucleocapsids are cut in three planes showing the hollow cores of the nucleocapsid tubules. ×110,000. (From Tellez-Nagel and Harter, 1966; reprinted with permission of the American Association for the Advancement of Science.)

1969; Payne et al., 1969). Such recovery is not invariable: using cultures derived from biopsy or autopsy tissue and cocultivation with highly susceptible cells, cell-free virus can be recovered in only about half the cases (Katz and Koprowski, 1973). Nonpermissiveness of human brain cells for measles virus appears to be a simple explanation, but these same explant cultures can be superinfected with wild strains of measles virus, and they release virus. Furthermore, some strains of measles virus recovered from the disease show altered growth in cell cultures and animals.

Subacute Measles Encephalitis with Immunosuppression

Before considering pathogenetic aspects of subacute sclerosing panencephalitis, the course of measles infections in immunocompromised patients needs consideration, because this third form of measles encephalitis can develop in patients with defective cell-mediated immune responses. Children with hypogammaglobulinemia recover normally from acute measles and subsequently can develop subacute sclerosing panencephalitis (Hanissian et al., 1972;

White et al., 1972). In contrast, children with defects in cell-mediated immunity may develop fulminant measles infections with giant cell pneumonia and signs of acute encephalitis.

A subacute measles encephalitis has also been described in children and adults receiving immunosuppressive drugs, most commonly for treatment of lymphoproliferative diseases (Aicardi et al., 1977; Wolinsky et al., 1977; Mustafa et al., 1993). A history of measles exposure precedes the neurologic disease by 1 to 6 months. The disease has a course of a few days to a few weeks, characterized by seizures, neurologic deficits, and stupor leading to coma and death. Seizures often are severe and may take the form of epilepsia partialis continua. The spinal fluid may show no abnormalities, and elevations of measles antibodies are not found. Pathologically, eosinophilic inclusions are found in neurons and glia, with varying degrees of necrosis, but a paucity of inflammation. Measles antigen is abundant in brain, and virus has been isolated directly from brain.

Despite the similar pathologic findings and the demonstration of measles virus in brain, the interval between initial exposure and disease, the temporal course, the serologic responses, and the ease of virus isolation clearly distinguish subacute measles encephalitis, which is an opportunistic infection of brain of an immunocompromised patient, from acute postinfectious encephalomyelitis and subacute sclerosing panencephalitis, both of which develop in immunocompetent children.

Pathogenic Aspects

How a ubiquitous virus causes a rare disease like subacute sclerosing panencephalitis in an otherwise normal child remains unknown. Almost all affected children have a history of uncomplicated measles years in the past. Certainly little similarity is evident in the clinical and pathologic features of this disease and those of acute postinfectious encephalomyelitis, a more frequent complication of measles (see Chapter 8), and no evidence exists that children who have had measles postinfectious encephalomyelitis are prone to develop subacute sclerosing panencephalitis. Three general categories of mechanisms have been postulated: an abnormality of the host response to measles virus, a combined effect of measles with a second agent, and modified replication and mutations in the measles virus (Johnson, 1970b). Furthermore, factors in initiation and maintenance of the persistent infection may be distinct from factors in expression of disease.

Abnormal Host Response

An immune-mediated pathogenesis of subacute sclerosing panencephalitis originally was suspected because of the high levels of antibody against measles found in serum and spinal fluid. Although immunoglobulins are found fixed to antigen-containing cells in brain (Sotrel et al., 1983), the development of the disease in children with hypogammaglobulinemia makes a pathogenetic role of antibody responses unlikely. Cell-mediated immune responses to measles virus are normal. A blocking factor was reported in the sera of some patients, but this is now thought to represent immune complexes, and it is not present in all patients.

Most data indicate that the increase in immunoglobulins simply results from ongoing antigenic stimulation. Furthermore, attempts at immunosuppression or immunoenhancement have not altered the course of the disease. Finally, virus remains cell associated, even after repeated passages of brain cells in culture where they have been totally removed from humoral and cellular immune responses. Therefore, immune responses do not appear to explain the difficulty in virus recovery.

Although immune responses have not been implicated in disease expression, they may play some role in the initiation or maintenance of persistence. Subacute sclerosing panencephalitis is more frequent in children who have had a history of measles prior to 2 years of age. This suggests that persistence in some way depends on the immaturity of immune responses, on the immaturity of target cells, or on infection while residual maternal antibody is still present. A child was reported who received immune serum globulin to modify measles at 2 years of age and who developed the disease 5 years later (Rammohan et al., 1982).

Acute measles in mice also can be modified from acute to subacute disease or persistent infection by antibody administration after infection. Experimentally, neonatal hamsters develop a fatal acute encephalitis when inoculated with measles virus. However, when born to mothers previously immunized with measles, the neonates develop persistent CNS infection (Wear and Rapp, 1971). Persistent infection and chronic disease can also be induced in hamsters with strains of measles virus from subacute sclerosing panencephalitis if inoculated into weanling animals. These viruses produce fatal encephalitis in neonates and no disease in adults. Persistence of infection only at a specific age and the conversion to susceptibility with immunosuppression suggest that maturation of the immune response may be an important factor in the pathogenesis of this persistent hamster infection (Byington and Johnson, 1975).

Chronic expression of cytokines by the inflammatory response may be important in disease symptoms or the pathogenesis of lesions such as the demyelination and gliosis. Elevated levels of cytokines in spinal fluid and within inflammatory and neural cells of brains of patients with subacute sclerosing panencephalitis have been reported (Mehta et al., 1992; Nagano et al., 1994).

The Second-agent Hypothesis

The role of a second agent was postulated on the basis of both epidemiologic and morphological studies. Epidemiologically, the higher rate of disease in rural males suggests a zoonotic infection. Subacute sclerosing panencephalitis might develop in children who have dual infections; alternatively, because the disease is more common if measles occurs during infancy, measles may persist in some children after initial infection, possibly in hematogenous cells, and then at age 7 or 8, during the course of a second infection, some synergistic effect may lead to initiation of the chronic CNS disease. The observations of papovavirus-like particles in cultures derived from brains of ferrets infected with subacute sclerosing panencephalitis virus have not been confirmed and may have represented glycogen particles or another virus unrelated to the disease (Katz et al., 1970).

Whatever the factors involved in the initiation or maintenance of persistence, at the time of disease the gene expression is impaired because the measles virus remains cell associated. Nevertheless, all of the essential genes appear to be present, at least in the patients from whom extracellular virus can be rescued. The explanation does not appear to be a different infecting virus strain, because the disease occurs without striking geographic or temporal clustering.

The Defect in Transcription of Envelope Proteins

In normal replication of measles virus, the RNA is replicated in the cell cytoplasm while still encapsulated in the nucleocapsid protein. The two major glycoproteins—the hemagglutinin that determines absorption and the fusion protein that leads to cell fusion or cell penetration—are inserted into the cytoplasmic membrane. The matrix protein attaches to the nucleocapsid and the inner surface of the membrane, where it probably stabilizes the location of glycoproteins. This alignment and budding sequence is not seen in subacute sclerosing panencephalitis (Fig. 10.2). Electron-microscopic studies show no virions

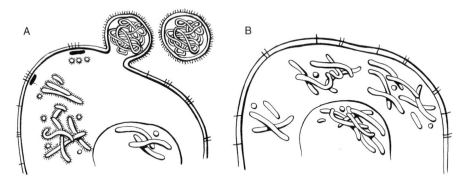

FIG. 10.2. Diagram of normal replication of measles virus and apparent defect in subacute sclerosing panencephalitis. Nucleocapsids are assembled in the cytoplasm, and viral glycoproteins are inserted in the membrane **(A,** *left).* The M protein shown (*heavy line*) stabilizes the envelope glycoproteins and directs the alignment of nucleocapsids to allow budding. Some nucleocapsids are seen in the nucleus, but these lack the normal fuzzy appearance that may represent M protein on the nucleocapsid surface. In defective infections in cell culture and presumably in subacute sclerosing panencephalitis **(B)**, nucleocapsids in the cytoplasms lack the normal fuzzy appearance. Few glycoproteins are inserted in the cell membrane. Alignment and budding fail to occur, and nucleocapsids accumulate in the cytoplasm and the nucleus, leading to inclusion bodies. (Adapted from Dubois-Dalcq et al., 1974.)

in the brain. Nucleocapsids concentrate in both the cytoplasm, where they are assembled, and in the nucleus. The three membrane proteins are often undetectable, particularly the matrix protein. When cultures of these brains are maintained in the laboratory, similar phenomena are seen. Nucleocapsids accumulate within the cell, and budding of virions does not occur.

Acute measles virus infection in CNS is limited to vascular endothelial cells (Esolen et al., 1995), and by the time postinfectious encephalomyelitis develops several days after the rash, measles antigens and RNA are not found in the CNS in any cell type (Moench et al., 1988). Since subacute sclerosing panencephalitis develops in only one per million children and after a lag of 5 to 10 years, the site of measles persistence is unknown. Persistence could occur in a rare child who has CNS infection or in extraneural tissues, with later invasion of the CNS. There is evidence of measles virus in extraneural tissues in patients with subacute sclerosing panencephalitis (Brown et al., 1989). Sequence analysis of mRNA from various parts of the brain of a patient who died of subacute sclerosing panencephalitis suggests that the virus is clonal (Baczko et al., 1993), but this does not clarify whether a single strain arose in brain, with subsequent spread, or whether a single strain invaded at multiple sites early or late in the infection.

Viruses recovered from brain show abnormal translation of envelope proteins and many mutations in sequences coding for these proteins (Sidhu et al., 1994). Measles virus genome is a nonsegmented RNA strand of negative polarity from which mRNAs are translated. A gradient of translation is seen, with messages for nucleocapsid and phosphoproteins being more plentiful than the downstream messages for matrix, fusion, and finally hemagglutinin proteins. In brains of patients and in cell lines harboring subacute sclerosing panencephalitis isolates, very steep expression gradients are found, so the 4 to 1 ratio of nucleocapsid to hemagglutinin transcripts seen in cell cultures is reduced to as much as 4,000 to 1 in infected brain cells (Cattaneo et al., 1987). This can, in large part, explain the failure to detect one or more of the envelope proteins in brain sections of patients (Baczko et al., 1986).

Viruses recovered from subacute sclerosing panencephalitis also contain many mutations (most frequently in the region coding for the matrix protein), have truncations and bicistronic messages, and have deletions particularly for the cytoplasmic domain of the fusion protein (Billeter et al., 1994). The biased hypermutation events predominantly in the matrix gene may be due in part to a cellular unwinding/modifying activity found in the cytoplasm of cultured human brain cells (Ecker et al., 1995). Matrix protein may be dispensable in persistent brain infection, but partial preservation of the fusion protein seems required to allow cell-to-cell spread of virus in brain (Cattaneo and Rose, 1993).

A possible model for the induction of the persistent infection at the time of measles infection is seen with a neuroadapted strain of measles virus that kills newborn rats after intracerebral inoculation. Passive transfer of neutralizing antibodies against the hemagglutinin protein modifies the infection, and a prolonged infection occurs. In these young rats, a transcriptional restriction of viral mRNAs, particularly for envelope proteins, is found, and this leads to a steep expression gradient (Liebert et al., 1990).

In summary, the presence of maternal or administered antibodies (or conceivably cross-reacting antibodies to a zoonotic agent) is important in some way as an initiating event leading to subacute sclerosing panencephalitis. Virus persists in neural tissues or extraneurally, and mutations accumulate. These mutations that block normal maturation would be eliminated in person-to-person infection but may be essential to persistent infection in the brain, because the paucity of membrane proteins and virions hinders normal immune clearance. The onset of clinical symptoms may depend on virus load or cytokine release by neural or inflammatory cells.

Treatment of Subacute Sclerosing Panencephalitis

When cases of subacute sclerosing panencephalitis were initially reported after measles vaccination, there was concern that the attenuated virus might have a heightened potential to cause chronic infection. However, the disease has virtually disappeared in populations with universal immunization. Prophylactic immunization with attenuated measles virus can reduce radically the incidence or prevent subacute sclerosing panencephalitis.

Therapeutically, few diseases have been subjected to such intensive and heroic efforts at treatment. Immunosuppression with varied modalities, attempts at immunoenhancement using transfer factor and cell transfer between identical twins, a variety of antiviral agents, interferon inducers, and plasmapheresis have shown no definite effectiveness in altering the course of this slow infection. Only the use of isoprinisine and intrathecal or intraventricular interferon has generated promising but inadequately controlled results (Gascon et al., 1993; Anlar et al., 1997). The claims of stabilization and remission are unconvincing, since this occurs in the natural course of disease in a significant group of patients. The time interval before entry into a study skews the study group toward long-term survivors. In this disease, treatment delay biases a study group toward that group which has a more prolonged course and more spontaneous remissions. Placebo-controlled studies are essential with the highly variable course.

PROGRESSIVE RUBELLA PANENCEPHALITIS

A slow progressive panencephalitis caused by rubella virus also has been recognized. Four children were reported in 1975 who had stable stigmata of congenital rubella and who developed a chronic neurologic disease during adolescence (Townsend et al., 1975; Weil et al., 1975).

This is a rare disease: fewer than 20 cases have been recognized during the past 20 years. The majority had stigmata of congenital rubella, but a few followed acquired rubella (Lebon and Lyon, 1974; Wolinsky et al., 1976). All patients have been males. The boys developed normally or within the limits of their congenital defects, which included mental retardation, hearing loss, growth retardation, microcephaly, cataracts, and cardiac murmurs. This development continued until ages 8 to 19, when deterioration in school performance and behavior signaled the insidious onset of intellectual deterioration similar to the early phase of subacute sclerosing panencephalitis. In addition to global dementia, ataxia has been a prominent neurologic sign. Spasticity and dysarthria usually develop late. Some patients have had myoclonus, but myoclonus is not as consistent as in subacute sclerosing panencephalitis. Optic atrophy is seen, and in some patients a retinopathy develops similar to the salt-and-pepper retinopathy of congenital rubella. The course appears to be very slow, extending over many years, with periods of stabilization and remission. Fever, headache, nuchal rigidity, and other findings to suggest infection are not evident (Wolinsky, 1978).

The electroencephalogram shows slowing, and the high-voltage suppression bursts of subacute sclerosing panencephalitis occasionally are seen. Computerized axial tomography or magnetic resonance imaging may show cerebellar atrophy, and high-density signals in white matter or spin-density and T2-weighted images. Spinal fluid may be acellular or show a modest pleocytosis. The protein is generally elevated, with strikingly elevation of IgG in an oligoclonal pattern. Serologic studies show the elevated levels of rubella virus antibodies in the serum and in spinal fluid, and a distortion of the normal spinal fluid to serum ratio indicates intrathecal antibody synthesis (Wolinsky et al., 1982b).

Pathologic studies have been limited but have shown gross atrophy of the cerebellum and greater involvement of white matter than gray matter. Inflammatory reactions found in meninges and perivascular spaces contain many plasma cells. Demyelination and leukomalacia with gliosis may be prominent. Inclusion bodies are absent, and perivascular periodic acid-Schiff–positive material is prominent, indicating mineralization similar to that found in congenital rubella encephalitis (Fig. 10.3). Vasculitis is present (Townsend et al., 1976 and 1982). Virus has been isolated from brain biopsy specimens (Cremer et al., 1975) and from peripheral blood mononuclear cells (Wolinsky et al., 1979).

The pathogenesis of progressive rubella panencephalitis is not understood. No immune deficit is evident in these patients; they have normal cell-mediated immune responses, excessive antibodies against rubella virus, and normal cell-mediated immune responses to mitogens and antigens.

The pathogenesis of lesions may relate to the immune complexes found in the serum and occasionally in the spinal fluid of patients with progressive rubella panencephalitis. These complexes have been dissociated and found to contain antirubella antibodies and rubella virus antigen. However, the antigen portion of the complexes is less dense than whole virus, so apparently only a portion of the complete virus is included (Coyle and Wolinsky, 1981). The unique vascular abnormality in the CNS might stem from the deposition of complexes, just as circulating complexes are found for prolonged periods in children with symptomatic congenital rubella and may relate to the similar cerebrovascular abnormalities in that disease (Coyle et al., 1981) (see Chapter 13).

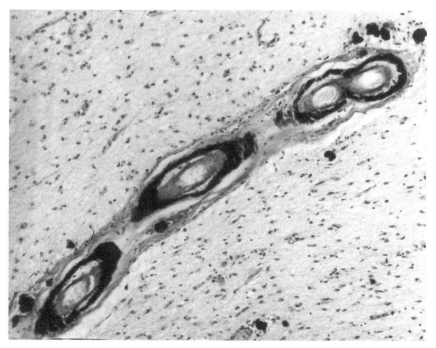

FIG. 10.3. Cerebrovascular changes in progressive rubella panencephalitis. Blood vessels in gliotic white matter of the cerebellum show deposits of periodic acid–Schiff-positive material in vessel walls. ×160. (From Johnson KP et al., 1978, with permission.)

In an editorial accompanying the first reports of this encephalitis, I commented on the timeliness of the report to alert physicians to prepare for the "legacy of the giant 1964 epidemic" (Johnson, 1975b). This predicted outbreak of progressive rubella panencephalitis never occurred, however, possibly because of interepidemic strain variations of rubella virus. No cases have been recognized related to the attenuated vaccine virus.

PROGRESSIVE MULTIFOCAL LEUKOENCEPHALOPATHY

Progressive multifocal leukoencephalopathy is a subacute demyelinating disease originally described with the subtitle of "a heretofore unrecognized complication of chronic lymphocytic leukemia and Hodgkin's disease" (Astrom et al., 1958). The histopathologic findings in this disease include inclusion bodies in large distorted oligodendrocyte nuclei surrounding the demyelinated foci and bizarre changes in astrocytes within the areas of demyelination. Because of the association with illnesses known to suppress cell-mediated immunity and the presence of the inclusion bodies, an opportunistic noninflammatory viral infection of the nervous system was postulated (Cavanagh et al., 1959; Richardson,

1961). The viral origin of this disease was established in the 1960s and 1970s with demonstration of virions within the lesions and consistent recovery of the JC papovavirus from the disease. From the biologic standpoint, it was the first chronic human demyelinating disease for which a viral cause had been firmly established.

Progressive multifocal leukoencephalopathy was an extraordinarily rare disease during these initial virologic studies. When we studied autopsy and biopsy tissues of 13 patients in 1973, we scoured freezers of 12 institutions in three countries (Narayan et al., 1973). In the 1970s, more cases were seen with more intensive immunosuppression to treat diseases, such as systemic lupus erythematosus, rheumatoid arthritis, and polymyositis, and to maintain allografts. Abruptly in the 1980s, the incidence increased with the eruption of HIV infection. Prior to 1982, many institutions, such as Columbia-Presbyterian Medical Center, Albert Einstein College of Medicine and affiliated hospitals, and the Johns Hopkins Hospital, had recorded only single cases of progressive multifocal leukoencephalopathy over the preceding 20 years; now about 4% of all AIDS deaths are complicated by this opportunistic demyelinating infection.

Disease Description

Progressive multifocal leukoencephalopathy has a worldwide distribution. Most of the patients are adults, although children with primary immunodeficiency disorders have developed the disease.

The neurologic disease can occur at any time during the course of the underlying immunodeficiency disorder. The onset usually is insidious, with symptoms and signs that suggest multifocal disease. Paralysis, mental deterioration, visual loss, and sensory abnormalities are common. Ataxia is less common, as are focal signs of brainstem or spinal cord involvement. The patients remain afebrile, and headaches are infrequent. The disease usually follows an ingravescent course to death in 3 to 6 months. Occasionally, patients survive for years, with stabilization or prolonged remissions (Price et al., 1983; Berger and Mucke, 1988).

The spinal fluid is generally normal, with no pleocytosis, no elevation of protein content, and no increase in abnormality of immunoglobulins. In patients with HIV infections, however, cells and protein elevations may be found as part of the primary infection. Electroencephalograms show only nonspecific changes. Serologic studies of serum and spinal fluid are of no help, because antibody against the major virus involved in progressive multifocal leukoencephalopathy is ubiquitous. Furthermore, the immune deficits of the patients usually abrogate antibody increases, and antibody is not found in spinal fluid. Computerized tomography may show radiolucent areas in white matter, but magnetic resonance images show characteristic multifocal lesions involving subcortical white matter without enhancement. Recent descriptions of polymerase chain reaction (PCR) for JC virus DNA on spinal fluid report sensitivities of 82% to 92% (Weber et al., 1994; McGuire et al., 1995).

A definitive diagnosis of progressive multifocal leukoencephalopathy can be made only pathologically. Gross inspection of the brain shows obvious areas of demyelination ranging from the size of pinheads to large confluent areas of leukomalacia. The multifocal areas of demyelination are most prominent in the subcortical white matter, and many become confluent, forming multilobulated lesions (Fig. 10.4A). Histologically, these demyelinating foci show a relative sparing of axons and a loss of both oligodendrocytes and myelin. The oligodendrocytes surrounding the foci often are greatly enlarged and may contain large intranuclear inclusion bodies. Within the demyelinated foci, the astrocytes are also enlarged and often contain bizarre mitotic figures, multiple nuclei, and multilobulated nuclei. In the original description of the disease, the authors stated that "astrocytes of this sort are ordinarily met with only in neoplastic processes" (Astrom et al., 1958). Indeed, several patients have had coexistent cerebral tumors, including one young patient with multifocal gliomas that topographically corresponded to areas of demyelination (Castaigne et al., 1974). In about half of the cases inflammation is absent, but in others some perivascular collections of mononuclear cells are found.

Staining for specific myelin proteins shows a wider perimeter of myelin-associated glycoprotein loss than myelin basic protein loss, indicating a "dying back process," since myelin-associated glycoprotein is concentrated in the distal extension of the myelin sheath adjacent to the axon (Itoyama et al., 1982). Unlike the concordant myelin protein loss characteristic of postmeasles encephalitis and experimental autoimmune encephalomyelitis or the variable extent of different myelin protein loss in multiple sclerosis (Gendelman et al., 1985b), the pattern in progressive multifocal leukoencephalopathy signals a primary disease of oligodendrocytes.

Recovery of Papovaviruses

Following the speculation in the early 1960s concerning a viral cause, no virus was recovered by inoculation of cell cultures, small laboratory rodents, or embryonated eggs or by inoculation and long-term holding of primates (ZuRhein, 1969). In retrospect, it is unlikely that the causative virus would have been recovered without the morphological clue as to which type of virus to look for. In 1964, ZuRhein, at the meeting of the Association for Research in Nervous and Mental Diseases, presented electron micrographs of formalin-fixed brain in which she showed crystalline arrays of viruslike particles within the oligodendrocyte inclusion bodies (Fig. 10.4B). Because the particles resembled icosahedral virions with a diameter of approximately 39 nm, she postulated that these were papovaviruses (ZuRhein and Chou, 1965). This conclusion was met with great skepticism and some overt hostility (Sabin, 1968). Known papovaviruses were tumor viruses, and the only known human papovavirus was wart virus. The drollness of warts in the brain was not lost on the audience. Nevertheless, the ultrastructural finding was confirmed in virtually every known case of progres-

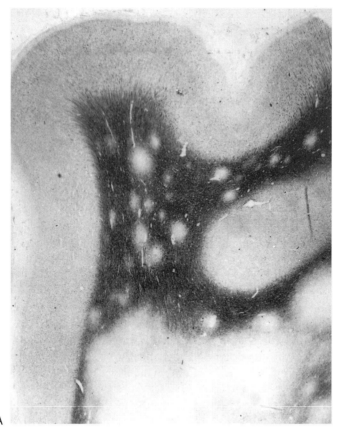

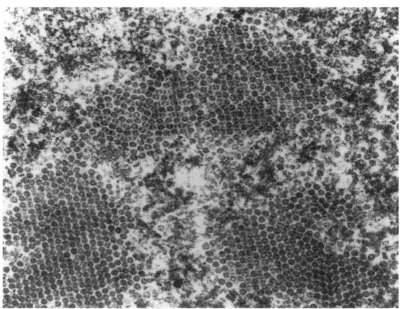

sive multifocal leukoencephalopathy, and the size range of the virions, 33 to 45 nm, clearly placed them not with the papilloma group of papovaviruses but with the smaller polyomaviruses, which then included only polyomavirus of mice, simian virus 40 (SV40), and a variety of nonprimate viruses. At that time, no polyomavirus had been recovered from humans.

Utilizing methods specifically directed toward the recovery of papovaviruses, two laboratories in 1971 recovered viruses from brain tissue of patients with progressive multifocal leukoencephalopathy. Padgett and her associates (1971) employed human fetal brain cultures that contained oligodendrocyte precursor cells previously shown to be susceptible to SV40; Weiner, in our laboratory, grew cells from the brain and fused them to rhesus monkey cells, a method used to rescue SV40 from nonpermissive tumor cells. Investigators in the two laboratories met and exchanged agents and reagents only to discover they had two different viruses. The virus obtained in Wisconsin was clearly a new virus, whereas our initial isolate was clearly SV40, a virus indigenous to rhesus monkeys and, in retrospect, possibly rescued by complementation with JC sequences (Penney et al., 1972; Weiner et al., 1972).

An additional papovavirus, BK virus, was then reported in England from the urine of a patient undergoing therapeutic immunosuppression, a virus that proved to be related to but distinct from both JC virus and SV40 (Gardner et al., 1971). Thus, within 1 year, three closely related polyomaviruses with 69% to 75% sequence homology were reported to be recovered from humans.

The virus isolated in Wisconsin was designated JC, the initials of the patient. In retrospect, this was an unfortunate choice, because subsequent confusion with the unrelated but transmissible Jakob–Creutzfeldt disease has been frequent. Subsequent to the isolation of these viruses, monospecific sera have been made that allow rapid identification by immunofluorescence staining of brain tissue and electron-microscopic agglutination of particles from brain and that avoid the tedious culture methods employed in the initial isolation. Subsequently, studies of hundreds of patients with progressive multifocal leukoencephalopathy have established that JC virus is the cause of all or almost all cases. SV40 has been reported in six cases, and BK virus has not been associated with any cases (Narayan et al., 1973; Walker, 1978).

Pathogenetic Aspects

These polyomaviruses have not been convincingly associated with any other human disease. The majority of persons develop antibody to JC virus when they

◀———————————————————————————

FIG. 10.4. Abnormalities in progressive multifocal leukoencephalopathy. Discrete and confluent demyelinating lesions in the subcortical white matter are in section stained with Luxol fast blue and cresyl violet **(A)**. ×5. The electron micrograph of glial nucleus in the periphery of a demyelinated focus shows viruslike particles in orderly crystalline arrays **(B)**. ×43,000 (From ZuRhein and Chou, 1968, with permission of the Association for Research in Nervous and Mental Diseases.)

are between 1 and 14 years of age and, by middle age, 70% to 75% have anti-body (Padgett and Walker, 1973b). This primary infection, in general, has not been related to any clinical disease. A single instance of severe encephalitis and paraplegia, followed by a fluctuating course of neurologic disease, was reported in a 13-year-old girl coincident with seroconversion to JC virus (Blake et al., 1992). Seroconversion and disease could be coincidental or could represent the precipitation of an initial attack of multiple sclerosis by an intercurrent infection.

BK virus is also a ubiquitous, human symbiote to which the majority of people develop antibody at an even younger age, with seroconversion between ages 3 and 6 in over 50% of the population (Gardner, 1973; Shah et al., 1973). Transmission is probably by respiratory spread or by urine, since intermittent urinary excretion of both JC and BK viruses occurs normally and excretion is increased during pregnancy, with increasing age, or with immunosuppression.

Human infections with SV40 do occur but under very specific circumstances. The virus is common among Asiatic macaques, and antibody is common in persons exposed to these monkeys. However, the major exposure of people to SV40 was between 1955 and 1961, when over 10 million persons were injected with killed poliovirus vaccines contaminated with live SV40; serologic studies indicate that active infection occurred in a large percentage of these vaccine recipients (Shah and Nathanson, 1976). In addition to these exposures, 3% of people who have no known exposure to monkeys and who never received contaminated vaccines have antibody to SV40, but the origin of this antibody is unknown.

Latency is known to occur in kidney, but JC virus also has been identified in spleen and marrow and some B cells (Tornatore et al., 1992). In HIV-infected patients, JC and BK sequences frequently are found in blood leukocytes (Azzi et al., 1996; Dubois et al., 1996). Spread to brain is presumably from the blood, but two questions remain unanswered: Is progressive multifocal leukoencephalopathy due to reactivation of latent virus in an immunodeficient host or is it due to primary infection of the rare immunodeficient adult who escaped primary infection in childhood? The answer is yet to be determined. The other question is whether JC virus is latent in brain (Lipton, 1991). There are reports of *in situ* hybridization and PCR detection of JC virus DNA in normal or aged brains (Mori et al., 1991; White et al., 1992; Vago et al., 1996), but other reports refute these findings (Aksamit et al., 1986; Wiley et al., 1988). Virus recovered from urine of nonimmunocompromised individuals (archetypal strains) differs in regulatory sequences from brain isolates, but sequence analyses of multiple isolates clearly show that brain isolates are derived from individual archetypal strains and do not constitute a unique lineage (Iida et al., 1993).

The pathogenesis of the demyelinating disease appears straightforward (Johnson et al., 1974b). First, the evidence linking virus to disease is compelling: (a) JC virus is present in unprecedented quantities, over 10^{10} particles per gram of brain, in progressive multifocal leukoencephalopathy (Dorries et al., 1979). (b) Virions are found in appropriate locations, primarily in oligodendrocytes that show cytopathic changes. (c) Although JC virus does not produce a disease in experimental animals, spontaneous progressive multifocal leukoencephalopathy due to SV40 has been found in immunocompromised monkeys (Holmberg et al., 1977).

The mechanisms by which these viruses produce unique cytopathologic changes in the brain are suggested both by histologic studies and by studies of cell cultures. In cultures of human fetal glial cells, two cell types predominate: large translucent vesicular cells that stain for glial fibrillary protein; and smaller dense cells, termed spongioblasts, that appear to represent populations of neuron and oligodendrocyte precursors. Inoculation of these cultures with JC, BK, or SV40 produces primarily infection and lysis of the spongioblasts (Shein, 1967; Oster-Granite et al., 1978). Some astrocytes may also be lysed, but in the case of SV40, surviving astrocytes proliferate rapidly and contain intranuclear T (tumor) antigen by immunofluorescent staining (Shein, 1967). Thus, within these cultures of human fetal glial cells, there are both permissive and nonpermissive populations of cells. In the human brain, the neurons show no evidence of disease and do not contain virus particles. In the white matter, the oligodendrocytes in the foci of demyelination are destroyed, and those at the border show marked cytopathic changes, with arrays of virions packing their nuclei. The oligodendrocytes appear to be permissive cells that are lysed. Within the areas of demyelination, the astrocytes are large and distorted and often contain multiple nuclei and resemble malignant cells (Fig. 10.5). They often contain JC virus DNA but only occasionally contain virions or viral antigen (Aksamit et al.,

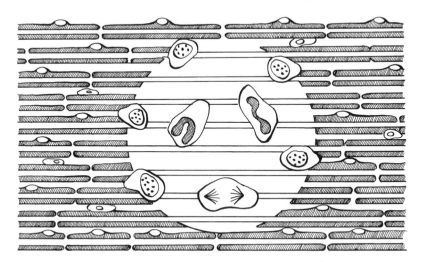

FIG. 10.5. Schematic diagram of progressive multifocal leukoencephalopathy. Neurons (not shown) are unaffected, and their axons (*open lines*) are intact through the demyelinated focus. Oligodendrocytes are absent within the focus and enlarged, with intranuclear inclusion filled with virions at the periphery of the area of demyelination. Astrocytes within the focus are enlarged and multinucleated, have dumbbell-shaped nuclei, and show abnormal mitotic figures. (Adapted from Johnson et al., 1974b.)

1986). Although sections of the brain may fail to show T antigen, putative astrocytes grown from the brains of patients with progressive multifocal leukoencephalopathy show T antigen by immunocytochemistry and may yield virus when fused with permissive cells (Weiner and Narayan, 1974).

The remarkably higher incidence of progressive multifocal leukoencephalopathy in AIDS than in other immunodeficiency disorders has suggested that HIV in brain may augment JC virus replication. Indeed, the *tat* protein of HIV increases the activity of the JC virus late promoter, which may, in part, explain the extraordinary increase in this disease (Tada et al., 1990).

JC, BK, and SV40 viruses all produce tumors when inoculated into hamsters. SV40 does produce progressive multifocal leukoencephalopathy in monkeys, and one of the murine polyoma strains causes rather diffuse myelin disruption in nude mice (McCance et al., 1983). Transgenic mice that have been generated with JC virus regulatory and early coding regions develop severe tremors at 2 weeks of age and show CNS hypomyelination. In the mice, T antigen of JC virus is expressed primarily in oligodendrocytes, rates of production of multiple myelin proteins are diminished, and myelin is not appropriately assembled (Trapp et al., 1988).

Several therapeutic approaches to progressive multifocal leukoencephalopathy have been advocated. To restore immunocompetence by the cessation of immunosuppressant therapy is reasonable, if possible. Cytosine arabinoside has now undergone a controlled study in AIDS patients, and no survival benefit was seen. Interferon α has been thought to slow disease and prolong survival in an observational study. Topisomerase inhibitors have been shown to inhibit JC virus replication in glioma cells (Kerr et al., 1993), and clinical trials are in progress (Sacktor and McArthur, 1997).

POSSIBLE VIRAL CAUSE OF MULTIPLE SCLEROSIS

Speculation on a viral etiology for multiple sclerosis has recurred for over 100 years. Pierre Marie (1884) postulated an infectious cause, and because rabies vaccine had recently been introduced by Pasteur, he also predicted that a viral isolate and a vaccine would soon be in hand for multiple sclerosis. Over the next century, a plethora of claims of recovery of infectious agents and of disease transmission have been proposed and refuted (Johnson, 1985b and 1994b).

Over the past 50 years, three areas of investigation have given credence to a viral etiology of multiple sclerosis. First, epidemiologic studies have indicated a childhood exposure factor (possibly an infectious agent) in the genesis of multiple sclerosis and have also shown that "viruslike" illnesses are related temporally to acute exacerbation of the disease (Sibley et al., 1985; Andersen et al., 1993; Panitch, 1994). Second, studies of a wide variety of animal models and human illnesses have shown that virus diseases can have prolonged incubation periods with remitting and relapsing courses and cause myelin destruction mediated by a variety of mechanisms. Third, studies of patients with multiple sclerosis have shown higher levels of antibody against a variety of viruses (particularly measles) in serum and spinal fluid of patients than in specimens of controls, have reported viruslike particles in tissues, and have claimed recovery of a variety of different agents.

Epidemiologic Studies

Geographic Distribution

National and regional death rates in over 300 prevalence studies have shown an uneven geographic distribution of multiple sclerosis (Kurtzke, 1993). These differences are not due to variances in clinical sophistication or quality of health care delivery, as previously believed. Data collected largely since World War II have demonstrated in Europe and North America a north–south gradient and prevalence, with rates of 30 to 100 cases per 100,000 in northern Europe, south-ern Canada, and northern United States, in contrast to rates below 30 in most of southern Europe and the southern United States. Prevalent rates in equatorial areas approaches 1 per 100,000. The Southern Hemisphere is less well delin-eated, but multiple sclerosis reaches moderate prevalence rates in South Africa, appears more common in the southeastern Australia and Tasmania than northern Australia, and is more prevalent in the southern than northern island of New Zealand. This is not, however, a smooth latitudinal gradient. There are foci of exceedingly high prevalence, such as in the Shetland and Orkney Islands, where they have been reported in excess of 200 per 100,000, and relatively high rates have been reported in Italy and Cyprus. Asia and Africa have uniformly low rates.

The rate is higher for women than men and half as frequent in blacks as in whites, although the north–south gradient in the United States is seen in both races. Disease also correlates, to a lesser extent, with higher socioeconomic class and urbanization.

The incidence appears to be stable over time in many studies, but others have shown in increasing rate. This is particularly notable in Rochester, Minnesota, where a stable rate was noted for many years, with a striking rise in incidence dur-ing a recent survey (Wynn et al., 1990). In the United States, the rates are uni-formly high in all states above the 37th parallel, with lower rates in most states below the 37th parallel. These are not consistent in states of the Southwest that have had sizable immigrations from north and south. Correlations also have been drawn with high rates in states with the larger populations of Scandinavian origin.

Multiple sclerosis is clearly tied to geography; this distribution has been inter-preted as a latitude gradient but can also be viewed as three high-risk zones including northern Europe and southern Scandinavia, northern United States and southern Canada, and New Zealand and southeast Australia. Each of these regions with prevalence rates of 30 to 100 is bounded by an area of medium fre-quency with prevalent rates between 5 and 29 per 100,000. This suggests that multiple sclerosis may have arisen in northern Europe, with subsequent establishment of foci among the descendants of migrants to these loci (Kurtzke, 1993).

Migration Studies

Following World War II, Dean found that the majority of patients with multiple sclerosis in South Africa were immigrants from the United Kingdom or northern Europe, even though they made up less than 10% of the total population. He determined a prevalence rate for white, Afrikaans-speaking natives of 3 per 100,000, for white English-speaking natives of 11 per 100,000, and for migrants from northern Europe of 50 per 100,000, the same order of magnitude seen in northern Europe (Dean, 1970). Further analysis indicated that migration prior to 15 years of age led to the same risk as that of native-born English South Africans, whereas migrants who came after that age carried the risk of their birthplace (Dean and Kurtzke, 1971). Recently, the rate in Afrikaans-speaking South Africans seems to be approaching that of the English-speaking South Africans. Similar risk of early life environment has been reported among immigrants to Israel, Australia, Hawaii, and the Antilles. Data are less complete for migrants from low-risk to high-risk areas but again tend to support the observation that migration after adolescence tends to transport the risk of the country of origin, whereas early life migration leads to a risk resembling that found in the new home.

In matched controlled studies of veterans of World War II, residence of birth and military induction showed a sharp north to south differential in risk for multiple sclerosis. Residents after induction and at the onset of disease showed no significant correlation (Beebe et al., 1967). Virtually all studies support the relation to an early childhood exposure occurring before the age of about 15 or necessitating repeated exposures during childhood up to the age of puberty. This is followed by a latency period for a number of years before the onset of clinical disease.

Familial Aggregation

Genetic susceptibility appears to be an important, but not overriding, factor in the cause of multiple sclerosis. There is a clear increase in risk of multiple sclerosis among siblings of affected persons and the children of the parents with multiple sclerosis. Recent twin studies have shown a higher concordance rate among monozygotic than dizygotic twins. In a long-term population-based study of Canadian twins, monozygotic twins had a concordance rate of 30.8%, whereas the dizygotic-sex-like twins had a concordance rate of 4.7% (Sadovnick et al., 1993). Nevertheless, nearly 70% of monozygotic twins were discordant even after correction for age. Kurtzke (1993) questioned whether the greater common exposure in the lifestyle of monozygotic twins might be sufficient to explain these differences. The Canadian collaborative group evaluated adopted, and thus nonbiologic, relatives and concluded that familial aggregation is genetically determined; they failed to find any effects of shared environment (Ebers et al., 1995).

Apparent Epidemics

The geographic gradients appear reasonably smooth, and the overall incidence of multiple sclerosis appears reasonably stable, but important exceptions have appeared in the settlements of the Norse Vikings in the North Atlantic. The Shetlands and Orkneys, with the highest prevalence rates in the world (in excess of 200 per 100,000), have recently shown a marked decrease in prevalence, suggesting these extraordinary rates may have represented a post–World War II epidemic (Cook et al., 1988 and 1995). The observations in the Faroe Islands, where multiple sclerosis was alleged to be exceedingly rare, have been even more dramatic. There has been a question of any cases, documented with an onset prior to 1943, yet prevalence in 1977 was 34 per 100,000 (Kurtzke and Hyllested, 1979). Onset of disease in 16 patients was documented between 1943 and 1949 and in an additional 16 patients between 1950 and 1973. No cases were documented with onsets between 1973 and 1981. This appears to be waves of a point-source epidemic, and the unique antecedent event prior to 1943 was the 1941 to 1945 occupation of the Faroes by the British. This led to the speculation that the disease was introduced by the British military troops or their baggage. Furthermore, a spatial relationship was shown between the villages where cases of multiple sclerosis occurred and where the troops were quartered. Canine distemper virus appears to have been introduced by the officers' dogs and was postulated as a factor (Cook et al., 1988). Subsequent studies of antibodies in patients, lack of spatial relationship between canine distemper outbreaks and multiple sclerosis, and veterinary observations of patients' contacts with sick dogs have failed to show correlations (Kurtzke et al., 1988).

Multiple sclerosis has long been recognized in Iceland, but reexamination of their rates shows a low level until a sudden rise in 1922, which then plateaued until 1945, when there was a second rise. Again, Iceland was occupied during World War II by Canadian and American as well as British troops (Kurtzke et al., 1982). These findings of apparent epidemics in the North Atlantic suggest that multiple sclerosis is not only related to a childhood exposure but is transmissible.

Epidemiologic Evidence of a Specific Virus

Although a viral cause could explain most of the epidemiologic data, there is a paucity of epidemiologic evidence to implicate any specific agent. In some studies, the epidemiologic data may reflect the age of acquisition of a common human infection, whereas other studies have stressed possible exposure to exotic or zoonotic viruses.

Age of acquisition may influence clinical manifestations. For example, poliomyelitis viruses seldom cause disease in infants but cause more frequent and more severe paralysis in older age groups. Thus, improved sanitation that delays acquisition of this enteric infection increases risk of paralysis. Parallels between the epidemiology of multiple sclerosis and poliomyelitis have been made (Poskanzer et al., 1963). However, travel from high-risk to low-risk areas increases incidences of paralytic poliomyelitis, a phenomenon that is not seen with multiple sclerosis, and disease associated with improved sanitation should have a later and later onset over the decades.

Age of acquisition of viral infection may also alter clinical manifestations, such as Epstein–Barr virus, where early childhood infection in developing countries is not associated with clinical disease, whereas delayed infection in adolescence and young adults is related to infectious mononucleosis. Indeed, patients with multiple sclerosis recall a history of infectious mononucleosis more frequently than do controls (Martyn et al., 1993), and documented heterophile antibody-positive mononucleosis is commoner in multiple sclerosis patients than in controls (Haahr et al., 1995). Several studies have shown the age of acquisition of measles is later in patients with multiple sclerosis than in controls, and there also has been a higher frequency of bronchitis, sinusitis, and early-life tonsillectomy in multiple sclerosis patients. The acquisition of infectious mononucleosis, late measles, and increased tonsillectomies may all simply reflect the higher socioeconomic level and consequently more sheltered childhoods of patients who later develop multiple sclerosis (Gronning et al., 1993). A north–south gradient of clinical chickenpox also has been noted and compared with the geographic distribution of multiple sclerosis (Ross and Cheang, 1995). In addition, there appears to be an excess of births in early spring of patients with multiple sclerosis (Templer et al., 1992), and infection was suggested as a possible explanation. This correlation would implicate maternal or neonatal infection, which is not consistent with the migration studies.

Animal exposure has been confronted in a number of studies. In the past, there was interest in the possible relationship to sheep, household birds, and dogs. Canine distemper virus in dogs has been implicated in the Faroe Islands and also in a cluster of cases of multiple sclerosis in Sitka, Alaska, 4 to 5 years after an outbreak of canine distemper (Cook and Dowling, 1982). Canine distemper virus is closely related to measles, giving possible serologic cross-reactions. Recent studies of sera of multiple sclerosis patients and controls for immunoprecipitation of canine distemper polypeptides showed no reactions to the unique canine distemper virus polypeptides (Krakowka et al., 1983). Thus, although the epidemiologic investigations point to an environmental exposure, these studies give little indication of what that exposure might be.

Virologic Studies

Studies of patients with multiple sclerosis have implicated poxviruses, herpesviruses, rhabdoviruses, orthomyxoviruses, paramyxoviruses, coronaviruses, flaviviruses, picornaviruses, retroviruses, and a variety of uncharacterized agents. Thus, almost the full gamut of viruses associated with neurologic diseases have, at one time or another, been suspected in multiple sclerosis. Viruses have been incriminated by immunologic studies of patients, morphological demonstrations of viruslike particles in tissue, reports of virus isolation, or demonstration of laboratory effects on tissue cultures or animals thought to indicate the presence of a virus.

Serologic Studies

In 1962, Adams and Imagawa reported that complement-fixing and neutralizing antibody titers against measles virus were higher in patients with multiple sclerosis than in a control group. The same antibodies were present in cerebrospinal fluid of over 75% of the patients with multiple sclerosis and absent in controls. These unlikely findings have been confirmed in over 30 subsequent studies (Norrby, 1978). With less consistencies, other studies have found higher levels of serum antibodies and disproportionately high levels of cerebrospinal fluid antibodies to a wide variety of other viruses (Table 10.3). In one study, 23% of patients with multiple sclerosis had disproportionately high spinal fluid antibodies to two or more viruses (Norrby et al., 1974); in another study, intrathecal antibody synthesis was found against 11 different agents in a single patient (Salmi et al., 1983). Twin studies, in general, show higher levels of serum and/or spinal fluid antibody in the affected twin than in the healthy co-twin (Kinnunen et al., 1990). These findings might suggest that multiple viruses can precipitate multiple sclerosis, or that preprogrammed B cells are nonspecifically activated (Cremer et al., 1980).

Some studies indicate otherwise. For example, antibodies are elevated to the surface glycoprotein E2 of rubella virus but not the core protein. The divergence

TABLE 10.3. *Higher antiviral antibodies in multiple sclerosis than in controls*

Serum	CSF
Measles	Measles
Parainfluenza 3	Parainfluenzas 1–3
Influenza C	Influenza A, B
Varicella	Varicella
Herpes simplex	Herpes simplex
Rubella	Rubella
Epstein–Barr	Epstein–Barr
	Mumps
	Respiratory syncytial
	Coronaviruses
	Adenoviruses
HTLV-I (gag)	HTLV-I (gag)
HTLV-II	Simian virus 5

HTLV, human T-cell lymphotropic virus.

in antibody response suggests that the antibody elevation is not simply a non-specific B-cell activation (Nath and Wolinsky, 1990).

The finding of higher serum antibody titers to measles is not specific to multiple sclerosis. Similar findings have been reported in lupus erythematosus, Reiter's syndrome, and chronic liver disease. Furthermore, antibody levels are not of the magnitude seen in a known chronic measles virus infection, subacute sclerosing panencephalitis, where conspicuously high levels of antibody are present in serum and spinal fluid in all patients. Indeed, the disproportionate levels in multiple sclerosis patients are found only by statistical analysis of many patients; patients with multiple sclerosis often have levels lower than controls, and some patients with multiple sclerosis have not acquired their primary measles virus infection until after the onset of their neurologic disease. Furthermore, the antibodies to measles and other viral antigens represent only a small proportion of the total antibody increase found in the spinal fluid of patients with multiple sclerosis. The viral antibodies in the serum and spinal fluid of multiple sclerosis do fluctuate over time, but this cannot be correlated with clinical disease (Arnadottir et al., 1982), and interferon fails to appear in serum or spinal fluid (Salonen, 1983). The major portion of antibody to measles virus found in the spinal fluid is directed against the nucleocapsid and fusion proteins and lack of response to the core phosphoprotein seen in subacute sclerosing panencephalitis (Pohl-Koppe et al., 1995).

A variety of reports have implicated defects in cell-mediated immune responses in multiple sclerosis, but these may correlate with disability rather than specific disease (Cook and Dowling, 1980). Again, the T-cell abnormalities are most striking with measles virus, since there does appear to be an expanded measles virus-specific T-cell population in patients with multiple sclerosis (Greenstein et al., 1984) and a significantly lower measles virus-specific cytotoxic T-cell response. This latter response was not found with influenza virus, so it did appear to be virus specific (Jacobson et al., 1985).

Morphological Studies

The loss of specific myelin proteins varies in different virus-induced demyelinating diseases. The myelin-associated glycoprotein is localized to the outermost lamina of periaxonal myelin, whereas myelin basic protein is distributed throughout the sheath. Therefore, in progressive multifocal leukoencephalopathy, a cytolytic infection of the oligodendrocyte causes a dying back of myelin, so there is a wider perimeter of myelin-associated glycoprotein loss than myelin basic protein loss (Itoyama et al., 1982). In contrast, in measles virus encephalomyelitis and in experiment autoimmune encephalomyelitis where there is a direct attack on myelin, a concordant loss of the two myelin proteins is seen (Itoyama et al., 1982; Gendelman et al., 1984). Multiple sclerosis follows neither the pattern of a virus-induced demyelinating lesion seen in postmeasles encephalomyelitis nor the primary disease of oligodendrocyte but shows both concordant and disconcordant losses of the two myelin proteins in acute lesions (Gendelman et al., 1985b). This suggests some alternate mechanism.

Electron-microscopic studies of autopsy and biopsy tissue of patients with multiple sclerosis have reported a variety of different particles. These include ovoid membrane bodies 30 to 200 nm in diameter, which are now thought to represent myelin breakdown products; dense intracytoplasmic osmiophilic granules of 60 to 80 nm in diameter surrounded by membrane, which are thought to be nonspecific changes in reactive astrocytes (Andrews and Andrews, 1973; Kirk, 1979); and intranuclear structures in inflammatory cells, which were initially thought to represent myxovirus nucleocapsids and are now believed to be nonspecific alterations of nuclear chromatin (Lampert and Lampert, 1975). None of these particles is specific for, or consistent in, multiple sclerosis, and none has been identified as viral in nature.

Virus Recoveries

There were many early claims of the transmission of multiple sclerosis to primates and smaller animals, but none either recovered a characterizable virus or could be confirmed by other laboratories (Innes and Kurland, 1952) (Table 10.4). Interest in specific viruses began with the report from Moscow in 1946 that viruses from two patients with multiple sclerosis had been isolated in mice: one virus from the blood of a patient and the other from cerebral tissue of a patient with acute multiple sclerosis (Margulis et al., 1946). These viruses, however, were identified in laboratories outside of the Soviet Union as rabies virus, and no antibody could be found against the agent in the sera of patients with multiple sclerosis (Dick et al., 1958). Nevertheless, the same laboratory later reported further isolates of similar agents (Bychkova, 1964).

TABLE 10.4. *Viruses recovered from patients with multiple sclerosis (MS)*

Rabies virus	1946
	1964
Herpes simplex virus, type 2	1964
Scrapie agent	1965
MS-associated agent	1972
Parainfluenza virus 1	1972
Measles virus	1972
Simian virus 5	1978
Chimpanzee cytomegalovirus	1979
Coronavirus	1980
SMON-like virus	1982
Tick-borne encephalitis flavivirus	1982
HTLV-I	1986
LM7 (retrovirus)	1989
Herpes simplex virus, type 1	1989
Human herpesvirus 6	1994

HTLV, human T-cell lymphotropic virus; SMON, subacute myelo—optico—neuropathy.

Various herpesviruses have been repeatedly recovered. The ubiquitousness of latent infections and the frequency of reactivation give rise to frequent isolations and nonspecific antibody responses. In 1964, a strain of type 2 herpes simplex virus was recovered from an Icelandic patient dying of multiple sclerosis (Gudnadottir et al., 1964). Despite lack of confirmation and many negative reports over subsequent years, a recent report noted immunoreactivity specifically with herpes simplex virus type 2 antisera in the lesions of three multiple sclerosis patients (Martin et al., 1988), and another report described a type 1 virus obtained from spinal fluid during the first attack of multiple sclerosis (Bergström et al., 1989). A recent detailed search for DNA of both type 1 and type 2 herpes simplex viruses was carried out in 77 plaques of 23 patients, all of which were negative (Nicoll et al., 1992). In contrast, a study using PCR reported herpes simplex type 1 or type 2 in 46% of multiple sclerosis cases and 28% of control samples (Sanders et al., 1996). The report of a simian cytomegalovirus was from a chimpanzee inoculated neonatally with brain cells from a multiple sclerosis patient, but the clinical disease that developed in the chimpanzee suggested an acute polyneuritis that may or may not have been related to the simian agent (Wrobleska et al., 1979).

The arguments surrounding Epstein–Barr virus have been more complex. In addition to the aforementioned serologic studies in serum and spinal fluid, there have been several reports of patients with neurologic complications of primary Epstein–Barr infection who subsequently developed progressive or relapsing neurologic deficits, leading to a diagnosis of multiple sclerosis (Shaw and Alvord, 1987; Bray et al., 1992a, 1992b). A 6-year-old child who had 11 episodes of relapsing disease beginning at 10 months of age had elevated Epstein–Barr virus antibodies and a clear-cut pathologic diagnosis of multiple sclerosis; Epstein–Barr virus was subsequently demonstrated in this tissue by PCR (Pedneault et al., 1992). Subsequently, an *in situ* hybridization study for Epstein–Barr-specific RNA was carried out in the brains of 10 patients with multiple sclerosis, and the results were entirely normal (Hilton et al., 1994). These contrasting data might suggest that Epstein–Barr virus can be a precipitating factor in some cases but is not a universal cause.

The implication of human herpesvirus 6 is based on even more curious conflicting data. PCR detection of DNA of this virus was reported in the spinal fluid of 3 of 21 patients with multiple sclerosis (Wilborn et al., 1994), but a subsequent study reported that 30% to 40% of spinal fluids with mononuclear cell responses were positive, irrespective of whether the diagnosis was multiple sclerosis or AIDS (Liedtke et al., 1995). More recently, antihuman herpesvirus 6 IgM was reported in serum of 70% of multiple sclerosis patients and only 13% of controls, and DNA was detected in serum of 8 of 23 multiple sclerosis patients and not in sera of controls (Berti et al., 1997). Antigen was reported in the nuclei of subependymal cells of CNS tissue in 70% of patients and controls, but in multiple sclerosis patients the antigen was found in oligodendrocytes particularly in the area surrounding demyelinating plaques (Challoner et al., 1995).

This would suggest a common virus that may spread during the disease process but may not be causally related to disease.

Measles and related viruses have also been implicated, but the sole reported recovery of measles from the brain of a single patient was interpreted in an initial report as a probable laboratory contamination (Field et al., 1972). Measles genomes also appear to be identified by *in situ* hybridization, occasional scattered cells in the brain in some patients with multiple sclerosis (Haase et al., 1981), but a variety of other studies using *in situ* hybridization and more recently PCR have failed to confirm the presence of measles virus in the brains of multiple sclerosis patients (Cosby et al., 1989; Godec et al., 1992). Isolation of parainfluenza type 1 virus from tissue culture derived from two patients dying of multiple sclerosis was pursued extensively and unsuccessfully. Simian virus 5 was reportedly obtained from marrow and spinal fluid of patients (Mitchell et al., 1979), but serologic studies show consistent relationship to multiple sclerosis (Goswami et al., 1987).

The recovery of a coronavirus in mice inoculated with brains from patients dying of multiple sclerosis is of interest because of the observation that a coronavirus causes relapsing and remitting demyelinating disease in mice. Subsequent studies of these isolates, however, suggested that they are murine coronaviruses (Weiss, 1983). Nevertheless, *in situ* hybridization studies done by the laboratory originally isolating the agent reported *in situ* hybridization of coronavirus RNA and antigen in 12 of 22 brain samples of multiple sclerosis patients (Murray et al., 1992). Another laboratory probing for the human oncornavirus OC43 failed to confirm this finding (Sorensen et al., 1986).

The report of the induction of scrapie in Icelandic sheep 16 to 20 months after the intracerebral inoculation of multiple sclerosis brain now appears to have stemmed from the contamination of a shipping container. The tie between the scrapie and the multiple sclerosis was again raised by the report of a decrease in polymorphonuclear cells after inoculation with multiple sclerosis tissue and scrapie material, but these findings were not verified in controlled studies (Brown and Gajdusek, 1974; Carp et al., 1977).

Since the description of visna virus, with its long incubation period, progressive or relapsing and remitting course, and demyelinating lesions, there has been interest in a retrovirus etiology, but no evidence of a visnalike virus has been found. The association of human T-cell lymphotropic virus type I (HTLV-I) with chronic myelopathy in humans, and the occasional finding of cerebral symptoms such as retrobulbar neuritis and the imaging of cerebral white matter lesions, have heightened the interest in retroviruses. In 1985, HTLV-I sequences were reported in spinal fluid cells from some multiple sclerosis patients, and antibodies were reported in a majority of patients (Koprowski et al., 1985). Partial confirmation was reported by several laboratories, but an array of subsequent reports of serology, *in situ* hybridization of cells and tissue, and PCR for viral sequences and sensitive reverse-transcriptase assays have been negative (Ehrlich et al., 1991; Hackett et al., 1996). An as yet uncharacterized retrovirus was recovered from a line of meningeal cells obtained from spinal fluid, and retrovirus-like particles have been shown in a cell line derived from a multiple sclerosis patient's blood (Haahr et al., 1991; Perron et al., 1991). The results of a variety of studies including PCR for spumiviruses and oncoretroviruses have been normal. Although some endogenous retrovirus-like sequences have been reported more often in the mononuclear cells of multiple sclerosis patients than in healthy controls (Rasmussen and Clausen, 1997), these sequences have been found with about equal frequency in the brain tissue of multiple sclerosis patients and controls (Lefebvre et al., 1995; Rasmussen and Clausen, 1997).

Inoculation of multiple sclerosis tissue into chimpanzees, followed by long-term holding, has not resulted in disease (Gajdusek, 1978). That is not, however, a definitive test, because neural tissue from patients with subacute sclerosing panencephalitis and progressive multifocal leukoencephalopathy was also inoculated into these primates without producing disease. In summary, to date there have been no consistent data to suggest a single viral agent as the cause of multiple sclerosis. However, the failure to isolate or detect virus does not rule out a virus. To apply a quote from physics, "Absence of evidence is not the same thing as evidence of absence" (Dyson, 1982).

Virus could be a cofactor interacting with the immune system, leading to multiple sclerosis, but, as in the case of postmeasles encephalomyelitis, the virus might no longer be present at the time of the onset of clinical neurologic disease. The virologic data could be interpreted as indicating that a variety of viruses on occasion precipitate the disease, just as it has been shown that nonspecific viral infections are temporally related to acute exacerbations of established disease. It may be that the childhood exposure is not the infectious agent at all, but that some other factor leads to demyelinating disease and abnormal production of viral antibodies. Even in this case, however, virus infections and multiple sclerosis are somehow linked.

POSSIBLE VIRAL CAUSES OF OTHER CHRONIC INFLAMMATORY DISEASES

Kozhevnikov's Disease and Rasmussen's Disease

Continuous focal epilepsy, or Kozhevnikov's epilepsy, was originally described in a Russian youth who developed focal seizures in his right leg 1 year after encephalitis; seizures accentuated over time, accompanied by progressive neurologic disability. The disease was seen often in Siberia following encephalitis and, following the isolation of a tick-borne encephalitis virus, serologic studies confirmed that patients with continuous focal epilepsy had antibodies to the virus more frequently than did controls.

Evidence that epilepsia partialis continua in Russia represents a persistent infection includes the presence of a chronic inflammatory reaction, high levels of antibody in spinal fluid of patients, and the recovery of virus from brain tissue removed from surgically resected epileptogenic foci of two patients 9 and 13 months after the acute encephalitis (Brody et al., 1965). In a further patient, virus was recovered from spinal fluid 3.5 months after the encephalitis, although in the majority of patients virus isolation has not been successful (Ilienko et al., 1974).

Most strains of tick-borne encephalitis virus kill rhesus monkeys with acute encephalitis. However, a few strains cause nonfatal disease, and many of these monkeys develop chronic choreoathetosis and show the chronic inflammatory reaction in brain similar to the human disease (Asher, 1975; Frolova and Pogodina, 1984).

Chronic encephalitis with focal intractable seizures and progressive neurologic deficits in North America are usually referred to as Rasmussen's encephalitis. Most patients are children, and only a minority of these patients have an antecedent history of acute encephalitis (Aguilar and Rasmussen, 1960). Attempts to isolate viruses from surgical resected tissue of the majority of these patients have been unsuccessful. Epstein–Barr virus or cytomegalovirus DNA has been demonstrated by *in situ* hybridization in some tissue sections (Walter and Renella, 1989; Power et al., 1990), but the detection of DNA from different herpesviruses by PCR in brains of patients with other inflammatory diseases or even without inflammatory changes must be interpreted cautiously, because DNA could reflect the passing presence of latently infected B cells not present in normal brains (Vinters et al., 1993; Jay et al., 1995).

An interesting twist to the mystery of Rasmussen's encephalitis recently arose when rabbits immunized against glutamate receptor, GluR3, developed focal seizures and CNS inflammation. Antibodies against GluR3 protein were then sought and found in some patients (Rogers et al., 1994), but they have not been found in the great majority of patients. Nevertheless, improved neurologic function has been reported after plasmapheresis and steroid treatment, irrespective of the presence of anti-GluR3 antibodies (Andrews et al., 1996; Krauss et al., 1996). Therefore, whatever the inciting event that explains the initial focal nidus, the pathogenesis of the ongoing encephalitis may be autoimmune (Farrell et al., 1995).

Recurrent Meningitis and Encephalitis

Claims of virus isolation have been made in several recurrent inflammatory diseases of the CNS, including Mollaret's meningitis, Behçet's disease, the Vogt–Koyanagi–Harada syndrome. These are rare diseases, but they are of particular interest because of their relapsing and remitting courses.

Mollaret's meningitis is a rare disease characterized by recurrent episodes of headache, fever, and nuchal rigidity. The episodes usually begin abruptly and last for 2 to 3 days. Patients are well for the weeks or months between attacks. At the time of the attack, the spinal fluid shows a pleocytosis of 200 to thousands of cells that are predominantly mononuclear cells, but polymorphonuclear cells and large, poorly staining epithelial cells are found during early hours of the attack (Hermans et al., 1972). Mollaret, who initially described the disease, reported the isolation of an agent in chick embryos and mice and fevers in baboons inoculated with spinal fluids of two patients. The results of these studies are unconfirmed, and Mollaret himself concluded that the cause remains undetermined (Mollaret, 1977). Recently, herpes simplex virus type 2 has been detected in many of the patients with recurrent benign meningitis (Tedder et al., 1994; Monteyne et al., 1996). The origin of the large epithelial cells in some cases remains a mystery, but these cells have been described in cases with herpes simplex, type 2 (Picard et al., 1993). Intermittent chemical meningitis induced by leaking epidermoid cysts can reproduce the syndrome, and in these cases the origin of the large epithelial cells is obvious (Chadarevian and Becker, 1980; Achard et al., 1990).

Behçet's disease is more common and is most prevalent in Mediterranean Europe, the Near East, and Japan. The disease is characterized by the triad of recurrent oral aphthous ulcers, recurrent genital ulcers, and inflammatory disease of the eye usually characterized by uveitis with hypopyon or iridocyclitis and occasionally chorioretinitis. In addition to the classic triad, lesions of the skin are common, including erythema nodosa, subcutaneous thrombophlebitis, and folliculitis. Arthritis, ulceration of the ileum and cecum, recurrent epididymitis, and vascular and renal lesions are occasionally seen (Inaba, 1989). In approximately 10% to 25% of patients, recurrent or progressive cerebral involvement develops as the most life-threatening feature of the disease (Wolf et al., 1965). The neurologic disease may be recurrent, with dispersed lesions that are most frequently localized to the diencephalon, pons, and thalamus. The course of disease can simulate multiple sclerosis, but unlike multiple sclerosis, the disease is more common in men, with a male-to-female ratio as high as 9 to 1. The spinal fluid generally shows a pleocytosis, an elevation of protein, and increases in IgG without oligoclonal bands (Inaba, 1989). Magnetic resonance imaging may show major venous occlusions and multiple or confluent high-density lesions on T2-weighted sequences that are most prominent in white matter. Unlike multiple sclerosis, lesions do not show a periventricular predilection and often include deep gray matter structures (Wechsler et al., 1993). Pathologic studies have shown meningeal and perivascular inflammation and multiple foci of necrosis in gray and white matter (Sugihara et al., 1969).

Virologic studies of Behçet's disease have been colorful. There have been claims of transmission of the disease to rabbits with spinal fluid and sputum and claims of repeated recovery of a virus in embryonated eggs from vitreous and subretinal exudates and from sera of the majority of patients. Filtration and electron-microscopic studies of the putative agents have been reported, as well as serologic studies of complement-fixing and neutralizing antibody against the agent in the majority of patients in Egypt (Sezer, 1956). These claims have allegedly been confirmed in a British paper, with a putative virus isolated on chorioallantoic membranes of embryonated eggs (Evans et al., 1957). However, the published photograph resembles an inoculation artifact, the scar made on that chorioallantoic membrane by the inoculation needle. Other laboratories in Japan and Egypt have reported isolations of virus from ulcers, ophthalmic fluid, and blood, causing lesions on chorioallantoic membranes of eggs and deaths of inoculated guinea pigs and mice. Despite all of these alleged virus recoveries, the putative agents have never been identified, and the laboratories reporting the isolations have not successfully maintained the agents in order to send them to other laboratories. Most laboratories, including my own, have failed to find agents by using the same methods, which casts doubt on an established viral cause of Behçet's disease (Dudgeon, 1961; Johnson and Herndon, 1974).

The Vogt–Koyanagi–Harada or uveoencephalitis syndrome is characterized by depigmentation of the skin and hair, inflammatory ocular lesions (iridocyclitis) or exudative retinal detachment, sensorineural hearing loss, and meningitis. In contrast to the situation with Behçet's disease, the CNS is involved in all cases, and this often precedes ocular involvement. The course usually is benign, however, with only headache, nuchal rigidity, and pleocytosis (Inomata and Kato, 1989). Major neurologic deficits are rare, and consequently there have been no neuropathologic studies. Here again, there have been a number of reports of virus recoveries in chick embryos, rabbits, mice, and HeLa cells, but, as in Behçet's disease, the nature of these agents is elusive, and other investigators have failed to recover viruses by using the same methods (Johnson and Herndon, 1974). The detection of Epstein–Barr virus sequences in the vitreous of a patient with Vogt–Koyanagi–Harada syndrome may represent nothing more than detection of a latently infected lymphocyte (Bassili et al., 1996), but application of contemporary methods to detect viruses in the uveoencephalitic syndromes might be fruitful.

Viluisk Encephalomyelitis

Viluisk encephalomyelitis is a progressive neurologic disease of the Jakut population of Siberia (Goldfarb and Gajdusek, 1992). The disease affects primarily young and middle-aged adults, with onset in the spring. Acute fever, headache, nuchal rigidity, and malaise are accompanied by multifocal neurologic signs, the most strikingly of which are bradykinesia, rigidity, and dysarthria. Some patients die during the first months of this early phase, but the majority survive for several years and develop slowly progressive disease, with apathy, somnolence, dementia, and an array of neurologic abnormalities. A mononuclear cell pleocytosis and elevated spinal fluid protein are seen during the acute phase. In subacute or progressive cases, focal necrotizing encephalomyelitis is found pathologically; in chronic cases, multifocal lytic lesions with gliosis, but without inflammation, are found predominantly within gray matter (McLean et al., 1997). A putative causative agent recovered in mice has proved to be a picornavirus, probably of murine origin (Lipton et al., 1983), and antibodies to this virus are not found in patients.

The biphasic nature of the disease, with an acute encephalitis followed by a chronic progressive disease with hydrocephalus *ex vacuo*, resembles the curious neurologic disease in rodents with infection with Borna disease virus.

Borna Disease

Borna disease is a naturally occurring encephalomyelitis of horses, sheep, cattle, cats, and ostriches. The Borna disease virus causes varied diseases in a wide range of experimental animals, including chickens, carnivores, lagomorphs, ungulates, and primates, and these have been touted as experimental models of uveoencephalitic syndromes, Viluisk disease, and behavioral disorders (Narayan et al., 1983a). The findings of antibodies in human sera have led to speculation of some link with acute or chronic inflammatory diseases of the CNS (Bode et al., 1992), and the virus has been isolated from peripheral blood mononuclear cells of patients with depression of bipolar disease and chronic obsessive–compulsive disorder (Bode et al., 1996).

Borna disease virus is a nonsegmented, negative-stranded RNA virus with the unique property of replication and transcription of its genome in the host cell nucleus (Briese et al., 1994; Schneemann et al., 1995). It, therefore, remains unclassified but will probably become the prototype of a new virus family. Experimental infection of some species, such as the horse, leads to acute fatal encephalitis, whereas infection of others, including a nonhuman primate (tupaiaias), leads to persistent infection, with behavioral abnormalities. Infection of adult rats has been studied in greatest detail.

In rats, infection is limited to the nervous system, with invasion along olfactory and neural roots and initial infection primarily of neurons of olfactory and limbic systems, spinal cord, or retina dependent on the route of inoculation (Gosztonyi and Ludwig, 1995). An acute meningoencephalitis and retinitis with frenzied and aggressive behavior occurs concurrent with the cell-mediated immune destruction of the neurons. This acute phase is followed by clearing of the inflammatory response, a persistence of virus in astrocytes and Schwann cells, and the clinical syndrome of passivity, blindness, and often morbid obesity (Narayan et al., 1983a and b; Carbone et al., 1989). Infection of neonatal rats causes persistent infection without disease, similar to persistent lymphocytic choriomeningitis virus infections of mice. Unlike that natural murine persistent infection, acute Borna disease cannot be induced by adoptive transfer of immune spleen cells, but immunopathologic disease could be induced by bone marrow cells (Carbone et al., 1991).

The wide experimental host range of Borna disease virus has raised the question of possible human infection. The unique biphasic disease in rats, with behavior changing from frenzy to apathy, and the predilection for the limbic and hypothalamic regions of brain stimulated studies of patients with affective disorders. Of 165 patients with depressive illnesses, 12 had antibodies by an indirect immunofluorescent focus assay, in contrast to 0 of 105 healthy volunteers

(Amsterdam et al., 1985). Viral RNA and antigen have been found in blood mononuclear cells of neuropsychiatric patients more frequently than in healthy controls (Sauder et al., 1996). Recently, Borna disease virus was reported to have been isolated from peripheral blood mononuclear cells of three patients with mood disorders, and sequence data document the uniqueness of each isolate, which argues against contamination (Bode et al., 1996; Bode and Ludwig, 1966). The same authors, however, had shown more frequently detectable antibodies in a spectrum of chronic inflammatory diseases (multiple sclerosis, HIV infection with lymphadenopathy, infectious mononucleosis, schistosomiasis, and malaria) than in healthy controls (Bode et al., 1992) which suggests a nonspecific activation of a human Borna disease virus.

SUPPLEMENTARY BIBLIOGRAPHY

Björnsson J, Carp RI, Löve A, Wisniewski HM. Slow infections of the central nervous system: the legacy of Dr. Björn Sigurdsson. *Ann NY Acad Sci* 1994;724:1–495.

11

Retroviruses

> As long as there are diseases of unknown aetiology there will be suggestions that viruses are responsible. Not because viruses are the last resort in the search for aetiological agents, but because of the unique and fascinating things that viruses can do.
> C.A. Mims,
> *Viral Aetiology of Diseases of Obscure Origin,* 1985

Retroviruses are the most unique and fascinating viruses. In the first edition of this book, it is stated that the retrovirus family includes "no known human pathogens," but now the roles of human T-cell lymphotropic viruses (HTLVs) and human immunodeficiency viruses (HIVs) in an array of neurologic diseases dominate neurovirology.

Although retroviruses were late entries on the stage of human virology, equine infectious anemia virus, recently classified as a lentivirus (the same genus of retrovirus as HIV), was the first animal virus recovered. Blood from a horse with a recurrent hemolytic crisis was passed through a filter, and the cell-free filtrate was inoculated into an unaffected horse, transmitting the disease (Vallee and Carre, 1904). There is an odd irony in this historical note, considering the recent caval about the ability of retroviruses to cause chronic disease and the argument that the relationship of AIDS and HIV fails to meet Koch's postulates (Duesberg, 1991) (see Chapter 18). A cousin was the first virus to fulfill the postulates!

The next retrovirus to be recovered was avian sarcoma virus; in 1911, Peyton Rous transmitted chicken sarcomas with cell-free filtrates. The subsequent recognition of similar oncogenic viruses in murine sarcomas, leukemias, and mammary tumors kindled excitement in the potential role of similar agents in human malignancies. During the War on Cancer declared in the 1960s, great emphasis was placed on the Virus Cancer Program in the hope that specific viruses would be related to specific cancers and that this, in turn, might lead to new vaccines and treatments. These hopes were largely unfulfilled, but the studies of RNA tumor viruses led to discoveries that revolutionized modern biology and laid the groundwork essential to the subsequent recovery of HIV. The recognition that these viruses could reverse the flow of information from RNA to DNA not only challenged biologic dogma, but provided the enzyme critical to much of our current DNA technology and engineering. In addition, the recognition that the "onc" genes, which gave most retroviruses their oncogenic properties, were of host cell origin led to the recognition of oncogenes and suppressor genes now central to the new advances in understanding cancer (see Chapter 15).

The discovery of reverse transcription from RNA to DNA not only overthrew a central principle of molecular biology, it posed intriguing questions about the Darwinian evolution of viruses and about the pathogenesis of chronic and relapsing diseases. Modern biology is founded on the orderly replication of informational DNA from DNA and an orderly flow of information from DNA by transcription of an RNA message that is translated to protein. Two disorderly exceptions to this residue-to-residue transfer can occur in virus-infected cells (Fig. 11.1). Nevertheless, Francis Crick's Central Dogma that "once sequential information has passed into protein, it cannot get out" has not been overridden (Crick, 1970). (The possibility that prions may affront the pith of the Central Dogma is addressed in Chapter 14.)

Most acute viral infections are caused by RNA viruses (see Chapter 5) in which genomic RNA is replicated from RNA. Within animal populations, this mode of replication has a survival advantage, because DNA proofreading and repair enzymes are bypassed. Errors or mutations in DNA replication are kept to a level of about 1 in 10^9 per incorporated nucleotide by these enzymes, whereas in RNA replication error rates occur at about 10^4—a 100,000-fold greater rate (Steinhauer and Holland, 1987). This facilitates mutations and the evolution of viruses that circumvent herd immunity against the original virus. DNA viruses counter population immunity by sequestering their genetic information in the host cell (latency), where they can await a new generation of susceptible hosts (see Chapter 6).

Retroviruses have evolved a survival strategy within animal populations and within the individual host that combines these strategies to elude immune

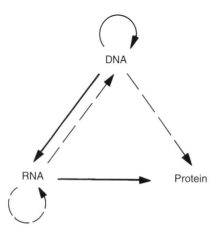

FIG. 11.1. Crick's central dogma of biology. The *solid arrows* show general transfers, and the *dotted arrows* show special transfers.

responses. By establishing latency with integration into host DNA and by achieving high mutational rates, retroviruses can persist in the population and in the individual, where ongoing infection and exacerbations of disease occur. In addition, retroviruses often capture host genes, and they seldom impair, but often potentiate, the growth of host cells (Varmus, 1988). As the most elusive viruses to host defenses, retroviruses are optimally adapted for everlasting survival within animal hosts.

NATURE OF RETROVIRUSES

Structurally, retrovirus are not unusual: they are positive-sense single-stranded RNA viruses with an icosahedral nucleocapsid and an envelope with viral-coded glycoproteins. They are the only viruses, however, that have diploid genomes (which may facilitate recombination and virus variability), that use cell messenger RNA (mRNA)-processing mechanisms to synthesize and process viral RNA, and that do not utilize their plus-sense, single-stranded RNA as mRNA soon after infection.

All nondefective retroviruses contain three major genes. They are arranged, from the 5′ end, as gag (group-specific antigen), which codes for capsid proteins; pol, which codes for the RNA-dependent DNA polymerase (reverse transcriptase) and integrase; and env, which codes for the envelope proteins. Most oncogenic retroviruses contain an onc gene, but the human oncogenic retrovirus, HTLV-I, has no onc gene, and a regulatory gene tax is thought to be central in cell transformation. Lentiviruses have a number of regulatory genes (HIV has six). The env mRNA of all retroviruses and messengers of some lentivirus regulatory proteins are spliced, making it possible to distinguish segments of mRNA from genomic RNA in polymerase chain reaction (PCR) studies.

Most retroviruses require dividing cells for infection, because integration of the proviral DNA is an essential step in their replication. Lentiviruses, however, are adapted to integrate into the host DNA and replicate in nondividing, terminally differentiated cells (Clements and Zink, 1996). Retroviruses adsorb to cells by attachment of the surface glycoprotein that attaches to receptors on the cell membrane; entry is by receptor-mediated endocytosis or by fusion mediated by the transmembrane glycoprotein with the plasma membrane. After uncoating, a minus-sense copy DNA is made that serves as the template for the plus-sense DNA, and the double-stranded DNA moves to the nucleus, where integration takes place via a viral integrase. Virus may then remain latent or produce progeny virus. In productive infections, virus assembly occurs by budding from plasma membranes into which the viral envelope glycoproteins have been inserted. Infection may be cytocidal, noncytocidal, or transforming.

Retroviruses have been classified into three groups: oncoviruses, lentiviruses, and spumaviruses (foamy viruses). The oncoviruses have now been reclassified into five separate genera that differ in morphology, gene regulation, and replication. Only three retrovirus genera are known to infect humans (Table 11.1).

TABLE 11.1. *Retroviruses that infect humans*

Genus	Virus	Systemic disease	Neurologic disease
BLV-HTLV	HTLV-I	Adult T-cell leukemia	Spastic paraparesis
	HTLV-II	?Hairy cell leukemia	Spastic paraparesis
Lentivirus	HIV1, HIV2	AIDS	Dementia, myelopathy, neuropathy, and others
Spumavirus	Human foamy virus	?	?

BLV-HTLV, bovine leukemia virus–human T-cell lymphotropic virus.
Modified from White and Fenner (1994).

The five groups of oncoviruses have been associated with a variety of tumors in their natural hosts, but curiously these naturally occurring tumors do not include CNS tumors, even though many of these viruses readily induce brain tumors experimentally (see Chapter 15). Chronic, nonneoplastic, neurologic degenerative disease has been associated with strains of murine leukemia virus.

The lentiviruses do not transform cells in culture or cause tumors in natural or experimental hosts. All infect macrophages and cause multisystem diseases; some also infect T cells, with resultant immunodeficiency. All cause persistent CNS infections, with inflammation, demyelination, and/or degenerative changes.

The spumaviruses infect a variety of species, probably including humans. They are common in subhuman primates and were found in monkey tissue cell culture many years ago. When I first worked in a diagnostic laboratory, these viruses represented a major obstacle, causing vacuolated giant cells and obscuring the cytopathology of the viruses we sought. Despite this dramatic cytopathic effect *in vitro*, they have not been associated with any disease in animals. Several putative isolations of foamy viruses from humans include recovery of a spumavirus from the brain of a young man thought to have dialysis encephalopathy (Cameron et al., 1978), but some have questioned the human origin of this virus and the validity of serologic studies indicating widespread human infection (Neumann-Haefelin et al., 1993). Nevertheless, it is tantalizing that transgenic mice expressing human foamy virus genes develop myopathy and severe neurologic disease, with ataxia, spastic paresis, and blindness leading to death in 4 to 6 weeks. Neuropathologic findings include selective neuronal degeneration and a mild inflammatory response (Bothe et al., 1991), with spumavirus antigens expressed primarily in hippocampal and cortical neurons (Aguzzi et al., 1993).

HUMAN T-CELL LYMPHOTROPIC VIRUSES

HTLV-I was the first retrovirus associated with human disease. After years of reported sightings of retrovirus-like particles in human tissues, of detection of reverse-transcriptase activity in patient specimens, and of unconfirmed claims of virus recoveries from neoplasms, in 1980 HTLV-I was isolated and convincingly related to acute human T-cell leukemia and lymphoma. The importance of this discovery was never fully appreciated, however, because AIDS emerged the next year and overshadowed this landmark discovery.

T-cell leukemias are highly aggressive malignancies of CD4 cells; the nuclei of the leukemic cells on blood smears are characteristically lobulated and indented. This leukemia was first described by Japanese hematologists in Kyoto (Uchiyama et al., 1977), who noted that many of their patients originated from Kyushu, the southern island of Japan. In addition to the geographic clustering, morphological suggestions of viral particles led to a hypothesis that this might be a virus-induced leukemia. Gallo's laboratory in Bethesda first recovered HTLV-I from a patient with a T-cell lymphoma invading the skin, a patient initially diagnosed as having mycosis fungoides (Poiesz et al., 1980). From serologic studies, it is apparent that HTLV-I infection is essential, but not sufficient, in the causation of T-cell leukemia; in areas such as Kyushu, 15% of the population is infected with HTLV-I, but all patients with T-cell leukemia are infected. In addition, virus can be isolated more readily from these patients with T-cell malignancies, but the strongest evidence for causation is that the provirus of HTLV-I is found within the same patient integrated at the same site in the host DNA, whereas patients infected with HTLV-I without leukemia have proviral DNA integrated at random sites. This not only establishes a monoclonal origin of the disease, but because integration sites differ from one leukemia patient to another, the provirus itself is implicated in malignant transformation rather than its adjacency to a host oncogene.

T-cell leukemias/lymphomas are unusual malignancies with frequent generalized lymphadenopathy, hepatosplenomegaly, bone marrow involvement, unexplained hypercalcemia, and involvement of the skin. The latter causes confusion with the Sézary syndrome and mycosis fungoides. T-cell leukemias and non-Hodgkin's T-cell lymphomas are seen primarily in the southern islands of Japan, the Caribbean Islands, the Seychelles, areas of Africa, and the southeastern United States, where infection with HTLV-I is the most prevalent. The disease comes on in middle life, is refractory to present therapies, and usually causes death within 10 months (Table 11.2).

In 1985, during a survey of HTLV-I seroprevalence in Martinique, the serendipitous finding was made that nearly 60% of patients with tropical spastic paraparesis (TSP) were seropositive for HTLV-I, whereas only 4% of the general population had antibodies (Gessain et al., 1985). Within months, similar associations of antibody to HTLV-I with TSP were made in Jamaica and Columbia, and high levels of antibody were also found in spinal fluid of these patients (Rodgers-Johnson et al., 1985). The following year, many chronic myelopathy patients in Kyushu, the southern island of Japan, were found to be infected with HTLV-I, and there the disease was named HTLV-I-associated myelopathy (HAM) (Osame et al., 1986). Similar patients were soon found among Caribbean immigrants in England and among native populations in Africa, many South American countries, and the southeastern United States (Roman et al., 1987).

TABLE 11.2. *HTLV-I-associated leukemia/lymphoma and myelopathy*

	Leukemia/lymphoma	Myelopathy
Demographic		
Male–female ratio	1.4:1	1:1.4
Mean age onset	40–45	40–45
Place of birth	Southern Japan	
	Seychelles	
	Caribbean basin	Same
	Equatorial Africa	
	Southeastern USA	
Risk factors		
Risk in seropositive	2–4%	0.25%
Blood transfusion (HTLV-I+)	No observed effect	Increases risk to 20%
Concurrent infections	No observed effect	HIV infection may increase risk
Disease	Aggressive: mean survival 10 months	Indolent: long life expectancy
Virology		
Viral DNA	CD4+ lymphocytes	CD4+ lymphocytes (?astrocytes)
Integration	At same site in malignant cells of individual (clonal origin)	Random sites (polyclonal)
Immune responses	Immunosuppression	Enhanced humoral and some cellular responses

HTLV, human T-cell lymphotropic virus.

The presence of abnormal lobulated lymphocytes in the spinal fluid and the recovery of virus from the spinal fluid provided further evidence of the association of HTLV-I with these cases of chronic spastic paraparesis (Bhagavati et al., 1988). In the patients with TSP/HAM, however, the origin of these T cells is polyclonal, without evidence of transformation and with integration of provirus at random sites in different lymphocytes of the individual patient. Nevertheless, viruses recovered from leukemia and from TSP/HAM fail to show significant sequence differences (Greenberg et al., 1989; Xu et al., 1996). The two very different clinical diseases and the rarity of clinical expression of either disease appear to be due to host and environmental factors. The presence of TSP/HAM in one identical twin and not in his seropositive sibling and the finding of both leukemia and TSP in several patients indicate that the diseases are not due solely to a genetic predisposition or to a mutually exclusive mode of pathogenesis.

Epidemiology

HTLV-I is distributed worldwide but with focal concentration: some districts of Kyushu and Okinawa have 30% prevalence of seropositivity compared with less than 1% on Hokkaido; 2% to 10% are infected in the Caribbean Islands and less than 1% in the southeastern United States. There is a high seroprevalence in a Jewish population from Marhad, Iran, and a high rate among the Zulus in South Africa (Montgomery, 1993). The high rates also are seen in the Tumaco district on the southwestern coast of Columbia and in the Seychelles Islands in the Indian Ocean.

The modes of transmission include perinatal transmission, sexual transmission, and transmission by blood, either from transfusion or by the contaminated needles and syringes. Breast-feeding seems to be the major mode of perinatal transmission, and discouraging breast-feeding by seropositive women in Japan had led to a decrease in the transmission rate. Sexual transmission is greater from infected men to women than from infected women to men, leading to slightly higher rates of infection in women than men. Transmission by breast milk generally requires breast-feeding for more than 7 months, and wives of seropositive husbands reach 50% seroconversion only after 1 to 4 years of marriage; these findings suggest inefficient transmission and the need for multiple exposures (Xu et al., 1996). In contrast, transmission by blood transfusion appears far more efficient, and 25% of the patients with TSP/HAM in Japan have had a transfusion (Osame et al., 1990). Data indicate that most patients seroconvert after receiving contaminated blood and that up to 20% of those receiving contaminated blood develop a myelopathy (Gessain and Gout, 1992). This is an extraordinary percentage and suggests either that an infection by this route of inoculation (with greater dosage of virus or greater numbers of infected cells) imposes particular risk for developing myelopathy or that reinfection causes activation or induces an immune response related to the development of spinal cord disease. I recently consulted on a case in which a young woman from Wisconsin had developed TSP/HAM 5 years after blood transfusions in the cosmopolitan community of Madison; the likelihood of her having been previously infected is minuscule, and her illness supports the former hypothesis.

Clinical Manifestations of Myelopathy

The onset of TSP/HAM is most frequent in the fourth and fifth decades of life, although it has been described in children as young as 6 years of age. Those with an onset before 15 years of age have short stature and a slower progression of disease (Nakagawa et al., 1995). It is more common in women than men, consistent with a greater female seroprevalence of HTLV-I antibody. The onset is usually insidious, but occasionally abrupt. Fever and systemic symptoms are not present. Dorsal and lumbar backache, stiffness and weakness of the legs, and male impotence develop early in the course of the disease. Incontinence is common. Dysesthesias in the lower extremities are frequent, and beltlike sensations may be experienced similar to the dysesthesias described during attacks of transverse myelitis.

Physical findings include weakness in the legs, with spasticity, hyperreflexia, and extensor plantar responses. Strength in the arms is relatively spared, but deep tendon reflexes tend to be brisk in the upper extremities and even in the jaw. Despite the sensory symptoms, sensory findings are usually subtle or absent. Some loss of position and vibratory sense in the lower extremities may be evident, but actual sensory levels are rare. A small number of patients lose their Achilles tendon reflexes, which suggests peripheral nerve involvement. Cranial nerve function is usually normal, but rare patients have been reported with retrobulbar neuritis, nerve deafness, seizures, or cerebellar ataxia. Progression continues for 1 to 3 years but then appears to slow or stabilize (Araújo et al., 1995; Kuroda et al., 1995). Even after the patient is wheelchair bound, reasonable function in the arms remains, and cognition is preserved.

Peripheral blood may show the lobulated nuclei in lymphocytes. Early in disease, the spinal fluid usually shows a mild pleocytosis, with abnormal cells, elevation of protein, increased immunoglobulin G (IgG) synthesis, and oligoclonal bands. Levels of antibody to HTLV-I in spinal fluid are higher than can be explained by permeability of the blood–brain barrier, indicating intrathecal synthesis of antiviral antibody. Spinal fluid also has been shown to have increased levels of interferon and neopterin (Ali et al., 1992; Kuroda and Matsui, 1993).

Magnetic resonance imaging of the thoracic cord during early disease may show cord swelling, with enhancement simulating a tumor; late in disease, cord atrophy may be the only finding. Imaging of the brain is normal in the majority, but some patients show subcortical bright foci on T2-weighted images. In patients with long-standing disease, these foci are more frequent (Kira et al., 1988), but long-standing disease correlates with increasing age when unidentified bright objects become more common in the general population.

Cytotoxic T lymphocytes are more frequent in the blood of patients with myelopathy than in the seropositive asymptomatic patients, and both have much higher levels than do patients with T-cell leukemias (Kannagi et al., 1994). In addition, there appears to be a greater viral load in blood, suggesting a more productive infection in patients with myelopathy (Kira et al., 1991). The virus, however, by sequence comparisons is not different from that seen in T-cell leukemia or asymptomatic infected spouses of patients with myelopathy, which argues against a role for specific neurotropic strains of virus (Gessain and Gout, 1992; Nishimura et al., 1993).

Pathology and Pathogenesis

Autopsy studies show thickened meninges and gross atrophy of the cord. Histologically, a mild to severe mononuclear inflammatory response is found in the meninges and in the perivascular spaces. Inflammatory cells may involve the vessel wall itself with a vasculitis (Fig. 11.2), and hyalinization of vessels and perivascular gliosis may be present (Akizuki et al., 1988; Rosenblum et al., 1992). These findings are most intense in the lateral columns of the thoracic spinal cord where demyelination and axon loss is most profound. Significant neuronal loss has not been found. The pathologic correlate of the periventricular lesions found by magnetic resonance imaging consists of ill-defined areas of myelin decrease, astrocytosis, and hyaline thickening of vessels; these lesions do not resemble the plaques of multiple sclerosis (Ogata et al., 1993). Most agree

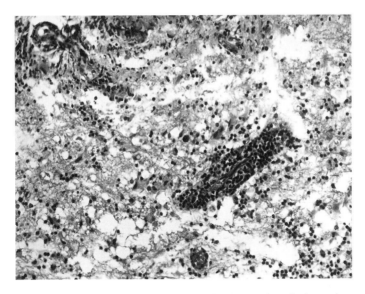

FIG. 11.2. Spinal cord biopsy specimen 6 months after onset of tropical spastic paraparesis. Vasculitis, perivascular cuffing, tissue necrosis, and proliferative change in pial vessel (*top left*) are shown. ×255. (From Johnson et al., 1988a, with permission.)

that the predominant inflammatory cells in the spinal cord are CD8 lymphocytes and activated microglia (Wu et al., 1993; Levin and Jacobson, 1997).

Patients with HAM/TSP have greater numbers of infected CD4 cells and greater quantities of proviral DNA in peripheral blood than do asymptomatic carriers, indicating that virus load may have a role in pathogenesis. HTLV-I antibody levels in serum are higher in patients with myelopathy (Kira et al., 1991). Possibly of greater importance has the finding of high levels of circulating HTLV-I-specific cytotoxic (CD8) T cells in patients with paraparesis but not in HTLV-I-seropositive individuals without neurologic disease. Furthermore, these cells predominantly recognized the gene products encoded by the regulatory region pX (Jacobson et al., 1990). The pX region lies between the *env* gene and the 3′ long terminal repeat, is unique to HTLV, and codes for tax and rev regulatory proteins. The tax protein induces production of tumor necrosis factor α and interleukin 6 in cultured human microglia (Dhib-Jalbut et al., 1994). Tax sequences directly transactivate a number of cytokine promoters (Wigdahl and Brady, 1996).

CD8+ T-cell lines were generated from biopsy tissue of a patient with TSP/HAM, and cells were cytotoxic, HTLV-1 specific, and major histocompatibility antigen restricted (Levin et al., 1997). CD4 T cells expressing pX mRNA have been shown in the thoracic spinal cord of patients with HAM/TSP. These infected cells were found in perivascular infiltrates predominantly in thoracic cord and in areas with myelin and axon destruction. Furthermore, they were more numerous in patients with disease of shorter duration, and pX expression was not found in cellular infiltrates in the spinal cord of a patient with acute T-cell leukemia (Moritoyo et al., 1996). Another study using similar methods and double staining for cell identification found pX gene expression in glial fibrillary acid protein–positive cells (Lehky et al., 1995), so a consensus on cellular localization of HTLV-I-infected cells in the cord lesions is still lacking.

The greater virus load and immune responses in blood, the expression of pX in CD4 T cells in cord, and the prominence of CD8 cells in the inflammatory response all suggest an immunopathogenesis in which HTLV-I-infected T cells enter the lateral columns of the midthoracic spinal cord. CD4 T cells from patients with TSP/HAM show heightened transmigrating activity *in vitro* across reconstituted basement membrane; CD8 T cells from these patients do not (Furuya et al., 1997). Infected CD4 cells, and possibly astrocytes, presumably express gene products to which susceptible individuals have or develop an intense specific CD8 cytotoxic cell response (Levin and Jacobson, 1997). Myelin and axon destruction may result from direct cytotoxic activity or release of cytokines (Fig. 11.3).

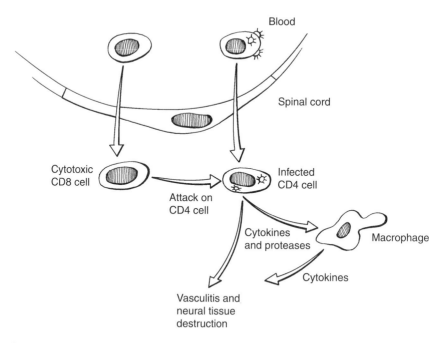

FIG. 11.3. Schematic of proposed pathogenesis of human T-cell lymphotropic virus myelopathy. Both infected CD4 lymphocytes expressing pX protein and cytotoxic T cells sensitized to pX protein enter. Reaction leads to cytokine or protease release, which indirectly causes vasculitis, demyelination, and tissue necrosis.

The localization to lateral columns of the midthoracic cord may be explained by the hemodynamics of this site (Osame et al., 1997). The single anterior and two posterior vertebral arteries originate from intracranial branches of the vertebral arteries with caudal flow; intercostal branches arising from the aorta contribute, but a major artery of variable origin (the artery of Adamkiewicz) enters at the lower thoracic level and gives rise to rostral flow. Thus, flow is caudal above the fourth or fifth thoracic segments and rostral below, making this a watershed with compromised blood flow. In addition, blood to the anterior two-thirds of the cord is supplied by the anterior spinal artery and blood to the posterior one-third of the cord is from the smaller posterior arteries, placing the lateral columns at similar risk. Greater expression of vascular cell-adhesion molecules (V-CAM1) on endothelium in thoracic cord segments was found in patients with HAM/TSP than in control patients, but different cord levels were not compared (Umehara et al., 1996). Whether decreased velocity of flow, differential expression of adhesion molecules, or compensatory attenuation of the blood–brain barrier at these sites modifies T-cell trafficking is not known. The lack of involvement of 99% of those infected, the long clinical latency, the failure to spread throughout the neuraxis, and the events that trigger the process still remain mysteries.

Recently, a chronic myelopathy has been reported in one specific strain of rats inoculated with rat T cells immortalized with superinfection by HTLV-I. After a long incubation period, some rats developed hindlimb paralysis. The pathologic changes showed demyelination centered in the thoracic cord but with little inflammation (Yoshiki, 1995). Expression of pX mRNA and an increase in tumor necrosis factor α were found in the same localization (Tomaru et al., 1996).

Other Neurologic Diseases

Polymyositis was initially associated with HTLV-I in Jamaica (Mora et al., 1988). Over 80% of patients with polymyositis were seropositive as opposed to 7% to 18% of the healthy population. Studies of seropositive Jamaican patients have shown the presence of HTLV-I DNA in muscle biopsy specimens and HTLV-I antigen in invading inflammatory cells (Sherman et al., 1995). In Japan, the association has been less compelling.

A United States resident who developed polymyositis 4 years after multiple blood transfusions was found to be seropositive for HTLV-I and HIV. On muscle biopsy, however, HTLV-I viral antigen was reported in muscle fibers with fiber atrophy and in areas of inflammation, but no HIV antigen was found (Wiley et al., 1989). Most studies, however, have found antigen limited to inflammatory or endomysial cells (Cupler et al., 1996).

Involvement of the eyes has appeared in several reports, including a retinal vasculitis (Sasaki et al., 1989) and uveitis (Sagawa et al., 1995). Two studies of antibody prevalence and a subsequent study using PCR implicated the virus in multiple sclerosis, but numerous subsequent studies have failed to confirm this association (see Chapter 10).

Treatment

Several treatments have been tested with limited responses. Value of zidovudine is uncertain (Gout et al., 1991). Plasmapheresis (Matsuo et al., 1988), α interferon (Izumo et al., 1996) and intravenous gammaglobulin (Kuroda et al., 1991) have all been reported to give transient improvements. Steroids have been most efficacious and used most widely (Nakagawa et al., 1996). The Japanese showed improvements with steroid treatment when given soon after diagnosis, whereas studies where investigators began therapy in long established disease showed little or no therapeutic response. My personal experience is that during the early phase of disease when there is ongoing clinical deterioration and a significant pleocytosis, a striking improvement can be obtained with steroids. In one patient followed over 20 years, we observed marked improvement in weakness and dysesthesias with steroids during the initial two to three years of disease and had great difficulty weaning him from steroids. Over the years his disease stabilized, the pleocytosis cleared, and steroids had no effect whatsoever. Curiously, though the clinical disease appeared to "burn out" intrathecal antibody synthesis against HTLV-I continued suggesting ongoing antigenic stimulation within the nervous system (Johnson et al., 1988a).

Human T-cell Lymphotropic Virus, Type II

HTLV-II has been isolated from two patients with hairy-cell leukemia, but this virus has not been definitely related to malignancies. HTLV-II has a 60% sequence identity with HTLV-I and is difficult to distinguish by usual serologic studies. HTLV-II appears to be an endemic infection in Amerindians, where virus is thought to spread primarily by sexual contact and breast milk (Khabbaz et al., 1991). The virus has been spread into the injecting drug users in the United States and is now widespread in this population.

About 25% of New York injection drug users are infected with HTLV-II, and a majority of these individuals are coinfected with HIV. Of those infected with only HTLV-II, a higher rate of neurologic disability and neuropathy is found than in those seronegative for HTLV-II and HIV, but no distinctive clinical syndrome is evident (Dooneief et al., 1996).

A disease resembling TSP/HAM has been associated with HTLV-II infection in several case reports (Harrington et al., 1993; Jacobson et al., 1993b). In a report of four cases of spastic paraparesis associated with HTLV-II, clinical and immunologic features closely paralleled those in TSP/HAM (Lehky et al., 1996). All four patients were African Americans, but three were also of Amerindian ancestry. In contrast, two seropositive American-Indian sisters were described with cerebellar ataxia and myelopathy (Hjelle et al., 1992). In a survey of seropositive blood donors, signs of myelopathy were ten times more frequent in those with HTLV-I infections than in those with HTLV-II infections (Murphy et al., 1997). HTLV-II sequences also have been reported in patients with chronic fatigue syndrome (DeFreitas et al., 1991) (see Chapter 8).

HTLV-II is assumed to be less neurovirulent than HTLV-I. Alternatively, the paucity of cases after intravenous exposure, where by analogy the risk may be greatest, may reflect a recent introduction of the virus into the drug-using population, and a bigger problem may be incubating.

NEUROLOGIC DISEASES OF ANIMAL RETROVIRUSES

Murine Leukemia Virus

In 1973, as part of the Virus Cancer Program, Gardner and his associates were monitoring wild rodent populations in southern California. While collecting mice in a pigeon farm, they found wild mice with hindlimb paralysis. The disease occurred only in middle-age mice and consisted of a slowly progressive motor neuron disorder with noninflammatory vacuolar degeneration of the spinal cord. The disease was transmitted with an incubation period of 5 to 6 months, and a strain of murine leukemia virus was recovered. The initial disease was also associated with a high rate of lymphoma. Subsequently, two viruses were found to be present (Hartley and Rowe, 1976): paralytic disease was due to an ecotropic virus (a virus that replicated in mouse cells but not nonmouse cells), whereas lymphoma was caused by an amphotropic virus (a virus that replicated in mouse cells and nonmouse cells).

Using clones and concentrated virus, the incubation period could be abbreviated to 2 to 4 weeks, but neurologic disease was still dependent on infecting suckling mice (Brooks et al., 1979). Sequential virologic studies showed initial virus replication in spleen and lymphoid tissues, followed by CNS invasion via the blood. Evolution of paralysis and pathologic changes correlated with the amount of virus in the brain and spinal cord and not with the length of the incubation period or the initial concentration of virus in the inoculum. The severe intracellular vacuolization, neuronal loss, and marked astrocytosis occurred in the absence of an inflammatory response, and an antibody response to the virus was not detected (Brooks et al., 1980). Electron-microscopic studies showed virus budding from cerebral and spinal vascular endothelial cells and pericytes (perivascular macrophages) within 12 days of inoculation. The polarity of infection was dramatic, with virus budding only from the abluminal surfaces of these cells (Fig. 11.4). Spongiform changes evolved in neural cells with membrane-lined vacuoles that often contained dense amorphous material of curled and fragmented membranes. Early in infection, these cells failed to show virus particles and thus mimicked the cytologic changes of prion diseases (Swarz et al., 1981). Later, aberrant particles were found budding into neuronal vacuoles, suggesting either that damaged neurons became susceptible to the exogenous virus or that an endogenous mouse virus was activated in these damaged cells.

This neurologic disease and the vacuolar changes are not unique to this strain of murine leukemia virus and have subsequently been described with a temperature-sensitive mutant of Moloney murine leukemia virus, in rats infected with

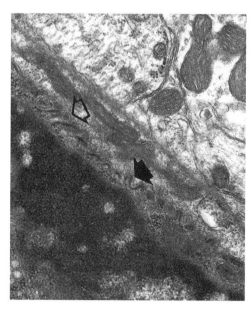

FIG. 11.4. Mouse spinal cord with spongiform encephalomyelopathy caused by neurotropic murine leukemia virus. Particles are budding exclusively from the abluminal surface of a perivascular macrophage (pericyte). Virus particles can be seen free between cells (*open arrow*) and budding from pericyte membrane (*filled arrow*). (From Johnson et al., 1979, with permission.)

rat-passaged Friend murine leukemia virus (Kai and Furuta, 1984), and in chimeras of the original wild-type virus and Friend leukemia virus (Lynch and Portis, 1993). With the original virus, molecular genetic analysis has localized neurovirulence to the env gene, but a second determinant in the long-terminal repeat region influences the incidence of disease and the regional distribution of spongiform lesions (Paquette et al., 1989). Transgenic mice harboring only the env gene of the wild-type neurotropic virus develop spongiform changes, indicating that the protein complex alone is sufficient to induce disease (Kay et al., 1993).

The cellular localization of virus has been a contentious issue. Some have reported viral antigen in neurons and glial cells, but this may be dependent on mouse strains, virus variants, or assay systems, particularly since gag antigens of endogenous and these exogenous viruses may cross-react (Wiley and Gardner, 1993). Curiously, infection of cerebellar granular neurons without pathologic changes have been reported by several groups, showing the lack of correlation between viral expression and neuronal damage (Kay et al., 1991; Lynch et al., 1991). All studies agree that vascular endothelial cells and pericytes and probably microglia are infected (Baszler and Zachary, 1990; Gravel et al., 1993). Indeed, a correlation has been shown between efficiency of virus growth in brain capillary endothelial cells *in vitro* and neurovirulence of multiple clones of virus *in vivo* (Masuda et al., 1993). The endothelial cells may also determine the age specificity of the disease, since inoculation of infected microglial cells into the brains of mice over 10 days of age leads to focal spongiform degeneration that colocalizes with the sites of the inoculated cells (Lynch et al., 1995).

Initially, this animal disease, with its clinical signs and noninflammatory pathology, excited interest as a model of amyotrophic lateral sclerosis. Subsequent focus on the ultrastructure of the vacuoles raised questions of a common mechanism of pathogenesis with prion diseases, although it has recently been shown that murine leukemia virus spongiform myelopathy develops in knockout mice with no prion gene (Jolicoeur et al., 1996). Now the interest has turned to the relevance to HIV-associated neurologic diseases, where the role of the blood–brain barrier and the indirect effects of the infection of microglia and macrophages are of interest in the disruption of neural structure and function.

Lentiviruses

Sporadic cases of chronic interstitial pneumonitis in sheep or hemolytic crises in horses, illnesses now recognized as lentivirus diseases, were recognized in the 19th century. Intense study of most of these animal diseases and recovery of viruses were spurred by outbreaks of the diseases—outbreaks that in most cases were precipitated by human interventions. These epidemiologic factors in animal diseases have parallels to the emergence of HIV infections and AIDS in humans.

All lentiviruses are remarkably species specific, with transmission only to closely related species and *in vitro* growth limited to cells of these species. No lentiviruses have been recovered from rodents (our best-monitored species), transmitted to rodents (our standard laboratory indicator), or grown in rodent cells. In cell cultures, some lentiviruses are cytolytic and are not "slow." In the complex interaction with the host animal, all are characterized by long incubation periods, slowly progressive or relapsing disease, and a fatal outcome. All cause multisystem disease, including combinations of lymphadenopathy, pneumonitis, arthritis, mastitis, hemolytic anemia, thrombocytopenia, and, in every case, chronic encephalitis (Table 11.3).

Lentiviruses can be generally divided into two groups: the ruminant and equine lentiviruses that infect macrophages and cause intense inflammatory diseases, and the lentiviruses of cats and primates that infect macrophages and T cells and lead to immunodeficiency and opportunistic infections. Both groups have the unique genetic devices to integrate their copy DNA (or proviral DNA) into the genomic DNA of fully differentiated, nonreplicating host cells and to regulate and modulate the output of virus. Variants are generated so that within a single host a divergent population (or viral swarm) develops (Clements and Zink, 1996). In some cases, these variants may lead to exacerbations or quicken the pace of disease.

TABLE 11.3. *Neurologic diseases with lentivirus infections*

Virus	Systemic disease	Blood cells infected	CNS signs	Neuropathology	Neural cells infected
Visna virus	Lymphocytic pneumonitis, arthritis, mastitis	Φ	+	Leukoencephalitis and demyelination	Macrophages, and microglia, ? vascular endothelium
Caprine arthritis–encephalitis virus	Arthritis, pneumonitis, mastitis	Φ	+	Leukoencephalitis and demyelination	Macrophages and microglia
Equine infectious anemia virus	Recurrent autoimmune hemolytic crises	Φ	+	Ependymitis, subependymal encephalomalacia, perivascular inflammation	Perivascular and meningeal cells
Bovine immunodeficiency virus	Lymphadenopathy, lymphocytosis, and wasting	?	+	Perivascular inflammation	?
Feline immunodeficiency virus	Immunodeficiency with opportunistic infections	Φ + T	+	Perivascular mononuclear cells, gliosis, and microglial nodules	Macrophages and occasional microglia
Simian immunodeficiency virus	Immunodeficiency with opportunistic infections	Φ + T	+	Perivascular and meningeal mononuclear cells and giant cells; minimal myelin pallor	Macrophages and microglia ? vascular endothelial
Human immunodeficiency virus	Immunodeficiency with opportunistic infections	Φ + T	+	Gliosis, microglial nodules, giant cells; diffuse myelin pallor; vacuolar myelopathy, axonal neuropathy	Macrophages and microglia; nonproductive infection of astrocytes

Φ, macrophages; T, T cells.

Visna Virus

Visna virus, the cause of the visna–maedi complex, was the first recognized lentivirus and is the prototype virus of the genus (see Chapter 10). The disease visna was first recognized in Iceland in 1935, following the importation of Karakul rams from Germany to be bred with the Icelandic sheep, the descendants of those brought in the Viking longboats in the 10th century. Several new diseases appeared after that importation. The most important was maedi, a chronic lymphocytic pneumonitis; another was an accompanying chronic paralytic disease called visna. The outbreak presumably resulted from introduction of a new virus into pristine sheep herds, the close penning of sheep during the severe winters, and the cointroduction of the etiologic agent of pulmonary adenomatosis that causes copious respiratory–pulmonary secretions (Narayan and Clements, 1989). The nature of housing and coinfection is of obvious importance in this outbreak, because in our sanitized and spacious animal facilities cohousing of infected and uninfected susceptible laboratory sheep has resulted in no cross infections in over 25 years. In Iceland, natural maedi and visna diseases were eliminated after extensive slaughter and prohibition of further sheep importation.

Natural visna, with the accompanying pneumonitis, was seen primarily in sheep that were more than 2 years of age. Experimental disease similar to the natural disease begins with paralysis of the hindlimbs or occasionally the forelegs. The disease progresses over a period of months to death. Trembling and blindness are also seen (Haase, 1975). Antibodies to the virus develop 1 to 3 months after inoculation, and antibody levels in spinal fluid may exceed those in serum (Griffin et al., 1978a). High levels of antiviral IgM and IgG persist in spinal fluid, and oligoclonal bands are found (Martin et al., 1982). Pathologically, the brain shows intense mononuclear inflammatory responses in the meninges and perivascular spaces within the first month after experimental intracerebral inoculation; over time, lesions accumulate preferentially in the white matter (Petursson et al., 1976). Primary demyelination is seen primarily in the periventricular white matter and in the subpial white matter of the spinal cord (Georgsson et al., 1982). Mononuclear cell inflammation also is found in synovial membranes, glandular tissue of the mammary glands, and in the spleen and lymph nodes.

Virus is found in macrophages and their precursors. Clusters of infected macrophage precursors have been found in bone marrow by *in situ* hybridization (Gendelman et al., 1985a). Monocytes are infected but produce little mRNA or viral protein, but when they mature into macrophages the latent infection becomes productive (Gendelman et al., 1986). Therefore, the monocytes in the blood are nonproductively infected, but when they enter specific tissues, such as lung and brain, they become macrophages and express virus. This infection, in turn, induces a cytokine produced by T cells that upregulates major histocompatibility complex antigens and enhances inflammation (Kennedy et al., 1985; Narayan et al., 1985).

Our initial experimental studies of visna were predicated on the hypothesis that the long incubation period, remitting and relapsing or progressive course, and demyelinating pathology might provide insights into multiple sclerosis (Narayan et al., 1974). These unique pathogenetic mechanisms have proved to have a more profound impact on our speculations regarding the pathogenesis of HIV-associated neurologic diseases, particularly in macrophage and microglial infection leading to disease by way of cytokines.

There is also an intriguing parallel to another rare human disease: lymphoid interstitial pneumonia. This disease resembles maedi, and a small percentage of patients with this disease develop neurologic illnesses. The pathologic study of a single patient showed intense inflammation and extensive demyelination in the brain that were reminiscent of the lesions of visna (Jefferson et al., 1971).

Caprine Arthritis–Encephalitis Virus

Caprine arthritis–encephalitis virus is closely related to visna virus. The virus was first recovered from dairy goats of the Northwest (Cork et al., 1974). Serologic studies indicate that infection is widespread among dairy goats of North America and Western Europe, but not in Asia and Africa. The transmission is primarily by the macrophage-rich colostrum, and some goat fanciers in endemic areas milk their goats and pool the milk for the hand-feeding of kids—a husbandry practice that spreads infections through the herd.

In the adult goats, the major disease is slowly evolving, crippling synovitis. Mastitis is also prominent. Some kids, usually between 2 and 4 months of age, develop progressive neurologic signs and have a leukomalacia with intense mononuclear inflammatory responses and demyelination (Norman and Smith, 1983).

The primary susceptible cells are monocytes and macrophages, and activation of virus expression with maturation of monocytes to macrophages, similar to the findings with visna virus, has been shown (Narayan et al., 1983c). The mode of transmission and the primary presentations of disease are different from visna, but the pathogenesis of disease appears similar.

Equine Infectious Anemia Virus

Equine infectious anemia virus has an epidemiology and clinical pattern distinct from other lentiviruses. It is the only lentivirus transmitted by arthropods, but transmission is mechanical (not biologic as occurs with arboviruses). Infected horses, mules, or donkeys develop a persistent plasma viremia, and blood-sucking flies act as vectors by their blood-contaminated mouthparts. Transmission is optimized by the crowding of animals during summer months at agricultural, sporting, or military events (Narayan and Clements, 1989), because crowding is needed to prevent drying of the blood on the fly between the biting of infected and susceptible animals.

The disease may be a single fatal episode of fever, cachexia, and hemolytic anemia within a month of infection, or there may be recovery over a few days, with subsequent acute relapses of crises weeks or months later. Relapses usually cease after three or four episodes, followed either by recovery or by chronic wasting. Thrombocytopenia may accompany the hemolytic episodes. Neurologic signs develop in some animals, and there are neuropathologic findings of chronic granulomatous ependymitis, meningitis, and encephalitis (McClure et al., 1982). Viral antigen has been found in perivascular and meningeal cells (McGuire et al., 1971).

Pathogenesis of the hematologic crises appears to be immunopathologic, but the recurrent crises appear to depend on the development of variations in the envelope gene sequences that allow an acute viremia with virus strains not neutralized by antibody formed against prior strains (Payne et al., 1987).

Bovine Immunodeficiency Virus

Bovine immunodeficiency virus is a recently recognized lentivirus about which little is known. The agent was originally isolated from a cachectic cow with persistent lymphocytosis and subsequently associated with lymphadenopathy and chronic encephalitis (Gonda et al., 1987). Virus can be isolated from peripheral blood mononuclear cells, spleen, lymph nodes, and brain. Serologic data indicate infection in many countries in a nonuniform distribution (Belloc et al., 1996). The mode of transmission is unknown, but it has been suggested that virus is spread within herds by hypodermic needles reused in immunizations or parenteral injections (Narayan and Clements, 1989).

Feline Immunodeficiency Virus

Feline immunodeficiency virus was originally isolated from sick cats in a cattery in northern California. In this dense population of homeless cats, an outbreak of chronic diarrhea, wasting, anemia, periodontal disease, and neurologic disease began in one pen in 1982. The virus was recovered and transmitted to kittens that subsequently developed a persistent lymphadenopathy (Pedersen et al., 1987).

Infections have been found to be common among cats but more common among males and among cats that are allowed to roam freely. Transmission is thought to be primarily by biting, although transmission from queens to kittens by milk has been reported. Experimentally, the virus can be transmitted by oral, vaginal, and rectal routes (Bennett and Hart, 1995).

Neuropathologic studies have shown diffuse gliosis, microglial nodules, and diffuse white-matter pallor with mild inflammatory changes (Boche et al., 1996), and vacuolar myelopathy has been reported (Abrama et al., 1995). Multinucleated giant cells characteristic of HIV encephalopathy are usually absent.

In addition to macrophages, CD4+ T cells are infected, and there are reports of infection in CD8 and B cells, as well as astrocytes (Bennett and Hart, 1995). Profound immunodeficiency does develop, and cats die of opportunistic infections.

Simian Immunodeficiency Virus

The first simian immunodeficiency viruses were isolated from rhesus macaques with lymphoma, at the New England Regional Primate Center in 1985 (Daniel et al., 1985; Kanki et al., 1985). The virus was transmitted to other rhesus monkeys, causing chronic lymphadenopathy, diarrhea, wasting, falling CD4 counts, and eventually lymphoid depletion, opportunistic infections, and death.

The origin of this virus proved to be complex. Studies of wild rhesus macaques of Asia showed no evidence of infection; studies of African primates uncovered a number of simian retroviruses, but none are known to cause disease in their natural host. Five lentiviruses have now been recovered from African primates: from African green monkeys (designated SIVagm), sooty mangabey monkeys (SIVsm), Syke's monkeys (SIVsyk), mandrills (SIVmnd), and chimpanzees (SIVchz). Each of these five primate lentiviruses has only 55% to 60% amino acid identities in their pol gene products to the other four viruses. The original macaque isolate (designate SIVmac) by sequence analysis has over 96% identity to sooty mangabey virus and is almost certainly an African virus introduced into captive Asian macaques in primate centers in the United States (Desrosiers, 1990). Furthermore, HIV-2 has a similar 82% to 100% identity to SIVsm, and the sooty mangabeys inhabit the coastal regions of West Africa where HIV-2 is endemic. HIV-1 shows a close relationship to the chimpanzee agent (SIVchz) (Huet et al., 1990) (Fig. 11.5). These relationships have caused concern among laboratory workers using SIVmac as a model for HIV, because a small number have become infected and harbor the virus, but evidence of immunodeficiency has not developed (Khabbaz et al., 1994).

Simian immunodeficiency virus (SIVmac) in rhesus macaques has become the major animal model for HIV infections of humans. The clinical signs, immunologic alteration, pathologic changes, and even the opportunistic infections mirror those in human infection. Unlike humans with HIV infections, however, monkeys infected with SIVmac do not lose CD4 T cells until the terminal phase of disease. A similar encephalitis develops in about 50% of monkeys, but cognitive and motor impairment has been demonstrated early in disease (Murray et al., 1992a). The major difference is the more rapid course of simian immunodeficiency disease: most macaques die within 2 years of infection, and one-third develop a rapidly progressive disease leading to death within a few months (Letvin and King, 1990).

Neuropathologic findings in the brain are remarkably similar to those in humans with AIDS, but lesions are more inflammatory. In severely affected animals, perivascular cuffing, microglial nodules, and multinucleated giant cells are prominent (Lackner et al., 1991; Clements and Zink, 1996). Neuronal loss in

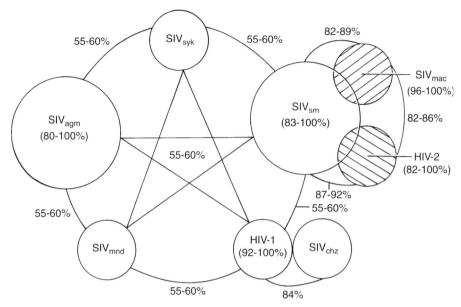

FIG. 11.5. Diagram of sequence relationships of primate lentiviruses. Percentages in the *lines* are amino acid identities in the pol gene product, whereas those in *parentheses* are the ranges of identities in the product in different isolates of each virus. (Data provided by Ronald C. Desrosiers.)

cortex and multifocal demyelination in white matter are also present. In lesser affected animals, focal demyelination in deep matter may be the most prominent finding, with only mild inflammation and few microglial nodules or giant cells (O. Narayan, *personal communication*). Vacuolar myelopathy is rare, and diffuse myelin pallor and peripheral neuropathies seen in HIV infections are not reported (Sasseville and Lackner, 1997).

Some strains of virus replicate productively only in CD4+ T cells, whereas others replicate in both macrophages and T cells (macrophagetropic strains). Infection in the CNS depends on both T-cell activation and macrophagetropic strains. Neuroinvasion depends on the intensity of T-cell activation, because only activated T cells cross the blood–brain barrier and deposit virus. These T-cell tropic viruses, however, cause immunodeficiency disease but not encephalitis (Sharma et al., 1992). Macrophagetropic variants will replicate productively in brain after the animal becomes immunosuppressed, but cloned macrophagetropic viruses are poorly neuroinvasive because they cannot activate T cells effectively. Thus, macrophagetropism has been shown to be essential, but not sufficient, for neurovirulence (Joag et al., 1995).

Virus in the brain is localized primarily in macrophages and microglia (Chakrabarti et al., 1991; Hurtrel et al., 1993). Infection of vascular endothelial cells has been reported (Mankowski et al., 1994), but this claim is controversial.

Interestingly, the same methods of double immunocytochemistry and reverse-transcriptase–*in situ* PCR used to detect simian immunodeficiency virus in rhesus macaque endothelium failed to find endothelial cell infection in human HIV infections (Takahashi et al., 1996). Vascular adhesion molecules and major histocompatibility complex class 2 molecules are upregulated on endothelial cells (Beilke et al., 1991; Sasseville et al., 1994). Several inflammatory cytokines and inducible nitric oxide synthase are found in brain (Lane et al., 1996; Sasseville et al., 1996), and DNA fragmentation indicative of apoptosis has been shown in neurons, endothelial cells, and glial cells of infected macaques (Adamson et al., 1996a). These findings suggest an indirect, possibly cytokine-mediated, effect on neuronal function and integrity. These mechanisms of pathogenesis are discussed further in the next chapter.

COMMENT

Emergence of the epidemic of HIV infections has led many to query where this virus came from and how the epidemic grew to global proportions. A look at family members may provide some biologic insights. Most lentiviruses have probably been endemic in their natural hosts, causing sporadic unnoticed disease; all are quite species specific and are not easily transmitted in natural settings. They have emerged due to crowding (visna, equine infectious anemia, feline immunodeficiency, and simian immunodeficiency viruses), pooling of secretions (visna and caprine arthritis–encephalitis viruses), injection of blood via needles or fly mouthparts (bovine immunodeficiency and equine infectious anemia viruses), coinfection (visna virus), or have been interjected into a pristine susceptible population (visna virus) or into a new, closely related species (simian immunodeficiency virus).

SUPPLEMENTARY BIBLIOGRAPHY

Roman GC, Vernant J-C, Osame M, eds. *HTLV-1 and the nervous system.* New York: Alan R Liss, 1989.
Rudge P, ed. *Neurological aspects of human retroviruses.* London: Baillière Tindel, 1992.

12

Human Immunodeficiency Virus

The rapid changes in modern society and the almost infinite genetic variability of viruses combine to promise a future changing scene of unpredictable events. We live in interesting times . . .

Johnson, R.T.
Viral Infections of the Nervous System, 1982

I wrote those closing sentences of the first edition of this book during the summer of 1981—the summer that the *Morbidity and Mortality Weekly Reports* noted the strange occurrences of *Pneumoncystic carinii* pneumonia and Kaposi's sarcoma among previously healthy gay men in New York and California (CDC 1981 a,b). At the time, my comments and the public health reports seemed unrelated, but the reports were the harbingers of the epidemic of the acquired immunodeficiency syndrome (AIDS). Over the past decade the causative virus, human immunodeficiency virus (HIV), has become the most prevalent infection of the nervous system worldwide and has been associated with the widest clinical spectrum of neurological syndromes ever associated with a single virus.

Nevertheless, my references to changing social mores and virus mutations were not evidence of foresight or even insight—simply a statement of facts. In 1981 greater sexual license had already led to the spread of genital herpes simplex virus which had become the first virus featured on the cover of *Time.* Diversity of many RNA viruses had been observed with the periodic new strains of influenza, the appearance of the neurovirulent La Crosse virus in the Midwest in the 1960s, and the epidemic of hemorrhagic conjunctivitis due to enterovirus 70 in Africa in 1969 (Johnson, 1994a). Mutations of a virus that allowed escape from antibody neutralization had been observed within a single host with visna virus infections in sheep in our laboratory (Narayan et al, 1985). Visna virus, the prototype lentivirus that causes chronic restricted infection and remitting and relapsing or progressive neurological disease, had been studied as a possible model for multiple sclerosis with no thought that a related lentivirus would emerge as a new human disease (Johnson, 1985a).

HUMAN IMMUNODEFICIENCY VIRUS INFECTIONS

In 1983 a virus was recovered from chronic lymphadenopathy syndrome in France (Barre-Sinoussi et al, 1983) and subsequently from AIDS patients in the United States (Gallo et al, 1984). It was initially thought by some that the virus was an oncovirus related to HTLV-I, hence the early designation HTLV-III. Eventually HIV proved to be a lentivirus. Lentiviruses are distinguished from other retroviruses by their complexity. They not only contain the three genes common to all retroviruses: *gag* (coding for internal proteins), *pol* (encoding for the reverse transcriptase), and *env* (coding for the glycosolated surface and trans-membrane proteins), but HIV codes for six additional regulatory proteins including several that require splicing for the formation of mRNA. The mature virion contains two identical strands of RNA along with a polymerase inside an inner shell made up of three gag proteins. One of the gag proteins, p24, is the most abundant structural protein and is often assayed as an indirect measure of virus quantity. The outer shell proteins include an inner surface protein and two gly-coproteins; gp41 is the transmembrane protein and gp120 is entirely external to the lipid bilayer of the virus envelope (Levy, 1994).

HIV interacts with the CD4 membrane antigen as a receptor, and this attachment is mediated by a segment of the gp120 envelope protein. Secondary receptors are important in defining macrophagetropic or T-cell line tropic strains and, in part, determine species specificity (Feng et al., 1996; Weiss, 1996). Secondary receptors may also enhance microglial infection in the CNS (He et al., 1997). Internalization of the virus occurs either by receptor-mediated endocytosis or by virus-mediated membrane fusion. Following the reverse transcription of the RNA, the proviral double-stranded DNA is integrated into the host genomic DNA, establishing latency. But in many cells a down-regulated production of virus continues with formation of the virions by budding from the cytoplasmic membrane as in T cells, or into cytoplasmic vacuoles, as is seen in macrophages.

Epidemiology

The initial reports of unusual opportunistic infections and neoplasms involved gay men who had severely depleted T cells with CD4 markers, and this syndrome became known as gay-related immunodeficiency or GRID. Within months the population at risk was found to include heterosexual men and women (most of whom were intravenous drug abusers or Haitian immigrants). Etiologic hypotheses at that time focused on an infectious agent, recreational drugs, or chronic antigen stimulation with spermatozoa exposure (Quagliarello, 1982). AIDS soon was recognized in subSaharan Africa, however, as a heterosexual disease with venereal spread. The disease was documented in infants born of infected mothers, in recipients of blood transfusions, and in hemophiliacs. This evidence of transmission by sex and blood was reminiscent of the transmission patterns of hepatitis B virus and supported a viral cause. Furthermore, the transmission to monogamous hemophiliacs with cell-free clotting factors VIII and IX tragically fulfilled Koch's third postulate of causation even before HIV was isolated.

The isolation of HIV in 1983 enabled tests to be developed for a serologic diagnosis of infection. This in turn allowed the determination of the prevalence of infection in different populations and demonstrated the long interval between infection and clinical AIDS; this interval ranges from months to greater than 15 years with an average of 8 to 10 years. Serological tests also allowed the testing of the blood supply greatly decreasing the likelihood of infection from transfusions or blood products. Testing for HIV antibodies still leaves a window of about 40 days in which a person who has been infected recently may not have detectable antibodies, but with new assays it is estimated that only 1 in 360,000 units of tested blood is contaminated (Lackritz et al., 1995).

About 75% of HIV infections worldwide are transmitted heterosexually, but communicability is remarkably low compared to other venereal infections. Even with anal receptive intercourse, it is estimated that transmission occurs in only about 1 in 100 contacts, male to female vaginal spread in about 1 per 500, and female to male vaginal spread in about 1 in 1000. A number of studies, however, have shown that these numbers are increased by partner numbers, by the presence of other sexually transmitted diseases (particularly those with penile ulcers in the male or venereal warts, chlamydia and other infections in the female), and by the lack of circumcision in the male. Each of these factors poses a greater risk of being infected and a greater threat of transmission (Simonsen et al, 1988). One study in Africa showed a remarkably high rate of seroconversion of uncircumcised men with penile ulcers after a single sexual exposure to an HIV-positive prostitute (Cameron et al., 1989).

Approximately 10% of infections worldwide are transmitted by contaminated syringes and needles. Rates of transmission among intravenous drug users are related to drug use behaviors. For example in "shooting galleries" in the Northeastern United States strangers may be admitted and "booting,", that is pulling up blood into the syringe before injection, is a common practice. Sharing of needles among tightly knit friendship groups poses a lower risk, since there is less chance of introduction of the virus into the group, although once introduced the entire group is at high risk.

In addition to the transmission across the placenta (see Chapter 13) transmission both from mother to infant and infant to mother via breast feeding has been documented in cases where there has been postpartum infection by transfusion of the mother or the neonate. Transmission of infection by needle sticks in hospital personnel occurs in about 1 per thousand exposures. Despite the public tempests about potential transmission by everything from communion cups to schoolyard scuffles, recovery of HIV from tears, saliva and urine has been rare and in very small quantities. Transmission by casual contact is virtually unknown. This has been dramatically shown in the households of infected hemophiliacs where sharing of beds, eating utensils, toothbrushes and all the intimacies of everyday family life are without risk, unless there is sexual contact or major contamination with blood (Lusher, et al, 1991).

With the explosive worldwide epidemic of HIV infection over the past decade, the natural question is, 'How could this occur with a virus that is so low in communicability?' A study of particular interest is one done over a 10 year period in rural Zaire where, despite the burgeoning rates in urban populations, the rate of infection in several villages was determined to be about 0.8%, and this rate did not vary over a 10 year interval (Nzilambi, et al, 1988). In these villages or, indeed, in small towns anywhere in the world, a low transmission rate might occur with a low rate of premarital promiscuity or marital infidelity. An occasional person in such a village dying with a strange disease might go unnoted. Indeed, if relationships were strictly monogamous, the virus would disappear entirely after the death of the infected conjugal pair and a percentage of their prepubescent infected progeny. Two important factors, urbanization and greater sexual license, appear important in the spread of this infection as well as the reuse of unsterile needles and syringes by intravenous drug users or medical personnel. It has been postulated that the introduction of syringes and needles with vaccines and antibiotics in the 1950s and 60s may have contributed to the initial kindling of the epidemic in Africa (Karpas, 1990).

The global magnitude of the epidemic is staggering. The World Health Organization estimated in mid 1996 that 21 million persons including several million children were infected with HIV (Piot, 1996). Half of these are in sub–Saharan Africa where the epidemic has caused the greatest loss of life and social disruption. In some areas 70 to 80% of the hospital beds are occupied by AIDS patients, and the epidemic has left over a million orphan children, has depleted the labor force, and has led to deterioration of the health systems. In sub–Saharan Africa, the number infected has tripled in the last five years, but there appears to be some stabilization.

In the United States greater than 1.5 million persons are infected and over 500,000 have developed AIDS, but in 1996 the number of AIDS deaths decreased for the first time since the onset of the epidemic. There has been a dramatic decrease in the rate of seroconversion among gay men. In certain sectors the infection rate has continued to rise, particularly in intravenous drug users, their sexual partners, and their progeny. The largest proportional increase has been among 13 to 29-year-olds in small towns and rural areas of the South and Midwest (CDC, 1995b). In 1992 HIV infection replaced unintentional injuries as the leading cause of death among persons 25 to 44 years of age in the United States (CDC, 1996c).

The largest increase in seroconversion rates have been seen in South and Southeast Asia where the epidemic has radically changed (Quinn, 1996). The introduction of HIV has been relatively recent, so the number of AIDS cases is still small. But rates of seroconversion as high as 5% per month have been seen among intravenous drug users in Thailand, rates that are previously unprecedented. It has been predicted that Asia, because of the size of its population at risk, will soon surpass Africa as the epicenter of AIDS. By the year 2000, it is estimated that between 40 to 100 million adults and 10 million children will be infected with HIV, with 12 to 15 million infections in India alone. Twenty million adults will develop AIDS within the next decade. The epidemic remains dynamic; its full economic and social impact has yet to be felt except in Africa (Mann, 1993).

Epidemiological studies are complicated by the genetic diversity of HIV. Sequence comparisons of the env gene of HIV isolates from different areas of the world show differences up to 50%. Viruses with more than 20% differences have been divided into 10 subtypes or clades. A, C, and D clades dominate sub-Saharan Africa, while the B clade is the cause of almost all infections in North America and Western Europe. The C clade dominates India and is established in Brazil as well as Central and South Africa and the E clade now is dominant in Thailand. In regions where multiple clades circulate simultaneously recombinants are found, and an A and E recombinant strain is involved in unprecedented rates of heterosexual spread in Thailand (Burke, 1997). This has raised the question as to whether these viruses have a genetic advantage in transmission. The recent demonstration of more efficient growth of Thai isolates in epithelial Langerhan's cells, a probable portal of entry in genital infection, has raised concerns about a greater societal threat of viruses of the E clade (Soto-Ramirez et al., 1996).

HIV-2 is a distinct virus closely related to the simian immunodeficiency virus (see Chapter 11). It has been associated with AIDS predominantly in West Africa (Clavel, et al, 1987). Most of the infections in North America have been in persons of West African origin, although the virus has become established in Brazil. The mode of spread appears to be the same as HIV-1 and the associated immunodeficiency and neurologic diseases are similar, but there are indications that HIV-2 may be less virulent than HIV-I (Sankalé et al., 1996).

Clinical Pathology of the Systemic Infection

In sexual transmission the relative importance of cell-free virus or virus-infected cells is unknown. Over a million cells are present in a single ejaculum, and large numbers of cells are present in vaginal secretions. On the other hand, transmission appears to be more likely during the initial period of infection and then later in infection after the onset of AIDS when cell-free virus is more plentiful, at least in serum. Initial sites of infection are similarly unknown. Cells susceptible to infection are present in the rectal epithelium and the mucosal surfaces of the nasopharynx (Frankel et al., 1996). Infection of the penile or vaginal epithelial cells is unlikely, and male to female transmission appears enhanced by the presence of cervical ectopy and during menses or immediately prior to restoration of the mucosal plug (Levy, 1994). The increased risk of both transmission and acquisition of infection in the presence of other sexually transmitted diseases is not surprising considering the increased numbers of infected mononuclear cells that may be present in semen or vaginal secretions of the transmitter and the greater risk of access to susceptible cells when genital lesions expose the recipient.

One to three weeks following transmission approximately half of those infected have symptoms of a mononucleosis-like illness characterized by fever, lymphadenopathy, laryngitis, maculo-papular rash, myalgia, thrombocytopenia, leukopenia, diarrhea, and headache. This clinical illness by definition lasts more than three days and usually is over within three weeks, but it may extend for months. Leukopenia and thrombocytopenia are found followed by an increase in the number of CD8 cells. HIV viremia is present until the development of antibody, which usually appears in two to six weeks, but antibody conversion may be delayed as long as six months or more in a rare case (Niu et al, 1993). The virus found in the blood at this time is relatively homogeneous in genotype and is quite uniformly macrophage-tropic; that is, it grows readily in macrophages as well as stimulated peripheral lymphocytes (Zhu et al, 1993). Studies of partners show that this transmitted virus is often a minor variant, and this implies a selectivity of certain strains in transmission. This supports the speculation that the macrophage may be a critical cell in transmission.

Following the development of antibody and virus-specific cytotoxic CD8 cells (Safrit and Koup, 1995), viremia becomes intermittent and predominantly cell-associated, and CD4 lymphocytes are reconstituted to near normal levels. CD4 numbers then slowly decline over subsequent years prior to the precipitous fall in CD4 counts with the development of AIDS (Fig 12.1). This long asymptomatic period has been referred to as a "latent period," but technically this is incorrect and the infected person remains capable of transmission during the long asymptomatic period. Although latency exists in some cells, infectious virus continues to be produced by others at high levels with evolution of a diversity of virus genotypes (Perelson et al., 1996). At one time this diversity was thought to result from HIV transcription being more error-prone; now it is recognized that up to 10^9 virions are produced daily and considering standard RNA mutation rate at 10^4 to 10^5 per nucleotide per replication cycle and an HIV genome size of 10^4 nucleotides, virtually all possible mutations are generated daily (Wain-Hobson et al., 1995; McKeating 1996).

Within the hemopoietic system CD4-positive lymphocytes produce the major portion of virus. Macrophages are also infected. Infected CD4 lymphocytes are prominent in the lymph nodes and HIV-infected cells have an upregulated surface lectin that induces homing to lymph nodes (Wang et al., 1997); macrophages are the predominant infected cells in the spleen. Within the blood, a very small number of mononuclear cells show the presence of viral antigen, but PCR studies suggest that as many as 1 in 10 to 1 in 1000 peripheral blood mononuclear cells contain viral DNA (Bagasra et al, 1992). The decline in CD4 cells over time does not appear to depend solely on the cytopathic effects of virus but also upon a decrease in the production of CD4 cells and possibly an autoimmune destruction of CD4 cells. With activation of CD4 cells, such as that produced by intercurrent infections with other agents, productive HIV replication

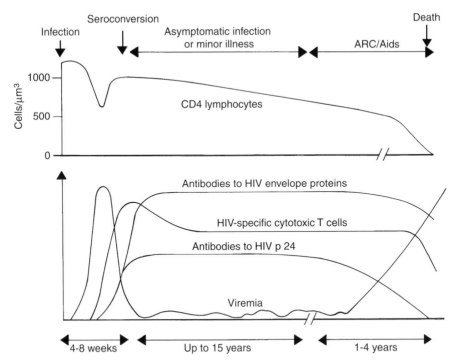

FIG 12.1. Diagram of HIV infection. In first weeks after infection a viremia occurs and CD4 cells decline abruptly in number. With the development of antibody and cytotoxic T cells, viremia declines or disappears and CD4 cells return to near normal numbers. Over the long asymptomatic incubation period CD4 cell counts slowly decline until clinical symptoms develop, antibodies and cytotoxic cells decline and plasma viremia returns. ARC, AIDS-related complex. (Modified from Weiss, 1996, with permission of the American Association for the Advancement of Science.)

occurs in these cells. There is evidence of a variety of dysfunction and deregulation of the immune system with decreased antigen presentation by macrophages, polyclonal activation of B cells, and even abnormal polymorphonuclear cell function during this time (Edelman and Zolla-Pazner, 1989). HIV infection is associated with marked changes in cytokine secretion by T cells, monocytes, and B cells. These cytokines can either up or down regulate other cytokine production, either stimulate or inhibit other immunocytes, and can increase or decrease HIV replication depending on the specific cytokine or mix of cytokines (Fauci, 1996).

The time to onset of AIDS is shorter in those who have symptomatic primary infections and in those who have more rapidly falling levels of CD4 cells and higher plasma levels of HIV-RNA (O'Brien et al., 1996). Genetic variations in several chemokine receptors also influence the time of progression to AIDS but not susceptibility to infection with HIV (Smith et al., 1997). Eventually in at least 90% of those infected, control of HIV replication collapses, and there is a recurrence of plasma viremia, widespread lymphadenopathy, and eventually signs and symptoms that have been designated as defining AIDS-specific opportunistic infections, specific tumors, dementia, or CD4 counts below 200. The mean time between infection and clinical AIDS is now estimated at almost 10 years. The rate of progression appears dependent on virus load, virus-specific cytotoxic T cell and binding antibody responses, and the genotype of host and virus (Haynes et al., 1996). Survival after the onset of the AIDS-defining disease was approximately 11 months, but this interval was increased to over 18 months with better treatment of opportunistic infections and the availability of azidothymidine (Zidovidine) therapy (Jacobson et al., 1993a).

Zidovidine has proved efficacious in controlled studies. Treatment results in an increase in CD4 cells, clearing of some symptoms of the disease, and longer survival. Drug resistant strains of the virus appear within approximately six months, so multiple nucleoside antiviral agents without common resistance patterns have been used. Dramatic decreases in virus replication and increased CD4 cell levels have now been achieved by administering HIV-protease inhibitors with the nucleosides (Collier et al., 1996). Survival with AIDS now may exceed two years in many patients.

The prevention of disease is straightforward, albeit difficult to achieve. Prevention can be accomplished by keeping blood supplies clean, using clean needles, and preventing sexual spread by limiting sex to a single partner. Those unable to practice partner limitation should use latex condoms as an alternative, less effective mode of prevention. Despite the apparent simplicity of preventive methods, rates of infection continue to increase in most countries of the world. Educational programs and condom use appear to have eased the epidemics in Thailand and Uganda, who have followed the lead of Australia, where AIDS was addressed from the outset as a public health problem rather than as a moral dilemma and where a major nonjudgmental and candid education campaign was combined with clean needle and condom distributions.

NEUROLOGICAL DISEASES

The recovery of HIV in cultures of activated lymphocytes in 1983 suggested a simple scenario: HIV infected cells in the immune system that expressed CD4 markers; this infection led to CD4 cell destruction and resultant immunodeficiency; this immunodeficiency permitted fatal opportunistic infections. Early neurologic interest focused solely on the opportunistic infections and tumors that affected the nervous systems of AIDS patients. These included the rather unique presentations of toxoplasmosis, cryptococcosis, and cytomegalovirus infections, the emergence of progressive multifocal leukoencephalopathy (which had previously been an extraordinarily rare disease) and the occurrence of primary CNS B cell lymphomas in relatively young patients (Table 12.1).

Patients were seen with progressive apathy, cognitive deficits and motor slowing and pathologic changes in these patients included cerebral atrophy, diffuse

TABLE 12.1. *Opportunistic neurologic processes in AIDS*

Infection	%	Present at autopsy	%
Toxoplasmosis	7	1984–89	10
		1990–94	5
Cytomegalovirus	19		
Cryptococcus	8		
Progressive multifocal			
leukoencephalopathy	4		
Primary B-cell lymphoma	11		

347 consecutive autopsies in the Johns Hopkins prospective study.

myelin pallor, and multifocal glial nodules. Because of the presumed restriction of HIV infection of lymphocytes, it was assumed that these represented an opportunistic infection by either cytomegalovirus or some unknown agent (Nielsen, et al 1984).

In 1985 focus was drawn to primary infection of the brain. In that year HIV was isolated from the brain, spinal cord, spinal fluid and peripheral nerves of patients who died with neurologic complications of AIDS (Ho et al, 1985; Levy et al, 1985). HIV RNA was demonstrated in the microglial nodules of the brain by *in situ* hybridization, and HIV DNA was found in the brains of children by Southern blot at levels even higher than those found in lymph node and spleen (Shaw et al, 1985). Finally, intrathecal synthesis of antibody against HIV was documented in patients with neurologic illnesses and AIDS (Resnick et al., 1985). These findings suggested primary HIV infection of the nervous system. Also, in 1985 the sequencing of the HIV genome was completed, and sequence comparisons with other known retroviruses showed unequivocally that HIV was not an oncovirus related to HTLV-I, as previously suspected, but was a member of the lentivirus family (Gonda et al., 1985). Lentiviruses are highly species-specific, infect macrophages that play a central role in their pathogenesis, and cause neurologic infection and chronic encephalitis (see Chapter 11).

The initial question was how frequently and early does the CNS become infected (Johnson and McArthur, 1986). Some thought that virus might infect the nervous system via inflammatory cells at the time of opportunistic infections. Under these circumstances, nervous system infection would be a preterminal event of little concern. The Multicenter AIDS Cohort Study, a prospective study of gay men, was initiated even before serological testing for HIV was available; with recognition of nervous system involvement, a subset of these men volunteered for periodic neurocognitive tests, neurological exams, and lumbar punctures. Some were seropositive, some were seronegative, but serologic status was determined after initial recruitment into the original program thus minimizing selection bias. Studies of spinal fluid of healthy men infected for less than two years showed that two-thirds had a pleocytosis, abnormal spinal fluid immunoglobulins, and/or recoverable virus (McArthur et al., 1988). This and similar findings by many others indicate that the CNS is infected early in the majority of asymptomatic seropositive persons, possibly during the period of initial plasma viremia. Since over 21 million persons are infected worldwide, we can assume that most currently have subclinical infections of the CNS.

The second issue, which arose as many different neurologic complications were being described with AIDS, was which complications resulted from direct or indirect effects of virus infection and which stemmed from immunodeficiency and opportunistic infection. The spectrum of these diseases associated with HIV infection continues to be defined, but a variety of clinical syndromes and pathologic findings affecting both central and peripheral nervous system as well as muscle are now thought to be due to HIV rather than an opportunistic infection (Fig 12.2) (Johnson et al, 1988c). Some are seen at the time of primary infection, such as acute encephalopathy, meningitis, and acute demyelinating polyneuritis resembling Guillain-Barré syndrome. Others are seen during the prolonged course of the asymptomatic infection such as recurrent headaches with pleocytosis or the mononeuritis multiplex in which vasculitis appears to result in multiple nerve infarctions (McArthur, 1987). The most devastating neurologic complications occur in the immunodeficient patients; dementia develops in 20 to 40%, a vascular myelopathy in 10 to 20%, and painful sensory neuropathy in 20 to 40%. About half of the patients with AIDS develop serious neurologic diseases apart from opportunistic infection (Glass and Johnson, 1996) (Table 12.2).

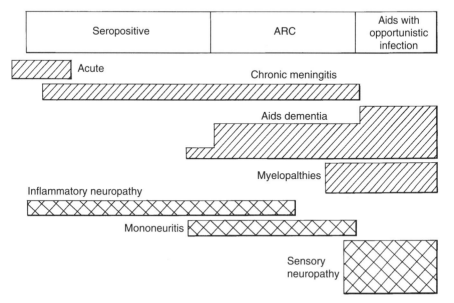

FIG 12.2. Schematic diagram of HIV-associated diseases. Diseases that affect central (diagonal lines) and peripheral (cross-hatched) nervous system evolve at different times in relation to stage of infection, and occur at different frequencies (vertical width). ARC, AIDS-related complex. (From Johnson et al., 1988c with permission.)

TABLE 12.2. *Major neurologic diseases attributed to HIV*

Clinical syndrome	%	Pathologic findings	%
Dementia	24	Multinucleated giant cells	18
		Diffuse myelin pallor	13
Myelopathy	9.4	Vacuolar myelopathy	39
Sensory neuropathy	20	Axonal neuropathy	80

325 autopsies in the Johns Hopkins prospective study.

Acute Meningitis and Encephalopathy

During the primary infection about half of those infected experience fever and headache, and in a small percentage of those nuchal rigidity, photophobia, seizures, and altered mental states may develop. On rare occasions ataxia, cranial nerve palsies, myelopathy, radiculopathies, acute demyelinating neuropathies and even a fatal encephalopathy have been reported (Paton et al., 1990; Jones et al., 1988; Cornblath et al., 1987; Silver et al., 1997). Although the symptoms usually clear, the development of neurologic manifestations with primary infection is associated with an accelerated progression to AIDS (Boufassa et al., 1995).

Acute aseptic meningitis, encephalitis, or Guillain-Barré syndrome also may occur prior to or after seroconversion during the long asymptomatic incubation period (Hollander and Stringari, 1987). Spinal fluid demonstrates a pleocytosis that mirrors the blood ratios of T cells so that CD8 cells often predominate, and virus can be recovered from the spinal fluid (McArthur et al., 1989).

Limited pathologic studies of the acute encephalopathies complicating seroconversion have shown multifocal demyelination resembling postinfectious encephalomyelitis (Silver et al., 1997). One patient who was inadvertently injected with HIV-positive blood during a scan died two weeks later, and virus was recovered from the brain and some perivascular cells contained HIV antigen (Davis, et al, 1992). In studies in Edinburgh and New York drug addicts, who died during the asymptomatic phase of HIV infection, lymphocytic meningitis and perivascular lymphocytic cuffs were found in over 20% of brains. Microglial nodules and macrophages were also found (Gray et al., 1996; Kibayashi et al., 1996). In about half of the Edinburgh patients HIV was detected by PCR in the area sampled, but virus was present at low levels (Bell et al., 1993). Vasculitis and myelin pallor suggesting blood-brain barrier damage were described in asymptomatic HIV-positive individuals who suffered accidental deaths in both studies.

HIV Dementia

This clinical syndrome is also known as AIDS-dementia complex, HIV encephalopathy, and more recently HIV dementia and refers to a progressive dementia seen almost exclusively in patients with AIDS. It is characterized by cognitive, behavioral, and motor deficits; cognitive abnormalities include mental slowness, forgetfulness, and poor concentration. Behavioral abnormalities include apathy, lethargy and a decrease in spontaneity and emotional responses.

The motor abnormalities include loss of fine motor control, unsteadiness of gait, and tremor. This clinical syndrome is the AIDS-defining disease in 3% of patients, but even in those, a CD4 count below 200 is usually noted which in itself would have defined AIDS. It is rare to see this syndrome in infected immunocompetent patients (Navia and Price, 1987). The frequency of this syndrome varies in different studies from 7 to 67% (Navia et al., 1986a, 1986b), but most studies show that approximately 20% of AIDS patients develop dementia before death. In one prospective study 7% of patients with AIDS developed dementia each year (McArthur et al., 1993). The course is usually rather abrupt over weeks or months and not insidiously over years. Most cases deteriorate to mutism, incontinence and generalized spasticity within a few months. Others dement and then remain stable for many months. Although survival from AIDS has been extended over the years, survival after onset of dementia has remained constant at 3 to 6 months (Harrison and McArthur, 1994).

When HIV dementia was first recognized in the mid 1980s, there was great concern that cognitive deterioration might begin at the time of initial infection and slowly progress to late stages of dementia. Most large studies including one with the Multicenter AIDS Cohort study have failed to document statistically significant difference in detailed neuropsychological studies between seropositive asymptomatic gay men and seronegative gay men (McArthur et al., 1989). Most longitudinal studies confirm that there is not a slowly progressive deterioration in cognition in seropositive persons prior to the onset of severe immunodeficiency (Selnes et al., 1990). A cohort study of active intravenous drug users has shown similar results, although the control levels of cognitive and motor-function examination were lower (Royal et al., 1991; Selnes et al., 1997). The spinal fluid examination in HIV dementia often shows a lesser pleocytosis than seen during the asymptomatic phase of the infection, although cells continue to be predominantly CD8 cells (McArthur et al., 1989). Imaging studies often show atrophy and white matter abnormalities characterized by white matter hypodensity, by computerized tomography, and hyperdensity sparing the U fibers on T2 images of magnetic resonance images. A relative decrease in the size of the caudate nucleus and putamen appears to correlate with dementia (Dal Pan et al., 1992; Aylward et al., 1993; Hall et al., 1996).

Neuropathologic changes do not correlate well with clinical deficits. A variety of neuropathologic changes have been described. HIV encephalitis is defined by multiple microglial nodules and multinucleated giant cells. When multinucleated giant cells are absent, the presence of viral antigen by immunocytochemistry has been used to fulfill this diagnosis. Diffuse myelin pallor frequently accompanies HIV encephalitis. Although the deep white matter stains poorly with myelin stains in these patients, individual myelin proteins are normal in staining, and the pallor appears to reflect a breakdown of the blood-brain barrier (Rhodes, 1991; Power et al., 1993). This is accompanied by reactive astrocytes and macrophages. Perivascular foci of demyelination are also seen resembling lesions of an antecedent postinfectious encephalomyelitis; this finding has no clinical correlate but could represent the residual lesions of an autoimmune reaction that might have occurred at the time of the neurologic symptoms associated with seroconversion. The third major form of neuropathology is referred to as diffuse poliodystrophy in which there is a diffuse, reactive astrocytosis and microglial activation particularly in the cerebral gray matter. All three of these neuropathologic groupings can occur together.

The findings of multinucleated giant cells and diffuse myelin pallor correlate best with dementia in patients who have been evaluated in prospective studies; but in half of the demented patients, neither multinucleated giant cells nor diffuse myelin pallor were found (Glass et al., 1993). Microglial nodules, in turn, have been found in some studies in 90% of patients, and therefore are common when there is no clinical evidence of dementia (de la Monte et al., 1987). It has been reported that the number of macrophages and microglia containing viral antigen correlates with clinical dementia (Achim et al., 1994), but studies of our prospectively evaluated patients have found these correlations weak (Glass et al., 1995). It is intriguing that some patients with severe HIV dementia have shown none of these pathologic changes, while other patients who have had detailed normal neuropsychologic examinations shortly before death have had marked neuropathologic abnormalities including astrocytosis, multifocal nodules, and multinucleated giant cells.

Routine neuropathologic examinations, even in patients with the most severe forms of dementia, rarely show recognizable neuronal loss on routine histopathologic sections. Using quantitative methods decreased numbers of neurons have been found in various regions of neocortex, hippocampus, substantia nigra, cerebellum and basal ganglia in HIV-positive individuals (Ketzsler et al., 1990; Everall et al., 1995). Somatostatin-immunoreactive neurons may be more vulnerable (Fox et al., 1997). A reduction of neuronal density can be seen by cytochemical studies (Wiley et al., 1991), and abnormalities of dendritic structures can be demonstrated by Golgi preparations and laser confocal microscopy. Dendritic simplification, arborization, and loss of presynaptic terminals have been described (Masliah et al., 1992).

Programmed cell death, or apoptosis, of cortical and basal ganglion neurons have been described in HIV-infected children and adults (Adle-Biasette et al., 1995; Gelbard et al., 1995). A recent study has also shown evidence of apoptosis in vascular endothelial cells as well, using both *in situ* detection of endonucleolytically cleaved DNA and morphological evidence of nuclear chromatin aggregation (Shi et al., 1996). This could provide an explanation for the changes in the blood-brain barrier.

Vacuolar Myelopathy

Approximately 20% of patients with AIDS develop a progressive myelopathy characterized by progressive spasticity and loss of proprioception predominantly in lower extremities. Bladder involvement may occur. A sensory level is not evident and the arms, aside from hyperreflexia, are usually spared. Pathologically, these findings correlate with vacuolar changes in the posterior and lateral columns most intense in the mid-thoracic spinal cord (Petito et al., 1985). Vacuoles in the cord are found in up to 50% of patients dying with AIDS, and, unlike the pathologic inconsistencies in HIV dementia, the severity of pathologic lesions do correlate with clinical severity of myelopathy (Dal Pan et al., 1994).

The vacuolization is characterized not by the intracytoplasmic spongiform changes seen with a variety of other diseases, but by intralaminar edema within myelin sheaths. The axon appears relatively intact and macrophages are observed within the vacuoles (Tan et al., 1995). By light microscopy lesions resemble the subacute degeneration of the cord with pernicious anemia and in some experimental viral infections (Tsukamoto et al., 1990). In posterior and lateral columns in AIDS patients there are increased numbers of macrophages and activation markers are evident on these macrophages (Tyor et al., 1993a). Vacuolar myelopathy appears to correlate with this macrophage infiltration, and it does not correlate well with virus recovery or numbers of virus antigen-positive cells. Indeed in many cases viral DNA cannot be detected in spinal cord by PCR despite the presence of severe clinical disease and intense vacuolar changes in cord (Johnson and Chesebro, unpublished). These findings suggest a unique mode of pathogenesis (Rosenblum et al., 1989; Petito et al., 1994; Tan et al., 1995). In a retrospective study of our patients vacuolar myelopathy was statistically associated with frequent opportunistic infections and with sensory neuropathy, but *not* with dementia (Dal Pan et al., 1994).

A more focal abnormality of the spinal cord in AIDS patients has been described with degeneration limited to gracile tracts with abnormalities of both axons and myelin sheaths. These changes are associated with signs and symptoms of peripheral neuropathy and are thought to represent a dying-back process from disordered dorsal root ganglia neurons (Rance et al., 1988). In rare patients necrotic lesions with proliferation of microglia, macrophages, and multinucleated giant cells have been found in the spinal cord reminiscent of HIV-encephalitis with a spinal cord localization (Geny et al., 1991a).

Clinical presentations of a wide variety of other CNS abnormalities have also been described including movement disorders of Parkinsonism, hemiballismus, spinal myoclonus, paroxysmal dystonia, rubral tremors, cerebral ataxia, and ocular flutter. Recurrent transient neurologic deficits composed primarily of hemiparesis, dysesthesia or dysphasia have occasionally been seen; their stereotyped pattern and resemblance of transient ischemia attacks suggest a vascular origin. Recently anticardiolipin antibodies and low protein S levels have been found in many of these patients (Brew and Miller, 1996).

Peripheral Neuropathies

Three distinct forms of peripheral neuropathy have been associated with HIV infections in addition to the severe lumbosacral radiculitis associated with cytomegalovirus infections in AIDS patients (see Chapter 6).

Inflammatory demyelinating polyneuropathies clinically resembling the acute Guillain-Barré syndrome and chronic inflammatory demyelinating polyneuritis have been described at the time of seroconversion and during the long asymptomatic phase of HIV infection. We have observed one case after the onset of AIDS. Patients develop rapid progressive weakness with areflexia and elevated spinal fluid protein. The major distinction from the typical Guillain-Barré syndrome is the presence of a pleocytosis often with over 20 mononuclear cells. Nerve biopsy shows inflammatory cell infiltrates and macrophage-mediated demyelination. The pathogenesis is, therefore, thought to be an autoimmune phenomenon precipitated by the immune deregulation associated with pre-AIDS HIV infections (Cornblath et al., 1987). The patients respond to plasmapheresis.

A mononeuritis has been seen both as single nerve lesions such as cranial nerve palsies, that have been described at varying times during the infection, as well as mononeuritis multiplex usually seen prior to the onset of AIDS. Nerve biopsies have shown a vasculitic process with centrofascicular degeneration suggesting nerve infarctions (McArthur, 1987).

The predominantly sensory polyneuritis that accompanies AIDS is the most frequent peripheral nerve complication of HIV infection. More than 20% of patients have severe symptoms with substantial morbidity. Patients develop a primarily sensory loss in the hands and feet often with painful dysesthesias. Stocking and glove sensory loss and depressed or absent deep tendon reflexes are found. The primary neuropathology is distal axonal degeneration involving both myelinated and unmyelinated fibers, and an admixture of sensory neuron loss in the dorsal root ganglia (de la Monte et al., 1988; Griffin et al., in press). Loss of fibers in the rostral gracile tract is found in some of the more severe cases.

Autonomic neuropathy also has been described with orthostatic hypotension, resting tachycardia, impotence, urinary dysfunction and cardiac conduction abnormalities. Axonal neuropathy does not complicate zidovidine treatment but didanosine (ddI), zalcitabine (ddC), and stavudine (d4T) all cause painful sensory neuropathies that clinically resemble the painful sensory neuropathy of AIDS. Since these toxic neuropathies are dose-dependent, onset of symptoms with initiation of drug or with an increase in dosage suggest the diagnosis, and these neuropathies are reversible with discontinuation of drugs (Simpson and Wolfe, 1991).

Myopathies

Myopathy also appears both as a complication of HIV infection and of its treatment with zidovudine. HIV myopathy can develop in patients in all stages of HIV infection. In both infection and drug-induced disease severe proximal muscle weakness may be seen, although myalgias appear to be more common in the patients receiving zidovudine. The clinical, neurophysiologic and pathologic features of HIV myopathy resemble those of polymyositis with predominance of CD8 cells invading the muscle. Immunocytochemical studies localize virus not to muscle fibers but to macrophages (Chad et al., 1990). In contrast, the disease associated with zidovudine is felt to be a toxic mitochondrial myopathy and shows appropriate declines in respiratory chain capacity. These myopathies may be difficult to distinguish, but myopathy induced by zidovudine may show the presence of ragged red fibers (Dalakas et al., 1986b and 1990; Grau et al., 1993) and remits with discontinuation of medication.

Summary of Clinical Syndromes

This array of distinct clinical syndromes associated with HIV infection is unique. Furthermore, there is not an evident linking of syndromes; any one of the complications can occur independently of the others. Lumping them clinically together as "neuroAIDS" is meaningless. Because complications develop at different times during the infection and because they show a unique spectrum of pathologic features including inflammatory, demyelinating and degenerative changes, multiple mechanisms of pathogenesis are almost certainly involved (Johnson et al., 1988a).

Two biases need to be highlighted. Most studies of HIV-associated neurologic diseases have been in populations of gay men infected with the B clade of virus, yet worldwide 75% of transmissions are heterosexual and the majority of infections are with other clades such as clade A in Africa, clade C in India and clade E in Thailand. HIV infections due to heterosexual transmission on this and other continents do show similar complications, but their frequency, pathology, and course may show important differences. It is evident that age is a major host determinant, since children have more severe encephalitis yet myelopathy and neuropathy are rare (see Chapter 13). Second, it must not be assumed that there is a common mode of pathogenesis among different complications. Most studies of virus localization and quantitation and of viral protein and cytokine toxicity have been studies of patients with HIV dementia or, more often, with the pathologic abnormality of HIV encephalitis. These findings may not apply to acute or chronic meningitis, vacuolar myelopathy, the varied neuropathies or HIV myopathy.

PATHOGENESIS OF NEUROLOGICAL DISEASES

HIV can be detected in the brain of over 90% of those who die with AIDS whether they have neurologic complications or not. Furthermore, the virus appears to be in the wrong cells to explain disease based on selective vulnerability of specific cell populations. These findings bring a cause and effect relationship under question.

Neuroinvasiveness, Neurotropism and Neurovirulence

HIV infection of the brain will be discussed in the terms of neuroinvasiveness, the ability of virus to enter the nervous system; neurotropism, the ability to infect neural cells; and neurovirulence, the ability to cause disease.

Neuroinvasiveness

HIV is highly neuroinvasive as discussed above; neuroinvasion occurs early in infection in a majority and is almost universal at time of death (Johnson, et al., 1996). It is assumed that the virus enters the brain from the blood across cerebral endothelium because of the presence of virus in cells of perivascular spaces and the presence of a prolonged viremia, but this assumption is not based on any observational data. It is unknown whether virus enters as cell-free virus during the plasma viremia of the primary infection or subsequently within infected mononuclear cells. Infection of endothelial cells has been reported in simian immunodeficiency virus infections (Ward et al., 1987), and infection of cerebral vascular endothelial cells have been reported in humans both *in vitro* and *in vivo* (Wiley et al., 1986). Recent studies of human autopsy specimens, however, question the infection of cerebral endothelial cells (Takahashi et al., 1996). Infected cells have been found in choroid plexus, and this could be an alternate route of CNS invasion by infected cells or cell-free virions (Falangola et al., 1995).

The virus could enter by passage of infected monocytes across the endothelial cells. Viruses recovered from the brain tissue are routinely macrophagetropic (Power et al., 1994). However, under normal circumstances monocyte traffic into the brain is minimal, unless some signal is released as in injury or infection. Macrophage inflammatory proteins are induced in HIV-infected monocytes, and the chemokines are expressed in microglia and astrocytes in HIV-infected brains. This could influence the trafficking of leukocytes and recruit uninfected lymphocytes and monocytes into the CNS (Schmidt-mayerova et al., 1996). Conversely, HIV-infected monocytes may have alterations of surface ligands causing attachment to adhesion molecules expressed on cerebrovascular endothelial cells. This could cause selective homing of HIV-infected mononuclear cells and macrophages into the brain. The question of how virus enters the CNS is not a trifling issue and could direct strategies to prevent viral invasion of the nervous system (Johnson, 1995). If HIV enters from plasma then early circulating antibody may be of prime importance to prevent CNS invasion; on the other hand, if HIV enters in monocytes blocking of ligands or adhesion molecules on cerebrovascular endothelial cells would be more effective.

Neurotropism

HIV can replicate in cell lines of neuronal and astrocytic derivation, and also in primary cultures of fetal astrocytes and cerebral endothelial cells. *In vivo*, however, infection is limited almost exclusively to cells of macrophage origin (Kure et al., 1990; Budka, 1990). These include microglia, macrophages and the perivascular macrophages which are located within the basement membrane. Identification of cells on purely morphologic grounds in studies localizing antigen or nucleic acid poses pitfalls. The site and shape of perivascular macrophages has caused difficulty in distinguishing them from microvascular endothelial cells (Gabuzda et al., 1986). Microglia and macrophages within tissue can assume shapes that are difficult to distinguish from astrocytes, oligodendroglia, and occasionally, even neurons. Several recent reports, however, show viral nucleic acids in cells stained for astrocyte-specific glial fibrillary acid protein (Saito et al., 1994; Tornatore et al., 1994) and one reports infection of cells with specific staining for neuron neurofilaments and with vonWillerbrand factor identifying vascular endothelium (Bagasra et al., 1996). In our own study using immunocytochemistry with specific cell markers combined with *in situ* PCR for DNA or RNA, the only infected cells containing viral antigen were macrophages and microglia, but viral DNA was found in some patients in cells staining for glial fibrillary acidic protein (Takahashi et al., 1996). Infected astrocytes in our experience were not found in all demented patients which casts doubt on their biologic significance.

Macrophage and microglial infection has been found preferentially in the globus pallidus, other basal ganglion nuclei and central white matter. The quantity of virus has not shown a clear cut correlation with clinical disease (Brew et al., 1995). Indirect measures such as determination of viral genomic material in spinal fluid have been tested and found to be positive more often in demented than nondemented AIDS patients (Goswani et al., 1991). In a prospective study, correlation was found between the level of p24 in blood and spinal fluid with the presence of HIV dementia. However, only 50% of the demented patients had detectable p24 in their spinal fluids (Royal et al., 1994). Higher levels of antibodies to HIV envelope protein also have been reported in spinal fluids of those AIDS patients with dementia (Trujillo et al., 1996).

Attempts to quantitate immunocytochemical staining have been done by counting antigen positive cells (Wiley and Achim, 1994). Some patients with severe HIV dementia, have shown little evidence of HIV infection of the brain by this methodology (Vazeux et al., 1991). PCR can potentially detect a single molecule of viral DNA. Methods of comparison of responses have been used to give rough quantitation and a more quantitative method using competitive quantitative PCR has been developed. In our study of patients who had cognitive testing on 2 or more occasions premortem, there was no correlation of molecules of viral DNA with dementia (Johnson et al., 1996). This could be explained, in part, by the problem of sampling within the whole brain or the problem that some strains may have mutations that interfere with primer recognition. Other studies using quantitative PCR have shown a statistically significant correlation between levels of HIV DNA and clinically defined HIV encephalopathy or encephalitis, but the overlap of values has been striking (Sei et al., 1995; An et al., 1996).

In the spinal cord and peripheral nerve there has been an even poorer correlation of virus load and clinical or pathologic changes. Sections of some areas of vacuolar myelopathy, although they contain activated macrophages, histologicly have been free of viral antigen and free of viral DNA by PCR (Johnson and Chesebro, unpublished data). In the peripheral nerves, once the perineurium is stripped away the affected nerves may be negative for viral DNA or RNA (Griffin et al., in press), although HIV RNA and protein has been reported in presumed macrophages in the endoneurium (Rizzuto et al., 1995).

Neurovirulence

Although macrophagetropic strains of HIV enter and infect the brain in virtually all infected individuals including those without neurologic complications, a possible explanation for dementia could be that specific substrains or quasispecies of macrophagetropic viruses are neurovirulent. To test this hypothesis we amplified a fragment of the envelope region directly from brains of 22 AIDS patients studied prospectively for dementia prior to death. The 430bp region of the envelope included the V3 loop and flanking regions and included the sequences determining macrophagetropism (Chesebro et al., 1992). Multiple clones recovered from the same patients showed a lack of the sequence diversity found in systemic isolates, and all brain-derived specimens had sequences characteristic of macrophagetropic viruses. Comparisons of sequences of these segments from demented and nondemented patients showed significant amino acid differences at 2 positions; this suggests that there may be specific neurovirulent strains of HIV (Power et al., 1994). Similar sequence changes have been found in macrophagetropic strains after passages in microglial cultures (Strizki et al., 1996). The long terminal repeat of retroviruses has also been associated with tissue tropism and may play a role in neurovirulence (Ait-Khaled et al., 1995).

The suggestion of neurovirulent strains of HIV leads to more questions. There are numerous precedences for neurovirulent versus nonneurovirulent strains of viruses. For example, in the case of measles and mumps in laboratory animals, neurovirulent strains of virus grow in neurons as opposed to the nonneurovirulent strains (Johnson, 1968; Griffin et al., 1974), but a change of host cell is not observed in the case of demented and nondemented patients with AIDS. Virulence of rabies virus is determined by a single amino acid substitution in the envelope protein and nonvirulent strains infect the same neurons; but a slowed spread of infection allows the immune response to prevent disease (Jackson, 1991). Observations of HIV are not consistent with either of these mechanisms of neurovirulence. An alternate explanation may be that specific strains in virus enhance or inhibit the release of soluble substances involved in the dysfunction or normal function of neurons.

Mediators of Toxicity

A wide variety of indirect mechanisms have been proposed to explain the neurotoxicity during HIV infections (Table 12.3). To relate any of these soluble substances to disease, it should be shown that 1) the substance itself is toxic directly

TABLE 12.3. *Indirect mechanisms of neurotoxicity in HIV infections*

Viral proteins	gp120
	tat
	nef
Macrophage factors	Low molecular weight toxic factors
	Quinolinic acid
	Arachidonic acid metabolites (prostaglandin and leukotriene)
	Platelet-activating factor
	Nitric oxide
Cytokines	TNFα
	IL-1β, IL-6, GM-CSF, IFN-α
Decreased neurotropic factors	Neuroleukin
Autoimmune mimicry	gp41
	Antibrain antibodies

GM-CSF, granulocyte-macrophage colony-stimulating factor; IFN, interferon; IL, interleukin; TNF, tumor necrosis factor.

or indirectly to neurons and 2) the levels of the soluble factor correlate with the presence of clinical symptoms or pathologic findings .

Toxicity of HIV Proteins

Most studies of toxicity have focused on gp120, which is released from cytoplasmic membranes of infected T cells, but this is less certain in brain macrophages and microglia where much of the virus budding appears to be into intracellular vacuoles. Free gp120 has not been demonstrated in cerebrospinal fluid. Multiple studies have shown that gp120 is toxic to neurons in cell cultures, and this toxicity may be direct or mediated through gp120 stimulation of macrophages or astrocytes. Cultures of rat retinal ganglial cells exposed to picomolar quantities of gp120 show a rise in intracellular free calcium presumably through activation of the dyhydropyridine-sensitive voltage-gated calcium channels (Dreyer et al., 1990). Antibodies against CD4 fail to block this effect indicating that the receptor is not necessary for the neurotoxicity. Several studies have demonstrated that the toxicity involves activation of neuronal excitory amino acid receptors (Lipton, 1991), and this neurotoxicity mechanism may involve generation of nitric oxide intermediates (Dawson et al., 1993).

An indirect mechanism of protein cytotoxicity has been suggested for the transmembrane glycoprotein, gp41. Nitric oxide has been proposed as a mediator of neuronal injury, and gp41 can induce the immunologic isoform of nitric oxide synthase in neuronal and glial cultures. Higher levels of gp41 and the synthase were found in severe HIV dementia (Adamson et al., 1996b).

A nonstructural protein of HIV, tat, has been shown to be cytotoxic to neurons at exceeding low concentrations, and this toxicity appears to be a direct effect on neuronal receptors. This trans-acting nuclear regulatory protein is released by infected mononuclear cells and stimulates HIV replication and tumor necrosis factor alpha (TNFα) release. Intracerebral injection of tat into mice is lethal, and tat is toxic to neuronal cell lines including human fetal cells by activation of excitatory amino acid receptors and heightening intracellular calcium (Nath et al., 1996). As with gp120 toxicity a correlation of levels of protein with clinical or pathologic changes has not been possible.

Macrophage Factors

One of the first recognized neurotoxic studies of HIV was the demonstration that infected monocytoid cells lines produced a very small heat stable and protease resistant diffusible factor that was able to kill neurons of ciliary ganglia and rat spinal cord (Giulian et al., 1990). A subsequent study suggested that this may be derived from a Mycoplasma contaminant (Bernton et al., 1992). In examination of the spinal fluid of demented versus nondemented patients, several factors have correlated with dementia; these include β-2 microglobulin (McArthur et al., 1992), neopterin (Brew et al., 1990), arachidonic acid metabolites, prostaglandins and thromboboxins (Griffin et al., 1994b). All of these substances are products of macrophage activation, and therefore heightened levels of macrophage activation appear to correlate with dementia. Other molecules associated with macrophage activation, such as platelet activating factor, quinolinic acid and nitric oxide, have demonstrated neurotoxicity and have been proposed as players in HIV dementia (Gelbard et al., 1994; Achim et al., 1993; Dawson et al., 1993).

Cytokines

Cytokines are regulatory molecules released by cells of the immune system. They have undergone extensive study in the pathogenesis of the systemic infection of AIDS and particularly in neurologic complications, since they had previously been implicated in the pathogenesis of the nervous system disease visna in sheep due to a related lentivirus (Kennedy et al., 1985) (see Chapter 11). Although all cells of the nervous system are capable of producing one or more cytokine, the majority of data demonstrate that macrophages, microglia and astrocytes are the most important cytokine producers (Merrill and Chin, 1991). Monocytes are capable of releasing TNFα, interleukin 1β and 6, and monocyte and granulocyte stimulating factors. TNFα has proved the most interesting of these, since this pro-inflammatory cytokine can help regulate the production of HIV-1, induce the proliferation of astrocytes (Barna et al., 1990), and influence the secretion of other cytokines by astrocytes (Benveniste, 1994). Furthermore, some strains of HIV induce TNFα in macrophage cultures while others do not (Le Naour et al., 1994); a difference that might explain virus strain specific neurovirulence. In the brains of patients who died with AIDS, macrophages and microglia appear to be the dominant cells producing TNFα (Tyor et al., 1992a). Although a difference in levels of TNFα in spinal fluid in demented and nondemented patients was not found, a striking correlation was found between the

TNFα mRNA in the brains of demented as compared to nondemented patients or seronegative controls (Glass et al., 1993; Wesselingh et al., 1993) (Figure 12.3). Expression of adhesion molecules on astrocytes also has been correlated with clinical dementia but TNF induces these molecules and this may or may not be a secondary affect (Seilhean et al., 1997). It is still not determined whether TNFα is an indirect marker, whether TNFα affects other cells that in turn influence neurons, or whether TNFα is directly neurotoxic. Studies of vacuolar myelopathy have given similar results with spinal fluid levels of TNFα failing to correlate with disease, even though there is greater immunostaining for TNFα in macrophages, microglia and endothelial cells in the spinal cords of patients dying with myelopathy (Tan et al., 1996).

A variety of other mechanisms have been proposed such as the possibility that cytokines or other factors released by monocytes inhibit neurotrophic factors necessary for normal function. The demonstration of common sequences between gp120 and neuroleukin suggests that the functional interaction between gp120 and neuroleukin might be important to the pathogenesis of HIV dementia (Lee et al., 1987a). A different mechanism has been proposed when sequence similarities were found between astrocytic transmembrane protein and the immunodominant domain of gp41. Anti-astrocytic antibodies are found in the spinal fluid of some AIDS patients with neurologic complications (Yamada et al., 1991; Spehar and Strand, 1995). Autoimmune mechanisms also have suggested that neurologic complications correlated with serum brain-reactive antibodies (Kumar et al., 1989) and antiganglioside antibodies (Sorice et al., 1995).

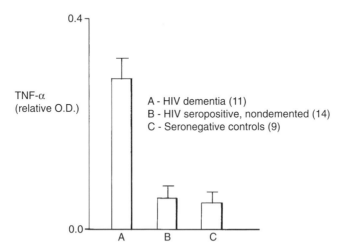

FIG 12.3. Relationship of relative quantities of tumor necrosis factor α (TNFα) with HIV dementia. A significant increase in TNFα messenger RNA in frontal white matter of demented patients is shown compared to non-demented HIV infected AIDS patients and noninfected controls. (Data from Wesselingh et al., 1993; graph from Glass and Johnson, 1996 with permission). From the Annual Review of Neuroscience vol. 19. ©1996 by the Annual Reviews, Inc.

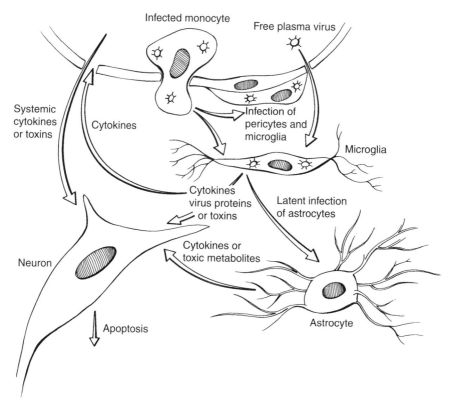

FIG 12.4. Schematic diagram of possible mechanisms of neuronal disruption in HIV-associated neurological disease. Virus may invade brain in infected monocytes or from plasma viremia during early infection. Perivascular cells and microglia are infected and may release viral proteins, cytokines or toxins that are toxic to neurons, affect astrocyte function, or alter the blood-brain barrier. Nonproductive infection of astrocytes may affect maintenance of neurons or the blood-brain barrier or may release cytokines.

Finally, the correlation of blood-brain barrier changes and dementia must not be overlooked. The neurotoxin affecting neuronal function could be generated by the systemic infection causing dementia only in those patients with the most compromised blood-brain barrier (Power and Johnson, 1995) (Fig 12.4). Our preoccupation with virus proteins, cytokines and neurotropic factors generated within the CNS could be misguided; if true our concern about drugs and the blood-brain barrier would be misdirected.

Animal Models

An animal model of HIV infection of the nervous system would be helpful to unravel the pathogenesis of the neurologic syndromes. HIV can infect chimpanzees, gibbons, and pigtail monkeys with persistent infection but without signs of immunodeficiency or neurologic disease. Chimpanzees have been infected even by the intracerebral inoculation of homogenates of brain of patients with HIV encephalopathy (Gajdusek et al., 1985), yet over a decade, although antibody persists and HIV sequences can be detected by PCR, no illness has been seen (Johnson et al., 1993). In chimpanzees studied sequentially during persistent infection no virus was isolated from spinal fluid, and no intrathecal antibody formed over several years of observation (Grimaldi et al., 1996). Pigtail monkeys show a similar persistent infection without clinical disease, pleocytosis or spinal fluid antibody synthesis, but limited pathologic studies are intriguing. The brain of 1 of 4 autopsied monkeys had focal white matter abnormalities with myelin loss, nerve fiber loss and gliosis; 2 of the 4 monkeys, not including the one with neuropathologic changes, had HIV-1 DNA detected in brain and *in situ* PCR localized DNA to vascular endothelial cells, microglia and possibly other glial cells (Frumkin et al., 1995). Although the histopathologic findings may be the result of unrelated disease, the PCR data are the first evidence of HIV in a nonhuman primate brain. Chimeric simian/human immunodeficiency virus has been derived that productively infect the CNS of rhesus macaques and produces microglial nodules, demyelinating lesions and multinuclear giant cells (Raghavan et al., 1997).

HIV-2 can cause lymphadenopathy, CD4 T cell loss, eventual lymphoid depletion and interstitial pneumonitis in baboons (Barnett et al., 1994b), but no neurologic disease has been reported. This disease is not surprising in view of the close relationship of HIV-2 to the simian immunodeficiency virus of mangebeys, but like the simulation of AIDS in macaque monkeys with simian immunodeficiency virus (see Chapter 11), it is not HIV-1 and this limits its value in the development of experimental drugs and vaccines.

Two interesting alternative methods have been utilized to study HIV-1 infections in rodents—the use of xenografts (both susceptible human fetal brain explants in rodents and infected human macrophages in rodent brain) and the use of transgenic mice with expression of HIV genes in mouse brain. Human fetal brain tissue injected into the anterior chamber of the eyes of rats can grow, vascularize, and form a semblance of a blood-brain barrier. Infections of this tissue shows giant cells development, neuronal loss and astrocytosis (Cvetkovitch et al., 1992). Alternatively in mice with severe combined immunodeficiency (scid) human lymphoid cells can be implanted. Human peripheral blood mononuclear cells inoculated into the brain of scid mice can be infected or infected human macrophages can be inoculated into brain (Tyor et al., 1993). These infected human cells can survive up to 5 weeks, and mouse brains show astrocytosis, microglial activation, and neuronal apoptosis (Persidsky et al., 1996). In strains of scid mice accepting human peripheral blood leukocyte engraftment, HIV infection can lead to viremia and invasion of the CNS (Koyanagi et al., 1997). Presence of antigen positive leukocytes in brain, however, was not accompanied by giant cells or astrocytosis.

A wide variety of transgenic mice expressing various HIV genes have been developed during the last decade. They have shown a wide spectrum of abnormalities including stunted growth, skin changes, mammary and kidney lesions, altered T cell function and neurologic diseases (Brady et al., 1994). Transgenic mice containing the long terminal repeats of two CNS-derived strains of HIV-1 showed expression in specific neuronal populations whereas similar genes from a lymphotropic strain of virus did not show CNS expression (Corboy et al., 1992). Transgenic mice expressing the entire HIV genome or the gene for the envelope proteins under the control of the human neurofilament gene promoter expressed the transgene in neurons of deep nuclei and motor neurons of the spinal cord leading to axonal swellings and peripheral nerve abnormalities (Thomas et al., 1994; Berrada et al., 1995). Since neurons are rarely, if ever, infected in human infection, the relevance of these trangenic models is dubious. The envelope protein (gp120) gene under the control of a promoter for astrocyte-specific glial fibrillary acid protein in mice is expressed predominately in astrocytes with astrocytosis and vacuolization of dendrites and neuronal loss (Toggas et al., 1994). The closest simulation of a human neuropathologic change is with transgenic mice that express the entire HIV-1 genome under regulation of oligo-dendrocyte-specific promoter; these mice develop a vacuolar myelopathy similar to that in AIDS patients (Goudreau et al., 1996).

TREATMENT

The pace of advances in AIDS research has been unprecedented in history. The clinical syndrome was first recognized in 1981, the virus was recovered in 1983, the virus was sequenced by 1985 and the first effective antiviral drug was tested and licensed in 1987.

The initial approved drug was azidothymidine (AZT aka zidovudine) and the definitive double-blind placebo-controlled trial was short lived. Between February and June of 1986 822 patients with AIDS or severe AIDS-related complex were recruited into the study, but abruptly on September 19 as several reports of death came in simultaneously, the drug was validated statistically with 19 deaths among individuals on placebo and only one death among individuals on drug (Fischl et al., 1987). The study was terminated and the drug approved. Those of us on the Data Safety Monitoring Committee were pleased with the clearcut efficacy but concerned in assuming that much data would be lost, since the brief 16 weeks of the study presumably would not allow for evaluation of effects on cognition. Even this abbreviated data, however, showed patients on zidovudine not only stabilized cognitive function, but they actually showed improvement in cognition compared with those receiving placebo (Schmitt et al., 1988). Early studies using continuous intravenous infusion of zidovudine in 21 children with symptomatic HIV infection over a six month period showed that those receiving zidovudine had improvements in both verbal and performance intelligence quotients (Pizzo et al., 1980). Thus in both of these studies it appeared the drug was not only effective in stabilizing patients but held promise that the dementia itself might be reversible. A subsequent European study suggested that zidovudine provided profound protection in preventing AIDS dementia (Portegies, 1989).

These early studies provoked excessive optimism, since it was soon realized that resistance to zidovudine developed within about 6 months (Larder et al., 1989), and subsequent studies have shown less efficacy of prophylactic zidovudine improving or preventing dementia. A placebo-controlled trial of zidovudine in already demented patients has shown improvement with drug, but this response was dose-dependent pushing the margin between tolerance and efficacy (Sidtis et al., 1993). Although zidovudine has prolonged the lives of patients with AIDS, it has not prolonged the abbreviated life expectancy of AIDS patients who develop dementia. Paradoxically, an effect on the pathologic changes in patients treated with zidovudine is seen. Patients with dementia who have died since the introduction of zidovudine have shown fewer multinucleated giant cells and less degree of diffuse myelin pallor (Gray et al., 1994a).

A number of other antiviral drugs are now available for treatment of HIV infections, but consideration must be given to brain-CSF penetration, systemic toxicity, neurotoxicity, drug resistance, cost and availability. No foreseeable drug can selectively excise the integrated provirus so no drug, as we know them, can "cure" HIV infection, but they can retard virus replication, prolong the time to AIDS and decrease transmission. The only available reverse transcriptase inhibitor other than zidovidine that crosses the blood-brain barrier is lamivudine (3TC) which is usually given in dementia when zidovidine resistance is suspected. However, since myelin pallor appears to represent a breakdown of the barrier and appears to be a marker for dementia; a circulating toxin may be important and CSF-brain penetration may not be the critical factor in drug choice. If microglial infection causes the barrier breakdown then penetration is an important consideration.

In addition to nucleoside analogue reverse transcriptase inhibitors, protease inhibitors now have been approved. A variety of other forms of reverse transcriptase inhibitors are undergoing evaluation. In addition to antiviral drugs, cytokine blockers (such as pentoxifylline and thalidomide that block TNFα), calcium channel blockers (such as nimodipine that protects rat neurons *in vitro* from toxicity of gp120), and antioxidants (that may inhibit apoptosis) have or are being studied in patients with HIV dementia (Sacktor and McArthur, 1997).

The improvement of cognitive function found with zidovidine was an encouraging finding indicating that the dementia is, at least in part, reversible. The development of drug resistance to zidovidine was disappointing and probably indicates the future need to design multidrug-therapy designed to block virus replication at multiple sites as well as to protect the neurons from cytokines or toxins.

Currently patients with HIV dementia generally are treated with high dose zidovidine and if cognition worsens or the patient cannot tolerate the drug, lamivudine (3TC), stavidine (d4T), didoxyinosine (ddI) or dideoxycytidine (ddC) are administered. The introduction of HIV-protease inhibitors to nucleotide antivirals appears to decrease viremia and increase CD4 counts and should further thwart drug resistance when given as a triple therapy. This should prolong life, but the effect on neurologic complications is yet to be determined.

CONCLUSION

The pathogenesis of disease in HIV infection is clearly different from that of other viral infections in the nervous system, where clinical signs tend to correlate with the selective vulnerability of specific neural cells to infection. For example, infection of meningeal and ependymal cells leads to the clinical syndrome of viral meningitis; infection of motor neurons by poliovirus leads to poliomyelitis; infection of oligodendrocytes by JC virus leads to progressive multifocal leukoencephalopathy. Furthermore, in experimental infections of the nervous system, the quantity of virus in the brain usually correlates with disease onset, severity, and outcome. In HIV-associated diseases none of these generalizations hold true. Infection is largely limited to macrophages and microglia, and damage to these cells has no specific clinical correlate. The relationship between disease or disease severity and virus load is unconvincing at present, and the presence of the neurovirulent strains do not correlate with an increased amount of virus or changes in the spectrum of susceptible host cells to explain the nature of neurovirulence. How neurovirulence is expressed is unknown; there are several indirect mechanisms that need further study, including the roles of viral proteins, cytokines, and other neurotoxins. Harking back to the period prior to 1985 we must not discard the idea that opportunistic agents, perhaps, unknown, play a role in some of the neurologic complications of AIDS.

HIV is the most prevalent nervous system infection in history, and the spectrum of neurologic diseases caused by this virus is remarkable. Of equal importance, however, may be the unique mechanisms of pathogenesis with interactions of virus and cells of macrophage origin, cytokine or neurotoxin release and noninflammatory damage to dendritic arbors and axons, myelin sheaths, and the blood–brain barrier. These novel mechanisms of pathogenesis may have implications in the pathogenesis of other diseases, not only infectious diseases but demyelinating, ischemic, and degenerative processes where signal molecules may mediate disease.

SUPPLEMENTARY BIBLIOGRAPHY

Harrison M and McArthur JC (1994): AIDS and the Nervous System. Churchill, Edinburgh.
Levy JA (1994): HIV and the Pathogenesis of AIDS. ASM Press, Washington.
Levy RM and Berger JR (Editors) (1995): AIDS and the Nervous System. Raven Press, NY.
Price RW and Perry SW (Editors) (1994): HIV, AIDS, and the Brain. Raven Press, NY.

13

Viral Infections of the Developing Nervous System

The remarkable frequency of the accompanying congenital defect of the heart and the apparent constancy in type of this (cataract) defect seem to me to indicate a common causative factor. Could this not be some toxic or infective process resulting in a partial arrest of development?

Sir Norman Gregg
Congenital Cataract following German Measles in the Mother,
report to the Ophthalmology Society of Australia, 1941

During the summer of 1941, Gregg personally examined 20 infants with congenital cataracts in Sydney; his Australian colleagues provided clinical information on 47 additional infants. Gregg noted that two-thirds of the infants also had microphthalmia, over half had congenital heart disease, and many had had low birth weights. Most important, almost all of their mothers gave a history of German measles in the early months of pregnancy during the preceding winter epidemic. His conclusion that viral infection might arrest or alter fetal development was a landmark in clinical observation.

In a subsequent study of children born after the same Australian epidemic, microcephaly, deafness, and mental retardation were also identified as consequences of maternal rubella (Swan et al., 1943). Over subsequent years, cytomegalovirus, herpes simplex virus, varicella-zoster virus, and human immunodeficiency virus (HIV) have been related to congenital nervous system infection, and many other viruses have been suspect.

The neuropathologic correlates of these fetal infections are predominantly inflammatory and necrotizing lesions. Because these lesions differ from classic malformations, it has been argued that viruses are not true teratogens (Mims, 1968). Teratogen means a cause of monsters, and congenital malformation means born with abnormal form. These terms usually pertain to defects in organ differentiation or cellular migration under genetic control, but similar defects can be caused by environmental factors. For example, if destruction of cerebral tissue by an infection results in microcephaly, which is present at birth, this represents a teratogenic effect of the causal agent and is a congenital malformation

315

irrespective of its pathogenesis or histopathology. Furthermore, in natural and experimental viral infections of animals, cerebral malformation that phenotypically mimic genetic disorders are caused by viruses.

PATHOGENESIS OF FETAL INFECTIONS

Infection of the mother is a prerequisite to fetal infection, but this infection may be clinically inapparent. Virus can reach the fetus by several routes: (1) by infection of the germinal cell or by genetic transmission of the viral genome; (2) from the blood across the placenta; or (3) by ascending infection from the birth canal. Although the first mechanisms are unknown in humans, lymphocytic choriomeningitis virus in mice has been shown to infect the germinal epithelium in the ovary and the ovum (Mims, 1966), and murine leukemia viruses can be transmitted as a provirus integrated with the parental chromosomes (Rowe, 1972). Spread of virus in the blood is the most common mechanism of fetal infection, and it necessitates that a viremia occur in the mother. Furthermore, the viremia must be of magnitude and duration sufficient to allow penetration of the barriers posed by the placental membranes. Ascending infection from the birth canal is a potential route of intrauterine infection, either across ruptured membranes, as in bacterial infections, or across the devitalized membranes overlying the cervical os. Infection can also occur during passage through the infected cervix and vagina, as in type 2 herpes simplex virus infections of newborns.

The Placental Barrier

The human placenta is formed from the chorion, the outer embryonic fetal membrane, and its intimate contact with the decidua, a modified portion of the mucosal coat of the uterus. This hemochorial placenta allows maternal blood to flow through an outer coat of trophoblasts arising from the fetal chorion into open intervillous spaces (Fig. 13.1). The fetal villi extending into these spaces contain the fetal blood vessels surrounded by trophoblasts of the fetal chorion. Thus, the fetal blood is separated from maternal blood by a layer of trophoblasts derived from the fetus, a basement membrane, and the endothelial cells of the fetal vessels. These membranes must be traversed or infected for a virus to gain access from maternal to fetal blood. Alternatively, penetration or growth of virus in the chorionic plate can lead to infection of the amniotic membranes. Shedding of virus into the amniotic cavity can give direct access of virus to the skin and to the respiratory and gastrointestinal tracts of the fetus.

Differences in placental structure at various stages of gestation and between different mammals may be important determinants of fetal infection. In contrast to humans, the maternal and fetal spaces in the murine placenta are separated by three layers of trophoblasts, two of which may be syncytial in character. This difference may account for the failure of transmission of viruses such as murine cytomegalovirus to the mouse fetus (Johnson, 1969). The placental barrier is

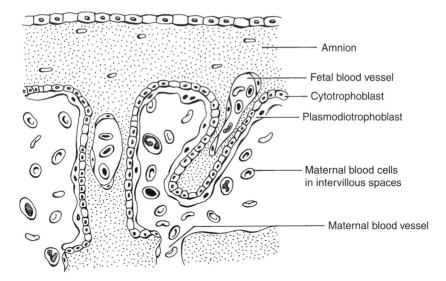

FIG. 13.1. Relationship of maternal and fetal blood within the human placenta. Maternal blood flows from maternal vessel (below) into open intervillous spaces. Fetal blood (with nucleated red cells) flows through vascular villi separated from the maternal circulation by the trophoblast cells and syncytia of fetal origin.

similar in some respects to the blood-brain junction because some substances are excluded, whereas other particles, such as ferritin, may pass even the complex rodent placenta with ease (Tillack, 1966). However, infection of the placenta per se may alter its barrier function. In human rubella virus infections, foci of cell damage are found in the chorionic epithelium and fetal vascular endothelium (Tondury and Smith, 1966), in human cytomegalovirus and varicella-zoster virus infections, intense inflammatory changes in the placenta have been found (Benirschke et al., 1974; Enders, 1984), and in HIV infections viral antigen and RNA have been demonstrated in trophoblasts and mesenchymal macrophages (Hofbauer cells) (Langston et al., 1995).

Mechanisms of Fetal Injury

The average pregnancy is accompanied by several viruslike illnesses. Most of these infections have no discernible effect on fetal development. However, the potential exists for fetal wastage or damage by a variety of mechanisms (Table 13.1). General maternal health or placental function can be adversely affected by infection and can cause fetal loss without fetal infection. The high rate of fetal loss observed during smallpox epidemics usually was not associated with recognizable fetal infection; a poxvirus of mice, ectromelia virus, causes placental infection and abortion without infection of the fetus but, in this instance, without serious illness in the mother. Similarly, mouse cytomegalovirus infects the

TABLE 13.1. *Possible effects of viral infections on the developing nervous system*

Indirect (maternal infection only)
    Constitutional effect on mother
    Infection of placenta

Direct fetal infection (acute or chronic)
    Generalized encephalitis with necrotic or inflammatory lesions or vasculitis
    Chromosomal damage
    Mitotic inhibition
    Infection of selected cell populations altering embryogenesis

Adapted from Johnson (1972a).

placenta of inapparently infected mothers and causes fetal death, but unlike human cytomegalovirus, the virus fails to infect susceptible fetal tissues (Johnson, 1969). Species differences can be seen with the same virus. Equine abortion virus, which crosses the equine placental membranes and infects the foal, fails to cross the placenta in the hamster, where the virus causes abortion secondary to a placentitis. In this infection the nongravid hamster uterine cells are not susceptible to infection, but the newly developed placental trophoblasts are the susceptible target cells (Burek et al., 1975).

If a virus does gain access to the fetal germinal cells, to fetal circulation, or to amniotic fluid, the effects on the fetus are dependent on the developmental stage of the fetus, on what fetal cell populations are susceptible to infection, and on what effect the viral infection may have on these cells. For example, a cytolytic virus like herpes simplex virus, that infects a wide range of neural cell types, leads to fetal death or severe retardation and microcephaly. On the other hand, if fetal cells are susceptible but the infection is noncytolytic, persistent infection may occur, as in lymphocytic choriomeningitis virus infections of mice, where even neurons are chronically infected for the lifetime of the animal (Mims, 1966).

Viruses, like irradiation and chemicals, are capable of causing cytogenetic abnormalities. In cell culture, a variety of chromosomal breakages, pulverization, and alterations of chromosome distribution and number can be produced (Nichols, 1970). The mechanisms of chromosomal damage are unclear, as is the biologic significance of these findings *in vivo*. Alleged temporal and geographic clustering of Down's syndrome with outbreaks of infectious hepatitis or epidemics of influenza have not been substantiated (Siegel, 1973). The theoretical potential exists, but no solid evidence implicates virus-induced chromosomal damage as a mechanism of teratogenesis in humans or animals.

Mitotic activity also can be inhibited by virus infection. This phenomenon may be a factor in the small size of infants with congenital rubella virus infections. A reduction in numbers of cells in organs has been documented in these infants (Naeye and Blanc, 1965), and infected cells grown from rubella-infected fetuses have shown depressed mitotic activity compared with normal fetal cells

(Rawls and Melnick, 1966). Human embryonic mesenchymal cells in culture infected with rubella virus show not only inhibition of cell growth and differentiation but a decrease in cell responsiveness to epidermal growth factor (Yoneda et al., 1986).

Finally, viral infections of selected cell populations can alter embryogenesis and produce symmetrical noninflammatory deficits that lack any pathologic features that suggest antecedent infection. In the CNS these abnormalities resemble malformations previously thought to have a genetic basis. They involve effects on organogenesis, the selective destruction of particular cell populations giving rise to abnormal cell differentiation and migration, or the destruction of differentiated cells in which the repair process leads to a histologic appearance of agenesis (Johnson, 1972a). Examples of these forms of teratogenesis are known in animals, but they may have counterparts in human disease.

FETAL AND NEONATAL INFECTIONS IN HUMANS

A variety of human viral infections have been implicated in congenital or neonatal neurologic diseases (Table 13.2). Only rubella virus, cytomegalovirus, and HIV infections of the fetus and herpes simplex virus infection of the newborn are common problems. The other associations are rare, and in some cases, they may represent chance association of malformations with common infections.

Rubella

Rubella virus and pestiviruses (hog cholera, bovine viral diarrhea, and ovine border disease viruses) represent the non-arthropod-borne togaviruses and flaviviruses respectively. All are associated with fetal infection, abortion, and malformations in their natural hosts.

Rubella virus in children and young adults causes an acute exanthematous disease called German or three-day measles. Half of adult infections are clinically inapparent. Epidemics of the disease occurred every 6 to 9 years, and major outbreaks occurred every 10 to 30 years. After licensure of the rubella vaccine in 1969 the incidence in the United States declined more than 99% by 1980, but a transient increase in rubella and the congenital rubella syndrome between 1989 and 1991 caused concern (Lindegren et al., 1991). Major outbreaks in the past may have been related to antigenic shifts of the virus, so reemergence of the disease is possible.

The major health problem caused by rubella virus is fetal infection. After recognition of the association between malformations and rubella in 1941, little further was learned until the virus was grown in the laboratory (Parkman et al., 1962, Weller and Neva, 1962). When a subsequent major epidemic struck in 1964, it provided the tragic opportunity to delineate the congenital rubella syndrome and to clarify the epidemiology and pathogenesis of fetal infection.

TABLE 13.2. *Viral infections of the nervous system in the human fetus or neonate*

Virus	Time of infection	Neurologic disease
Major importance		
Rubella virus	First trimester	Chronic encephalitis, microcephaly, retardation, diplegia, visual and auditory deficits
	Later gestation	Hearing loss and minor retardation
Cytomegalovirus	During gestation	Silent infection with minor mental and auditory deficits; cytomegalic inclusion disease with microcephaly, retardation, and motor, visual, and auditory deficits
Human immunodeficiency virus	During gestation and intrapartum	Chronic encephalopathy with acquired microcephaly, diplegia, and basal ganglia calcification
Herpes simplex virus	During parturition	Severe encephalitis
Minor importance		
Herpes simplex virus	During gestation	Encephalitis with congenital microcephaly
Varicella–zoster virus	First half of gestation	Cicatricial scar, limb hypoplasia, and encephalomyelitis
Coxsackie, group B viruses, and echoviruses	Neonatal (?late gestation)	Encephalitis associated with myocarditis
Polioviruses	Late gestation	Congenital or neonatal paralytic poliomyelitis
Influenza virus	First trimester	Possible relation to varied malformations including neural tube defects and hydrocephalus
Lymphocytic choriomeningitis virus	?	Hydrocephalus(?)
BK virus	?	Hydrocephalus, microcephaly(?)
Arboviruses		
Venezuelan equine encephalitis virus	Late gestation	Congenital or neonatal encephalitis
Cache Valley virus	?	Hydrocephalus and microcephaly
Tenshaw virus		
HTLV-1	?	Hydrocephalus(?)

HTLV, human T-cell lymphotropic virus.
Modified from Johnson (1988).

Pathogenesis of Fetal Anomalies

Primary rubella virus infections of adults are accompanied by viremia, even when infection is clinically inapparent. In symptomatic infection, virus may be found in the blood for 7 days before the appearance of rash, and it is present in 80% to 90% of patients at the onset of rash (Dudgeon, 1969). Reinfection with rubella can occur, but usually without rash or viremia. Congenital rubella after reinfection of the mother has been documented, but this is a rare phenomenon (Partridge et al., 1981). The frequency of congenital infection after maternal primary infection and rash is greater than 80% during the first 12 weeks of gestation, over 50% between 13 and 16 weeks, and 25% at the end of the second trimester (Miller et al., 1982). The rate of malformations also decreases with increasing fetal age. Almost all infants have congenital lesions if infected during the first trimester, 35% of infants infected between 13 and 16 weeks have deficits particularly hearing loss, and abnormalities are rare with infection after 16 weeks of gestation. Many babies who appear normal at birth are found to be excreting virus in throat, urine, feces, or cerebrospinal fluid, and babies infected late in gestation often fail to have detectable hearing loss until after 1 year of age (Hardy, 1973a, Menser and Forrest, 1974, Wild et al., 1989).

The pathogenesis of the malformations in the developing fetus appear to involve several mechanisms. In some cells, infection may lead to destruction, whereas in others the infection may be noncytopathic with mitotic inhibition (Singer et al., 1967). Children born with the rubella syndrome tend to be small for gestational age and tend to have an actual decrease in cell numbers. Cells grown from children with congenital rubella show a decrease in mitotic activity. Furthermore, this noncytopathic infection may be focal or multifocal; tissues from a child with the rubella syndrome have demonstrated scattered areas of histologically normal cells with viral antigen (Fig. 13.2), and cultures of cells from infants have shown that comparatively small numbers of cells are infected, but

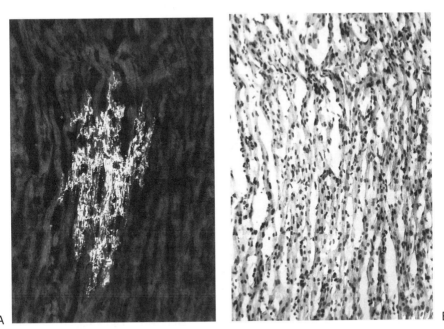

A   B

FIG. 13.2. Lack of cytopathic effects and focal nature of congenital rubella virus infection. The cardiac muscle of an infant dying with congenital rubella syndrome stained with fluorescent antibody shows a focal area of viral antigen (A), but the same section counterstained with hematoxylin and eosin shows no detectable cytopathic change in the chronically infected cells (B). ×100. (From Woods et al., 1966, with permission.)

in vitro these cells give rise to clones of infected cells with slower growth rates (Rawls and Melnick, 1966).

Clonal noncytopathic infection with mitotic inhibition could account for a number of the unusual phenomena observed in congenital rubella, such as asymmetrical noninflammatory lesions in some organs, the persistence of the infection despite the presence of transplacental maternal IgG and the fetal production of IgM antibody, and the ultimate apparent clearance of virus by the child (Rawls, 1974). After an initial transplacental infection of embryonic cells, maternal antibody may prevent further cell-to-cell spread of infection; because virus fails to lyse the infected embryonic cells, their cell division is slowed, but each daughter cell is infected. This mechanism could account for hypoplasia of one eye arising from an infected progenitor despite a normal eye on the other side arising from an uninfected progenitor. Cells with lower doubling time would eventually die out in most organs. This may explain why children congenitally infected with rubella eventually clear virus and why virus persists longer in organs with limited cell division such as the brain, lens, and inner ear.

Congenital Rubella Syndrome

The classic rubella syndrome usually follows infection during the first trimester. The newborn is small for gestational age and may have signs of early cataracts, microphthalmia, cardiac malformations, deafness, microcephaly, spastic diplegia, chorioretinitis, and glaucoma. In addition, transient acute meningoencephalitis, thrombocytopenia, hepatosplenomegaly, jaundice, bone lesions, pneumonitis, and lymphadenopathy are seen in the neonatal period (Cooper, 1975). Alternatively, babies may appear normal but may develop encephalitis or interstitial pneumonitis and a chronic rubelliform rash when several months of age, the so-called late-onset disease. Some abnormalities, such as deafness or psychomotor retardation, may be overlooked during the neonatal period and may be found only on subsequent examination. In some children neurologic and audiologic deficits definitely progress during early months of life (Table 13.3). Congenital rubella typically is a multiple deficit disease, although sensorineural deafness and pigmentary retinitis stand out as the most common solitary deficits (see Chapter 16).

In one study, neurologic abnormalities were found in 81 of 100 infants with the congenital rubella syndrome (Desmond et al., 1967). In the most frequent form, the child at birth or within the first few weeks was noted to be lethargic, hypotonic, and inactive, with a large full anterior fontanelle. Over the next 1 to 4 months, irritability became more evident, often with opisthotonic posturing while crying. Growth and motor development were slow, and a lack of response to sound was commonly noted. However, between 6 and 12 months of age, half of these children had an amelioration of signs. Another group of congenitally infected infants were relatively normal postnatally but failed to progress satisfactorily in weight gain, motor activity, or socialization. Increased deep tendon

TABLE 13.3. *Abnormalities in congenital rubella virus infections*

	Evident in neonatal period		May not be evident until months or years later
	Common	Rare	
CNS	Encephalitis, enlarged anterior fontanelle	Microcephaly	Mental retardation, language abnormalities, motor deficits, autism
Eye	Pigmentary retinopathy, cataract, microphthalmia	Glaucoma, cloudy cornea, iris hypoplasia	Pigmentary retinopathy
Ear	Sensorineural deafness		Sensorineural hearing deficits
Skeletomuscular	Low birth weight, postnatal growth retardation, bone radiolucencies, micrognathia	Dermal erythropoiesis	High palate, pes cavus, talipes equinovarus, finger abnormalities, dental abnormalities
Hematologic	Hepatosplenomegaly, thrombocytopenia, leukopenia, adenopathy	Hepatitis, immunologic dyscrasias, hemolytic anemia, hypoplastic anemia	
Cardiovascular–pulmonary	Pulmonary arterial hypoplasia, patent ductus arteriosus, coarctation of aortic isthmus	Septal defects, interstitial pneumonitis, myocardial necrosis	
Other	Undescended testes	Genitourinary malformations	Diabetes mellitus, growth hormone deficiency, hypothyroidism

reflexes and intermittent opisthotonus developed in some after 6 months of age. A third group had an abrupt onset of convulsions or a meningitis-like picture within the first few days of life.

In the majority of these infants, the spinal fluid protein concentration was increased at birth, and it decreased subsequently to normal levels. However, protein remained elevated for over a year in some cases. In most, a moderate pleocytosis was also present. Virus was frequently isolated from spinal fluid, and in some cases virus isolation was possible for over a year.

Despite the dire appearance of these children during the neonatal period, many showed striking improvement between 6 and 12 months of age. Follow-up at 18 months of age showed that 34 of 64 surviving children had few or no motor abnormalities; of the 30 children with severe involvement, 15 improved between 12 and 18 months of age, whereas 15 failed to improve or deteriorated. The majority had some hearing deficit. A large percentage had residual ocular abnormalities, with cataracts, glaucoma, or chorioretinitis. Indeed, only 9% of the 64 had no hearing, speech, or visual problems.

Several long-term follow-up studies of children with congenital rubella have provided an optimistic outlook, despite the frequent cerebral disease at birth, the persistence of infection of the brain, and the small head size that would portend a poor outcome. A follow-up of 50 patients with congenital rubella from the Australian epidemic of 1940 showed that 48% were deaf, 26% had cataracts or chorioretinitis, and many were small, with minor skeletal defects. Nevertheless, most had achieved remarkably good socioeconomic adjustment; mental deficiency was present in only 5 patients and was severe in only one (Menser et al., 1967). The small head circumference may be proportional to the general diminutive stature, and it does not correlate with intelligence. In one group of 92 children from the 1964 epidemic who had sufficient vision to take intelligence tests, the mean IQ was 99 (Macfarlane et al., 1975). In contrast, in the Baltimore study of children who survived congenital rubella, 29% were found to be mentally defective with IQs below 70 (Hardy, 1973b), and in the New York Rubella Project, 26% were mentally retarded. In the latter study, half of the children had some neuropsychiatric disorders at ages 8 to 10, with a 6% incidence of autism, a syndrome found in less than 0.05% of the general population (Cooper, 1975).

Although many of the lesions of the congenital rubella syndrome, such as patent ductus arteriosus and microphthalmia, resemble true malformations, the neuropathologic abnormalities appear to result primarily from inflammatory vascular disease. Walls of cerebral arteries and veins show focal destruction, and the internal elastic lamina may be defective with proliferation of subintimal fibrous tissue. Chronic perivascular collections of inflammatory cells are present, and mineralized debris is deposited along the vessels (Fig. 13.3). Focal areas of parenchymal necrosis, when present, are usually adjacent to damaged vessels or in their terminal field of supply (Rorke and Spiro, 1967). These lesions may be related to vascular injury by immune complexes, because circulating immune complexes that contain rubella virus antigens are found in children with congenital rubella. Furthermore, the levels of immune complexes are higher in children with severe clinical disease and in children who develop the

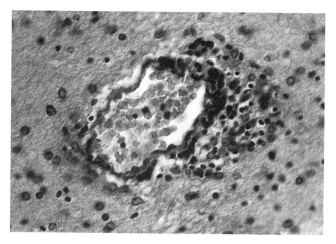

FIG. 13.3. Cerebrovascular abnormality in congenital rubella syndrome. Brain of an infant dying with congenital rubella syndrome shows perivascular inflammation and mineralization. ×320 (From Johnson and Johnson, 1969 with permission.)

late-onset disease (Tardieu et al., 1980; Coyle et al., 1981). They are also found in adolescents with progressive rubella panencephalitis (see Chapter 10).

In addition to these inflammatory changes, the brain tends to be small. This may results from mitotic inhibition or may be a result of the associated cardiac disease, effects of the placentitis, or other factors. Quantification of neuronal populations has not been reported. Delayed myelination has been seen (Rorke and Spiro, 1967). Abnormal patterns of gyri, with polymicrogyria, hydrencephaly, and aqueductal stenosis, have been found (Wolf and Cowen, 1972), but these malformations could be coincidental. A study of the offspring of 2,500 mothers with rubella uncovered 22 infants with gross malformations of the brain that included encephalomyelocele, meningocele, spina bifida, and hydrocephalus. However, statistical analysis of these data showed no relationship between maternal rubella and these malformations, with the possible exception of meningocele (Lundstrom, 1962).

Prevention

Once congenital infection has occurred, no intervention is known to clear the infection or modify its course. Prenatal diagnosis is possible in 85% of cases using PCR for rubella virus RNA in biopsies of chorionic villi, but false positive and false negative results can be obtained (Bosma et al., 1995). The principles of immunization are unique in rubella, because the objective is not to protect the vaccinee from disease but to induce immunity in girls prior to childbearing years to protect the next generation. Therefore, "rubella parties" intended to expose girls to another child with rubella were a time-honored and effective public health measure.

The introduction of a live attenuated virus vaccine has been more effective, but the strategy of vaccination has varied. In the United States, delivery of vaccine has been aimed at all preschool and elementary-school children in the hope of eliminating rubella from the population. Rubella has dramatically decreased, but this decrease in circulation of virus has led to the persistence of some non-immune young adults of childbearing age. In some other countries, preadolescent girls and high-risk nonimmune women have been targeted for vaccination in the hope of preventing infections during pregnancy.

Since the vaccine virus causes viremia and can infect the fetus, pregnancy has been considered a contraindication to immunization. Registries of inadvertent vaccinees were kept until 1989. No instance of the congenital rubella was found in over 200 live deliveries of mothers given the vaccine during pregnancy, and birth defects were no higher than found in uncomplicated pregnancies (CDC, 1989a).

Cytomegalovirus

Cytomegalovirus is the commonest cause of fetal infection. One percent of all newborns have serologic and virologic evidence of fetal infection, but only about

5% of these have classic cytomegalic inclusion disease. However, up to 20% of the "silent" infections lead to hearing loss or mental retardation, which makes cytomegalovirus the commonest known cause of mental retardation.

The finding of characteristic cytomegalic cells in autopsy tissues of 1% of infant deaths delineated the problem of cytomegalic inclusion disease prior to recovery of the virus. Diagnosis of infection during life became possible when cytomegalic cells were identified in urinary sediments. After isolation of cytomegalovirus from human tissues (Rowe et al., 1956; Smith, 1956), serologic tests became available that clarified the magnitude of the problem of fetal cytomegalovirus infections. Cytomegalovirus is an endemic virus in all populations of the world; consequently, congenital infections are not geographically clustered and occur sporadically throughout the year.

Prenatal and Postnatal Infections

Between 40% and 100% of adults have antibody to the virus with highest prevalence rates in lower socioeconomic groups and in underdeveloped countries. Transplacental, perinatal, childhood contact, transfusion and sexual contact all have been shown to transmit cytomegalovirus (Bale, 1984). Postnatal primary infection usually is subclinical, although the agent has been associated with heterophil-negative infectious mononucleosis, posttransfusion fever, and serious systemic disease in immunosuppressed patients (see Chapter 6). The pregnancy histories of mothers who have borne cytomegalovirus-infected babies show no differences in the reporting of clinical illnesses than do those of matched controls (Starr et al., 1970).

The frequency of the maternal infection is very high. Seroconversion occurs in 1% to 2% of pregnancies, and about half of these primary infections lead to fetal infection. The remainder of infections are reactivations which cause more common perinatal infections and less severe neurologic disease. Four percent to 5% of pregnant women have cytomegalovirus in their urine, and 3% to 28% have virus in cervical secretions. Cytomegalovirus also is common in breast milk. Forty percent of infants born to mothers who are secreting cytomegaloviruses near the time of delivery become infected. Thus, primary infections and reactivation are common in pregnant women, and pregnancy itself activates genitourinary excretion of virus. Reactivation and infection during parturition or in the neonatal period is generally benign and associated only with transient hepatomegaly.

Intrauterine infection can be detected by anticytomegalovirus IgM in cord blood, and 0.5% to 1.5% of all live births have evidence of fetal infection (Alford et al., 1990). A primary infection with viremia at any time during pregnancy may spread to the fetus (Davis et al., 1971), but an adverse outcome is more likely if infection occurs in the first 20 weeks of pregnancy (Stagno et al., 1986). However, intrauterine infection does not require primary maternal infection. A prospective study has shown that 3% of women who were seropositive before pregnancy have babies with evidence of infection, a rate similar to that for the nonimmune population. Furthermore, molecular epidemiologic studies of these infections indicate that endogenous virus is the most common source of fetal infection in immune mothers (Huang et al., 1980). However, fetal infections of previously immune mothers rarely cause cytomegalic inclusion disease which suggests that maternal immunity confers protection to the fetus from severe disease but not from infection (Stagno et al., 1977).

Cytomegalic Inclusion Disease

Florid cytomegalic inclusion disease of the newborn presents with hepatomegaly, splenomegaly, jaundice, petechiae, and cerebral and retinal disease (Table 13.4). During the neonatal period the spinal fluid shows a mononuclear cell pleocytosis, elevated protein content, and occasionally evidence of hemorrhage. Enlarged cells with inclusions have been seen in the fluid (Arey, 1954), but virus usually is not recoverable. In survivors cerebral infection results in microcephaly, with mental retardation and delayed psychomotor development in 70% (Alford et al., 1990). Mortality is as high as 30%. The hepatic and hematologic disease usually resolves leaving only neurologic and sensory deficits. Seizures are common. Ten to 30% have radiologic evidence of intracerebral calcifications. Deafness is common, and cytomegalic cells and virus are present in the endolymphatic structures of the cochlea (see Chapter 16). Chorioretinitis may result in blindness or severe visual impairment. Only about 15% of survivors of cytomegalic inclusion disease are normal later in childhood (MacDonald and Tobin, 1978).

TABLE 13.4. *Abnormalities in congenital cytomegalovirus infections*

	Cytomegalic inclusion disease in neonatal period		Silent congenital infection (late appearance)
	Common	Rare	
CNS	Microcephaly, periventricular calcification, severe psychomotor retardation, seizures	Hydrocephalus	Microcephaly, low intelligence
Eye	Chorioretinitis, strabismus, optic atrophy	Microphthalmia, cataract, retinal necrosis, optic disc malformations	Chorioretinitis
Ear	Sensorineural deafness		Sensorineural deafness
Skeletomuscular	Low birth weight, indirect inguinal hernia	Clubfoot, dislocations of hips, diastasis recti	
Hematologic	Hepatosplenomegaly, thrombocytopenia, hyperbilirubinemia	Hemolytic anemia	
Cardiovascular–pulmonary	Pneumonitis	Cardiovascular anomalies (but no consistent pattern)	
Other		Biliary atresia, gastrointestinal ulcerations	

"Silent" Fetal Infection

Over 95% of infants with congenital cytomegalovirus infection appear normal at birth, yet both severe and subtle neurologic deficits later are evident in 5% to 15% of these children. Some are small and fail to thrive; some later prove to be retarded and develop mild microcephaly (Alford et al., 1990). Slowly progressive encephalopathy has been reported with progressive calcification extending to thalamus, cerebellum and brainstem (Koeda et al., 1993). In institutionalized retarded children, cytomegalovirus antibodies are more prevalent in microcephalic children than in normocephalic children, despite the lack of a history of cytomegalic inclusion disease (Hanshaw, 1971).

Long-term follow-up studies of the majority of children with inapparent congenital infection show no obvious abnormalities of physical or mental development, although many excrete virus in urine for over 4 years (Kumar et al., 1973). Other prospective studies have detected subtle differences. A study in Alabama showed some degree of sensory neural hearing loss in 9 of 16 congenitally infected "normal" children and a trend toward subnormal intelligence (Reynolds et al., 1974). A study in upstate New York followed 44 normal newborns who had cytomegalovirus IgM antibody in cord blood. Testing 3.5 to 7 years later showed a statistically significant lower IQ as compared with control groups, over twice the risk of school failure, and a higher incidence of hearing defects (Hanshaw et al., 1975). These studies suggest that cytomegalovirus infections may be significant in determining mild degrees of mental and auditory impairment in the absence of the classic cytomegalic inclusion disease.

Diagnosis

The diagnosis of infection, but not necessarily disease, can be established by isolation of cytomegalovirus or detection of DNA by PCR from spinal fluid, urine or throat washings, by visualization of virus by electron microscopic study of urine, by the demonstration of characteristic inclusions or viral antigen in cells in urinary sediment or in biopsy tissues, by rising levels of antibody, or by the detection of anticytomegalovirus IgM in the newborn. The presence of periventricular calcification, while suggestive of *in utero* infection with cytomegalovirus, is not pathognomonic, because the clinical syndrome of microcephaly and chorioretinitis can occur with congenital toxoplasmosis, rubella, and probably other infections.

In most instances, the virus infects the fetus across the placenta, and a placentitis with a plasma cell infiltrate, persistence of Hofbauer cells, and edematous congested villi have been found, with characteristic large intranuclear inclusions in enlarged cells (Monif and Dische, 1972). In other cases of infected neonates, histologic changes may be absent, but antigen is found in villous stroma in cells identified by cell-specific staining as vascular endothelial cells (Muhlemann et al., 1992). As in mouse cytomegalovirus infections, placental infection without fetal involvement has been described in humans (Hayes and Gibas, 1971).

Infants dying of cytomegalic inclusion disease show widespread pathologic changes in the salivary glands, lungs, liver, spleen, kidney, pancreas, inner ear, and retina (see Chapter 16). Neuropathologic studies show periventricular necrosis and calcification. In some cases calcification of the convexities of gyri, cerebellar hypoplasia, hydrocephalus and porencephalic cysts are found (Perlman and Argyle, 1992). The presence or absence of inclusion bodies may be dependent on the stage as well as the severity of the infection, and if death occurs after the neonatal period, the characteristic inclusion-bearing cells may be absent. Microgyria has been reported in a number of cases (Wolf and Cowen, 1972). Hydranencephaly and porencephaly have been reported, and the localization of inclusion-bearing cells around a porencephalic cyst gives credence to a causal relationship rather than a chance association of a common malformation and a common infection in the same patient (Navin and Angevine, 1968).

Prevention and Treatment

About 1% of newborns excrete cytomegalovirus and 10% of these suffer significant CNS damage; therefore, cytomegalovirus is a major cause of neurologic disability. Two recently developed drugs, ganciclovir and foscarnet, are effective against cytomegalovirus *in vitro* and against chorioretinitis and gastrointestinal infections in immunocompromised patients (Balfour, 1990). The relapse of infections with discontinuation of treatment and thus the need for long-term treatment combined with the toxicity of these drugs do not make them promising agents for the treatment of infants. Several live attenuated virus vaccines have been developed. Problems may be posed by the antigenic heterogeneity of virus strains and by the uncertainty of whether or not immunization in childhood will prevent a viremia during a reactivation in pregnancy.

Human Immunodeficiency Virus

The first case of childhood acquired immunodeficiency syndrome (AIDS) apparently related to perinatal infection was diagnosed in 1982, before the isolation of HIV. The numbers of cases in the United States remained small until the infection became epidemic in intravenous drugs users and their sexual partners. With this shift in the epidemiology of HIV infections, the number of infected children increased dramatically and will increase further in the future. Childhood HIV infection due to the treatment of hemophilia or to blood transfusions is now decreasing, and 85% of the HIV infected children now are infected perinatally. The majority are from black and hispanic communities (Bertolli et al., 1995). In Africa and Asia where heterosexual transmission is the major mode of spread of HIV infections, more than 1.5 million children have been infected, more than 3 million women of childbearing age currently are infected.

Transmission from the infected woman to the fetus or newborn is not universal. Estimates of transmission rates vary from 13% to 60%, with the true incidence probably being about 25%. High maternal plasma concentration of virus is a risk factor for transmission to the infant (Sperling et al., 1996). Some data also suggest that women with lower CD4 counts or lower levels of antibody to the gp 120 surface protein may be more likely to transmit the virus, but this finding has not been consistent in all studies (MacDonald et al., 1991; John and Kreiss, 1996).

Pathogenesis

HIV can infect the fetus *in utero* as judged by finding virus in fetal tissues and documenting viremia at birth. Virus can infect the neonate intrapartum presumably by maternal blood contact with mucous membranes or damaged skin, and possibly by transfusion of maternal blood with disruption of placental barriers. Finally virus can infect the baby by breast milk, as documented in mothers infected by postpartum transfusions. Although infection in all 3 periods has been documented, the relative frequency is uncertain; intrapartum infection is probably twice as common as intrauterine infection and breastfeeding may add an additional 5% risk (John and Kreiss, 1996). Since potential methods of treatment are tied to mode and timing of infection, these missing data are critical in advising the first trimester seropositive mother regarding termination of pregnancy, deciding at term on cesarian section, drug treatment of pregnant women and advice regarding breast feeding.

By *in situ* hybridization and immunoperoxidase staining studies of placental tissue at the time of abortions as early as week 8 have shown infection of decidual leukocytes, villus trophoblasts and mesenchymal cells (the so-called Hofbauer cells, which are probably a form of macrophage) as well as embryonic blood cell precursors. Thus, it appears that the infection of maternal leukocytes can lead to infection of the trophoblasts, the Hofbauer cells, and ultimately the fetal blood cells (Langston et al., 1995). It has also been reported in cultures of placental tissues that the trophoblasts can express CD4 *in vitro* and when infected, have a decreased production of chorionic gonadotropin and progesterone. A decrease in placental hormones may impair fetal development (Amirhessami-Aghili and Specter, 1991).

In situ hybridization showed signal in parenchymal cells of the brain in 2 of 8 fetuses in one study and 1 of 4 in another, but precise identification of these cells was not made in either study (Lyman et al., 1990; Langston et al., 1995). PCR data from some studies have suggested a higher rate of fetal infection than from the epidemiologic studies, but contamination with maternal blood might lead to false positive results. PCR results from infants who ultimately prove to be infected show only about 50% are positive in the first week of life; presumably the other 50% are infected during delivery or postpartum (Courgnaud et al., 1991). An African study of babies with unequivocal later evidence of infection showed 30% had positive cord blood and 80% had positive blood at 3 months indicating that a majority are infected during delivery or postpartum (Simonon et al., 1994).

Exposure to infected maternal blood or cervicovaginal secretions during delivery may transmit virus to some neonates. This is supported by studies of the discordant infection of twins in which the first born is at greater risk, by prospective studies documenting a protective role of cesarian sections and by demonstration of greater risk of infection if fetal membranes have been ruptured more than four hours before delivery (Goedert et al., 1991; Esquilin and Hutto, 1995; Landesman et al., 1996). Transmission is also higher in vaginal deliveries in which episiotomy, scalp electrodes, forceps or vacuum extractors were used (European Collaborative Study, 1992).

Transmission to infants is more frequent with advanced clinical disease in the mother or when primary infection occurs during pregnancy or postpartum while breastfeeding. These clinical observations suggest that increased virus load is important in both *in utero* and intrapartum transmission, and this is supported by laboratory studies correlating infant infection with greater numbers of HIV DNA copies and with higher frequency of infected cells in the mother's blood (Roques et al., 1993; Borkowsky et al., 1994; Weiser et al., 1994). A small number of children have been reported who had perinatal infection documented by virus isolation and DNA detection over a number of weeks but who subsequently became HIV-seronegative with no clinical or virologic evidence of infection (Bryson et al., 1995).

The genotype of virus may be a factor in perinatal transmission. Virus isolates that replicate rapidly in human mononuclear cells, that grow in T cell lines and that resist neutralization by maternal serum tend to transmit (Kliks et al., 1994). The rate of transmission of HIV-2 is 20-fold less than HIV-1 in the same West African population (Adjorlolo-Johnson et al., 1994).

Clinical Syndromes

Infected infants appear normal at birth, and the subsequent systemic and neurologic abnormalities seem to show a bimodal distribution (Table 13.5). Thirty-three percent of those infected develop AIDS by 12 months of life; and more than 50% by 2 years of age. HIV hepatitis, interstitial pneumonitis and diarrhea are common in the first year of life. In this early onset group there is a high incidence of progressive encephalopathy and early death. In the second group the neurologic disease occurs more rarely and the median age of onset is 6 years of age. The reason for this disparate distribution is unknown; it may be that the first group is infected *in utero* but there also may be a difference in dosage, route of infection, or phenotype of the infant's virus. Children with encephalopathy usually have a normal size at birth, but failure of normal head growth leads to microcephaly. Loss of motor milestone, weakness and pyramidal tract signs usually develop with the variable presence of other findings, such as basal ganglia signs, ataxia, cortical blindness, myoclonic jerking and seizures. In those children who have a more static deficit, these tend to be more subtle, cognitive deficits with or without developmental microcephaly and some neurologic

TABLE 13.5. *Abnormalities in congenital human immunodeficiency virus infections*

	Evident in neonatal period	Appears in subsequent months to years	
		Common	Rare
CNS	0	Acquired microencephaly, progressive encephalopathy, basal ganglia calcification	Ataxia, movement disorders, myoclonus, seizures, opportunistic infections
Skeletomuscular	HIV dysmorphism(?)		
Hematologic	0	Generalized lymphadenopathy, hepatosplenomegaly	Thrombocytopenia, hepatitis, lymphomas
Cardiovascular–pulmonary	0	Interstitial pneumonitis	Cardiomyopathy
Other	0	Failure to thrive, chronic diarrhea, bacterial infections, oral candidiasis	Nephropathy, parotitis

impairment, but at 24 months of life two thirds of infected children without AIDS show delays in mental and motor functioning (Gay et al., 1995).

The vacuolar myelopathy commonly seen in adults is exceedingly rare in children (Sharer et al., 1990), and peripheral neuropathies also are unusual (Floeter et al., 1997). Cases are described of cerebral toxoplasmosis, cryptococcal meningitis and other opportunistic infections, but they are less common than in adults, as is CNS lymphoma. Thus, in children, there is a more intense cerebral disease due directly to HIV with fewer opportunistic infections. Cytomegalovirus encephalopathy may coexist in HIV-infected children, and the question has been raised as to whether the HIV may reactivate congenital cytomegalovirus infection (Curless et al., 1987; Belec et al., 1990).

The spinal fluid is often normal, but a mild pleocytosis or increase in protein content may be found irrespective of the clinical syndrome. Computerized tomography is abnormal in 86% of children with AIDS showing (in order of greatest frequency) increased ventricular size, cortical atrophy, white matter attenuation or cerebral calcification (DeCarli et al., 1993). Similar abnormalities may be shown in greater detail with magnetic resonance imaging (Belman et al., 1988).

The neuropathologic features include diffuse gliosis of the cortex and the subcortical nuclei and perivascular inflammation. Many microglial nodules and multinucleated giant cells are found in some cases whereas in others megalic cells indicate either a primary or a complicating cytomegalovirus infection. The major findings that differentiate these cases from those in adults are the vascular and juxtavascular mineralization in the frontal lobe white matter, and a true vasculitis with inflammatory cells within parenchymal blood vessel walls (Sharer, 1992).

Diagnosis

In contrast to rubella and cytomegalovirus, there are usually no obvious signs of infection at birth. Considering that only one quarter of children born of HIV-positive mothers are infected, diagnosis is difficult. A few have microcephaly at birth (Schmitt et al., 1991a); dysmorphic syndrome was described, with flattening of the nasal ridge, box-like forehead, hypertelorism, and abnormal lip formation (Marion et al., 1987), but this has not been consistently found or convincingly verified as a diagnostic image. Definitive serologic diagnosis can be made at 15 to 18 months of age, after the decline of maternal HIV antibody when evidence of the child's generation of IgG can be established by the usual methods. By this time, however, the children with the rapidly progressive disease have already developed AIDS, and a number have already died. It is clear that better methods of diagnosis in infants are needed. Assays for virus-specific IgA antibodies show high sensitivity, specificity and predictive value in children over 3 months of age (Quinn et al., 1991). Also it has been proposed that the production of antibody by the infant's lymphocytes *in vitro* can be used as a possible diagnostic method.

Neonatal diagnosis by virus isolation or p24 antigen detection has low sensitivity (Burgard et al., 1992). DNA detection has great sensitivity fraught with some false positive results, particularly since PCR can theoretically be positive by detecting a single molecule of viral DNA from the mother's blood in cord blood or in the neonate's circulation. With peripartum infection no viremia may be present in the first days of infection. An evaluation is needed to determine which primers are best to detect DNA, to determine which postpartum day to obtain sensitive and specific results and to determine what clinical specimen will give the greatest sensitivity and specificity in determining perinatal infection.

Treatment

All women in high risk groups should be tested during prenatal care, be advised of risks and options, and be monitored so that treatment can be started when indicated. Breastfeeding by seropositive mothers is not recommended in developed countries, but in developing countries the benefits of breastfeeding may outweigh the risk of transmission. One of the major social problems, particularly in the developing countries, is the combined social catastrophes of the infected infants and the two-thirds of infants who are not infected but whose parents are both infected. "AIDS-orphans" constitute an enormous problem in sub-Saharan Africa.

Zidovidine was noted to be especially effective in arresting the encephalopathy of children with AIDS. Indeed serial measurements of IQ after 3 and 6 months of therapy showed not a stabilization but an actual increase in scores (Pizzo et al., 1988). Unfortunately drug resistance evolves after about 6 months. In the future multidrug treatment such as adding another reverse transcriptase inhibitor such as lamivudine (3TC) or a protease inhibitor may extend this period of efficacy.

Zidovidine given to pregnant women can reduce the perinatal transmission by two-thirds (22.6% in placebo group; 7.6% in treated) (Sperling et al., 1996). Oral drug is given throughout pregnancy, intravenous loading dose and continuous infusion is given during labor, and the newborn is treated with oral medication for the first 6 weeks of life (CDC, 1994b). Since zidovidine at therapeutic doses can inhibit gamma DNA polymerase, required for mitochondrial replication, concern was raised about possible adverse affects on fetal development; however, malformation, premature birth, or fetal distress have not yet been observed with maternal treatment (Sperling et al., 1992).

Herpes Simplex Virus

Severe disseminated infections and encephalitis of the newborn can occur with both type 1 and type 2 herpes simplex viruses, but in three-quarters of infants these severe infections are related to type 2 or genital strains (Whitley et al., 1991). The incidence of neonatal herpes simplex virus infections has increased over the past 3 decades to approximately 1 per 3500 live births (Whitley, 1993). Mothers of affected babies are predominantly young primiparas; most are without signs or symptoms of genital herpes at the time of delivery, and 70% do not have a history of recurrent genital lesions or sexual partners with lesions (Whitley, 1993).

Almost half of the clinically affected infants are born prematurely, which indicates either that infection per se may induce premature labor or that premature infants are more susceptible to infection by the mother. Signs of systemic disease usually are not present at birth and begin 1 to 3 weeks postpartum. In about 40% of infants infection remains limited to skin, eyes or mouth, but in 25% wide dissemination occurs with respiratory distress, jaundice, bleeding, seizures, and signs of increased intracranial pressure. In 35% of infants, disease is localized to the CNS or retina (see Chapter 16). The electroencephalogram usually shows a characteristic multifocal periodic or quasiperiodic pattern (Mizrahi and Tharp, 1982). Computerized tomography shows patchy or diffuse areas of low attenuation in white matter (Noorbehest et al., 1987). In contrast to the situation with herpesvirus encephalitis in children and adults, virus readily can be recovered from spinal fluid.

Necrosis of the liver and adrenal glands is typical of disseminated infection, but lesions are also found in the spleen, lung, skin, and brain. In the brain eosinophilic intranuclear inclusion bodies are localized around the necrotic areas. When neonatal infection is localized to the brain, the brain lesions are diffuse, in contrast to the localized orbital-temporal lesions seen in herpes simplex virus encephalitis of children and adults (see Chapter 6).

The normal appearance of these babies at birth, the late development of signs in the perinatal period, the association with vaginal infection of the mother, and even the frequent vertex or breech sites of skin lesions that may correspond to obstetrical presentation all support the thesis that infection is acquired during transit through the birth canal. Risk is also increased by prolonged rupture of membranes prior to birth suggesting ascending infection. About half of the infections in babies result from primary infections of mothers acquired during pregnancy; about half result from reactivation (Arvin, 1991). Serologic testing of couples can identify those at risk; 10% of seronegative women have seropositive spouses and they are at high risk of primary infection (Kulhanjian et al., 1992); the seropositive women are at risk of recurrences. Prevention or at least reduction of risk can be provided by cesarean section, but the use of virus cultures and antigen detection tests are not sufficiently accurate or timely and indication for cesarian section is limited to finding infection on physical exam at the time of labor (Libman et al., 1991).

Herpes simplex virus encephalitis in infants is more severe than in children or adults, and does not show as dramatic a response to acyclovir. In babies with encephalitis a randomized, blinded study showed that both vidarabine and acyclovir reduced the mortality to about 15%, and nearly 50% of survivors showed normal development 3 years after treatment. In babies with disseminated disease, however, mortality was reduced only to about 50% with 60% of survivors showing normal development 3 years later (Whitley et al., 1991a). Infection with type 2 herpes simplex virus results in greater mortality and morbidity than type 1 infections in infants (Whitley et al., 1991b; Corey et al., 1988). Furthermore, relapse and progression of disease after antiviral treatment is seen in 8% in contrast to the rarity of relapses in children and adults with localized type 1 virus infections (see Chapter 6).

Primary infection of the mother during the first 20 weeks of gestation have been associated with increased frequency of abortion, stillbirths and rare congenital malformations (South et al., 1969; Nahmias et al., 1970; Montgomery et al., 1973; Hutto et al., 1987; Whitley, 1993). These children have had varying combinations of microcephaly, hydranencephaly, calcification of atrophic cerebral hemispheres, micro-ophthalmia, and chorioretinitis (Fig. 13.4). A vesicular rash is often present at birth or shortly thereafter, and type 2 herpes simplex virus has been isolated from these skin lesions. One infant has been reported with microcephaly and intracranial calcifications who had no skin lesions, but type 1 herpes simplex virus was recovered from spinal fluid and urine (Florman et al., 1973). Primary maternal infection during the second and third trimesters has been suspected as a cause of interuterine growth retardation (Brown et al., 1987).

Varicella-Zoster Virus

Varicella-zoster virus can cross the placenta during the final weeks of pregnancy. Maternal chickenpox 1 to 3 weeks before delivery has resulted in infants born with the characteristic but benign rashes of chickenpox or shingles. Mater-

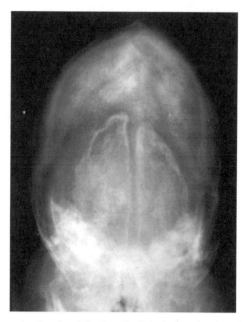

FIG. 13.4. Fetal herpes simplex virus infection. Radiologic examination of the skull of a 5-week-old microcephalic infant shows overlapping bones and a calcified atrophic brain. Type 2 herpes virus was recovered from skin lesions. (From South et al., 1969, with permission.)

nal chickenpox from 4 days before to 2 days after birth has been associated with severe and often fatal varicella in the 5 to 10 day old newborns (Enders, 1984).

Chickenpox during the first 20 weeks of gestation does have a 2% absolute risk of embryopathy above controls (Pastuszak et al., 1994). Less than 1% of newborns whose mothers had varicella between 8 and 19 weeks of gestation have been born with such a characteristic malformation that a cause-and-effect relationship seems self-evident. These infants have a cicatricial skin lesion in a zosterlike distribution associated with hypoplasia of the corresponding limb or cranial structure (Fig. 13.5). These children also may have severe ocular abnormalities that include optic atrophy, microphthalmia, cataracts, and chorioretinitis, and the majority have had evidence of severe brain damage (Nicola and Hanshaw, 1979). Autopsy findings have shown a necrotizing encephalomyelitis, cystic necrosis and dorsal radiculitis (Srabstein et al., 1974); in one case polymicrogyria and cerebellar heterotopias also were found (Harding and Baumer, 1988; Magliocco et al., 1992). Although varicella-zoster virus has not been recovered from these children, the distribution of the cutaneous lesions supports the view that this is a rare complication of maternal varicella. Maternal herpes zoster has not been incriminated in fetal damage (Paryani and Arvin, 1986; Enders et al., 1994).

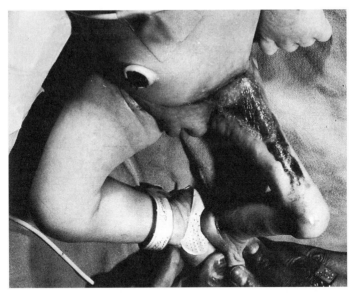

FIG. 13.5. Fetal varicella-zoster virus infection. The infant has a cicatricial scar on the thigh and hypoplasia of the leg. The mother had varicella between 13 and 15 weeks of gestation. (From Srabstein et al., 1974, with permission.)

Other Viral Infections

As with varicella-zoster virus, several other viruses can cross the placenta late in gestation and cause diseases in newborns similar to those in adults. Infants of infected mothers have been born with the characteristic cutaneous lesions of smallpox, vaccinia, and measles virus infections, hepatitis due to hepatitis B virus, flaccid paralysis of poliomyelitis virus infection, and acute encephalitis due to Western encephalitis virus (Copps and Giddings, 1959). Massive cerebral necrosis of fetuses associated with Venezuelan equine encephalitis virus infection of the mother (Wenger, 1967) has been reported, as has recovery of Japanese encephalitis virus from brain of an abortus of an infected mother (Chaturvedi et al., 1980). The roles of these and other viruses as true teratogens are less clear.

Enteroviruses can cause severe infections during the first 2 weeks of life suggesting infection in the immediate perinatal period. Group B coxsackieviruses cause an acute myocarditis, and echoviruses (particularly echoviruses 11) cause hepatitis. Both coxsackie and echovirus infections have been associated with encephalitis (Modlin, 1986; Abzug et al., 1995). Intrauterine infections with these enteroviruses have not been related to chronic CNS disease or to malformations. In an extensive prospective serologic study of over 22,000 pregnancies, no association of selected coxsackievirus and echovirus infections with musculoskeletal or nervous system malformations was detected, even though associations were suspected with anomalies of the cardiovascular, digestive, and uro-genital systems (Brown and Karunas, 1972). In a retrospective serologic study of 338 mothers of newborns with gross malformations of the CNS (anencephaly, meningomyelocele, and congenital hydrocephalus) and matched controls, a higher frequency of antibody to echovirus 7 was present in the study group, but no differences were found with 26 other microbial antigens, including group B coxsackie viruses and mumps and influenza viruses (Lapinleimu et al., 1972). Live poliovaccine during pregnancy has also been cleared of any untoward effects on the fetus, even though a viremia develops with the type 2 strain (Har-julento-Mervaala et al., 1993).

Influenza has been credited with causing increases in abortions, stillbirths, and some CNS malformations (Hardy, 1973a), but often such studies have accepted a clinical diagnosis of influenza, as did the Dublin study that associated influenza with anencephaly (Coffey and Jessop, 1963). An epidemiologic asso-ciation of epidemic influenza and CNS malformations was reported in Finland, but the authors cleverly noted that this increase correlated with increased phar-macists' sales during the same epidemic period, which suggests other potential teratogens (Hakosalo and Sacen, 1971). In Atlanta mothers reporting a flulike illness during pregnancy had a 3-fold increase in risk of having an infant with a neural tube deficit; if they took medications for their episodes of flu with fever the odds ratio increase to 4.3 (Lynberg et al., 1994). Most serologic studies have not supported a role for influenza viruses in the pathogenesis of malformations (Wilson and Stein, 1969; Elizan et al., 1969), and the usual absence of a viremia with influenza virus infections would make these viruses unlikely candidates. However, in one instance of fatal influenza pneumonia in a pregnant woman, viremia and transplacental passage of influenza virus has been documented (Yawn et al., 1971). Influenza A gene sequences in serum and spinal fluid were reported in 3 children with congenital CNS disease—one with hydrocephalus and 2 with progressive encephalopathy (Tentsov et al., 1989).

Two pregnant women with histories of exposure to hamsters and with sero-logic evidence of lymphocytic choriomeningitis virus infection delivered infants with hydrocephalus (Ackermann et al., 1974). Subsequently other case reports have accumulated with serologic evidence of maternal and fetal infection with lymphocytic choriomeningitis virus and a rather stereotyped syndrome of non-obstructive hydrocephalus with periventricular calcifications and chorioretinitis (Barton et al., 1995). A serologic survey of antibodies to lymphocytic chori-omeningitis virus in children with hydrocephalus has given further support to this occasional association (Sheinberg, 1975).

Because of the association of bunyavirus infections with hydrocephalus and arthrogryposis in lambs and calves a serologic survey for North American bun-yaviruses was done on the sera that had been collected between 1959 and 1964 in the NIH prospective study of the congenital rubella syndrome. Mothers of infants with macrocephaly or microcephaly had significantly greater frequency of antibodies to Cache Valley and Tensaw viruses, arboviruses known to infect humans but not previously associated with human disease. Two women who delivered macrocephalic babies had significant rises in antibody between the first and second trimesters. In contrast antibodies to La Crosse and Jamestown Canyon viruses, the bunyaviruses previously associated with human CNS disease in North America, showed no correlation with congenital abnormalities (Calisher and Sever, 1995). Antibodies to two animal pestiviruses (border disease virus and bovine viral diarrhea virus) have been shown in mothers of 6 of 129 newborns with microcephaly, suggesting the possible role of an antigenically related virus (Potts et al., 1987).

IgM antibodies to BK virus, a human papovavirus as yet unrelated to any human disease, have been found in 3 neonates with hydrocephalus, as well as individual children with microcephaly, mental retardation, and congenital ataxia (Rziha et al., 1978). Prospective studies of pregnancies have shown frequent activation of BK and related JC virus during pregnancy without evidence of virus transmission to the fetus (Coleman et al., 1980; Daniels et al., 1981). If fetal infection does occur, it presumably occurs during primary maternal infection. Hydrocephalus has also been described in two HTLV-1 seropositive infants born of mothers with infection and myelopathy, (Kawahara et al., 1990; Tohyama et al., 1992), but these two cases may represent chance occurrences.

Human parvovirus B19 is the cause of erythema infectiosum, a benign epidemic exanthem. This virus also causes hydrops fetalis and abortion or stillbirth (Anand et al., 1987). Virus has been demonstrated in many fetal tissues including brain (Schwarz et al., 1996; Jordan and Sever, 1994), and inflammatory lesions and hypoplasia of the fetal retina have been found (Weiland et al., 1987). The virulence of this virus in the fetus may preclude its role in neonatal abnormalities.

If an infection inciting a malformation is a self-limited infection early in gestation, IgM might be absent at birth. If self-limited infection is cleared prior to 20 weeks of gestation, when specific humoral immune responses develop, a total absence of fetal antibodies to the agent might be found. To address these problems, cell-mediated immune responses to viral antigens can be sought in umbilical cord blood lymphocytes. In a study of 23 infants with CNS anomalies, lymphocytes of 7 infants (2 with hydrocephalus, 2 with meningomyelocele, and one each with microcephaly, sacral agenesis, and hydranencephaly) showed heightened lymphoproliferative responses to mumps virus, and 1 infant with communicating hydrocephalus showed responses to herpes simplex type 2 (Thompson and Glasgow, 1980). This predominant and specific incrimination of mumps virus, freed from blame as a teratogen by serologic surveys, is of particular interest because the virus can produce hydrocephalus in experimental animals and probably young children, and a related paramyxovirus (Newcastle disease virus) can inhibit closure of the neural tube in chick embryos.

VIRAL TERATOGENESIS IN ANIMALS

In humans well-documented fetal and neonatal infections have been associated primarily with inflammatory cerebral lesions, but in animals a number of natural and experimental viral infections cause symmetrical noninflammatory malformations of the brain and spinal cord. These defects often lack the neuropathologic findings of inflammation, gliosis, calcification, or inclusion bodies to suggest antecedent infection. Indeed, they resemble malformations of humans that are assumed to have a toxic, genetic, or vascular basis. These include abnormalities in closure of the neural tube, encephalocoele, cerebellar hypoplasia, defective myelin formation, hydranencephaly, porencephaly, and hydrocephalus (Table 13.6).

Defects in Organogenesis

The first experimental teratogenic effect of a virus on nervous system development was described by Hamburger and Habel in 1947. They inoculated influenza A virus into the developing chick embryo and found abnormalities of the neural tube. Embryos infected at 48 hr of incubation showed collapse of the primitive brain (microencephaly) and abnormalities of neural tube flexion during the next 24 to 48 hr. Subsequently, failure of neural tube closure was also found in these infected embryos (Robertson et al., 1960). These embryos do not survive so these early experimental developmental failures do not lead to congenital meningomyelocele or spinal bifida.

Studies of this neural tube abnormality have failed to show any histologic abnormality of the neural ectoderm, notochord, or surrounding mesenchymal cells. The mitotic activity along the luminal surface of the neural tube appears normal. Immunocytologic studies indicate that the influenza virus infection does not involve the neural ectoderm or mesenchymal tissue but is limited to the chorionic and amniotic membranes, the nonneural ectoderm, and focal areas of the primitive myocardium and gut. Thus, infection of noncontiguous extraneural tissues appears to indirectly alter organogenesis (Johnson et al., 1971).

Interestingly, Newcastle disease virus, a natural virus of chickens, can produce the same abnormalities in chick embryos (Robertson et al., 1955). However, in this infection cells of the caudal neural tube are infected (Williamson et al., 1965). Therefore, the same teratogenic effects can result even when different cells are infected by different viruses. In mice, both a mutant of Semliki Forest virus and murine cytomegalovirus have been associated with neural tube defects when infected at 8 to 10 days of gestation (Mabruk et al., 1989; Baskar et al., 1987). The nature of the defect in organogenesis can be dependent on the ontogenetic stage at which the insult occurs, rather than on the specific target cells of the insults, a principle long recognized in the teratogenic effects of irradiation and chemicals.

Selective Destruction of Immature Cells Populations

Viral destruction of specific populations of immature cells in fetal or newborn animals can cause a variety of cerebellar or cerebral malformations. The basis of the selective vulnerability differs with different viruses and may change with maturation of host cells. The cell destruction may be a direct virus effect or may be mediated by immune responses.

TABLE 13.6. *Experimental cerebral malformations induced by viruses*

Malformation	Virus	Host species
Defects in neural tube closure	Herpesvirus	
	Mouse cytomegalovirus	Mouse
	Myxoviruses	
	Influenza virus	Chick embryo
	Newcastle disease virus	Chick embryo
Encephalocele	Flaviviruses	
	Semliki Forest (mutant) virus	Mouse
	St. Louis encephalitis virus	Mouse
	Bunyavirus	
	Aino virus	Chick embryo
Cerebellar hypoplasia	Parvoviruses	
	Rat virus	Hamster, rat, cat, ferret
	Feline panleukopenia virus	Cat, ferret
	Minute virus of mice	Mouse
	Arenaviruses	
	Lymphocytic choriomeningitis virus	Rat
	Tamiami virus	Mouse
	Flaviviruses	
	Hog cholera virus	Pig
	Bovine viral diarrhea virus	Sheep
	Border disease virus	Sheep
Hypomyelination	Flaviviruses	
	Hog cholera virus	Pig
	Bovine viral diarrhea virus	Sheep
	Border disease virus	Sheep
Hydranencephaly and/or porencephaly	Bunyaviruses	
	Aino virus	Chick embryo
	Akabane virus	Cow, sheep, chick embryo
	Cache Valley virus	Sheep
	La Crosse virus	Sheep
	Main Drain virus	Sheep
	San Angelo virus	Sheep
	Rift Valley fever virus	Sheep
	Orbivirus	
	Bluetongue virus	Cow, sheep
	Togaviruses	
	Venezuelan equine encephalitis	Monkey
	Wesselsbron virus	Sheep
	Flaviviruses	
	Bovine viral diarrhea virus	Sheep
	Border disease virus	Sheep
Hydrocephalus[a]	Herpesvirus	
	Herpes simplex, type 1 (mutant)	Mouse
	Poxvirus	
	Vaccinia virus	Cat
	Paramyxoviruses	
	Mumps virus	Hamster, monkey
	Parainfluenza virus types 1, 2, 3	Hamster, mouse
	Canine parainfluenza	Dogs
	Respiratory syncytia virus	Hamster, mouse
	Pneumonia virus of mice	Mouse
	Measles (mutant) virus	Hamster
	Newcastle disease virus	Mouse
	Orthomyxovirus	
	Influenza virus	Hamster, mouse, monkey
	Reovirus	
	Type I	Mouse, hamster, rat, ferret
	Togavirus	
	Ross River virus	Mouse
	Flaviviruses	
	St. Louis encephalitis virus	Mouse

[a]Includes communicating and noncommunicating hydrocephalus, but obstructive hydrocephalus due to virus-induced neoplasia and hydrocephalus *ex vacuo* due to chronic infection are not included (Johnson, 1975a).

Cerebellar hypoplasia

In 1964 Kilham and Margolis reported granuloprival cerebellar hypoplasia after intracerebral inoculation of neonatal hamsters with rat virus, a parvovirus. Sequential histologic studies showed selective viral destruction of the external germinal cells of the cerebellum prior to their postnatal migration to form the granular cell layer. This led to a small cerebellum, with abnormalities of foliation, total or subtotal absence of a granule cell layer and an abnormal synaptic organization (Margolis and Kilham, 1968; Herndon et al., 1971). This effect of rat virus also can be produced in neonatal rats, cats, and ferrets, and by other parvoviruses in both natural and experimental hosts. For example, feline panleukopenia virus has proved to be the cause of spontaneous ataxia of kittens, the commonest neurologic disease of the domestic cat, and a disease long thought to be a genetic disorder (Kilham and Margolis, 1966).

These and other parvoviruses, such as minute virus of mice, replicate only in cells involved in DNA synthesis. This determinant of susceptibility limits infection to dividing cell populations. Mitotic activity is not the sole determinant, however, because some mitotic cells within the brain and extraneural tissues are not susceptible to infection with parvoviruses (Lipton and Johnson, 1972). Nevertheless, this dependence on DNA synthesis explains why in adult cats feline panleukopenia virus infection causes leukopenia and diarrhea, because bone marrow and intestinal cells have high mitotic activity, whereas in the late-gestational fetal kitten the mitotic germinal cells of the cerebellum are also destroyed. In the fetal kitten, lysed hematopoietic or intestinal cells are replaced prior to birth, but the germinal neurons cannot be replenished. The kittens at birth appear normal, because neonates are normally ataxic, but as they fail to achieve smooth motor control, the deficit becomes increasingly obvious, giving the erroneous impression that this is a progressive, degenerative disease.

Lymphocytic choriomeningitis virus inoculated into newborn rats leads to a similar cerebellar hypoplasia (Monjan et al., 1970). This virus also selectively infects the external germinal cell layer, but the mechanism of cell destruction is dependent on immune lysis of infected cells, and the disease can be prevented by immunosuppression. A similar immunopathologic cerebellar hypoplasia with heterotopias can be induced in mice with Tamiami virus, a related arenavirus (Friedman et al., 1975b). Whether induced by cell lysis by parvoviruses or immune-mediated destruction by arenaviruses, the resultant cerebellar hypoplasia shows remarkable pathologic resemblance to cerebellar hypoplasia in man (Sarnat and Alcala, 1980), a disease in which the role of human parvovirus B19 should be sought. Since the inflammatory cells, parvovirus inclusion bodies, and debris of destroyed germinal cells are cleared before clinical ataxia is evident, no pathologic footprints persist to suggest the antecedent infectious process.

Cerebral Anomalies

Selective infection of germinal cells of the forebrain leads to different anomalies. Attenuated live bluetongue virus vaccine produces forebrain lesions in sheep and mice. Bluetongue virus is an arthropod-borne double-stranded RNA virus (orbivirus) that causes an acute respiratory and gastrointestinal disease of adult sheep (Howell and Verwoerd, 1971).

After the disease was recognized in the United States, a live virus vaccine was developed by attenuation of virus in chick embryos, and widespread immunization was carried out in 1955. The attenuated virus appeared to be an excellent vaccine that caused no clinical illness and conferred solid immunity. In the subsequent fall, however, a large number of ewes immunized during pregnancy delivered lambs with noninflammatory cavitary defects of the forebrain (Schultz and DeLay, 1955). Because bluetongue virus grows in the vascular endothelial cells of adult sheep, it was assumed that the vaccine virus produced a vasculitis in the fetus, with infarction of the developing brain and subsequent cavitation (Richards and Cordy, 1967).

Sequential experimental studies showed that this is not the case. Direct intramuscular inoculation of ovine fetuses with the vaccine virus produced consistent malformations. We found that fetuses inoculated at 50 days of their 150-day gestation period developed hydranencephaly, and those inoculated at 75 days of gestation developed porencephaly (Osburn et al., 1971a). Inoculation after 100 days of gestation caused no gross abnormalities, but only microscopic microglial nodules in the brain. The fetal animals cleared virus after this acute infection. Immunostaining showed that infection was localized to the subventricular zone of germinal cells in the forebrain. This cell population lying lateral to the ventricles proliferates and migrates outward, forming the neurons and glia of the cerebral hemispheres. In a first-trimester fetus, infection led to massive necrosis and cavitation of the cerebral hemispheres. By the time of birth, however, the inflammatory response resolved, and the necrotic material was cleared, leaving a noninflammatory cavity that resembled human hydranencephaly. By midgestation, most of the cortical plate has developed, and infection of the germinal cells led to focal encephalitis with resultant cavitation in the white matter. These cavities often communicated with the ventricular system or subarachnoid space, similar to human lesions of porencephaly. Thus, the age dependence of the lesion was determined by the availability of vulnerable immature cells (Osburn et al., 1971b).

Selective infection of the subventricular zone of the forebrain was confirmed in neonatal and late-gestational mice with a mouse-adapted strain of bluetongue virus. Infection of the immature murine nervous system led to symmetrical, partially cavitated forebrain lesions, with predominant involvement of the basal ganglia or olfactory bulbs (Narayan and Johnson, 1972). The germinal cells of the cerebellum were not involved. Cyclophosphamide treatment reduced the lesions, but this resulted from the antimetabolic effect of cyclophosphamide on the dividing and subventricular cells which inhibited virus replication. Thus, inhibition of disease by "immunosuppression" cannot always be glibly interpreted as evidence for an immune-mediated pathogenesis (Narayan et al., 1972).

Cavitary malformations of the forebrain also have been seen after several other natural and experimental arbovirus infections. Hydranencephaly has been related to naturally occurring bunyaviruses including Akabane virus in Australian and Asian cattle, Cache Valley in North American sheep and cattle and to vaccine strains of Rift Valley fever virus (Kurogi et al., 1975; Konno et al., 1982a; Edwards et al., 1989; Calisher and Sever, 1995). Similar lesions have been related to a flavivirus, Wesselsbron virus, in South African sheep (Coetzer and Barnard, 1977). Experimental cavitary lesions of the forebrain resembling porencephaly, as well as microcephaly and hydrocephalus, have been induced by inoculation of fetal monkeys with an alphavirus, Venezuelan equine encephalitis vaccine virus (London et al., 1977), and hydrancephaly or hydrocephalus often associated with arthrogryposis multiplex have been induced with an array of bunyaviruses including Akabane virus in cattle, goats, and chick embryos (Kono et al., 1982b; Kono et al., 1988); Aino virus in chick embryos (Kitano et al., 1996) and Main Drain, San Angelo and LaCrosse viruses in lambs (Edwards et al., 1997). The pathogenesis of the arthrogryposis multiplex or multiple fixed joints may have a central or peripheral basis, because both spinal cord lesions and a concurrent myositis are seen, or result from the restriction of fetal movement by oligohydramnios. The development of multiple fixed joints can result from any lesions that immobilizes the fetus. For example, in chick embryos, arthrogryposis can be produced by removal of spinal cord, infusion of neuromuscular blocking agents, or infection of muscle with a coxsackievirus (Drachman et al., 1976).

Other Anomalies

More widespread infection of immature and germinal cells has been found with fetal infections of the pestiviruses—hog cholera virus, bovine viral diarrhea virus, and border disease virus of sheep. Like rubella virus, these flaviviruses cause variable malformations in their natural host, with more severe lesions after early gestational infection and with persistent infection of the fetal CNS.

Hog cholera virus infections are generally lethal, but hog cholera vaccine virus given to pregnant sows leads to an increased rate of abortions, as well as malformed piglets with congenital tremors (Emerson and Delez, 1967). The brain shows moderate microcephaly, with simplified gyral pattern and marked cerebellar hypoplasia with both granular cell destruction and hypomyelination. Inflammation and necrosis are not found by the time of birth (Johnson et al., 1974a). Bovine viral diarrhea virus, when inoculated during the first trimester, also causes cerebellar hypoplasia in calves; but in sheep, hydranencephaly, porencephaly, hypomyelination, and arthrogryposis can be the outcomes (Barlow et al., 1980). Border disease virus infections of pregnant sheep lead to a congenital deficiency of CNS myelin without evidence of oligodendroglia or myelin destruction and without inflammation. Experimental inoculation of border disease virus into pregnant sheep during the first trimester can cause more dramatic lesions in the lamb, including hydranencephaly, porencephaly, cerebellar hypoplasia, cysts of the septum pellucidum, and arthrogryposis (Barlow,

1980; Potts et al., 1985). Thus, pestivirus infections during early gestation all appear to cause hypomyelination, with hypoplastic development of forebrain and cerebellum, and with each infection, arthrogryposis has been seen, presumably secondary to motor neuron infection.

Virus-induced Hydrocephalus

Hydrocephalus can be produced in experimental animals by a variety of viral infections. Some cause acute selective infection of ependymal cells leading to aqueductal stenosis; others obstruct meningeal spaces and cause communicating hydrocephalus; others cause chronic infections of the parenchyma of the brain, resulting in hydrocephalus ex vacuo (Johnson, 1975a). The aqueductal stenosis following ependymal cell infection is the form that mimics a true malformation.

Our observation that viruses can cause hydrocephalus in fetal or neonatal rodents was a serendipitous finding. In a study of a neuroadapted strain of mumps that caused acute encephalitis in suckling hamsters, wild strains were studied as controls (Johnson, 1968). Although animals inoculated with the wild-type mumps virus showed no evidence of acute clinical disease, virus replication was found in the brain during the first week after inoculation, and viral antigen was limited almost exclusively to ependymal cells lining the ventricular walls and choroid plexus. A perivascular inflammatory reaction accompanied this infection but resolved within 2 weeks. During this infection, the suckling hamsters appeared normal, but 3 to 6 weeks later these animals began losing weight and many showed cranial enlargement. Hydrocephalus with enlargement of the lateral and third ventricles and stenosis or occlusion of the aqueduct of Sylvius was found (Johnson et al., 1967) (Fig. 13.6). By the time clinical disease was manifest, no inflammatory reaction remained; small clusters of ependymal cells often persisted in the area of stenosis or occlusion and formed rosettes or aqueductules; the area normally occupied by the aqueduct was not replaced by glial tissue but contained normal brainstem parenchyma. Indeed, normal tissue appeared to extend between the clusters of residual ependymal cells (Johnson and Johnson, 1968b). Thus, at the time of clinical disease, virus was no longer recoverable, virus antigen was not detectable, the inflammatory response had resolved, and the stenotic aqueduct fulfilled all the histologic criteria proposed in human neuropathology to establish a diagnosis of primary agenesis of the aqueduct of Sylvius (Russell, 1949) (Fig. 13.6).

Subsequent studies of several paramyxoviruses, influenza virus, reovirus 1, an arbovirus (Ross River), and type 1 herpes simplex virus have shown similar selective infection of ependyma with resulting hydrocephalus in a variety of fetal and neonatal laboratory rodents (Johnson and Johnson, 1968b; Chew-Lim and Webb, 1976; Margolis and Kilham, 1969; Mims et al., 1973; Friedman et al., 1975a; Hayashi et al., 1986).

Hydrocephalus has also followed neonatal infection of hamsters and cats with vaccinia virus (Davis, 1981), fetal infection of swine with Japanese encephalitis

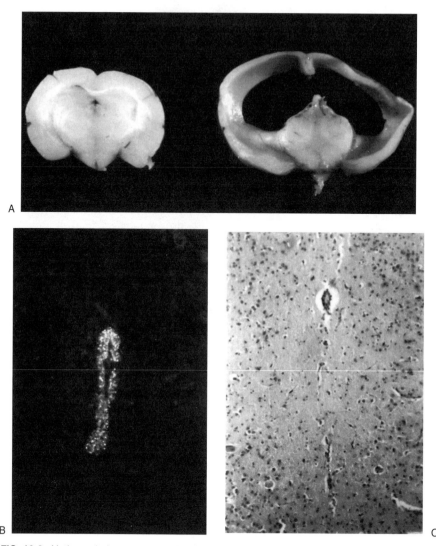

FIG. 13.6. Hydrocephalus as a sequela of viral infection. (A) Gross hydrocephalus shown in a 4-week-old hamster after neonatal infection with mumps virus (right) contrasted with normal brain from a hamster that received virus plus antiserum. (From Johnson et al., 1967, with permission. ©1967 by the American Association for the Advancement of Science.) This results from the selective infection of ependymal cells shown with fluorescent antibody staining of a section through the aqueduct of Sylvius 7 days after neonatal virus inoculation (B). ×100. (From Johnson and Johnson, 1968a, with permission.) Subsequent aqueductal stenosis is shown 4 weeks later (C). The lack of inflammation and gliosis and the small clusters of residual ependymal cells and aqueductules fulfill the criteria for primary agenesis of the aqueduct. ×100.

virus (Shimizu et al., 1954), rhesus monkeys with influenza virus (London et al., 1975), neonatal mice with St. Louis encephalitis virus, and dogs with canine parainfluenza virus (Anderson and Hanson, 1975; Baumgartner et al., 1982). The latter studies and sequential studies of murine paramyxovirus and human respiratory virus in hamsters and mice showed hydrocephalus preceded closure of the aqueduct suggesting that the ependymal infection may be the primary cause of hydrocephalus and the aqueduct closure may be secondary (Lagace-Simar et al., 1980, 1982).

Hydrocephalus can be produced in adult mice with influenza virus, and in contrast to the newborn mice, these animals showed a glial reaction in the area of the aqueductal stenosis that provided a histopathologic clue to the earlier destructive process (Johnson and Johnson, 1972). Thus, in the newborn animal the resemblance of the resultant aqueductal stenosis to a developmental defect apparently results from a different pathologic reaction of the immature animal to the ependymal destruction.

In adult rodents inoculated with mumps virus or small doses of influenza virus, only patches of ependymal cells are destroyed, leading to gaps in the ependyma, with a loose fibrous appearance and areas of gliosis. These histologic changes simulate the granular ependymitis seen as an incidental finding in the majority of adult human brains (Johnson and Johnson, 1972). Since mumps virus commonly invades the CNS even in patients with parotitis and no clinical signs of CNS involvement (Bang and Bang, 1943), mumps virus may well be a cause of this granular ependymitis. In occasional persons, sufficient ependymitis might lead to hydrocephalus.

Subsequent to the animal studies, a number of children were reported with hydrocephalus following mumps virus infections (Johnson, 1975a; Spataro et al., 1976; Thompson, 1979). These children have ranged from 6 to 11 years of age at the time of mumps infection and have developed aqueductal stenosis 5 weeks to 4 years thereafter. Further evidence that mumps virus may cause aqueductal stenosis has been obtained through electron microscopic examination of spinal fluid sediment in patients with mumps meningitis. The sediment contains numerous ependymal cells, and in many instances, these cells contain cytoplasmic tubules consistent with mumps virus nucleocapsids. In other diseases, ependymal cells in spinal fluid are rare (Herndon et al., 1974). The clinical observations and the demonstration that mumps virus selectively infects ependymal cells in man provide circumstantial evidence implicating mumps virus as a cause of acquired hydrocephalus in childhood. Whether mumps can cross the placenta and cause ependymal cell destruction of the fetus is unknown.

Problems Relating Similar Human Malformations to Viral Infections

The average pregnancy is attended by several viral infections, and attempts to associate such banal maternal infections with birth defects in the infant pose formidable problems (Johnson, 1979). The associations of rubella virus, cytomegaloviruses, and HIV with birth defects were relatively straightforward. Rubella is an epidemic disease with stereotyped clinical signs, the rate of malformations following maternal infection is high, and the newborn with the rubella syndrome presents a rather stereotyped constellation of abnormalities. Thus, Gregg's association of cataracts and heart disease in infants with early gestational epidemic rubella among mothers was feasible as an astute clinical observation. Cytomegaloviruses were recognized as causes of birth defects because of the high rate of disease among newborns, representing 1% of infant deaths, and the characteristic pathologic features, with cytomegalic cells, inclusion bodies, and inflammation that pointed to the viral cause. Because both rubella and cytomegaloviruses persist after fetal infection; recovery of virus and identification of virions or antigens in lesions of the newborn allow unequivocal association of the virus with the lesions. The epidemic nature of HIV and the immunodeficiency in mother and baby with fatal courses made the association possible even before the recovery of the virus.

Relating intrauterine herpesvirus infections with rare malformations has been possible because of very characteristic syndromes. The infants in whom intrauterine herpes simplex virus infections have been related to microcephaly, calcification of atrophic cerebral hemispheres, microophthalmia, and chorioretinitis have had postnatal vesicular rashes from which herpes simplex virus was recovered. The infants in whom intrauterine varicella-zoster virus infections have been related to malformations have had mothers with unmistakable histories of chickenpox during pregnancy, and the cicatricial lesion and limb hypoplasia in a unique zosteriform pattern.

From studies of natural and experimental viral infections in animals, we know that other mechanisms may produce malformations. In many of these infections, no persistence of virus and no pathologic features are present at the time of clinical disease to provide a clue to an antecedent infection. If, in humans, a single virus on rare occasions produces malformations, but these malformations are variable, depending on gestational age of infection (as in bluetongue vaccine virus infections in sheep), or if a single malformation is a rare complication of many different viral infections (as hydrocephalus due to many viruses), association of the malformation with the infection might defy present investigative methods.

SUPPLEMENTARY BIBLIOGRAPHY

Remington JS and Klein JO (Editors) (1995): Infectious Diseases of the Fetus and Newborn Infant. 4th Edition. W.B. Saunders, Philadelphia.
Johnson RT and Lyon G (Editors) (1988): Viral Infections and the Developing Nervous System. Kluwer, Dondrecht.

14

Degenerative Diseases and Prions

Sir,- While attempts to draw too close an analogy between diseases of man and lower animals are attended by numerous pitfalls, many valuable clues contributing to the understanding of the fundamental nature of a disease can be gained from a broad comparative viewpoint. . .

Thus, it might be profitable in view of veterinary experience with scrapie to examine the possibility of the experimental induction of kuru in a laboratory primate, for one might surmise that the pathogenetic mechanisms involved in scrapie—however unusual they may be—are unlikely to be unique in the problems of animal pathology.

William J. Hadlow,
Scrapie and Kuru, letter to the editor of Lancet, 1959

These statements open and close a modest letter directing attention to the remarkable similarities between the epidemiological, clinical, and pathologic features of scrapie and kuru. Hadlow also called attention to the experimental transmission of scrapie to the dairy goat and suggested the analogous use of subhuman primates to study kuru. These observations provoked the studies of Gajdusek and Gibbs that led to the transmission of the first slow infection of man. The contributions of comparative medicine and pathology to the seminal advances on slow infections of humans were further exemplified when the pathologic comparisons of the neuronal changes of kuru and Creutzfeldt-Jakob disease provided impetus to pursue transmission studies of the latter disease.

The agents of scrapie, kuru, and Creutzfeldt-Jakob disease are grouped under the name prions or subacute spongiform encephalopathy agents. Here we enter the "twilight zone" of microbiology to deal with agents that probably contain no nucleic acid, whose infectivity or expression is based on an abnormal isoform of a normal cell protein, and whose physicochemical properties boggle the traditional virologist. They probably should not be classified as viruses, and I considered editing them out of this volume; however prions are transmissible, their infectivity is amplified in the host animal, and they do produce fascinating diseases.

SCRAPIE

Shepherds have recognized this progressive degenerative disease of sheep for over 200 years. The disease is widespread among sheep in Europe, Asia, and the Americas and among goats co-habitating with affected sheep. Although it is known by many names, the Scottish term scrapie is now generally used. Scrapie is restricted to certain flocks, and new outbreaks often are related to the introduction of breeding stock from scrapie flocks; this led to the long-standing assumption that scrapie was a heritable disease.

The natural disease is seen in sheep over 2 years of age, the onset is insidious, with apparent cutaneous irritation that leads to the rubbing of fleece against a fixed object—hence the name scrapie. Affected sheep become hyperexcitable and show behavioral changes and tremors, but the most prominent sign is a relentlessly progressive ataxia that leads to death in 6 weeks to 6 months. During the course of the disease, the sheep remain afebrile, and no pleocytosis is found. Remissions are never seen. Pathologic changes are limited to the CNS, where neuronal loss, cytoplasmic vacuolization of degenerating neurons, and a striking astrocytosis are found in gray matter (Beck et al., 1964). In the natural disease these findings are most prominent in the cerebellar cortex, pontobulbar nuclei, midbrain, and diencephalon.

The "established" genetic nature of the disease was corroborated by elaborate genealogical studies that indicated an autosomal recessive transmission. Nevertheless, two French investigators (Cuille and Chelle, 1936) had the Gaulic audacity to transmit the disease, and they even showed the filterability of the transmissible agent. Thereafter, the mode of natural transmission was hotly debated for many years, with those supporting the genetic transmission of scrapie finally accepting the experimental transmission, but maintaining that natural transmission was vertical (Parry, 1962). Convincing evidence has been obtained that field transmission occurs with intimate contact of young sheep and infected flocks. In retrospect, clear-cut genetic differences in susceptibility between different breeds explain some of the early discrepancies.

Laboratory studies of scrapie have been facilitated since 1961, when Chandler experimentally transmitted the disease to mice. More recently, the hamster has been used because of a higher level of infectivity and a shorter incubation period, but the lack of a tissue culture assay system for quantitation has meant that mice and hamsters remain the mainstays of experimental work. The incubation period in these rodents is from 3 to 9 months, and considering the number of animals necessary for titrations, studies of pathogenesis and of the physicochemical properties of the agent have required heroic patience and effort.

Pathogenesis

The pathogenesis of scrapie has been investigated in sheep and goats, but is best delineated in mice. In naturally infected sheep, infectivity is found first in lymphatic tissue and intestines at about 1 year of age, which suggests infection of lambs by the alimentary tract. Infection of the nervous system is not found until 2 years of age, and thereafter infectivity increases until clinical disease evolves about 1 year later (Hadlow et al., 1979).

In mice, variations in incubation period, topography of pathologic lesions, and the infectivity titers depend both on the strain of the agent and on the genetic background of the host (Dickinson and Fraser, 1977). After experimental extraneural inoculation of mice, the earliest replication is found in the spleen and lymphoreticular organs (Eklund et al., 1967), and the incubation period is prolonged in splenectomized animals. After several months, infectivity is found in the CNS, where it slowly increases for 4 to 6 months until the development of clinical disease. Clinical disease appears to develop when a specific concentration of the agent is reached in the brain. Furthermore, after inoculation in the hind leg or foreleg, the lumbar or cervical cord will show initial infection, respectively, which suggests spread along neural pathways to the nervous system (Kimberlin and Walker, 1980). By manipulating the variables of genetic susceptibility of different mice and particular strains of the agent, "incubation periods longer than life" can be documented; that is, infectivity continues to increase into senescence without reaching the threshold for clinical disease before death from old age intervenes (Dickinson et al., 1975).

The pathologic findings in mice resemble those in sheep, with neuronal loss, astrocytosis, and total absence of an inflammatory response. Ultrastructural studies show that the vacuoles are in the cytoplasm of neurons and glial cells and contain only amorphous material or fragments and loops of membranes (Lampert et al., 1972). Neuronal death is probably due to apoptosis which may explain the absence of inflammation (Giese et al., 1995).

Neutralizing antibody is not detected in the natural or experimental disease, and the incubation period and disease cannot be altered with immunosuppression or immunopotentiation. B and T cell functions are normal in scrapie-infected animals. The responses to intercurrent infections in scrapie-infected animals are unaltered, and other infections fail to attenuate or interfere with the inexorable course of scrapie.

Properties of the Scrapie Agent

In addition to the extraordinarily long, genetically determined incubation period, the unique noninflammatory degenerative abnormality, the lack of demonstrable virions, and the apparent total lack of antigenicity, the physical-chemical properties of the infectious agent are highly unusual (Table 14.1).

The resistance of scrapie infectivity to UV irradiation, nuclease and extremes of pH had long led to heretical speculations that the scrapie agent might not contain a nucleic acid and a self replication protein had been suggested (Anonymous, 1967). In 1981 Prusiner colocalized infectivity with a 27 to 30 K protein and coined the term prion "to denote a small proteinaceous infectious particle which is

TABLE 14.1. *Stability of the scrapie agent*

Relative resistant to	Inactivated by
Formaldehyde	Autoclaving (121°C 2 kg/cm^2)
Ethanol	Extremes of pH (<2 or >10)
Alkylating agents (such as β-propiolactone)	Chaotropic agents (such as phenol)
Proteases	Inorganic salts (strong solution of soluble salts)
Nucleases	Detergents (such as sodium dodecyl sulfate)
Heat (80°C) (moderate stability at 100°C)	
Ultraviolet and ionizing radiation	

resistent to inactivation by most procedures that modify nucleic acids" (Prusiner, 1982). The resistance of this protein to digestion with proteinase K distinguished it from similar sized proteins in normal brain. The protein was also found to be the major constituent of the amyloid-like birefringent fibrils or prion rods that were specific to spongiform encephalopathies. The quantity of the novel protein in general correlated with titer of infectivity, the protein colocalized with plaques and astrocytosis, copurified with infectivity and was absent in uninfected brains; procedures that denature, hydrolyse or modify proteins decreased infectivity. Thus, it appeared that this proteinase resistant prion protein was the scrapie agent, or a major component of the agent (Prusiner, 1987). It was therefore a surprise to find that the prion protein was coded by a chromosomal gene (PRNP). The normal isoform (PrP^c) is a proteinase sensitive membrane glycoprotein; in the pathologic process it appears to undergo post-translational modification to a proteinase resistant isoform (PrP^{sc}) that can transmit disease (Oesch et al., 1985) (Table 14.2). PrP^c

TABLE 14.2. *Normal and abnormal forms of prion protein*

	Normal	Abnormal
Term	PrP^c	PrP^{sc}
Protease K	Sensitive	Resistant
Detergent extraction	Soluble	Amyloid fibrils or rods formed
Size	Monomeric (22–36 kD)	Macromolecular aggregates (>400 s)
Form	High α-helix content	High β-sheet content
Location	Cell surface glycoprotein	Intracellular vesicles and extracellular space
Tissue	Brain, heart, lung, activated lymphocytes	Spongiform brain and lymphoid
Concentration in normal hamster brain	~1–5 µg/g	0
Concentration in scrapie infected hamster brain	~1–5 µg/g	5–10 µg/g
Synthesis (t$_{1/2}$/hr)	<0.1	1–3
Degradation (t$_{1/2}$/hr)	~5	>24
Cell lines	Most positive	Scrapie-infected organs, neuroblastomas, and pheochromocytoma cells

PrP, prion protein.
Modified from Chesebro and Fields (1996), Prusiner (1991), and Prusiner et al. (1996).

has a secondary structure that contains 43% α helix and less than 1% β-sheets, whereas PrP^{sc} has a β-sheet content of 43% and an α helix content of 30% (Pan et al., 1993). The insoluable PrP^{sc} accumulates in brain and comprises the amyloid plaques, and accumulation correlates topographically with the astrocytosis.

The species barriers have been partially explained with transgenic mice expressing human or hamster PrP (Prusiner et al., 1996). Recent evidence that the conformation of PrP^{sc} functions as a template in the formation of nascent PrP^{sc} may explain strains of prions (Telling et al., 1996).

The conservation of PrP^c across species led to the assumption that this membrane protein was critical in neuronal function, yet knockout mice without PRNP appeared normal. More important scrapie can not be transmitted to these mice, unequivocally establishing that PrP is necessary for the development of scrapie. Furthermore, scrapie prions will not even spread along neural pathways to susceptible PrP^c expressing neuroectoclonal grafts in these knockout mice (Brandner et al., 1996). The question remains whether or not PrP^c is sufficient (Prusiner et al., 1993). Transgenic animals that overexpress PrP or that have mutations in PRNP develop spongiform changes, but fail to develop high titers of PrP^{sc} (Hsiao et al., 1991). Transgenic mice overexpressing PrP develop a curious complex of a necrotizing myopathy, a demyelinating polyneuritis and focal vacuolation of the CNS, and the development of disease is dependent on transgene dosage. The subsequent transmission of spongiform encephalopathy to hamsters with brain extracts of these transgenic mice is powerful evidence against the role of a foreign nucleic acid (Prusiner, 1996).

The recent *in vitro* conversion of PrP^c to PrP^{sc} in cell cultures further supports the "protein only" hypothesis, but eliminating any possibility of nucleic acid contamination is difficult (Bessen et al., 1995). Therefore, despite the growing weight of evidence for a "protein only" transmissible agent a persistent skepticism remains in some laboratories where nucleic acids, viruslike particles and other evidence for a more conventional agent continue to be sought (Özel et al., 1994; Manuelidis et al., 1995).

KURU

Kuru is a degenerative disease of the brain limited to a remote tribe of people in the mountains of eastern New Guinea (Fig. 14.1). It is a disease that most readers will never see, since it is disappearing even in its endemic focus. Nevertheless, kuru has had a unique impact as the first slow infection established in humans and as a disease that has overturned fundamental concepts in neurology and virology.

In the 1950s stories of a residual focus of von Economo disease with postinfectious parkinsonism had filtered out of the eastern highlands of New Guinea, an area where the Melanesian natives were just evolving from the Stone Age. Drawn by these stories, Carleton Gajdusek accompanied Vincent Zigas into this region inhabited by the Fore linguistic group, who still lived in barricaded vil-

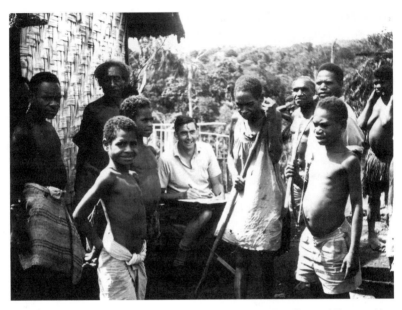

FIG. 14.1. Kuru among the Fore of New Guinea. A woman in the village of Osuna with severe truncal ataxia and little, if any, dementia. She is being examined by Dr. Richard Hornabrook in 1964. (Photograph by the author; reproduced from Johnson and Johnson, 1969 with permission.)

lages and practiced witchcraft and ritual cannibalism. There they found and described this extraordinary disease that had reached endemic proportions probably unequalled in history (Gajdusek and Zigas, 1957).

The population of the Fore district was just over 35,000, and the yearly incidence rate for kuru was approximately 1% of the entire population. Kuru affected all ages beyond infants and toddlers, but was most common in adult women. The disease was less common in children, but of equal frequency in boys and girls, and was least common in adult men. This excess of deaths among young adult females led, in some villages, to populations where men outnumbered women 3 to 1. A few cases were seen in neighboring tribal groups who had intermarried with the Fore.

Disease Description

Kuru means shivering or trembling in the Fore language. The disease followed a stereotyped pattern that began insidiously with truncal titubations and ataxia in an otherwise healthy person. Ataxia became increasingly severe, until the slightest voluntary movement led to violent uncontrolled atactic movements. Although these movements resembled chorea or myoclonus, they ceased when the patient was completely at rest. Nystagmus was generally absent, although disorders of conjugate gaze did appear late in the disease. In the terminal stage, muscle weakness and wasting and dementia were common, but sensory loss or prominent pyramidal tract signs were absent (Hornabrook, 1968). No remission or recovery was ever documented. Although patients were diligently cared for by their families, ataxia interfered with eating and all voluntary movement. Deaths occurred 3 to 24 months after the onset, not infrequently when slight movements during the night caused the victims to roll into the fire and suffer fatal burns.

During the course of the disease, the patients remained afebrile, and the spinal fluid showed no abnormalities. Electroencephalograms showed no specific abnormalities. Pathologic changes included gross cerebellar atrophy and microscopic neuronal loss, with neuronal vacuolization, astrocytosis, and no inflammation. Granular cell loss was most striking, but neuronal loss in brainstem, thalamus, basal ganglia, and cortex also was evident. Some patients had PAS-positive plaques of the abnormal isoform of PrP, so-called kuru plaques (Lampert et al., 1972; Hainfellner et al., 1997).

Transmission of Kuru

Although an infection or postinfectious process was initially suspected, the slow afebrile progression of the disease, the absence of abnormal laboratory findings, and the noninflammatory degenerative histopathologic abnormalities directed attention of toxic, dietary, or genetic causes (Gajdusek and Zigas, 1959). Hadlow's recognition of the similarities of kuru in humans and scrapie in sheep redirected investigations. Scrapie tends to be confined to a particular flock, but it occurs in other flocks with the introduction of breeding stock. Both diseases begin as progressive cerebellar ataxia that leads to death in the absence of any evidence of inflammation, and the pathologic changes are virtually identical. Therefore, a laboratory was established at the National Institutes of Health to inoculate tissues from patients with kuru and a variety of other chronic diseases into chimpanzees and other subhuman primates.

Transmission of kuru to the chimpanzee, the first demonstration of a slow infection of humans, was reported by Gajdusek and associates in 1966. Initial disease appeared in chimpanzees after an incubation period of 14 to 82 months, and serial transmission reduced the incubation period to 10 to 18 months. The disease was subsequently transmitted to a variety of New World and Old World monkeys. The disease in the chimpanzee recapitulates the disease in humans with remarkable fidelity. Furthermore, the agent can be transmitted by peripheral inoculation and is present not only in brain but also in kidney, lymph nodes, and spleen. The highest concentrations, however, are found in the brains of patients, which may contain more than 10^8 infectious doses per gram.

The properties of the kuru agent have been studied less extensively than those of scrapie. Filterability, lack of immunogenicity, inability to visualize the agent with the electron microscope, and resistance to ultraviolet light, gamma radiation, formalin, heat, etc., are similar to the findings for the scrapie agent. Sera from patients with natural disease or animals with transmitted disease have no neutralizing effect on infectivity.

Cannibalism and Kuru

In the early 1960s the incidence of kuru began decreasing, particularly among the children, and, indeed, children with kuru have not been seen since 1970. The decline in adults also became evident and has continued until the present time. In retrospect, this decline is clearly associated with the suppression of ritual endocannibalism (Gajdusek, 1977). Although transmission by cannibalism was suspected early, the discarding of the hypothesis for an infectious cause made it seem unimportant. Gajdusek (1963) did suggest the possibility of a hypersensitivity disease resulting from childhood consumption of human tissues. Glasse (1967), an anthropologist, documented the remarkable correlations of the practice of ritual cannibalism with the distribution of the disease. The body of a family member was consumed largely by female relatives, with adult males rarely participating. However, children, irrespective of sex, shared in the ritual with their mother. Furthermore, stories gleaned from the elders indicated that kuru had followed the introduction of cannibalism to the area, and the incidence of kuru varied between specific hamlets and correlated with the practice of cannibalism. Some neighboring groups who practiced endocannibalism only rarely had cases of kuru; these people regarded kuru as a contagious disease, however, and did not consume the victims; in contrast, the Fore believed kuru resulted from sorcery.

Children as young as 4 years of age had been seen with the disease in the late 1950s and early 1960s, and rare women have been seen with the disease during the past decade. Forty years have passed since the suppression of cannibalism, so the incubation period appears to range from 4 to more than 30 years. The absence of new childhood cases, despite the fact that women with the disease bore, suckled, and reared children, indicates a remarkable lack of communicability and a lack of vertical transmission. The actual inoculation of cells into conjunctiva, oral lesions, or topical sores during the ritual mourning rites may have been crucial in transmission.

CREUTZFELDT-JAKOB DISEASE

Creutzfeldt-Jakob disease is a presenile dementia characterized by rapidly progressive mental deterioration, myoclonic jerking, and other inconstant neurologic signs. The nosology of the disease is confused; the patient described by Creutzfeldt and 3 of the 5 patients described by Jakob would not meet present clinical or pathologic criteria for the disease (Masters and Gajdusek, 1982). Furthermore, differences in presentation, neurologic signs, and topographies of lesions have been described under an array of other eponyms. The transmission to experimental animals and the induction of a uniform clinical-pathologic syndrome in these animals have led to consolidation of clinical syndromes under the accepted misnomer of Creutzfeldt-Jakob disease.

The incidence of the disease is 0.5 to 1.0 per million per year with little annual, seasonal or geographic variation (Holman et al., 1995). Alleged clusters have usually been explained by familial cases, that account for 8 to 10% of the cases of Creutzfeldt-Jakob disease (Raubertas et al., 1989). A higher incidence has been reported for urban areas than for rural areas (Brown et al., 1987a).

Disease Description

Creutzfeldt-Jakob disease most commonly begins between 55 and 70 years of age, but it has been described in a patient of 16 years and several times in patients in their eighties. In general familial cases begin at an earlier age than sporadic cases (Roos et al., 1973). As in subacute sclerosing panencephalitis, the progression of disease can be divided into 3 stages. A prodromal period often occurs; one third of patients complain of vague nonlocalizing symptoms of fatigue, insomnia, and decreased appetite; one third begin with neurologic complaints of forgetfulness, confusion, or uncharacteristic behavior; and one-third begin with focal neurologic symptoms such as ataxia, aphasia or visual loss. In some patients, visual loss, aphasia, or hemiparesis may develop in less than a week, or even in less than 24 hrs, suggesting cerebrovascular disease.

The subsequent inexorable progression of the disease is fairly stereotyped. The dementia is remarkable, with dissolution of intellect from week to week, or even day to day, leading to severe dementia within 6 months of onset. This dementia is associated with a galaxy of abnormal signs. The most characteristic and constant sign is myoclonus, which is often stimulus-sensitive. In addition, ataxia, blindness, amyotrophy, choreoathetosis, and pyramidal tract signs are seen with variable frequency (Brown et al., 1994b). The typical case is readily recognized, but the patients with sudden onset of focal signs, the patients in whom amyotrophy is a prominent early feature and in whom dementia occurs later, and the patients in whom cerebellar ataxia or severe choreoathetosis mask the myoclonus pose problems in clinical diagnosis. In the late stage of the disease, the patient is mute and demented, and the myoclonic jerking may disappear with the dissolution of neural function. Mean survival is only 5 months; over 80% of patients die within 12 months of onset, although some patients have lingered for up to 8 years. The amyotrophic form of disease accounts for only about 5% of patients, poses the greatest difficulty in diagnosis, and accounts for most of the cases surviving over 2 years (Will and Matthews, 1984).

The spinal fluid usually is normal, although mild elevation of protein is occasionally found. Recently two proteins have been detected by immunoassay or electrophoresis of spinal fluids of patients with Creutzfeldt-Jakob disease which are relatively sensitive and specific, at least in differentiating the disease from other chronic noninflammatory dementing illnesses (Hsich et al., 1996; Zerr et al., 1996). The electroencephalogram shows diffuse slowing, and paroxysmal sharp-wave complexes are common and are characteristic, but not pathogno-monic, for the disease.

Pathologically, moderate to severe cerebral atrophy is evident, with widened sulci. The histopathologic hallmarks are the same as for other spongiform encephalopathies, neuronal loss, astrocytosis, and cytoplasmic vacuolization of neurons and astrocytes causing status spongiosis. Inflammation is absent at all stages. Prion protein immunoreactivity may be found in a diffuse synaptic pat-tern or in a patchy perivascular distribution or in plaques when present (Budka et al., 1995).

Topographically, the frontal cerebral cortex usually shows the most evident change, but in some cases neuronal loss is greater in anterior horn cells (amy-otrophic form), the cerebellum (Brownell-Oppenheimer variant), or the parietal and occipital lobes (Heidenhein's disease), which accounts for corresponding clinical symptoms. Plaques, similar to those seen in kuru and scrapie, are found in about 5% with sporadic Creutzfeldt-Jakob disease (Brown et al., 1994b). The degree of spongiform change is variable and appears to represent an early stage of pathologic change, because biopsies or autopsies early in the disease show more vacuolization than is seen in brains examined in later stages (Masters and Richardson, 1978). Vacuoles apparently collapse and disappear with neuronal loss. Electron microscopy shows the vacuoles to be intracytoplasmic and to con-tain proteinaceous granules and curled or fragmented membranes, as in scrapie and kuru.

Laboratory Transmission

The sporadic distribution of the disease, the familial forms, the absence of clinical signs of infection, and the histopathologic findings made a viral cause highly improbable. In 1968, Van Rossum, wrote that "exogenous factors play no part in this pathogenesis." However, in the original pathologic study of kuru, in which kuru was ascribed to a genetic error in metabolism modified by hormonal factors, the histopathologic charges were said to be "the closest in resemblance to Creutzfeldt-Jakob disease" (Klatzo et al., 1959). With the transmission of kuru, interest focused on Creutzfeldt-Jakob disease, despite its different epi-demiologic and clinical features.

In 1968, a chimpanzee developed ataxia, hemiparesis, and myoclonus 13 months after inoculation and died 2 months later (Gibbs et al., 1968). Brain tis-sues from more than 300 patients now have transmitted the disease with most exhibiting a somewhat shorter incubation period than kuru (11 to 17 months). Experimentally infected chimpanzees develop apparent confusion, myoclonic jerking, amyotrophy, and an unremitting progression to a moribund state. Fur-thermore, brain tissues from 36 members of familial pedigrees have induced the disease in primates. The disease has been transmitted to New World and Old World monkeys, the cat, the guinea pig, and the mouse but at lower frequency than chimpanzees; goats and sheep have been refractory to primary transmission. Transgenic mice with a human PrP sequence may prove to be the host of choice for isolation and treatment studies in the future (Telling et al., 1994). As in kuru and scrapie, infectivity is not limited to the CNS; infectivity is found in liver, spleen, lung, kidney, lymph nodes, cornea, and vitreous and lens but not in skin, muscle, urine, or sputum. Disease was transmitted twice from human spinal fluid and from blood of experimentally infected guinea pigs and mice. No humoral or cell-mediated immune responses against the agent have been found.

Mode of Natural Transmission

The mode of natural transmission of Creutzfeldt-Jakob disease remains a mystery. A cluster of cases among Libyan Jews in Israel originally was ascribed to their practice of eating eyeballs of sheep, but this is now recognized as a familial clustering. Case-controlled studies have variably (and weakly) implicated consumption of hog brains (Bobowick et al., 1973), surgery and trauma (Kondo and Kuroiwa, 1982); pork, ham and hot dogs (Davanipour et al., 1985b); tonometry (Davanipour et al., 1985a); and (my favorite advice) abstinence from alcohol, eating tripe and keeping pet ferrets (Harries-Jones et al., 1988). In sum, these studies provide scant evidence for a common risk factor (Wientjens et al., 1996). The development of Creutzfeldt-Jakob disease in one prominent neurosurgeon led to anxiety regarding the occupational hazards of caring for patients with the disease, but little correlation with occupation, particularly the lack of excess cases in health workers, butchers, abattoir workers or housekeepers subject to knife wounds during food preparation. Lack of communicability, in the usual sense, is also evidenced by the lack of temporal or geographic clustering of cases and by the lack of confirmed conjugal cases (Matthews, 1975; Hainfellner et al., 1996).

Familial Cases

About 10% of persons with Creutzfeldt-Jakob disease have a family history consistent with an autosomal dominant inheritance. In most, but not all, of these kindreds point mutations or insertions are found in the gene (PRNP) coding for the prion protein. In humans the gene is located on the short arm of chromosome 20. Twenty different insertions or mutations have been associated with human prion diseases (Fig. 14.2). The phenotypes of the familial cases vary but, in general, have an early age of onset and in some cases a distinctive clinical presentation and prolonged clinical course with longer survivals.

The Gerstmann-Sträussler-Scheinker syndrome is an example of a variant so unlike Creutzfeldt-Jakob disease that it was considered a distinct disease. This autosomal dominant illness is characterized by chronic cerebellar ataxia with many amyloid plaques throughout the brain. Dementia, pyramidal tract signs and spongiform changes are frequent but not invariable (Masters et al., 1981). The prominent cerebellar and pyramidal tract signs have led to its classification as a

51			
	insertions	CJD 5, 6, and 7 repeats	US, England, Spain
		GSS 8 repeats	French - Breton
91			
102		GSS with prominent ataxia	Hungary, France, Germany, US, England, Italy, Japan
105		CJD with spastic paraparesis	Japan
117		GSS with prominent dementia	France, Japan, US
129		Normal silent polymorphism (homozygocity determines susceptibility and phenotype)	
145		GSS	Japan
178		FFI and FCJD (dependent on 129)	Italy, France, Finland, US, Japan, Australia, Spain, Netherlands, Venezuela
180		CJD	Japan
183		CJD	Brazil
198		GSS	US and Sweden
200		FCJD (and FFI)	Israel, Chile, Slovakia, France, Japan, Spain, England, US, Canada
208		CJD	United States
210		CJD	France, Italy, United States, Canada, Taiwan
217		GSS with neurofibrillar tangles	US
232		CJD	

(Note: left column labeled vertically "5 octapeptide repeats" spanning 51–91)

FIG. 14.2. Diagram of the PRNP gene showing sites of insertions and mutations found in human prion diseases. CJD, Creutzfeldt-Jakob disease; FCJD, familial with sufficient subjects for linkage; GSS, Gerstmann-Sträussler-Scheinker disease; FFI, fatal familial insomnia. Bold face are those discussed in text. (Data from Mastrianni et al., 1996 and Larisa Cerveakova and C.J. Gibbs, Laboratory of CNS Studies, National Institute of Neurological Disorders and Stroke.)

spinocerebellar degeneration, and the occasional presence of numerous neurofibrillary tangles along with the plaques (albeit, plaques immunoreactive to prion protein) can lead to confusion with Alzheimer's disease (Ghetti et al., 1989). Mean age at death is only 48 years, and mean duration of disease is 5 years with survivals up to 11 years. Clinical and pathologic heterogeneity is found even within an affected family (Hainfellner et al., 1995). The disease has been transmitted to subhuman primates and rodents. In 1989 a mutation at codon

102 of the prion protein gene was linked to the disease (Hsiao et al., 1989). Subsequently mutations at other codons have been associated with this phenotype; PrP amyloid plaques are common with mutations at codon 102 and neocortical neurofibrillar tangles with mutations at codon 217 (Hsiao et al., 1992).

In the same year an insertion of 5 extra copies of the octapeptide repeats was reported in a family of typical familial Creutzfeldt-Jakob disease (Owen et al., 1989). Since then an array of insertions and point mutations have been described in kindreds with varied phenotypes and geographic origins (Fig 14.2). Insertions in the unstable region of 5 variant tandem octapeptide coding repeats, in general, has correlated with typical Creutzfeldt-Jakob disease, but the number of repeats (5 to 9 extras) has not been correlated with disease course (Goldfarb et al., 1991a). Persons with 4 octapeptide inserts have been described without neurologic disease and with typical disease (Campbell et al., 1996).

The mutation at codon 200 has clarified several prior epidemiologic studies. Clusters of disease among Libyan Jews in Israel, and in populations in Slovakia and Chile, had all been investigated for possible dietary or other explanations. Each of these clusters now is explained by familial disease due to this mutation (Hsiao et al., 1991; Goldfarb et al., 1991b).

A single amino acid shift at codon 178 has been associated with several kindreds with fatal familial insomnia and with numerous kindreds of Creutzfeldt-Jakob disease, characterized by long courses and an absence of typical periodic bursts on the electroencephalogram. Fatal familial insomnia is a curious prion disease; characterized by progressive insomnia, dysautonomia and dementia leading to death in 7 to 15 months. At autopsy atrophy of the ventral and mediodorsal thalamic nuclei indicate this is a variant of thalamic dementia. Because of the variable presence of spongiform changes brains were examined and found to be immunoreactive to prion protein, and a point mutation in the prion protein gene at codon 178 was found (Medori et al., 1992).

Familial thalamic dementias have been divided into those with and without multiple system atrophy. Three of 4 families with selective thalamic dementia showed the mutation at codon 178, and none of the kindreds with multiple system atrophy had the defect (Petersen et al., 1992). Tissues of some kindreds of fatal familial insomnia have been transmitted to rodents. To explain the same genetic alteration in two very different phenotypes the polymorphism at codon 129 was examined; the methionine allele segregated with fatal familial insomnia and the valine with familial Creutzfeldt-Jakob disease. Thus, two distinct phenotypes linked to a single mutation may be determined by a common polymorphism (Goldfarb et al., 1992).

The polymorphism at codon 129 also is important in sporadic Creutzfeldt-Jakob disease. The sporadic cases are not associated with mutations in the prion protein gene but almost 90% of cases are homozygous at the polymorphic amino-acid residue 129, whereas half of the normal population is heterozygous at this site. Homozygosity appears to be an important determinant of susceptibility to sporadic and iatrogenic disease, and the nature of the homozygosity may modulate the phenotype of disease (Palmer et al., 1991; Parchi et al., 1996; MacDonald et al., 1996).

Iatrogenic cases

Creutzfeldt-Jakob disease is clearly transmissible, not only in the laboratory but in the clinic. Inadvertent transmission of the disease to patients by physicians has occurred with tissue transplantation, contaminated instruments, and the administration of hormones prepared from contaminated human pituitaries (Table 14.3).

The first report of iatrogenic transmission was that of a corneal transplant recipient who also developed rapidly progressive Creutzfeldt-Jakob disease 18 months after receiving a cornea from a patient who had died of the disease, which was undiagnosed premortem (Duffy et al., 1974). Only one subsequent transmission by corneal transplant has been reported. In contrast, since 1988 more than 60 cases of Creutzfeldt-Jakob disease have been seen 16 months to 12 years after dural grafts of cadaveric origin were placed (Clavel and Clavel, 1996), and two cases have been reported after extracranial injection of dura mater for embolization (Antoine et al., 1997).

Instruments probing cerebral tissue have been implicated. Two young patients developed the disease about 2 years after stereotactic electroencephalography during surgery for excision of epileptogenic foci (Bernouilli et al., 1977); silver recording electrodes, previously implanted in a patient with Creutzfeldt-Jakob disease, had been sterilized with 70% alcohol and formaldehyde vapor (techniques now known to be ineffective for inactivation of the agent); later retrieval of the same electrodes and placement into chimpanzees led to transmission. A number of other patients have had prior cranial surgery; in one review of the disease, three of the patients had been operated on by the same neurosurgeon in the same unit within a period of 8 months (Nevin et al., 1960). Thus, the physicians' concern in managing these patients should not be focused on his or her risk of contracting the disease but on his or her risk of transmitting it to other patients.

TABLE 14.3. Transmission of spongiform encephalopathy from human to human

Transmission mode	Examples
Intracranial transplant or inoculation	Dural grafts
	Inadequately sterilized surgical instruments
	Stereotactic electrodes
Extracranial transplant	Corneal graft
Extraneural inoculation of neural tissue	Human growth hormone and gonadotropin
Extraneural inoculation or oral exposure to neural and extraneural tissue	Ritual cannibalism (kuru)

Modified from Johnson (1996c).

In 1985 three young adults developed Creutzfeldt-Jakob disease in the United States; each had been the recipient of multiple injections of human growth hormone extracted from cadaveric pituitary glands. Reports of similar cases soon appeared from the United Kingdom and New Zealand. In the United States alone 10,000 children received the human product between 1963 and 1985; lots of the growth hormone and gonadotropin contained 500 to 20,000 human glands per lot. The potential for a major outbreak of disease was alarming (Brown et al., 1985). The growth hormone and gonadotropin made from human glands was withdrawn, and a recombinant growth hormone was quickly approved for use. Only 16 cases have been reported in the United States, 25 in the United Kingdom, 53 in France and scattered cases elsewhere (Bilette de Vilemeur et al., 1996), but reports are becoming less frequent suggesting the peak of the outbreak is past (Markus et al., 1992). The minimum incubation periods of these cases has been 4 to 19 years; the maximum is unknown (Brown, 1988). The clinical illness has been dominated by early cerebellar signs rather than dementia; and the pathology shows prominent cerebellar atrophy and, in some cases, amyloid plaques. It is intriguing that the agent injected into a peripheral site results in a clinical and pathologic features more reminiscent of kuru.

Each lot of growth hormone retained on file at the National Institutes of Health was inoculated into three squirrel monkeys; one of three monkeys inoculated with one of 76 lots developed disease 5.5 years after inoculation which suggests a rare, random and low level of contamination (Gibbs et al., 1993). This and the peripheral inoculation presumably explain why the numbers of cases have remained low. Genetic factors also play a role in susceptibility. A study of iatrogenic cases resulting from transplants, electrodes and growth hormone injection showed no patient had a point or insert mutation resembling those in familial disease, yet allelic homozygosity at the polymorphic codon 129 has been found in 92% of patients and only 50% of controls (Brown et al., 1994a).

Sporadic cases

Persons with sporadic Creutzfeldt-Jakob disease fail to show insertions or mutations in the gene for the prion protein. Somatic mutation has been postulated, but 3 factors argue against this explanation. First, sporadic Creutzfeldt-Jakob disease shows a unimodal age-specific onset curve peaking at about 60 years of age. Random somatic mutation should lead to increasing incidence with age, yet the incidence of disease decreases sharply at 70 years of age. Mutation at a specific age or a cofactor determining middle age onset would be necessary to explain this curve. Second, the phenotype of sporadic cases is more stereotypical than the variable familial cases; random somatic mutations in the prion protein gene should lead to a more variable phenotype of sporadic cases. Third, most prion diseases are laterally transmitted (Table 14.4) even though a mode of lateral transmission of most cases of sporadic Creutzfeldt-Jakob disease remains a mystery.

TABLE 14.4. *Modes of transmission of prion diseases*

	Lateral transmission	Vertical transmission or inheritance
Animal diseases		
Scrapie	+	
Transmissible mink encephalopathy	+	
Bovine spongiform encephalopathy	+	
Human diseases		
Kuru	+	
Creutzfeldt–Jakob disease		
Iatrogenic	+	
Familial		+
Sporadic	?	

In view of arguments against somatic mutation and the lack of epidemiologic evidence for transmission a third explanation of sporadic Creutzfeldt-Jakob disease has been proposed: spontaneous conversion of PrP^c setting off a cascade of conversion leading to disease. This would be consistent with the stereotyped phenotype of sporadic cases and the higher levels of infectivity and greater ease of transmissibility in sporadic cases; the age-specific onset curve still would remain unexplained. Further insights into lateral transmission may come by revisiting animal disease and the relationship of "mad cow disease" and "variant Creutzfeldt-Jakob disease."

BOVINE SPONGIFORM ENCEPHALOPATHY

In April, 1985 a dairy farmer in the south of England observed a previously healthy cow that became apprehensive, hyperesthetic and ataxic and developed aggressive behavior. Progressive ataxia resulted in falling and the animal was sacrificed. Tissues were sent for diagnostic evaluation to the nearby Central Veterinary Laboratory. Over the ensuing months specimens of other Holstein-Friesian dairy cattle between 3 and 6 years of age with similar illnesses were submitted from disparate geographic areas of England. Histologically these animals had a spongiform encephalopathy with a consistent pattern of bilateral symmetrical lesions in the gray matter particularly involving the brainstem. There were intracytoplasmic vacuoles of neuronal perikarya and neurites. The resemblance to scrapie in sheep and goats was striking (Wells et al., 1987).

Over the next few years the numbers of cases grew rapidly; 16 cases were found in 1986 and more than 7,000 cases in 1989. In addition to the explosive nature, the two other remarkable features of the epidemic were the random distribution of affected cattle throughout the United Kingdom and the scattered distribution on dairy farms with many farms having only a single case. These data pointed to a common source epidemic, and the disease appeared to be related to the supplementation of the diet with meat and bone meal obtained from commercial rendering plants. It was assumed in Britain that the epidemic was initiated when scrapie-infected sheep products were fed to calves; subsequent rendering and recycling of cattle with spongiform encephalopathy sustained and augmented the outbreak. The incubation period in cattle appeared to be $2^{1}/_{2}$ to 8 years. Not only is more meat and bone meal given to dairy herd calves to enhance milk production, but beef cattle are often killed between 12 and 36 months of age before the end of the incubation period.

Meat and bone meal from the rendering plants has been used as supplement for young calves for many years in many countries. The new epizootic appeared to have resulted from changes of the rendering process. During the oil crisis of the early 1970s, in order to conserve energy many rendering plants had changed from batch heating to continuous heating which could have resulted in unequal heating of material. Of greater importance, however, appears to be the collapse of the tallow market in the late 1970s with the dietary shifts from lard to vegetable oils. This led to the inclusion of greater amounts of fat in meat and bone meal and the removal of hydrocarbon solvents from the process, solvents that might have been important in stripping away the high lipid content long known to provide protection to the infectious agent of scrapie.

A statutory ban on feeding ruminant-derived protein to ruminants was imposed in the United Kingdom in 1988, and it was predicted that numbers of cases would fall following the long incubation period (Wilesmith, 1994). This indeed occurred; after the peak years in 1992 and 1993 with in excess of 36,000 and 34,000 cases respectively, a drop of approximately 40% of cases per year has been recorded.

By January 1997 over 165,000 cases of bovine spongiform encephalopathy were confirmed distributed to over 34,000 herds in the United Kingdom. France, Ireland, Portugal and Switzerland had diagnosed cases in native cattle assumed to have been fed bone meal of British origin. About 300 cases of bovine spongiform encephalopathy have been observed in Ireland, Portugal, France, Germany, Italy, Canada, Denmark, the Falkland Islands, the Sultanate of Oman and Portugal in cattle imported from the United Kingdom. After destruction of these cattle no contact cases were seen in native cattle (Collee and Bradley, 1997a, 1997b).

Nervous system tissues of cows with spongiform encephalopathy have transmitted disease to mice, sheep, goats, cattle and mink by both intracerebral and oral inoculation and to pigs, marmosets and squirrel monkeys by intracerebral inoculation (Patterson and Dealler, 1995). A curious feature that distinguishes the bovine disease from scrapie is that only the brain and spinal cord of natural disease have consistently transmitted disease; muscle, milk, udder, placenta, kidney, bone marrow, spleen, lymph nodes or semen have not been found to contain infectious material.

There was early concern that because the infectious agent was presumed to have crossed species barriers from the sheep to the cow by the oral route that it might pose a human hazard. In 1989 cattle offal including nervous system, glandular tissue, lymph nodes and intestines, were banned from human food in the United Kingdom, although about 450,000 infected cattle had entered the human food chain before this ban was imposed (Anderson et al., 1996). Further apparent cross-species transmissions did occur. A Nyala at a zoo developed spongiform encephalopathy at the outset of the bovine epidemic, and subsequently the disease was described in further species of exotic ruminants in British zoos (gemsbok, Arabian oryx, greater kudu, eland, Scimitar [horned oryx], bison, and ankole cows). Because of the temporal and geographical coincidence of these diseases with the emergence of bovine spongiform encephalopathy and because these animals had been fed with bone meal supplement, they were considered a portion of the epidemic. Solace was taken, however, in the possibility that transmission resulted from the unnatural feeding of meat products to ruminants.

This comfort was soon cast away by the development of apparent food-borne transmission of spongiform encephalopathy to carnivorous felines. In 1990 several domestic cats in the United Kingdom developed ataxia with a histologic diagnosis of a scrapie-like spongiform encephalopathy, and by 1996 there had been 70 cases in domestic cats in the United Kingdom and one in Norway. The disease has also occurred in wild felines in zoos; pumas, cheetahs, ocelots, and a tiger. Again these illnesses appeared to have come from the feeding of meat or commercial food containing products from the rendering process. In addition, a 9-year-old rhesus monkey in a zoo in Marseille, who spent his first 4 years in a zoo in the midlands of England before being purchased by the French, developed lethargy and abnormal aggressive behavior and typical spongiform encephalopathy. The monkey had been fed protein supplement of bone meal (Bons et al., 1996).

The tabloid press in Britain had dubbed the disease mad cow disease early in the epidemic, and it whipped up hysteria with the possibility of human transmission. By 1990 the Germans had banned beef from the United Kingdom, many of the schools within England had banned beef in the children's lunches, and the consumption of beef in the United Kingdom had dropped precipitously. Stories captured the headlines as to whether foods, pharmaceuticals, or cosmetics derived from animal tissues might pose a danger to human health.

In April of 1996 the National Creutzfeldt-Jakob Disease Surveillance Unit in Edinburgh reported 10 patients identified in the United Kingdom with a clinicopathologic variant of the disease. All occurred after February 1994 and had the unusual clinical features of young age (under age 42), of early psychiatric and behavioral abnormalities and sensory symptoms preceding a prominent cerebellar ataxia. The disease's course was greater than 14 months in contrast to 6 months for sporadic Creutzfeldt-Jakob disease. Neuropathologic examination of all 10 cases showed spongiform changes, and striking plaques resembling the protease resistant prion protein plaques of kuru (Will et al., 1996). This variant of Creutzfeldt-Jakob disease has been subsequently described in a young man in France (Chazot et al., 1996) and 12 further British patients (Will et al., 1997); the mean age is 27 years (mean for sporadic disease 65 years) and disease duration averaged 14 months; all had eaten meat although one had become a strict vegetarian in 1991, but none had knowingly eaten brain. None had insertions in the prion protein gene but all were homozygous for methionine in the polymorphism at codon 129. Surveillence in the United States gives no evidence of variant cases (Holman et al., 1996). It was felt that the most plausible explanation for this cluster of cases was that they are causally linked to bovine spongiform encephalopathy related to oral intake of contaminated beef prior to the food ban in 1989 (Cousens et al., 1997). Others held strongly to the belief that these cases were an artifact of intense surveillance.

Several new laboratory studies provide powerful evidence that the causative agent of the new variant of Creutzfeldt-Jakob disease has a common origin with the agent of bovine spongiform encephalopathy. Studies of both glycosolation patterns of PrP and mouse susceptibility show that material from sporadic Creutzfeldt-Jakob disease and iatrogenic disease (pituitary hormone injections and dural transplants) yield similar patterns, and these are quite distinct from the glycosolation pattterns and mouse susceptibility of the new variant human disease and bovine spongiform encephalopathy which are indistinguishable (Hill et al., 1997). In varied inbred mouse strains different strains of scrapie give distinctive incubation periods and topographic lesion distributions, interim results of these studies indicated that the same strain of agent caused the variant Creutzfeldt-Jakob disease, bovine spongiform encephalopathy and the spongiform encephalopathies in cats and exotic ruminants; these signature patterns were readily distinguishable from those of sporadic Creutzfeldt-Jakob disease (Bruce et al., 1997).

The World Health Organization has recommended the worldwide ban of ruminants being fed with tissue of ruminants, that no animal with signs of spongiform encephalopathy enter any food chain, that offal not be included in human foods, and that active surveillance occur of cattle worldwide (CDC, 1996d).

Another Viewpoint

Not all investigators agree with the British scenario or with the tenet that the cattlemen and consumers in North America need not worry. Bovine spongiform encephalopathy may not have begun in the 1980s. The index case may have been a Gascon cow described years ago. She developed apparent itching at the base of her tail so intense that she rubbed against fixed objects resulting in a decubitus ulcer. Within two months she had become emaciated, and held her head low against the wall pushing "in the manner of a dizzy horse." She began to fall and over the next three days paralysis became progressive to the point that she could no longer stand. The attending veterinarian's diagnosis was scrapie, a disease of sheep with which he was familiar, and in his opinion the disease appeared to be more serious and rapidly progressive in the cow. He told this to the farmer who immediately sold the cow to the butcher. The year was 1881 and the case was reported as "Un cas de tremblante sur un boeuf" (Sarradet, 1883).

There are other hints that spontaneous cases of spongiform encephalopathy may occur in cattle. In 1947, 1961, and 1963 there were outbreaks of a spongiform encephalopathy on mink ranches in Wisconsin resulting in the combined deaths of several thousand mink. Evidence again implicated the feed sources and the possibility that sheep carcasses may have been included at some stage in the preparation of the mink food was not ruled out. However, in April 1985 a mink rancher in Wisconsin reported a debilitating neurologic disease in his herd; a diagnosis of transmissible mink encephalopathy was made by histologic findings, and the disease was transmitted to mink and squirrel monkeys. The rancher was a "dead-stock" feeder using "downer" and dead dairy cattle and a few horses; he maintained that neither sheep nor bone meal had ever been fed to the mink. Rare sporadic cases of spongiform encephalopathy in cattle again was posited (Marsh et al., 1991).

Another spongiform encephalopathy in North America is the wasting disease of mule deer and elk. This disease was initially described in the 1970s in captive herds in northeastern Colorado but has subsequently been reported in wild deer and elk in Colorado and Wyoming. Tens of thousands of mule deer are killed by hunter and on the Western highways each year. A portion of these continue to go to rendering plants and may enter the food chain.

The media circus and economic catastrophe over the last decade in the United Kingdom was originally generated without conclusive evidence of a risk to human health. With potential import of disease, possible endemic sporadic bovine disease, the known endemic spongiform encephalopathy of deer and elk and the mounting evidence of human risk, a proactive approach might be appropriate in this country.

POSSIBLE VIRAL CAUSES OF HUMAN DEGENERATIVE DISEASES

The transmission of Creutzfeldt-Jakob disease heightened interest in the possible viral cause of other forms of dementia particularly Alzheimer's disease. Speculation regarding a viral etiology of amyotrophic lateral sclerosis originated in clinical case reports in the nineteenth century, and speculation about a viral etiology of Parkinson's disease and schizophrenia stem from observations of von Economo encephalitis and the Spanish flu in the era of the first World War. Although these four major chronic non-inflammatory diseases have been the focus of numerous studies, no compelling data link any of these diseases to viruses or prions.

Alzheimer's Disease

Alzheimer's disease represents the major form of presenile or senile dementia and is characterized by the loss of neurons and abnormalities of dendritic processes in cerebral cortex, particularly the frontal and temporal lobes. The histologic hallmarks of this disease are senile plaques (abnormal neurites associated with extracellular amyloid).

The interest and intensive investigations of the possible role of a virus or prion in Alzheimer's disease was stimulated by several similarities to infectious processes. First, the recovery of measles and rubella viruses from chronic dementias of subacute panencephalidities and the transmission of the noninflammatory subacute dementia of Creutzfeldt-Jakob disease suggested a possible similar pathogenesis for the most common dementing illness of humans. This led to the search for a variety of conventional viruses and to the attempts to transmit Alzheimer's disease tissues to subhuman primates and hamsters. Second, topographic and histopathologic comparisons were cited as possible evidence for a viral etiology of Alzheimer's disease. The localization of neuronal loss of basal forebrain and hippocampus in Alzheimer's disease bear some similarity to the localization of cell destruction in herpes simplex virus encephalitis, and the birefringent amyloid plaques of Alzheimer's disease bear histologic resemblance to plaques in transmissible spongiform encephalopathies, particularly in certain strains of scrapie in mice, in kuru, in Gerstman-Sträussler-Scheinker syndrome and in the variant of Creutzfeldt-Jakob disease temporally and geographically associated with bovine spongiform encephalopathy. However, these plaques in prion diseases and Alzheimer's disease are composed of different proteins both of which happen to form beta-pleated sheets.

The search for herpes simplex virus proteins and genomes in tissue of patients with Alzheimer's disease recounts the story of the refinements of methods for virus detection. Herpes simplex virus antigens or DNA were inconsistently reported in brains of patients dying with Alzheimer's disease, but with more discerning methods of Southern blotting or spot hybridization, most reports were negative (Taylor et al., 1987; Pogo et al., 1987; Kittur et al., 1992). Exquisitely sensitive PCR results, however, are sometimes positive but positive for both demented patients and normal controls (Jamieson et al., 1991). Herpes simplex virus does not appear to play a primary role in dementia except in those patients with a static dementia as a sequela of herpes simplex virus encephalitis.

The reports of transmission of a spongiform encephalopathy to chimpanzees and hamsters are more difficult to resolve. Following the transmission of kuru and Creutzfeldt-Jakob diseases extensive efforts were made at the National Institutes of Health laboratories to transmit sporadic and familial Alzheimer's disease, Pick disease, parkinsonian-dementia syndrome of Guam, and Huntington's chorea. All were unsuccessful, with the exception of specimens from two patients from two separate pedigrees with clinical and pathologic diagnoses of Alzheimer's disease and single patients with progressive supranuclear ophthalmoplegia and Leigh disease. Of the patients with diagnoses of Alzheimer's disease, one had dementia, seizures, spasticity, and probable myoclonus. The other patient, whose father had died of the progressive dementia, had a rapid progressive dementia without myoclonus. In both cases, neurofibrillary tangles and plaques were found histologically without spongiform changes. In both cases, subhuman primates, after typical intervals developed classic clinical and pathologic findings of Creutzfeldt-Jakob disease without neurofibrillary tangles or plaques (Goudsmit et al., 1980). One interpretation of these findings is that some pedigrees of familial Alzheimer's disease represent a form of Creutzfeldt-Jakob disease with abundant plaques, little spongiosis, and some tangles. Alternatively, the two patients may have had Alzheimer's disease but incidentally harbored the agent of Creutzfeldt-Jakob disease, the latter disease being transmissible. Tissues from numerous patients with sporadic disease and several others with familial disease failed to induce disease.

Subsequently a spongiform encephalopathy was reported in hamsters after passage of hamster brains injected with white blood cells of patients with Alzheimer's disease and their relatives (Manuelidis et al., 1988). No neurologic disease was found in initial passage but only a systemic illness. The fighting of hamsters in cages and the second passage of brains enhanced the possibility of cross-contamination (Rohwer, 1992), and the neurohistologic changes in hamsters was undistinguishable from Creutzfeldt-Jakob disease. Attempts to repeat this finding have been unsuccessful (Godec et al., 1994).

Amyotrophic Lateral Sclerosis

Speculation concerning a viral etiology of amyotrophic lateral sclerosis arose from three very different observations: 1) a putative higher rate of disease after paralytic poliomyelitis, 2) Russian claims of the transmission of the disease to monkeys, and 3) analogies to the progressive paralysis found in wild mice infected with a neurotropic strain of murine leukemia virus (Johnson and Brooks, 1984) (see Chapter 11).

Amyotrophic lateral sclerosis is a chronic noninflammatory degenerative disease of motor neurons of the brain and spinal cord. The disease usually begins in middle life with muscle atrophy and spasticity and follows an ingravescent course until death. Sensory and cognitive abnormalities are absent.

The incidence of the disease is similar to that of multiple sclerosis in North America and Europe, but its geographic distribution is worldwide with an apparently constant incidence except for foci of high incidence in Guam, the Kii Peninsula in Japan and an area in southern West New Guinea. In Guam in addition to the motor neuron loss and corticospinal tract degeneration seen in classical amyotrophic lateral sclerosis neurofibrillary tangles resembling those of Alzheimer's disease are found in the hippocampus, selected brainstem and cerebellar nuclei (Garruto and Yanagihara, 1991). In classical amyotrophic lateral sclerosis inflammatory cells of the suppressor/cytotoxic T-cell subset and macrophages as well as increased expression of major histocompatibility complex products and human leukocyte antigens are found in corticospinal tracts and anterior horns suggesting an autoimmune or infectious process (Troost et al., 1990).

Speculation that a virus might cause amyotrophic lateral sclerosis originated from analogies to poliomyelitis, because selective destruction of motor neurons is seen in both diseases, and because progressive motor weakness and fasciculations may develop in patients many years after recovery from paralytic poliomyelitis (see Chapter 9). The hypothesis has been proposed that amyotrophic lateral sclerosis might represent a chronic form of poliovirus or other enterovirus infection or that prior infection predisposes motor neurons to etiologic factors in amyotrophic lateral sclerosis. In the patients with motor neuron disease following paralytic poliomyelitis, poliovirus antibody is not present in spinal fluid, and serum levels of antibody are not higher than those in controls (Kurent et al., 1979). Hybridization studies have failed to demonstrate evidence of persistent poliovirus RNA in neural tissue (Roos et al., 1980; Miller et al., 1980) although one study reported enteroviral sequences in CNS tissue of 1 of 5 amyotrophic lateral sclerosis patients and 1 of 6 controls (Brahic et al., 1985). Using a wide range primers for non-poliovirus enteroviruses PCR studies were positive for sequences in 8 of 11 cases of sporadic amyotrophic lateral sclerosis, 1 of 2 familial cases, and none of 6 matched controls (Woodall et al., 1994). Although intuitively it seems unlikely, the possible role of an enterovirus in the pathogenesis of amyotrophic lateral sclerosis remains unresolved.

In the Soviet Union, progressive atrophy considered to be amyotrophic lateral sclerosis was described as a sequela of both acute tick-borne encephalitis and Viluisk encephalitis (see Chapter 10). Tick-borne encephalitis virus and other flaviviruses involve neurons of the cervical spinal cord, and after tick-borne encephalitis progressive atrophy of the musculature of the shoulder girdle is seen during convalescence. However, evidence of a progressive motor neuron disease is lacking. Largely because of these observations, Soviet scientists initiated attempts to transmit amyotrophic lateral sclerosis to primates in the 1950s. In 1963, a progressive neurologic disease was reported in rhesus monkeys 1 to 3 years after intracerebral inoculation of medulla and spinal cord from patients dying of amyotrophic lateral sclerosis (Zil'ber et al., 1963). Furthermore, the disease was transmitted from monkey to monkey. The agent has never been characterized, and whether it originated from the patients or in the primate colonies was unclear (Brody et al., 1965). Although unconfirmed in other laboratories, subsequent further transmissions were reported in the same Soviet laboratory (Gardashyan et al., 1970).

Additional positive reports include the apparent recovery of a flavivirus (Muller and Schaltenbrand, 1979) and an adenovirus 26 (Delsedime et al., 1974) from spinal fluids of patients with amyotrophic lateral sclerosis, but these isolations also remain unconfirmed. One serologic study of patients with amyotrophic lateral sclerosis showed decreased prevalence of adenovirus antibodies and elevation of antibodies to adeno-associated parvovirus with parvovirus recovered from CNS explants from 2 patients (Kascsak et al., 1982).

The bulk of serologic studies and routine virus isolation studies, however, have uncovered no clues for a viral cause of amyotrophic lateral sclerosis (Kennedy, 1990). Furthermore, the primates at the National Institutes of Health after inoculation with homogenates of neural tissue from the affected Soviet monkeys, from sporadic cases in the United States, and from patients from the Guamanian focus, exhibited no disease (Gibbs and Gajdusek, 1972). Studies of explant cell cultures of brain and of isolated motor neurons from amyotrophic lateral sclerosis patients have also produced no evidence of a virus (Cremer et al., 1973; Weiner et al., 1980).

Subsequent to the observation of an amyotrophic-lateral-sclerosis-like disease in mice due to a retrovirus (see Chapter 11) evidence for a possible retrovirus infection was sought in the human disease. An apparent particle-associated RNA-instructed DNA-polymerase was found in the brain tissue of some patients from Guam and failed to show activity in patients in the continental United States (Viola et al., 1975). The subsequent finding of a terminal deoxynucleotidyl transferase in normal brain that could be confused with a reverse transcriptase weakens the evidence for retrovirus activity in humans (Viola et al., 1979). Recently serologic studies for human foamy virus were reported to be positive in almost half of patients with sporadic motor neuron disease (Westarp et al., 1992), but a subsequent report failed to confirm the findings using several serologic methods (Rösener et al., 1996).

Parkinson's Disease

Parkinson's disease is a common progressive neurologic disease of late life characterized by slow resting tremor, rigidity, and hypokinesis. There is a loss of neurons in the substantia nigra and a deficiency of their dopamine transmitter in the basal ganglia.

The hypothesis that Parkinson's disease may be the sequela of an acute viral infection or may represent an ongoing slow infection of the nervous system stems from the World War I era when the pandemic of von Economo disease (encephalitis lethargica) spread across the globe. A parkinsonian syndrome developed as a sequela in about one-third of survivors, and this often developed after a latent period of 6 months to 20 years. This syndrome, however, differs from the idiopathic or typical Parkinson's disease by its occurrence in a younger age group, its slower progression, and a characteristic abnormality of eye movement in the form of oculogyric crises.

Von Economo encephalitis was assumed to be a viral disease on both clinical and pathologic grounds. The disease had a febrile course, with lethargy or stupor as a prominent sign; external ophthalmoplegia, bradykinesia, mutism and hallucinations were also described. An inflammatory response was evident in spinal fluid, and pathologic studies showed perivascular mononuclear cell infiltrates, with greatest intensity in the midbrain.

First appearing in the Balkans in 1915, the disease spread through Europe in 1916 and 1917 and was first seen in North America in 1918. Pandemics were reported in various parts of the world until late 1928 when they decreased, and only sporadic cases of the disease were reported after 1930 (Yahr, 1978). More than a million cases of severe encephalitis occurred causing over one half a million deaths. The occurrence of the disease in the United States at the same time as the pandemic of influenza has led some to postulate that a neurotropic strain of swine influenza was the cause (Ravenholt and Foege, 1982). In Europe, however, von Economo disease appears to have preceded the influenza epidemic and in both continents it lingered long after. Sporadic reports still appear of acute encephalitis resembling von Economo encephalitis (Howard and Lees, 1987). Further nosologic confusion resulted from use of the term encephalitis A. Thereafter, the virus recovered from encephalitis in Japan was called encephalitis B, and von Economo disease was often listed as an arbovirus encephalitis, even though the winter and spring seasonal occurrence in temperate zones precludes an arthropod vector.

Cases of parkinsonism following von Economo encephalitis are disappearing, and little has been done to determine if the disease might represent a chronic infection. there is, however, an alleged endemic focus to the disease in Outer Mongolia, and the clinical descriptions sound very much like the disease described by von Economo. A tantalizing story has been told that the initial European appearance of the disease coincided with the movement of Mongolian troops into the Balkans during the unrest preceding World War I (P. Yakovlev, personal communication).

Although no virus has been recovered from Parkinson's disease and no transmission to animals has been reported, immunologic studies have implicated both influenza and herpes simplex viruses. Immunofluorescent staining of tissues from several patients with postencephalitic parkinsonism was reported using antisera against a neuroadapted strain of type A influenza virus (Gamboa et al., 1974). The virus specificity of this reaction is in question, however, because antisera against the prototype strains of influenza from which the neurotropic strain was derived failed to react, which suggests that the antigenic determinant may have originated from mouse brain and not from the influenza virus. Serologic studies of influenza and arbovirus antibodies in patients with idiopathic Parkinson's disease show no differences between patients with idiopathic Parkinson's disease and controls. Serologic studies have reported an increased antibody response in patients with Parkinson's disease against several antigens of type 1 herpes simplex virus (Marttila et al., 1982). In general autopsy tissues from patients with idiopathic Parkinson's disease have been thoroughly examined by electron microscopy, immunocytochemistry and nucleic acid hybridization for evidence of both herpes simplex type 1 and influenza, and no evidence was found to incriminate persistence of either virus (Schwartz and Elizan, 1979; Wetmur et al., 1979).

Parkinsonian syndromes do occur as a rare complication of documented infections with Western St. Louis, and Japanese encephalitis viruses and with group B coxsackieviruses. An acute parkinsonian syndrome also has been described after encephalitis in eastern Europe (Bojinov, 1971). However, in each case these abnormalities have tended to be transient or nonprogressive, have not been associated with oculogyric crises, and have not developed after a long latent period. Thus, these cases appear to be different from both the parkinsonism observed after von Economo encephalitis and the usual idiopathic form of Parkinson's disease.

Schizophrenia

The 1918 pandemic of influenza and possibly von Economo disease also launched the speculation regarding a viral causation for some cases of schizophrenia. The famous Karl Menninger noted the strange behavior, catatonia, mutism, and hallucinations resembling schizophrenia associated with the pandemic of "influenza" (Menninger, 1926). He noted, however, that the schizophrenia or dementia precox following influenza often improved or recovered completely.

Recent studies have given credence to cytopathic origin of schizophrenia by showing structural abnormalities of the hippocampus, hippocampal gyrus and amygola with decrease in volume by antatonic and imaging data and decrease in cell density by histologic data. Genetic factors evidently play a significant role, since concordance in identical twins is over 60%, but environmental factors must play a role to explain the level of discordance. Those factors that might selectively cause temporal lobe damage included perinatal or fetal anoxia, trauma or infection. The seasonality of schizophrenia births favors the infectious hypothesis. Studies in Northern Europe and United States has shown births of schizophrenics to be higher between December and April, and this appears to be reversed to winter months in South Africa (Torrey et al., 1977). Laboratory data implicating viruses is limited and contradictory. Considerable excitement was evoked in the 1970s when a "virus-like agent" causing cytopathic effect in cell culture was reported to be detectable in spinal fluid in 40% of patients with schizophrenia (Tyrrell et al., 1979). Cytopathic effects, however, occurred with inoculation of spinal fluid of about the same percentage of patients with a variety of chronic neurologic diseases (Crow et al., 1979). Further characterization of the "agent" was not forthcoming.

Serologic studies have reported greater prevalence of antibodies to type 1 herpes simplex virus and cytomegalovirus in spinal fluids from patients with schizophrenia (Albrecht et al., 1980; Torrey et al., 1982; Bártová et al., 1987). The finding of hepatitis B surface antigen in spinal fluid (Libíková et al., 1981), the detection of a novel sequence in the brain of a patient resembling the gene for reverse transcriptase of a primate type D retrovirus, and the detection of Borna virus sequences in cells from some individuals with schizophrenia (Yolken, 1996) represent fragmentary evidence. Borna virus has also been implicated by the finding of antibodies in 14% of schizophrenic patients that react with one or more viral proteins of Borna virus on Western blot assays; none were found among controls (Waltrip et al., 1995). To date extensive molecular hybridization and PCR studies of brain and spinal fluid for a number of common viruses including herpes viruses, influenza virus, and Borna viruses have been negative or failed to show differences from control tissue (Sierra-Honigman et al., 1995; Gordon et al., 1996; Carter et al., 1987) as have attempts to transmit disease to subhuman primates with longterm holding, behavioral observations, and histological studies of brain (Kaufmann et al., 1988).

SUPPLEMENTARY BIBLIOGRAPHY

Gibbs CJ Jr. (editor) (1996): Bovine Spongiform Encephalopathy: The BSE Dilemma. Springer, New York.

Prusiner SB (editor) (1996): Prions Prions Prions. Current Topics Microbiol Immunol Vol. 207. Springer, Berlin.

PART IV

Other Perspectives

These final chapters present different viewpoints. The possible role of viruses in human cerebral tumors has been diminished except for the very specific recent demonstrations of Epstein–Barr virus in cerebral B-cell lymphomas and simian virus 40 in ependymomas and choroid plexus papillomas. The impact of viral investigations on the discovery of oncogenes and tumor-suppressor genes has been critical, and the experimental induction of cerebral tumors in animals remains an important tool in studies of pathogenesis and treatment.

In Chapter 16, acute and chronic diseases are reconsidered from the vantage of different anatomic sites. In clinical medicine, blindness, deafness, vertigo, and muscle pain and weakness often are ascribed to viral infections, and limited clinical and experimental evidence gives credence to these speculations.

Environmental control, immunization, and antiviral drugs revisit the epidemiologic, immunologic, and virologic principles introduced in Chapters 5, 4, and 2, respectively. The future methods of immunization and drug design promise a new era in the prevention and treatment of virus infections.

The postscripts are simply personal essays on the importance of animal studies, the issues of causation, and the ever-changing landscape of viral infections of the nervous system.

15

Cerebral Tumors

Tumours produced by the inoculation of a cell-free tumour agent must be produced by
malignant transformation of the brain's own cellular elements, and not by survival and
multiplication of implanted cells, as occurs with grafts. Our knowledge of the extracellular agents of filterable tumours suggests that their action is exerted on cells of mes-
enchymatous origin and especially on young, undifferentiated types which are prone to
proliferation.

Enrique Vazquez-Lopez,
On the Growth of Rous Sarcoma Inoculated into the Brain, 1936

This Spanish investigator was the first to report the induction of cerebral tumors
with a virus. Adopting the techniques with which Peyton Rous had first related
viruses to tumors 25 years earlier (1911), he inoculated cell-free filtrate from a
Rous sarcoma into young chicks by the intracerebral route and observed the
development of sarcomas in the brains after 9 to 39 days. As a protégé of Rio-
Hortega, his primary focus was the probable mesenchymal origin and the
microglial reaction to these tumors, but he noted that tumors arose from undifferentiated cells and only in young animals. Most subsequent experimental studies of cerebral tumors in animals have necessitated intracerebral inoculation of
large numbers of viruses. Most have also required the use of young animals
whose neural cells still are undergoing mitosis.

The pathogenesis of human cancer is proving to be a complex multistep
process involving both oncogenes and tumor suppressor genes that over time are
activated or suppressed culminating in deranged cell growth and unbridled cell
proliferation. Cancer is fundamentally a genetic disease due to inherited predisposition, DNA rearrangements during cell cycle, viral infection and integration,
and exposure to carcinogenic agents or radiation (Batra et al., 1994).

In reviewing Rous' initial experiments, his first transmission among chickens
was carried out using whole cells among closely related animals presumably
because of the barrier of histocompatibility antigens. Only later was the tumor
transmitted with some difficulty by extracts, and later still it was transmitted
over a wide range of species even including the production of the glioblastoma
model in dogs. In retrospect, it may be that the cancer cell came first; subsequently under the intense selective pressure imposed by histocompatibility anti-

gens, cell genes responsible for the cancer were transferred to a virus, which could then circumvent the barrier moving freely from one animal to another. As Cairns (1978) stated, "The possibility that certain tumor viruses are simply artifacts makes them in some respects more interesting rather than less, because it means that they may be offering us a way of isolating and studying genes responsible for the cancer state. This seems to be the real justification for putting so much effort into investigating tumor viruses." Indeed the studies of the genome of Rous sarcoma virus showed that a cell gene named *sarc* induced transformation, and this was the first virus gene that was shown to be derived from a normal protooncogene of the natural host. Subsequently a variety of oncogenes of viruses were found to have parallel series of homologous host genes. The host genes termed protooncogenes are normal growth promoting genes, and over 100 have been identified. They include growth factors, growth factor receptors, transducers, and transcriptional factors and are important during development and repair. Tumor suppressor genes are pivitol in normal development and cellular differentiation (Gutmann, 1995). The loss of the tumor suppressor genes (antioncogenes) appears to be fundamental in the development of many CNS tumors in humans (Batra et al., 1994).

Viruses are recognized as contributing factors in some natural tumors by indirect or direct mechanisms: indirectly by inducing immunosuppression (e.g. the development of Kaposi's sarcoma and other neoplasms in HIV-infected patients), by modification of the host cell genome (e.g. chromosomal damage), or by an acute infection without requiring persistence of viral DNA. Viruses have a direct effect by either introducing oncogenes (e.g. the sarc gene in Rous sarcoma virus) or by altering expression of host cell proteins at the site of viral DNA integration (e.g. some retroviruses lack oncogenes but integrate DNA adjacent to a host protooncogene causing activation) (ZurHausen, 1991).

In humans there is no definitive evidence linking a virus as the sole and direct cause of cancer. There is strong evidence that Epstein-Barr virus plays a role in Burkitt lymphoma and in nasopharyngeal carcinoma, that papilloma viruses are related to anogenital carcinoma, and that HTLV-1 infection is a prerequisite for T-cell leukemia. Only in the latter is infection found in all persons with the tumors, so it may be essential. On the other hand HTLV-1 infection per se is not sufficient, since there is an extraordinarily long incubation period between infection and the development of leukemia, leukemias develop in less than 5% of these infected, and the leukemia cells are monoclonol suggesting they have derived from the single transform cell. Thus, even in HTLV-1 infections there appears to be additional affects of other genetic, physical or chemical carcinogens (see Chapter 11).

Genetic predisposition or other alterations of host cell DNA virus has been causally linked to naturally occurring brain tumors in humans or animals. Several viruses, however, have been suggested as important factors in human brain tumors. These include Epstein-Barr virus in cerebral B-cell lymphomas and papovaviruses in chorioid plexus papillomas and possibly other tumors. In experimental animals an array of tumors can be produced by viruses, virus-induced tumors are more readily generated in brains than in extraneural sites, and these experimental brain tumors have been useful in the study of the biology of cerebral tumors and in testing therapeutic methods.

PATHOGENESIS OF CELL TRANSFORMATION BY VIRUSES

The Transformed Cell

In cell cultures, cell growth can be altered by tumor viruses, and most of our insights into viral oncogenesis have come from these studies. Normal cells in culture grow, as in the host, in an orderly fashion. They tend to maintain specific orientation toward one another and grow to form a uniform monolayer demonstrating contact inhibition. They can be subcultured for a finite number of times, and then they die. After infection with oncogenic viruses, the cells tend to round up. They lose their orderly alignment and develop irregular and interlacing patterns of growth. They lose contact inhibition and pile up; they often lose the need for surface attachment and therefore can grow in agar. They will grow in excess or deficient amounts of nutrients, and sugar and nutrient transport across the plasma membrane is accelerated. Studies of these cells show changes in chromosomes, changes in doubling time, and alterations in their cell surfaces, with differences in glycoproteins and lectin binding. Surfaces often express fetal antigens, tight junctions may be lost, and, most important, the cells do not grow through finite subcultures but become immortal (Tooze, 1973). Cells from these cultures can produce tumors when inoculated into histocompatible animals.

Mechanisms of Transformation

DNA and RNA viruses vary in their mechanisms of oncogenesis. DNA viruses tend to be lytic in cells of the natural host. Transformation occurs primarily in unnatural hosts, and the host range is limited, in most cases, to rodents. For example, SV40 produces asymptomatic infection in its natural host, the rhesus monkey, and the human adenoviruses produce benign respiratory disease in man, but these viruses are oncogenic in hamsters. In contrast, RNA tumor viruses, retroviruses, tend to produce tumors in their natural host as well as in unnatural hosts, and the range of unnatural hosts susceptible to oncogenesis is much wider.

These differences are dependent on the molecular events during viral transformation. The papovaviruses and adenoviruses are the two families of DNA viruses that can cause experimental brain tumors most readily and reproducibly. They transform nonpermissive cells. These cells are infected and translate early proteins, but they fail to transcribe messenger RNA for late proteins, and they fail to produce progeny virus.

Permissive replication of retroviruses does not require the killing of the host cells. These viruses mature and spread by budding from the host-cell membrane; so cell destruction is not a prerequisite for virus release. Thus, in oncogenic retrovirus infections the virus is capable of both transforming the cell and producing progeny virus concurrently, and this is the usual mode of infection in tumors induced in the natural host. The integrated, complementary, double-stranded DNA may transcribe the messages for oncoproteins or activate an adjacent host protooncogene.

Tumor Induction

These differences in the mechanisms of replication of DNA and RNA tumor viruses explain in part their varied efficiencies of tumor induction. DNA tumor viruses are not amplified in the hosts in which they produce tumors. Furthermore, they are inefficient in cell transformation; usually 10^4 to 10^6 infectious virus particles are required to result in a single focus of transformation in cell culture, and 10^6 to 10^8 infectious virus particles are required to produce 50% tumor induction in animal hosts. In contrast, the RNA tumor viruses are more efficient in transforming cells in their natural hosts or cell cultures derived from natural hosts, because progeny virus particles are continually being released from the transformed cells. However, in unnatural hosts, where infection is nonpermissive, this efficiency is lost.

EXPERIMENTAL INDUCTION OF CEREBRAL TUMORS

Virus-induced cerebral tumors must be viewed both as viral infections of the brain and as neoplastic diseases. Because of the relatively sequestered nature of the brain, tumor induction is most efficiently accomplished by direct intracerebral inoculation of virus. With the DNA viruses and RNA sarcoma viruses in their unnatural hosts, failure of infectious virus replication in brain cells makes inoculation of large concentrations of virus mandatory. An infectious virus within the inoculum must reach a susceptible cell and produce a stable transforming event, and the altered cell must escape immunologic surveillance. The barriers to immunologic clearance in the CNS probably explain why many viruses produce tumors more readily in the brain after intracerebral inoculation than in extraneural tissues after peripheral inoculation (Wikstrand and Bigner, 1980).

Most intracerebral inoculations of oncogenic viruses lead to tumors that originate from fibroblasts or ependymal cells (Table 15.1). This is not surprising, because in small animals colloidal particles in the inoculum flow back along the needle track and flood the spinal fluid, rather than being deposited in the brain parenchyma (Mims, 1960). Inoculated virus particles follow the same path. Because most oncogenic agents do not replicate in brain cells, with liberation of progeny virus to enter the neuropil, cells at risk of transformation are largely

TABLE 15.1. *Experimental cerebral tumors induced by viruses*

Virus family Virus	Tumor type	Experimental host
Papovaviruses		
Bovine papilloma virus	Meningioma Meningeal fibroma	Hamster, calf
Mouse polyoma virus	Anaplastic fibrosarcomas	Hamster, rat, rabbit
Simian virus 40	Ependymoma, choroid plexus papilloma	Hamster, marmoset
Human JC virus	Medulloblastoma, meningioma, pineocytoma, gliomas, meningeal sarcoma, choroid plexus papilloma	Hamster
	Glioma	Owl, monkey
Human BK virus	Choroid plexus papilloma	Hamster
Adenoviruses		
Human adenovirus, type 12	Sarcoma	Hamster
	Medulloblastoma	Mouse
	Neuroblastoma	Rat, hamster
Human adenovirus, type 18	Sarcoma	Hamster
Simian adenovirus, SA7	Sarcoma	Hamster, rat
	Ependymoma, glioma, medulloblastoma, choroid plexus papilloma	Hamster
Simian adenovirus, SV20	Undifferentiated	Hamster
Bovine adenovirus, type 3	Choroid plexus papilloma, giant cell glioblastoma	Hamster
Avian adenovirus, CELO	Ependymoma or choroid plexus papilloma	Hamster
Retroviruses		
Avian sarcoma virus	Sarcoma	Chicken, turkey, rabbit, guinea pig, dog, rat, marmoset, rhesus monkey
	Glioma	Hamster, mouse, rat, rabbit, dog, cat, marmoset, rhesus monkey
	Meningioma, ependymoma	Dog
Murine sarcoma virus	Sarcoma	Rat, mouse
	Meningioma, hemangioma	Rat
	Glioma	Rat, mouse
Simian sarcoma virus	Glioma	Marmoset

those that line the ventricles and subarachnoid spaces. Furthermore, these cells continue to undergo mitosis in the postnatal animal and therefore constitute populations more susceptible to transformation. Proliferating cells along the needle tract may also be subject to nonpermissive infection. In parenchymal tumors of neonatal mice caused by adenovirus 12, the early colonies of transformed cells appear to arise from cells of the subventricular zone of the lateral ventricles, a population of cells still proliferating postnatally (Murao, 1972). In larger animals, such as the dog, the inoculum can be placed more specifically. Inoculation of avian sarcoma virus over the cortical surface leads to sarcomas, whereas inoculation deep in the parenchyma of the dog s brain leads to gliomas that presumably arise from subventricular-zone cells (Bigner et al., 1972).

The latency between inoculation and the clinical or gross pathologic evidence of cerebral tumor ranges from 9 to 200 days. The nature of the tumor usually is dependent on the virus, but this can be altered by a variety of manipulations. SV40 in hamsters causes only ependymomas or choroid plexus papillomas; however, SV40 can transform hamster astrocytes in culture, and the inoculation of these transformed cultured cells into neonatal hamsters will cause gliomas (Shein, 1968). The related JC virus has different oncogenic properties, because this virus produces a variety of different tumors in neonatal hamsters, sometimes with tumors of several morphologies within the same brain (Walker et al., 1973). Some strains of JC virus produce medulloblastomas almost exclusively, and one strain causes a preponderance of pineal tumors (Padgett et al., 1977). BK virus is clearly the least oncogenic of the primate polyomaviruses. In our studies, only choroid plexus papillomas were produced, and only in neonatal hamsters that had been immunosuppressed. This weak oncogenicity of BK virus does not appear to reflect inability of the virus to transform cells, because transforming events are readily induced in cultures of hamster embryo fibroblasts. Instead, the low yield of brain tumors appears to be due to the immunogenicity of the BK virus-transformed cells, with attendant rejection by the host animal. This hypothesis is supported by the findings that the tumors were induced only in hamsters treated with antithymocyte serum and that the tumor cells were more readily transplanted in recipients treated with antithymocyte serum or when cells were deposited in the cheek pouch, an immunologically privileged site (Greenlee et al., 1977).

Several adenoviruses readily produce cerebral tumors, but the tumors have not been studied extensively, because they have been difficult to classify. Electron microscopy of some tumors induced by adenovirus type 12 showed a single cilium with 9+0 tubules (9 double tubules without an axial tubule pair), an ultrastructural configuration characteristic of sensory neurons suggesting that they are neuroblastomas (Mukai and Kobayashi, 1973).

Avian sarcoma viruses have the widest host range for cerebral tumor induction and can cause a variety of tumors in fowl, rodents, canines, and primates. The best-defined astrocytomas have been induced in dogs and rats (Wilfong et al., 1973). With the exception of tumors in chickens, virus particles usually are not seen in these tumors.

The mouse sarcoma viruses are unusual because they are defective and replicate only with the help of the endogenous rodent leukemia viruses. Therefore, the host range is restricted to rats and mice that have complementary viruses. With the helper virus, mature C-type particles are produced by tumor cells (Duffy, 1970).

The induction of brain tumors in marmosets with simian sarcoma virus (Wolfe and Deinhardt, 1975) is of particular interest, because these tumors appear to bear the greatest resemblance of any virus-induced experimental brain tumors to the human glioblastoma multiform (Bigner and Pegram, 1976). Virus-induced tumors in animals can provide models for testing of therapeutic modalities. For such a model, a consistent tumor-type resembling the human counterpart is needed, and the tumor must occur at a high rate and have a uniform latency. Anaplastic astrocytomas caused by avian sarcoma viruses have provided the best model because 100% induction is possible in dogs and rats, microscopic tumors evolve within 2 to 4 weeks, and median survival in the rat is 70 to 100 days (Bullard and Bigner, 1980). In hamsters, some strains of JC virus give high rates of medulloblastomas, SV40 and avian adenoviruses consistently produce choroid plexus papillomas, and human adenovirus 12 predictably induces neuroblastomas. These agents in the specific species can provide practical models for therapeutic studies.

EVIDENCE FOR VIRUSES IN HUMAN BRAIN TUMORS

There is no definitive evidence linking any virus causally with a cerebral neoplasm in humans. A number of studies have suggested the possibility of viral transformation of neural cells (Table 15.2) but the strongest evidence relates to Epstein-Barr virus and the papovaviruses.

TABLE 15.2. *Viruses implicated in human brain tumors*

Virus	Tumor type	Evidence[a]
Epstein-Barr virus	Primary cerebral B-cell lymphomas	Presence of viral DNA in tumor cells; consistent demonstration in AIDS patients where the tumor is common
Papovaviruses		
SV40	Medulloblastomas	Epidemiologic association with maternal immunization with contaminated poliovaccine
	Meningiomas Ependymoma Choroid plexus papillomas	Staining for T antigen and/or DNA hybridization
	Ependymomas Choroid plexus papillomas	PCR probes for T antigen and capsid sequences
BK virus	Reticulum cell sarcoma Glioblastoma Neuroblastoma Astrocytoma Meningioma Oligodendroglioma	Virus isolation Rescue of viral DNA by transfection of tumor DNA into human embryonic fibroblasts
	Meningiomas Neuromas Gliomas Ependymoma	Southern blot analysis with virus-specific probe
Adenovirus, type 3	Pituitary adenoma	Virus isolation
Retroviruses	Varied	Reverse transcriptase activity in cultured cells and spinal fluid

PCR, polymerase chain reaction.
[a]Virus recoveries from tumor-derived cell cultures not included.

Epstein-Barr Virus

Epstein-Barr virus is the virus most convincingly implicated in Burkett lymphoma and nasopharyngeal carcinomas, and recently data have linked the virus to primary cerebral lymphomas. Epstein-Barr virus was first demonstrated in tumor cells of a primary cerebral lymphoma by in situ hybridization (Hochberg et al., 1983). Subsequent studies confirmed viral DNA in 10% to 50% of both extraneural and primary cerebral B cell lymphomas, and by using biotinylated probes it has been possible to localize the virus genome within tumor cells and not in neighboring reactive lymphocytes (Geddes et al., 1992). In patients with AIDS this rare cerebral tumor is common, and the role of Epstein-Barr virus is more convincing. In 18 consecutive primary cerebral lymphomas in AIDS patients at our institution, all had evidence of Epstein-Barr virus infection using in situ hybridization with a nonprotein coding transcript (MacMahon et al., 1991). The consistent presence of this latency transcript in nuclei of tumor cells and absence in nontumor cells suggest a causal relationship. The absence of the virus in a majority of primary cerebral lymphomas in immunocompetent patients indicates that Epstein-Barr virus is not the sole cause of primarily cerebral lymphomas.

Since Epstein-Barr virus is an almost universal infection and is activated in AIDS patients, infection of transformed B cells in lymphomas might represent nothing more than an opportunistic infection of the tumor cells, but the absence of virus transcripts in most extraneural lymphomas in AIDS patients does not support this explanation. Primary cerebral B cell lymphomas develop in about 10% of AIDS patients; the oncogenic role of Epstein-Barr virus in these patients with crippled immune surveillance remains unsettled.

Papovaviruses

Studies of the possible role of SV40, BK and JC viruses in brain tumors have given complex and contradictory results. SV40 virus, a common infection of macaque monkeys, was first isolated as a contaminant of batches of human poliovirus vaccines in 1960. When SV40 proved to cause tumors in hamsters concern was generated for the hundreds of millions of people who had received killed or oral polio vaccines. Nowhere was this concern more intense than in Cleveland, where a study had been carried out in over 1000 children less than 3 days of age with live attenuated monovalent poliovirus vaccine orally or in activated poliomyelitis vaccine intramuscularly to determine whether newborn infants would respond to vaccination. Neonatal infection theoretically put these children at greater risk of any oncogenic effect, but follow-up of these children 17 to 19 years later showed no excess risk of cancer. Indeed no case of cancer was found, although one would have been expected by chance (Mortimer et al., 1981).

Studies of fetal exposure were carried out by examining the progeny of 50,000 pregnancies between 1959 and 1965, and a higher incidence of neural tumors was found in children of mothers who had received inactivated poliovirus (7 of 18,342) than in children of nonimmunized mothers (1 of 32,555). Immunization with influenza or live poliovirus vaccine and spontaneous viral infection during pregnancy were not associated with increased tumor rates. The significant differences in the tumor rates in children of women potentially exposed to SV40 were limited to neural tumors but included minor histologic abnormalities in adrenal glands in three patients. If these were discarded, the data would be less compelling (Heinoen et al., 1973). A subsequent study of the Connecticut tumor registry showed an increase in brain tumors in children born between 1955 and 1960, the period when inadvertent exposure of pregnant mothers to SV40 was higher. This case-control study suggests that intrauterine exposure to SV40 was associated with increased incidence of childhood medulloblastoma and possibly glioma (Farwell et al., 1979).

Demonstration of papovavirus tumor antigen within cells of brain tumors have been varied. There have been a number of reports of T antigens in meningiomas (Weiss et al., 1975). Both antigen shown by indirect immunofluorescence as well as DNA hybridization have suggested SV40 or a closely related virus in a variety of different brain tumors (Geissler, 1990). Our studies of brain tumors and the T antigen common to cells transformed by SV40, BK and JC virus did not support these findings (Greenlee et al., 1978). Antigen was often difficult to demonstrate in SV40-induced hamster choroid plexus tumors, but cell cultures derived from these tumors were found to consistently express antigens in 95% or more of tumor cells, and this expression persisted and intensified in subsequent passages (Becker et al., 1976). Therefore, cell cultures were established from 80 human brain tumors including 14 meningiomas and examined at different passage levels; no evidence was found for T antigen (Greenlee et al., 1978). These negative studies were confirmed in Japan in a study of 69 brain tumors and cells cultured from tumors at various passage levels (Kosaka et al., 1980).

More recently using PCR amplification of polyoma virus T antigen gene sequences, 10 of 20 choroid plexus tumors and 10 of 11 ependymomas showed hybridization to probe specific for SV40 viral DNA but not for BK and JC viral DNA (Bergsagel et al., 1992). A subsequent study by the same laboratory performed DNA sequence analysis showing authentic SV40 regulatory region and major capsid sequences in 14 of 17 tumors tested. It showed the sequences were distinguishable from laboratory strains of SV40 (Lednicky et al., 1995).

In a conflicting study, a variety of types of human brain tumors were analyzed by Southern blot analysis for the presence of JC, SV40 and BK virus. No positive hybridization was found with JC and SV40 virus specific probes, but 11 of 14 indicated the presence of BK virus DNA and the DNA-associated sequences were associated with high molecular weight cellular DNA suggesting a chromosomal location (Dörries et al., 1987). BK DNA and RNA and BK virus recovery were reported in a portion of gliomas, meningiomas and ependymomas in several studies (Corallini et al., 1987; Negrini et al., 1990). The recovery of BK virus from reticulum cell carcinoma from the brain of a child with Wiscott-

Aldrich syndrome is of dubious significance, since the child also had virus in the urine. Virus may have represented blood contamination of the specimen or an innocuous infection of susceptible neoplastic cells. Unfortunately tumor cells were not successfully grown in culture, so expression of T antigen or the search for virus genes was not possible (Takemoto et al., 1974).

It is odd that JC virus, the established human pathogen of this group, has not been implicated in these studies despite the fact that aberrant tumorlike astrocytes have been seen in progressive multifocal leukoencephalopathy (see Chapter 10). In three patients with that disease multifocal astrocytic neoplasms have been found, which seemed to localize to white matter in proximity to the demyelinating lesions (Castaigne et al., 1974; Sima et al, 1983; Gullotta, 1992).

Other Claims of Viral Infections

A variety of ultrastructural examinations of human brain tumors have shown "viruslike particles" but these have been of dubious significance (Johnson, 1982). Several claims have been made of visualization or isolation of viruses from cells serially passed from tumors. The recovery of a type 3 adenovirus from a pituitary adenoma (Cooper, 1967) was a solitary finding, and because this is a relatively ubiquitous human agent that often persists in the posterior nasopharynx, this isolation is of doubtful significance.

Reverse transcriptase activity was found in materials sedimented at 70S from human glioblastoma tissues in culture and also from spinal fluid from patients with a variety of brain tumors (Cuatico et al., 1977), but this is similar to unconfirmed findings in a variety of human neoplasms.

No single methodological approach has provided convincing evidence that a virus is involved in the pathogenesis of a human cerebral tumor. Epidemiologic data of clustering, common exposure or increase in antibody to tumor antigens have not be found that are both specific and selective. The strongest epidemiologic data is the finding of tumors in the progeny of pregnant women exposed to the SV40 virus, but this clearly has been a very rare occurrence. Laboratory data of consistent recovery of viral DNA or demonstration of viral antigens or nucleic acids in tumor cells can form a reasonable argument for a role in pathogenesis. This has not been the case with papovaviruses with the divergent results from different laboratories, but does appear to be the case of Epstein-Barr virus in primary cerebral B cell lymphomas, specifically those in patients with AIDS. Nevertheless, it does not appear to be a sole factor because only about 10% of patients with AIDS develop primary cerebral lymphomas even though the majority harbor the virus.

16

Neurovirology Afield

I don't know. It must be a virus.
Physicians, 1881–present

Over the past century invoking of viruses to explain diseases of cryptic etiology has become a timeworn tradition in clinical medicine. This ploy now seems less absurd, with the linking of CNS viral infections to chronic inflammatory disease, malformations, demyelinating and degenerative processes, neoplasms, and diseases of previously assumed genetic and metabolic causes. However, apart from the diversity in clinical courses and pathologic features, the variety of anatomic sites of potential diseases warrants consideration.

Peripheral nerve viral infection is not a recognized health problem in humans, except in HIV infections (Chapter 12), but studies of Marek's disease in chickens have presented the intriguing possibility of direct infections of peripheral nerve leading to polyneuritis (see Chapter 8). Other neural tissue have remained relatively neglected in clinical and experimental virologic investigations. Although the retina is a part of the CNS, it has been overlooked in many investigative studies, despite the recognition of retinitis in congenital cytomegalovirus infections over 40 years ago. Viral infection of the neural cells of the membranous labyrinth of the inner ear has been the subject of extensive anecdotal clinical reports, but there have been limited clinical or experimental virologic studies. Inflammatory muscle disease has recently attracted the attention of virologists, and even asymptomatic muscle infection may have significance, because the motor endplate and the muscle spindle are possible sites of virus ingress or egress in CNS infections. Vasculitis is recognized in several viral infections of human and animals, but experimental studies of virus-induced vasculitis are sparse. The autonomic nervous system remains largely unexplored. A few reports have related human autonomic neuropathy to viral infections (Pavesi et al., 1992), and rabies virus in animals has been shown to infect autonomic ganglion cells in Auerbach's plexus and Meissner's plexus of the gut and the neuroinnervation of hair follicles and tongue papillae. This chapter will not emphasize different clinical courses or pathologic lesions, but different anatomic sites of infection relevant to neurologic diseases.

RETINITIS

The retina is sequestered from most acute and chronic CNS infections. Viral retinopathies in humans have been recognized, primarily with congenital or neonatal viral infections with rubella virus or herpesviruses. However, the mature retina is vulnerable to virus invasion and susceptible to infection, because herpesviruses and measles virus do cause acute or subacute retinitis in adults. The clinical spectrum of viral retinopathies may be broader, however, since natural and experimental retinal infections of animals can lead to retinal dysplasias and chronic retinal degeneration.

Pathogenesis

As a rostral extension of the CNS, the retina lies within the blood-brain barrier (Fig. 16.1). The arteries that accompany the optic nerve and supply the retinal layers give rise to capillaries that have a continuous endothelium joined by tight junctions as well as a continuous basement membrane, and are tightly

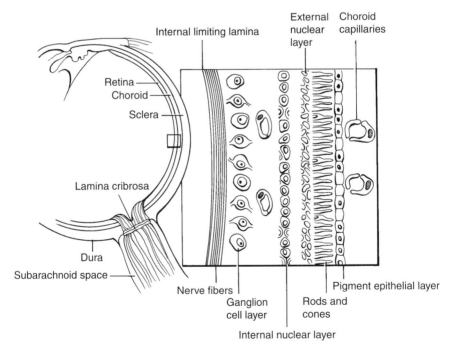

FIG. 16.1. The retina. General relationships and closure of the subarachnoid space at the lamina cribrosa are shown in diagram (left). Schematic of the retina (right) shows capillary system of the neuroretina with tight junctions and those of the choroid below the pigment epithelial layer with fenestrations.

apposed by glial processes similar to the capillaries of the brain. Little, if any, vesicular transport is seen in these vessels. In contrast, the choroid capillaries have fenestrated endothelium and a discontinuous basement membrane, and they lie in a loose stroma, similar to the capillaries of the choroid plexus. However, the retinal pigment epithelial cells of the outer retina and the ciliary epithelium anterior to the vitreous have tight junctions like those of choroid plexus epithelial cells and the cells of the pia on the surface of the brain. Thus, the blood-vitreous and retinal barriers structurally resemble the blood-brain and spinal fluid-brain barriers (Rapoport, 1976).

Viral spread to the retina encounters the same restraints as does spread to other portions of the CNS (see Chapter 3), but some of the same potential pathways exist. Virus can invade the retina from the brain along the neural pathway via the optic nerve. Since the subarachnoid space is obliterated at the lamina cribrosa, viruses must pass through limited extracellular spaces, infect the oligodendrocytes or astrocytes of the optic nerve, or enter within axons. Axonal transport of viruses to the inner ganglion cell layer may occur, but because the termination of all of these axons is on the small lateral geniculate ganglia, infection of these precise nuclei will be necessary to permit entry via axonal transport, a small window through which to gain access to the retina. Infection can also extend from intraocular structures across the pigment epithelial cells posteriorly or across the ciliary epithelium anteriorly into the peripheral retina. Direct hematogenous spread of virus to the retina can occur either directly by penetration across the capillaries in the neuroretinal layers or indirectly across the fenestrated choroidal vessels and then across the pigment epithelial cell layer.

It is tempting to conclude that major involvement of the inner ganglion cell layer implies a neural pathway, that retinopathy adjacent to the ora serrata indicates spread from an iridocyclitis, or that involvement of outer retinal layers suggests invasion from the choroidal capillaries. However, such localization of cytopathologic findings may also be explained by selective vulnerability of different cells within retinal layers or areas.

Herpesviruses

Herpes simplex virus and cytomegalovirus have been associated with retinopathies of congenital or neonatal infections and with retinitis of later life. Cytomegalovirus, herpes-zoster virus and herpes simplex viruses all cause retinitis in patients with low CD4 counts induced by HIV (see Chapter 12). Disseminated herpes simplex virus infections of the neonate are complicated by inflammatory ocular lesions, including retinitis in a small percentage of infants. Retinitis has also been reported in neonatal herpes simplex virus infections localized to the skin or cornea. The retinal lesions may evolve with the acute disease or after its resolution. Funduscopic examination shows a necrotizing chorioretinopathy with hemorrhages and exudates, and histologic examination shows disintegration of the retina, with later proliferation of the pigment epithelium.

The optic nerve may be involved as well as the cornea. The delayed onset, the symmetry of the lesions, and the absence of inflammation in adjacent nonneuroepithelial structures led to speculation that the retinal disease might be immune-mediated (Cogan et al., 1964). The absence of inclusion bodies and failure to recover virus were cited by others to support this hypothesis.

Retinitis is a rare complication of localized herpetic encephalitis of adults. In autopsy studies, a severe chorioretinitis has been seen with intranuclear inclusion bodies in all retinal cell layers and intranuclear viruslike particles. The greater involvement of the ganglion cell layer of the inner retina and the absence of inclusions in endothelial cells have led to the proposition that virus spreads along nerves from the CNS (Johnson and Wisotzkey, 1977). However, in one patient, herpesvirus-like particles were identified primarily in the outer pigment epithelial cells (Minckler et al., 1976). A similar chorioretinitis was seen in 1 of the 4 patients who survived herpesvirus simiae encephalitis (Roth and Purcell, 1977).

Cytomegalovirus is a more frequent cause of retinitis, both in congenitally infected children and in immunocompromised adults. The retinitis of congenital cytomegalovirus infections is clinically similar to that of herpes simplex virus infections. Involvement may range from irregular sheathing of retinal vessels, with no retinal necrosis, to patchy retinal necrosis, with pigment epithelial damage causing a white scar, to total bilateral retinal necrosis, with only small islands of identifiable retina. Lesions can be unilateral or bilateral, peripheral or central, focal or multifocal. The retina may be normal until several weeks of age, when chorioretinitis can evolve. Histologically, inclusion-bearing cytomegalic cells may be seen in the endothelial cells of both retinal and choroidal vessels, as well as diffusely throughout the areas of retinal necrosis (Nicholson, 1975).

Cytomegalovirus retinitis in adults was originally described in those receiving cytotoxic drugs to maintain renal allografts. Retinal lesions develop in 1% to 5% of these patients and in 20% to 25% of patients with AIDS (Jabs, 1995). The patients may complain of blurred vision, scotomata, or decreased visual acuity, and this can progress to total visual loss that may be unilateral or bilateral. Branch vessel occlusions, vascular sheathing, retinal edema, scattered hemorrhages, and exudates are seen in small foci, and these may enlarge and coalesce to involve the entire retina. Bilateral retinal detachment can occur (Meredith et al., 1979). Pathologic findings include retinal necrosis, with cytomegalic cells in all layers and only a mild attendant inflammatory response. Other signs of reactivation of cytomegaloviruses, such as pneumonitis, hepatitis, or encephalitis, need not be present (Murray et al., 1977).

Direct involvement of the retina by varicella-zoster virus also occurs. In patients with ophthalmic zoster, swelling of the disc with retinal hemorrhage and exudates has been observed. One patient with ophthalmic zoster who received systemic steroids developed a necrotizing retinopathy in the ipsilateral eye. An autopsy 7 weeks later showed extensive retinal necrosis, with inclusion bodies in sensory neurons and pigment epithelial cells. Electron microscopy showed herpesvirus-like particles (Schwartz et al., 1976). In patients with AIDS an acute retinal necrosis occasionally occurs associated with zoster eruptions. Inflammation of the anterior segment is associated with peripheral necrosis with central progression toward the posterior pole. Progression to blindness occurs in the majority usually with retinal detachment (Batisse et al., 1996).

The direct role of HIV in retinopathy is still unclear (Kennedy et al., 1986; Faber et al., 1992). Although the virus has been isolated from retinal specimens and antigen and RNA have been demonstrated in vascular or perivascular cells (Pomerantz et al., 1987; Reux et al., 1993); the coexistent herpesviruses appear to be the primary pathogenic agents.

Measles Virus

The protean clinical manifestations of measles virus infections with acute, subacute, and chronic CNS disease are accompanied by a variety of retinopathies. A mild retinopathy with vascular sheathing has been described during acute uncomplicated measles, and papillitis and retrobulbar neuritis may occur in the postinfectious perivenular demyelinating disease complicating acute measles. Retinitis is more commonly seen, however, with the subacute fatal measles encephalitis of immunocompromised patients and with the chronic infection of subacute sclerosing panencephalitis. In one patient with subacute measles encephalitis during chemotherapy, retinal changes developed 2 months after onset of measles. Postmortem examination showed intranuclear inclusion bodies in neurons and glia with a paucity of inflammation. The demonstration of viral antigen and paramyxovirus nucleocapsid-like structures in retinal cells of this patient indicated direct involvement of the retina with measles virus (Haltia et al., 1977).

In subacute sclerosing panencephalitis, a retinitis is seen in approximately 50% of patients (Green and Wirtschafter, 1973). This retinitis can develop prior to other clinical signs or can evolve during the course of disease. It may be unilateral or bilateral and may involve the periphery or the macula with significant visual loss. On funduscopic examination, edema, hemorrhage, an inflammatory preretinal membrane, retinal folds, gliotic scars, and changes in the retina pigment epithelium all have been described. The acute retinitis may subside, leaving a gliotic retinal scar that resembles a retinal dystrophy. With contraction of the internal limiting membrane, a macular hole may develop. Pathologic studies have shown diffuse chorioretinitis, with prominent involvement of the chorioid capillaries. Viral antigen and nucleocapsid-like structures have been found in varied cells of the retinal epithelium (Font et al., 1973).

Rubella Virus

Congenital rubella is complicated by a retinopathy, and the appearance and histopathology of the retinal lesions are distinct from those seen with herpesvirus and measles virus infections. Along with microphthalmia and cataracts, retinitis is one of the three common ocular manifestations of the congenital rubella syndrome (see Chapter 13), and it occurs in 13% to 60% of children with the syndrome. Retinopathy can also be the sole stigmata of congenital rubella virus infection. Clinically it tends to be a stationary abnormality manifest by irregular spotty pigmentation that gives a "salt-and-pepper" or "Scotch-tweed" appearance to the retina. The retinopathy does not significantly interfere with vision. Irregular degeneration of the retinal pigment epithelium is found, with areas of increased and decreased pigmentation. These changes are not associated with inflammation, and serious retinal dysplasia, necrosis, and detachment are not found (Zimmerman, 1968). A similar retinopathy is seen in progressive rubella panencephalitis.

Viral Retinopathy in Animals

Retinal lesions observed in natural and experimental infections in animals involve a wider spectrum of viruses and diverse pathologic changes (Table 16.1). Several experimental studies have given insights into the sequential pathogenesis of these lesions. The retinal dysplasia in newborn sheep that follows fetal infection with bluetongue virus shows rosettes of cells, disorganization of cell layers, retinal folds, and absence of pigment epithelium, similar to human dysplasias believed to result from abnormalities of histogenesis. Sequential studies, however, have shown that a necrotizing retinitis occurs *in utero*, and the disorganization of retinal layers seen in the neonatal lamb results from abortive repair rather than dysgenesis (Silverstein et al., 1971). Similar destructive inflammatory lesions of the retina, with sequelae bearing the hallmarks of retinal dysplasia, have been seen after the inoculation of fetal cats with feline leukemia virus (Albert et al., 1977), newborn puppies with canine herpesvirus (Albert et al., 1976), and mice with type 2 herpesvirus (Love et al., 1993). Defective repair of retinitis in the mature retina can also lead to apparent retinal dysplasia, as shown in adult hamsters inoculated with strains of measles virus (Parhad et al., 1980; Khalifa et al., 1991).

Some animal viruses cause retinal disease similar to the related human viruses. Canine distemper, a virus closely related to measles, causes a retinitis in dogs similar to that complicating measles infections in humans (Fischer and Jones, 1972). Fetal infection of calves with bovine viral diarrhea virus, a pestivirus similar to rubella, can mimic the major congenital malformations of the eye seen with the congenital rubella syndrome, including microphthalmia, cataracts, and retinal abnormalities. However, bovine viral diarrhea virus can cause a more intense retinitis, which results in retinal atrophy and migration of pigment cells into other neuronal layers (Bistner et al., 1970).

The route of virus invasion of the retina has been investigated with several viruses. Bornavirus, an unclassified virus that causes a slowly progressive encephalomyelitis in horses and sheep, causes a subacute encephalitis in several experimental hosts. After intracerebral inoculation of rabbits, encephalitis and

TABLE 16.1. *Viral retinopathies*

	Fetal or neonatal	Adult	Retinal lesion
Humans			
Herpesviruses			
Herpes simplex virus	+	+	Retinitis
Herpes simiae virus		+	Retinitis
Cytomegalovirus	+	+	Retinitis
Herpes zoster virus		+	Acute retinal necrosis
Paramyxovirus			
Measles virus		+	Retinitis
Togavirus			
Rubella virus	+		Pigment epithelium loss
Animals			
Herpesvirus			
Herpes simplex, type 2 (mouse)		+	Retinitis
Canine herpesvirus (dog)	+		Retinal dysplasia
Paramyxoviruses			
Measles virus (hamster)	+	+	Retinitis and retinal dysplasia
Canine distemper virus (dog)		+	Retinitis
Retrovirus			
Feline leukemia virus (cat)	+		Retinal dysplasia
Arenavirus			
Lymphocytic choriomeningitis virus (rat)	+		Acute retinal degeneration
Coronavirus			
JHM virus (mouse)		+	Acute retinitis and chronic degeneration
Reoviruses			
Reovirus, type 3 (mouse)	+		Retinitis
Bluetongue virus (sheep)	+		Retinal dysplasia
Togavirus			
Bovine viral diarrhea virus	+		Retinitis
Unclassified agents			
Borna virus (rabbit)	+		Retinitis
Scrapie agent (hamster and mice)	+		Retinal degeneration

retinitis develop after about 3 weeks, with antigen in the retina detectable first in the inner ganglion layers, followed by sequential involvement of outer layers. This suggests spread along axonal pathways to the eye and then from ganglion cells to bipolar cells to sensory nuclei (Krey et al., 1979a). Coagulation of one optic disc without disruption of retinal or choroidal vessels prevents retinal infection on the treated side supporting the hypothesis of virus transport via optic nerve fibers (Krey et al., 1979b). Sequential histologic studies of mice infected with reovirus type 3 also suggest neural spread, because inclusions develop in the optic disc, followed by inclusions in the ganglion cell layer. Conversely, after infection of neonatal hamsters with rat virus, inclusions develop primarily in the outer receptor cells, even though no sequela is evident after this infection (G. Margolis, personal communication). Considering the restriction of parvoviruses by host-cell DNA synthesis, this localization is probably explained by later maturation of receptor cells rather than by a particular route of virus dissemination. Studies of retinitis after intracerebral inoculation of several strains of measles virus into hamsters have used parallel growth curves of virus in retina and brain and early involvement of all retinal layers to argue for hematogenous spread of virus to the retina (Parhad et al., 1980).

In each of these experimental studies, retinal lesions appear to result from direct viral lysis of retinal cells. However, in lymphocytic choriomeningitis virus infections in rats, a retinopathy develops that appears to be immune-mediated. Retinal lesions are not found in acutely or chronically infected natural murine hosts, but when newborn rats are inoculated, necrosis is found in the pigment epithelial cell layer and all neuronal layers, with greatest involvement in the outer nuclear layers. Very little virus or viral antigen is found in the retina, and inflammation is minimal. Nevertheless, prevention by immunosuppression with cytotoxic drugs or antilymphocyte serum suggests an immune-mediated pathogenesis (Monjan et al., 1972). Intraocular inoculation of murine coronavirus led to an acute retinitis with vasculitis but after virus antigen and inflammation was cleared a progressive degeneration of photoreceptors and pigment epithelial cells continued and was associated with antiretinal autoantibodies and a persistence of viral RNA in retina and pigment epithelium (Robbins et al., 1990; Hooks et al., 1993; Komurasaki et al., 1996).

A novel slow progressive degeneration of the retina also has been described in hamsters and mice inoculated with scrapie. In mice the severity of the retinopathy is dependent on both the strain of scrapie and the genotype of the mouse (Foster et al., 1986). The sequence of involvement is interesting, because there is a gradual loss of the rod outer segments, followed by progressive loss of the rod inner segments and photoreceptor nuclei. Thus, the degeneration slowly progresses from outer to inner layers. Vacuolization, the hallmark of this infection in the neurons and glia of the brain and spinal cord, is sparse (Hogan et al., 1981). In mice infected with the prion of Creutzfeldt-Jakob disease the abnormalities are more pronounced and include vacuolization and astrocytosis of the optic nerve (Hogan et al., 1983).

The spectrum of viruses that can produce retinal lesions are probably more diverse than the limited studies to date would indicate. The retina often has been overlooked in virologic studies of CNS infections; yet the retina, with its well-defined laminar structure, unidirectional and focused axonal projection, and compartmentalized vascular supply, provides an interesting, accessible, and relevant site for investigations of the pathogenesis of CNS infections.

LABYRINTHITIS

In clinical medicine, deafness and disorders of equilibrium often are ascribed to viral infections of the inner ear with scant justification. Congenital hearing deficits have been clearly associated with rubella and cytomegalovirus infections, and, in the latter, pathologic and immunocytochemical studies of temporal bones have established viral infection within cells of the cochlear duct. Acquired acute hearing loss has been temporally related to the characteristic rash or parotitis of measles, varicella-zoster, and mumps virus infections. On the other hand, the widely accepted view that acute labyrinthitis or vestibular neuronitis is a viral disease is based entirely on temporal relationships of nonspecific respiratory or gastrointestinal complaints to the onset of labyrinthine dysfunction. Over 20 viruses have been tentatively related to inner ear disease on the basis of clinical signs, serologic conversions, or antibody prevalence (Davis, 1989b; Pyykkö et al., 1993). The speculations that Meniere disease or otosclerosis have a viral cause are even more tenuous. Thus, the incrimination of viral infections in the pathogenesis of varied inner ear diseases is based on clinical observations, a limited number of pathologic studies of temporal bones (most carried out long after the acute infection), and rare recoveries of cytomegalovirus and mumps virus from the inner ear. Experimental studies of inner ear infections have been limited (Table 16.2). The paucity of clin-

TABLE 16.2. *Viral infections of inner ear*

	Fetal or neonatal	Children or adult	Lesion
Humans			
Rubella virus	+		Cochleosaccular degeneration and strial atrophy
Cytomegalovirus	+		Endolymphatic cells in auditory and vestibular system
Measles virus		+	Hair cell degeneration and loss of ganglion cells
Mumps virus		+	Atrophy organ of Corti and stria vascularis
Varicella–zoster virus		+	Inflammation perilymphatic structures and sensory end-organs
Experimental animals			
Cytomegalovirus			
Mouse	+		Perilabyrinthitis
Guinea pig	+		Ganglion cell infection
Influenza A virus			
Hamster	+		Infection of mesenchymal cells in perilymphatic channels
Mumps virus			
Hamster	+		Infection of endolymphatic cells
Measles virus			
Hamster	+		Infection of neural end-organ and ganglion cells
Herpes simplex virus			
Hamster	+		Infection of perilymphatic and endolymphatic cells
Rabbit		+	Inflammation in membranous labyrinth and degeneration of organ of Corti and stria vascularis
Reovirus, type 3	+		Infection of neurons of cochlear and vestibular ganglia

ical and experimental studies does not stem from a lack of interest in or importance of these infections, but from the fact that the inner ear is buried within the temporal bone, posing a formidable obstacle to pathologic and virologic investigations.

Pathogenesis

Four routes of virus invasion of the inner ear have been postulated: direct extension from infection in the middle ear through the round window, spread of virus from the cerebrospinal fluid through the cochlear aqueduct into the perilymph, spread via the internal auditory canal into the modiolus of the cochlea, and hematogenous spread to the labyrinth. The first of these mechanisms has been considered in variola and varicella-zoster virus infections, where middle ear infections occur (Bordley and Kapur, 1972).

The cochlear aqueduct provides a potential direct connection between the subarachnoid space and perilymph (Fig. 16.2). The aqueduct is patent during development, but it is believed to be nonfunctional after infancy. However, red blood

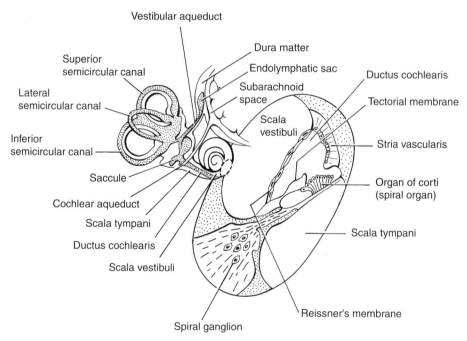

FIG. 16.2. The inner ear. The relationship of the subarachnoid space to the perilymph is shown at the top with connection via the cochlear aqueduct. The endolymph (shaded) is probably generated from the stria vascularis in the ductus cochlearis and may be absorbed in the endolymphatic sac lying adjacent to the subarachnoid space. Enlarged diagrammatic view of the one turn of the cochlea is shown at the right. The perilymph ascends in the scala tympani and descends in the scala vestibuli. The organ of Corti lies within the ductus cochlearis containing the endolymph.

cells have been found in the inner ear after subarachnoid hemorrhage (Holden and Schuknecht, 1968), and polymorphonuclear cells have been found in perilymph during bacterial meningitis (Perlman and Lindsay, 1939). Therefore, in infections such as mumps, where infected cells are numerous in cerebrospinal fluid, virus or virus-infected cells may pass through this channel into the perilymph of the membranous labyrinth.

Hematogenous spread of virus has been assumed to be the mechanism of invasion in cytomegalovirus, rubella, measles and mumps virus infections because pathologic changes are found in cells lining the endolymphatic space. The endolymph has a composition similar to that of intracellular fluid and is believed to be produced in the stria vascularis of the cochlear duct. Endolymph either travels in a linear fashion, with reabsorption in the endolymphatic sac, or circulates, with reabsorption through the stria vascularis. The assumption that infection of cells of the stria vascularis, organ of Corti, or sensory organs of the cochlear or vestibular apparatus or cells lining the cochlear duct must result from hematogenous spread is not justified in view of experimental studies that will be described later, demonstrating localization to selectively susceptible cells irrespective of the route of inoculation.

Congenital Hearing Deficits

Rubella Virus

Following the Australian epidemic that resulted in Gregg's recognition of congenital abnormalities due to fetal rubella virus infections, deafness was noted as part of the congenital rubella syndrome (Swan and Tostevin, 1946). However, detailed studies of rubella virus-induced hearing loss were not possible until the 1964 epidemic. Those studies showed that approximately one-half of the progeny of mothers clinically or subclinically infected with rubella virus during the first trimester of pregnancy had some hearing impairment. Progeny of mothers infected during the second trimester of pregnancy were less frequently affected, but some had hearing loss as the sole stigmata of fetal infection (Hardy et al., 1969). Furthermore, clinically inapparent maternal infection can lead to the birth of infants with severe sensorineural hearing loss (Karmody, 1969). Surprisingly, in approximately 25% of those affected, hearing loss appears to be progressive in the postnatal period (Bordley et al., 1972). In one report rubella in an adult was followed by hearing loss (Joachims and Eliachar, 1982).

Temporal bones have been studied from numerous children who have died at birth or within the first year of life with congenital rubella virus infections (Brookhauser and Bordley, 1973). A relatively uniform finding is collapse of Reissner's membrane, with adherence of the membrane to the stria vascularis and organ of Corti. The tectorial membrane usually is abnormal. The saccule may be collapsed, and the stria vascularis may show abnormal development and hypoplasia. Few, if any, abnormalities are found in the organ of Corti, utricle, semicircular canals, or spiral ganglia.

The pathogenesis of these lesions is unknown. Virus may continuously seed into the perilymph from the chronically infected cerebrospinal fluid. Alternatively, early hematogenous spread of virus may lead to chronic infection of cells of the membranous labyrinth. Abnormal development of the stria vascularis may lead to a defective formation of endolymph, resulting in collapse of the cochlear duct, or this collapse may result from infection of cells that line the duct. The asymmetry of the deafness and its progressive nature suggest chronic persistent clonal infection similar to that seen in the developing eye and other organs after early embryonic infection with the rubella virus (see Chapter 13). Because studies of inner ear infections in experimental animals with rubella virus have not been successful, and because virologic and pathologic studies of early fetal infections or studies in children with progressive auditory defects have not been carried out, many questions remain unanswered.

Cytomegalovirus

Although deafness was not included among the original cardinal signs of neonatal cytomegalic inclusion disease, cytomegalovirus infection of the fetus or newborn now is recognized as a major cause of childhood hearing impairment. histologic studies of temporal bones of infants dying with cytomegalic inclusion disease have shown cytomegalic cells in the epithelium of the cochlea, saccule, utricle, and semicircular canals. The localization is highly specific for endolymphatic cells; for example, in the two cell layers of Reissner's membrane, the cells on the endolymphatic side, which are of epithelial origin, are involved, and the cells on the perilymphatic side, of mesenchymal origin, are not (Myers and Stool, 1968; Davis et al., 1977a). Electron micrographs have shown typical herpesvirus particles within these distorted cells, immunocytochemical studies have demonstrated cytomegalovirus antigen within these cells, and virus has been recovered from perilymphatic fluid (Davis et al., 1981).

Long-term follow-up studies of "normal" infants with silent congenital cytomegalovirus infection, detected only by finding IgM antibody against cytomegalovirus in umbilical cord blood, have shown a high incidence of hearing deficits (Hanshaw et al., 1976). Considering that 0.5% to 1% of all liveborns are symptomatically infected with cytomegalovirus, involvement of the inner ear accounts for over 4000 cases of sensorineural hearing loss per year in the United States alone.

Sudden Acquired Deafness

Prior to the introduction of measles virus vaccine, measles caused 3% to 10% of deaf-mutism. Deafness usually occurs suddenly and usually is bilateral, and in some cases it occurs without any signs of CNS involvement. One pathologic study of a child who died 4.5 months after measles complicated by deafness showed degenerative changes in both the cochlear and vestibular systems. Hair cell degeneration was complete in both cochlea, and a reduction in the number of ganglion cells was evident, particularly in the basal coils. Multinucleated cells and inflammatory cells were still present, despite the long interval after the infection (Lindsay, 1973).

Mumps virus also is a common cause of deafness, but it accounts for less than 1% of profound deafness because the hearing loss usually is unilateral. Prior to vaccine programs mumps virus infections were estimated to account for 5% of cases of unilateral deafness (Everberg, 1957). Again, histologic studies have been limited. In a 6-year-old child who had developed acute deafness with a mumps virus infection at age 2, histologic abnormalities were limited to the structures within the cochlear duct, with collapse of Reissner's membrane, abnormality of the tectorial membrane, and degeneration of the stria vascularis. Changes in the organ of Corti were interpreted as representing secondary changes (Lindsay, 1973). A woman who had had a stapedectomy for otosclerosis developed mumps, with sudden deafness, and a surgical exploration was done to rule out a perilymph fistula. None was found, but a sample of perilymph was cultured, and mumps virus was recovered. This represented the first isolation of a virus from the inner ear (Westmore et al., 1979).

Varicella-zoster virus has been associated with a small number of cases of hearing loss and disequilibrium complicating chickenpox or herpes zoster oticus. Temporal bone studies in chickenpox have shown evidence of viral infection primarily in the middle ear (Bordley and Kapur, 1972). However, temporal bone studies after herpes zoster oticus have shown rather extensive inflammation in the perilymphatic structures and sensory end organs. Studies of the inner ears of a patient who died almost 2 years after herpes zoster oticus, with mild hearing loss but severe disruption of oculovestibular reflexes, showed severe changes in the ipsilateral semicircular canal receptor organ and nerve, with complete absence of the cupula (Proctor et al., 1979).

Lassa fever in West Africa is a major cause of acute sensorineural deafness. Audiometric evaluation showed 29% of patients hospitalized with Lassa fever virus infections developed hearing deficits (Cummins et al., 1990). The pathogenesis of this acute hearing loss has not been investigated.

Seroepidemiological studies of patients with acute hearing loss in North America have given varied results. One study of 39 patients reported 10 patients with a history of symptoms of upper respiratory infections prior to sudden deafness, but only one of these patients had serologic evidence of a recent viral infection; the virus was mumps (Rowson et al., 1975). In contrast, another study of 47 patients with sudden deafness reported the recovery agents from the nasopharynx in 37% [parainfluenza viruses 1 and 3, adenoviruses (7), herpes simplex (2), *Mycoplasma pneumoniae* (7)] and an even larger number of patients with fourfold or greater antibody increases to a similar spectrum of infectious agents (Maassab, 1973). Although this study gave credibility to an association of parainfluenza and adenoviruses with acute hearing loss, the frequent recovery of adenoviruses and herpesviruses from nasopharyngeal washings of normal persons or patients suffering other illnesses must be kept in mind.

Recently measles virus has been implicated in some cases of otosclerosis, a common bone dyscrasia of the endochondral layer of the human temporal bone. Ultrastructural descriptions of nucleocapsid-like structures, immunocytochemical demonstration of measles virus antigens, detection of measles virus RNA sequences in surgically removed stapedes, and anti-measles antibodies in perilymph have all been reported to support this seemingly unlikely association (McKenna and Mills, 1989; Niedermeyer and Arnold, 1995).

Labyrinthitis

Acute labyrinthitis or vestibular neuritis is widely regarded as a viral disease, but this assumption is based largely on the observation that the disease often occurs at the time of, or within a few days after, an upper respiratory illness. In a review of 443 patients, 43% gave a history of antecedent or concomitant infection that usually was flulike, although hepatitis, gastroenteritis, nephritis, infectious mononucleosis, and inflammations of the ear, nose, and throat were reported (Clemis and Becker, 1973). Some authors differentiate acute "viral" labyrinthitis or epidemic vertigo from vestibular neuritis by the normal caloric responses, associated neurologic signs, and epidemiologic clustering in the former disease. However, "lumped or split," there is not an established viral cause. Pathologic studies of 4 patients with prolonged vestibular neuritis showed atrophy of nerve trunks and their associated sense organs similar to findings after herpes zoster oticus (Schuknecht and Kutamura, 1981).

Viruses have been proposed in Ménière's disease based on the finding of abnormalities of the epithelium in the endolymphatic sac (Arenberg et al., 1970; Pulec, 1972). The viral hypothesis is based on presumed regulation of endolymphatic pressure and reabsorption of endolymph within the sac. If an antecedent viral infection alters these cells, their dysfunction could cause intermittent abnormalities of pressure regulation and lead to attacks of vertigo and the ultimate development of endolymphatic hydrops. Herpesvirus infections have been implicated in Ménière's syndrome on the basis of clinical observations (Adour et al., 1980) and of higher herpes simplex virus type 1 antibodies in patients with Ménière's disease (Bergström et al., 1992).

Experimental Studies in Animals

Experimental studies have been limited. Davis and his colleagues (Davis and Strauss, 1973; Davis and Hawrisiak, 1977) produced cytomegalovirus infections of the inner ear of newborn mice by intracerebral inoculation of the murine cytomegalovirus. Virus appeared to spread from the subarachnoid space into the connective tissue of the temporal bone via the cochlear duct and along the perineurium of the acoustic nerve into the modiolus. A perilabyrinthitis developed, in contrast to the endolabyrinthitis seen in the human temporal bone studies of congenitally infected infants. The investigators postulated that the human cytomegalovirus infection resulted from hematogenous spread of virus across the stria vascularis to explain the endolymphatic channel infection, in contrast to the direct extension of infection into the perilymph of the mouse. Guinea pig cytomegalovirus infection of pregnant animals led to auditory deficits in 28% of progeny with viral replication localized to spiral ganglion cells (Woolf et al., 1989).

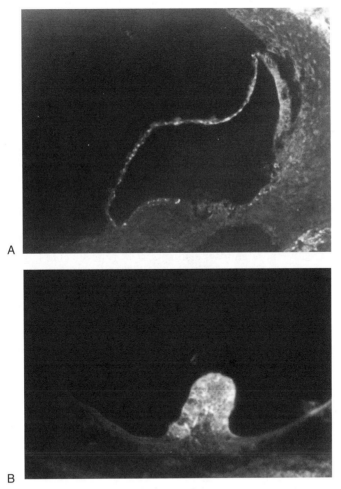

FIG. 16.3. Experimental viral infections of the inner ear. Fluorescent antibody-stained structures show selective vulnerability of specific cells in acute infections with mumps (A) and herpes simplex viruses (B). Mumps antigen is limited to the epithelial cells on the endolymphatic surface of Reissner's membrane and the stria vascularis. Herpes simplex virus antigen is shown in the crista of the semicircular canals.

In our laboratory (Davis et al., 1975; Davis and Johnson, 1976), acute infections of the inner ear of newborn hamsters were studied after intracerebral inoculation and after percutaneous inoculation through the temporal cartilage into the endolymphatic and perilymphatic spaces of the labyrinth. Selective vulnerability of the inner ear structures differed with different viruses (Fig. 16.3). Influenza virus infected only mesenchymal cells throughout the perilymphatic channels of the cochlea, mumps virus infected principally the cells lining the endolymphatic spaces, measles virus preferentially infected neural end organs and ganglion cells, and herpes simplex viruses infect both perilymphatic and endolymphatic cells. The route of inoculation did not influence the localization of infection in hamsters, which casts doubt on the assumption made in human temporal bone studies that the site of infected cells delineates the route of virus invasion. For example, in mumps virus infections where deafness is usually unilateral and frequently associated with meningitis, inner ear involvement may result from movement of virus down the cochlear aqueduct, even though the study of human temporal bones after mumps shows degenerative changes of endolymphatic structures, with relative preservation of the organ of Corti and spiral ganglia. However, in drawing analogies to human disease, it must be recognized that the newborn hamster is extremely immature at birth, having inner ear development equivalent to that of a 15-week-gestational human fetus.

Involvement of the inner ear in mature animals has been described in rabbits inoculated with herpesvirus through the stylomastoid foramina into the facial nerve to produce facial nerve paralysis (Kumagami, 1972). The cochlea in these animals showed marked inflammatory changes in the inner wall of the membranous labyrinth, degeneration of the organ of Corti, and changes in the stria vascularis. Clinically, these animals also appeared to have acute labyrinthine dysfunction with nystagmus and circling.

MYOSITIS

Viruses can cause acute myositis and may, at times, be related to chronic polymyositis. A variety of viruses, particularly alphaviruses, influenza viruses, and coxsackieviruses, have a specific affinity for muscle in some experimental hosts. These same viral infections in humans are accompanied by severe myalgias, and it has been postulated that these myalgias may represent direct growth of virus in muscle cells rather than the "toxic" effect traditionally invoked to explain the malaise of viral illnesses (Johnson, 1965b). The tenuous relationships of viruses to the muscle weakness or asthenia of chronic fatigue is discussed in Chapter 9. The association of infection with acute and chronic inflammatory disease of muscle is addressed here. The evidence relating viruses to human myositis has been largely electron microscopic data, which are inconclusive and serologic data, which at times are difficult to interpret. However, coxsackieviruses and influenza viruses have been recovered directly from muscle of patients with inflammatory myopathies.

Coxsackieviruses

In the acute encephalomyocarditis of neonates, group B coxsackieviruses have been recovered from both cardiac and skeletal muscles. However, it is uncertain whether or not coxsackieviruses can grow in mature muscle. In mice, the affinity of coxsackieviruses for muscles is age-dependent. Intense acute polymyositis occurs in newborn mice, but virus fails to grow in adults muscle, although dennervation or blocking acetycholine release with botulinum toxin does render adult muscle susceptible (Andrew et al., 1984). Using coxsackievirus B1 the time course of myositis in neonatal mice has been studied, virus could only be recovered for 2 weeks and viral RNA was detected for only 4 weeks. Nevertheless, histologic signs of myositis persisted for at least 16 weeks suggesting that virus initiated myositis but that virus did not persist even though inflammatory changes continued (Zoll et al., 1993).

In humans with hypogammaglobulinemia persistent enterovirus infections do occur often causing chronic meningoencephalitis and occasionally an accompanying chronic polymyositis. Echoviruses 3 and 11 have been isolated from muscles of these patients (Crennan et al., 1986). Evidence of chronic infection of muscle with enteroviruses in immunocompetent individuals is unconvincing. Many electron micrographs have been presented showing putative pseudocrystalline arrays of picornavirus-like particles in skeletal muscle of patients with myositis. Interpretative problems arise because the size of picornaviruses is similar to that of glycogen, which is normally abundant in muscle, and of ribosomes. Although the crystalline pattern is suggestive of virus arrays, ribosomes of chick muscle form crystalline patterns when muscle is cooled (Byers, 1966). In human tissue similar crystallization of organelles may accompany the pathologic changes or may occur as artifacts during tissue preparation.

Serologic evidence for chronic picornavirus infections, such as reported increasing levels of antibodies to B3 and B4 coxsackieviruses in 4 patients with dermatomyositis or polymyositis (Travers et al., 1977), is difficult to interpret. These patients had been symptomatic for at least 2 months before the first serum was obtained so rising levels are of dubious significance.

One study reported signal over muscle macrophages in biopsy specimens of 3 of 5 patients with adult-onset dermatomyositis using a probe derived from a murine picornavirus (Theiler's virus). Adjacent sections showed no reactions with probes to human enteroviruses (Rosenberg et al., 1989). This raises the question that an as yet unidentified enterovirus might be involved in some cases. Several extensive series have failed to demonstrate human enterovirus RNA in muscle biopsy specimens of inflammatory myopathies using PCR (Leff et al., 1992; Leon-Monzon and Dalakas, 1992; Fox et al., 1994).

In a widely cited case, coxsackievirus type A9 was isolated from the muscle of an 11-year-old child who had lifelong muscle weakness and retardation and who died of pneumonia secondary to atrophy of the diaphragm and intercostal muscles. Almost no inflammation was found in the atrophic muscles. However, collections of picornavirus-like particles were found, and coxsackievirus A9 was recovered from diaphragmatic muscle (Tang et al., 1975). This unusual case may represent a congenital or neonatal myopathy with persistence of virus and survival to 11 years of age, or it may represent an opportunistic infection of abnormal muscle as a terminal event. The case does little to confirm or refute the possible role of enteroviruses in the usual cases of chronic myositis.

Influenza Viruses

Malaise, cramps, fatigue, and electromyographic findings of myopathy are found during influenza virus infections and as an aftermath of the disease. Furthermore, human muscle cells are susceptible to infection with influenza viruses in culture (Armstrong et al., 1978). In acute and chronic myositis, nucleocapsid-like structures have been found in both vascular endothelial and sarcolemmal nuclei that have been interpreted as myxoviruslike particles. However, these structures resemble those abnormalities seen in reactive cells in multiple sclerosis and a variety of other diseases, and they probably represent nonspecific changes in nuclear chromatin.

A distinctive benign myositis sometimes called myalgia cruris epidemica occurs in some children with influenza virus infections. As the fever and respiratory symptoms are resolving, there is an abrupt onset of pain and weakness, primarily in the calves. Influenza virus has been implicated by epidemiologic data, isolations of virus from throat, and antibody increases (Ruff and Secrist, 1982). Both influenza A and influenza B viruses have been isolated from muscle in rare patients (Paisley et al., 1978; Farrell et al., 1980; Kessler et al., 1980) but the abrupt, brief clinical course, the fiber degeneration without inflammation, and the rarity of virus isolation simulate the nonpermissive infection of mouse muscle fibers after intramuscular inoculation of influenza B virus (Davis, LE, *personal communication*).

In adults, acute rhabdomyolysis with myoglobinuria can complicate influenza, (Singh and Scheld, 1996). Influenza B was recovered from muscle of an elderly man who had had several months of myalgia followed by an episode of acute myoglobinuria (Gamboa et al., 1979). Muscle biopsy showed polymyositis. Whether this virus was related to the antecedent myalgias or was an acute infection at the time of the myoglobinuria is uncertain.

Thus, influenza viruses are associated with an acute distal myopathy in children and with rhabdomyolysis in adults, and influenza viruses have been isolated from muscle in each syndrome.

Other Viruses in Humans and Animals

A viral etiology has been suspected in inclusion body myositis because of eosinophilic nuclear and cytoplasmic inclusions in myofibers. Abnormal 15- to 18-nm wide filaments are seen ultrastructurally in inclusions, and this led to claims of mumps virus antigens in inclusions (Chou, 1986). A subsequent *in situ* hybridization study of 20 cases has refuted this finding (Nishino et al., 1989). Report of isolation of type 2 adenovirus from two successive muscle biopsy specimens has been reported in another case of inclusion-body myositis (Mikol et al., 1982). In a fatal case of polymyositis with hepatitis B antigenemia muscle showed deposits of gamma globulin and complement that suggested an immune-complex disease (Mihas et al., 1978) and in a similar case deposits of complexes along the sarcolemma were shown (Damjanor et al., 1980). The strongest link-age of viruses with chronic myositis is the association of retroviruses with polymyositis in humans and other primates (Dalakas et al., 1986; see Chapters 11 and 12). Nevertheless, the pathogenesis remains obscure. Electron microscopy, immunocytochemistry, *in situ* hybridization and PCR have shown HIV in muscle specimens of seropositive patients with polymyositis. In most cases, the virus has not been found in muscle fibers but in interstial mononuclear cells. The predominant endomysial cells are CD8+ cells which are not suscepti-ble to the virus. The prevalent hypothesis is that infected macrophages release some cytokine that triggers a T-cell-mediated cytotoxic process against unin-fected myosites (Dalakas, 1991).

We addressed the role for immune responses in the pathogenesis of viral polymyositis in studies of Ross river virus, an alphavirus, that is a human pathogen causing epidemic polyarthritis in Australia and South Pacific Islands. The virus in mice causes an age-dependent polymyositis (Murphy et al., 1973b). Four-week-old animals develop no clinical signs, but 1-week-old animals develop severe weakness and polymyositis. Immunosuppression does not alter this age-dependent resistance, and immunosuppression of 1-week-old mice pro-longs clinical signs and reduces inflammation but fails to alter the pattern of muscle necrosis and regeneration. Thus, immune responses in this disease do not appear to determine either the age dependence or the muscle necrosis. These findings do not imply that other virus-induced polymyositis is not immune-mediated, but because the histopathology of this myositis resembles that of experimental autoimmune myositis and human polymyositis, these findings do underscore the principle that the histologic changes alone cannot differentiate myositis caused by viral cytotoxicity from myositis induced by immune responses (Seay et al., 1981).

VASCULITIS

Infection of vascular endothelial cells was addressed in earlier chapters as it relates to seeding a viremia and to penetration of the blood-brain barrier, but some infectious agents appear to cause primary vascular disease. This vascular disease may occur by several mechanisms which have been discussed in previ-ous chapters: (1) direct swelling and lysis of endothelial cells leading to occlu-sive or hemorrhagic disease, as occurs in rickettsial infections (see Chapter 5); (2) infection of vascular endothelial cells with a probable immune-mediated component, as in the cerebral granulomatous arteritis that may complicate oph-thalmic zoster and cytomegalovirus infection of cerebrovascular endothelial cells in immunocompromised patients (see Chapter 6); (3) immune-complex dis-ease, as postulated in the vascular lesions seen with congenital rubella and pro-gressive rubella panencephalitis (see Chapters 9 and 10).

The role of viruses in cerebrovascular disease may need to be expanded, par-ticularly with the recognition that febrile illnesses is a significant risk factor prior to ischemic brain infarction in patients under 50 years of age (Syrjänen et al., 1988). Furthermore, herpesvirus-like particles have been seen in cerebral granulomatous arteritis in the absence of herpes zoster (Reyes et al., 1976) and hepatitis B and parvovirus B19 have been associated with periarteritis nodosa and necrotizing angiitis. Herpes simplex virus messenger RNA and cytomegalovirus antigen have both been reported in arterial smooth muscle cells in atherosclerosis (Benditt et al., 1983; Melnick et al., 1983).

Hepatitis B Virus

Hepatitis B virus has been associated with acute arteritis; approximately 30% of patients with periarteritis have circulating hepatitis B surface antigen (HbsAg). Circulating immune complexes in this disease can be identified by ultrastructural analysis of clumps that contain 20-nm spheres and rods repre-senting the surface coat protein and 40-nm particles with dense cores (Dane par-ticles) that represent the intact virus. Studies have shown the presence of the antigen, immunoglobulins, and complement in the walls of inflamed vessels (Gocke et al., 1970). These presumptive complexes may have been deposited from blood or may have formed in the vessel wall. In either case, the activation of complement may lead to tissue injury.

Clinical signs of arteritis can develop at any time during the course of the infection; the arteritis is unrelated to the severity of liver disease, and once arteri-tis is cleared, it has not been observed to recur, even though there may be pro-gressive liver disease or persistent antigenemia (Sergent et al., 1976).

Numerous patients with hepatitis B develop neurologic abnormalities that may take the form of altered mental state, seizures, movement disorders, acute hemiparesis, myelitis, mononeuritis multiplex, or Guillain-Barré syndrome (Apstein et al., 1979). These complications may appear in the pre-ecteric stage, or liver involvement may be subclinical; so assays for hepatitis B antigen may be of value if there are any signs of liver dysfunction in a patient with acute vas-culitis or unexplained acute neurologic disease. Spinal fluid often is normal or may show an elevation of protein; pleocytosis is unusual. Several patients have died with cerebrovascular accidents, and autopsies have shown multiple areas of infarction, with evidence of healed vasculitis (Duffy et al., 1976; Sergent et al., 1976).

Focal CNS signs and mononeuritis multiplex are thought to be related to deposition or formation of complexes in small arterial vessels of brain and peripheral nerve, with resultant necrotizing arteritis and vascular occlusion (Brooks, 1977; Rosenberg et al., 1977). The symmetrical peripheral neuropathy and Guillain-Barré syndrome probably are unrelated to arteritis, and the role of circulating or deposited antigen in this illness is unknown. In one patient with Guillain-Barré syndrome, hepatitis B antigen was found in spinal fluid when absent in serum. This suggests virus replication in the CNS because hepatitis antigen usually does not cross into cerebrospinal fluid (Huet et al., 1980).

Parvovirus B19

Systemic necrotizing vasculitis resembling periarteritis and Wegner granulomatosis has been described in 3 children with parvovirus B19 DNA detected in serum and tissue samples by PCR and by presence of IgM antibody to the virus (Finkel et al., 1994). Onset of periarteritis nodosum with mononeuropathy in an adult has been reported with serologic evidence of acute parvovirus B19 infection (Corman and Dolson, 1992). A possible association of parvovirus B19 with temporal arteritis was reported in an adult who had similar evidence of chronic infection after transfusions (Staud and Corman, 1996). The infections and vasculitis may have been coincidental and CNS lesions were not described, but further investigations of this agent in vasculitis are needed.

Cerebrovascular Disease in Animals

Vascular disease manifest by intracerebral hemorrhage or arteritis with vascular occlusion has been described in several natural and experimental viral infections of animals. Infection and lysis of vascular endothelial cells appear to cause a hemorrhagic encephalopathy in chick embryos infected with the neurotropic strain of influenza virus (Hook et al., 1962), as well as a hemorrhagic encephalopathy in rats caused by a rat parvovirus (Nathanson et al., 1970). Ultrastructural studies of the latter disease, however, showed that alterations in vascular endothelium were found only at sites where aggregates of platelets and fibrin were attached to infected endothelial cells which suggests that the hemorrhages may have resulted from disseminated intravascular coagulation (Baringer and Nathanson, 1972).

Arteritis with infiltration of vessel walls with inflammatory cells and necrosis of vessel walls is found in several natural animal diseases: in horses infected with equine arteritis virus, a coronavirus (genus arterivus); in cattle infected with malignant catarrhal fever virus, a herpesvirus; in sheep infected fetally or postnatally with border disease virus, a pestivirus; in mink infected with Aleutian mink disease virus, a parvovirus. The lesions in equine arteritis are most prominent in large arteries with well-developed muscular coats, and they are characterized by necrosis of smooth muscle, lymphocytic infiltration of the vessel wall, and ultimately vascular occlusion and infarction (Jones et al., 1957). Electron microscopic studies show virions within damaged endothelial cells, with degeneration of apparently uninfected underlying smooth muscle cells (Estes and Cheville, 1970). Unfortunately, studies have not examined cerebrovasculature.

The periarteritis of border disease in sheep also involves the arterial circulation, almost exclusively arterioles. The disease is seen in sheep infected after 80 days of gestation or in the neonatal period. Lesions develop in 15 to 20 days and may run a protracted course to 180 days. There is an interesting predilection for CNS vessels (Zakarian et al., 1975). Viral antigen has been demonstrated to persist in vessel wall, and it has been postulated that the nodular periarteritis may represent a cell-mediated immune response to the persistent infection (Gardiner et al., 1980).

Malignant catarrhal fever virus causes a disease in cattle in which necrotizing vasculitis of cerebral vessels has been considered a pathognomonic finding, and fibrinoid degeneration of vessel wall, with cellular infiltrates is present in the cerebral vessels even in mild cases (Fig. 16.4).

Aleutian disease is a naturally occurring persistent parvovirus infection of mink. The infection results in enormous increases in immunoglobulin levels and specific antiviral antibody. Pathologically, hepatitis, arteritis, and glomerulitis are associated with a widespread proliferation of plasma cells (Porter, 1986). The necrotizing arteritis affects muscular vessels, and lesions are found of varying age. Extracellular deposits of immunoglobulin, complement, and viral antigen have been demonstrated in the areas of fibrillary necrosis and between prolifer-

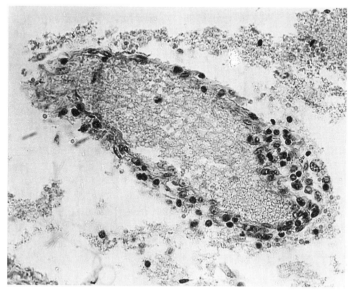

FIG. 16.4. Cerebral arteritis in natural malignant catarrhal fever virus infection of a cow. Meningeal artery shows inflammation within vesel wall (From Johnson and Narayan, 1974 with permission).

ating endothelial cells (Porter et al., 1973). There are persistent high levels of circulating immune complexes. The vasculitis can be attenuated by immunosuppression or infection *in utero* and can be accentuated by inactivated vaccine. All these findings suggest a vasculitis secondary to the chronic deposition or formation of immune complexes in vessels. In naturally and experimentally infected mink, arterial lesions are found in brain, associated with both intracerebral hemorrhages and focal areas of infarction.

These animal diseases support the contention that a variety of acute or chronic inflammatory vascular diseases may be related to viral infections.

17

Prevention and Therapy

A hundred thousand persons, upon the smallest computation have been inoculated in these realms. The number who have partaken of its benefits throughout Europe and other parts of the globe are incalculable; and it now becomes too manifest to admit to controversy, but the annihilation of the Small Pox, the most dreadful scourge of the human species, must be the final result of this practice.
  Edward Jenner,
  The Origin of the Vaccine Inoculation, 1801

Jenner's ebullient optimism about the annihilation of smallpox with his cowpox virus was not widely shared. Although vaccinia proved to be the first effective vaccine, the human spread of smallpox appeared too widespread to ever envision universal immunization. One hundred years later, yellow fever became the first disease for which worldwide eradication seemed possible. Walter Reed's commission had shown that yellow fever was spread by a mosquito vector, and they succeeded in eradicating the disease in Cuba by quarantine, screening, and mosquito control (Reed, 1902). An international commission decided that it would be possible to eliminate yellow fever, because the virus in its intermediate host appeared susceptible to environmental control.

In the 1970s we saw the first eradication of an important human disease, and it was smallpox, not yellow fever. Smallpox does not persist; it has no animal reservoir, it is antigenically stable, and it spreads slowly. With an effective vaccine that gave long-term immunity, the World Health Organization was able to mount a massive cooperative program of quarantine and immunization that has eliminated smallpox from the face of the earth, except for several vials of virus deposited in designated laboratories. Polioviruses and measles viruses have the epidemiologic characteristics to make them similar candidates for annihilation.

In contrast, Walter Reed's hopes will never be realized. Yellow fever can be eliminated from urban areas and island populations by the control of *Aedes aegypti* and can be prevented by an effective vaccine, but the virus has sylvatic cycles. In both Africa and South America, mosquitoes of the jungle canopy and arboreal monkeys circulate the virus, which leaves yellow fever forever in the treetops awaiting the nonimmune worker entering or clearing the forests. With-

411

TABLE 17.1. *Impact of vaccines*

Disease	Number of cases in the United States	
	Prevaccine peak years	1995
Paralytic poliomyelitis	57,000	0
Congenital rubella	20,000	7
Measles	900,000[a]	309
Mumps	150,000	804

[a]Estimated 900 cases of encephalomyelitis.

out continuing control of urban mosquitoes, the patient with sylvatic disease poses a constant threat of reinitiating an epidemic cycle in his community.

Enormous successes have been made with vaccines introduced during the past generation (Table 17.1), and new methods of vaccine development promise major future successes in prevention. However, each will be individualized and can be developed only with full cognizance of the natural history of the individual viral infection, from its natural ecology to its molecular biology.

Hopes for antiviral chemotherapy became widespread with the introduction of bacteriostatic and bacteriocidal agents in the 1940s and 1950s. The recognition that virus synthesis is intimately linked to the cell's normal metabolism caused hopes to dwindle. Even the laity felt frustration, asking why a society that can put a man on the moon cannot cure the common cold. However, with further knowledge of the molecular biology of virus replication, it has become evident that in the replicative cycle of each virus, virus-coded functions occur that potentially can be blocked without irreparable damage to the host cell. New approaches to drug design now promise effective new treatments for a wide variety of viral infections.

ENVIRONMENTAL CONTROL

Selective intervention into the ecologic cycle in many cases can interrupt the spread of viruses from animals to humans or between arthropods and humans. Interruption of human to human respiratory, enteric, or venereal dissemination is the more difficult.

The earliest method devised to control human to human spread was quarantine. Quarantine of the infected individual has proved remarkably ineffective for most viral infections, because a large number of infections are subclinical and because infectivity often is maximal prior to the development of typical clinical disease. In the 1930s, when a public health nurse nailed a scarlet chickenpox quarantine sign on our front door, probably all my classmates had been exposed before my eruption; even if exposure was avoided, quarantine only delayed their inevitable encounter with this ubiquitous and highly infectious virus. In contrast, international quarantine combined with vaccination was effective during smallpox eradication.

Improvement in public sanitation can decrease the dissemination of enteric viruses. Sewage abounds with picornaviruses and adenoviruses, and proper control of drinking and irrigation waters can decrease the spread of these agents. The major virologic impacts of improved sanitation have been the decrease in hepatitis A virus infections in developed countries and the fostering of poliomyelitis epidemics, presumably because of the delay in the age of contracting infection (see Chapter 5).

The transmission of HIV infections by blood products has been almost eliminated in many countries by routine testing, and in some populations significant successes in slowing the spread of HIV infections have been made through education, needle exchanges, and condom distribution (see Chapter 12).

Zoonotic infection can be controlled by immunization, containment, or slaughter of infected animals. In rabies control, all three have been successful. Immunization of pet dogs and cats or killing of feral dogs and quarantine of imported animals have eliminated rabies from some island countries. The required vaccination of dogs and the killing of strays have been the major factors in decreasing rabies to its present low level in the United States, but total eradication is not possible with these methods because of the sylvatic cycles of the virus. The control of wild carnivore and bat populations poses far greater obstacles. Wildlife reduction has been used, and a live attenuated virus vaccine in bait has shown promise in the reduction of sylvatic rabies (see Chapter 7). Containment also has been effective in reducing the risk of herpesvirus B infections in laboratory workers by quarantine of rhesus monkeys and routine examination of monkeys for both oral lesions and antibody.

Environmental control of arboviruses can employ a variety of strategies, including elimination of the arthropod, elimination or immunization of the natural or amplifying host and protection of man with immunization as well as screening, netting and repellents. Different strategies are necessary with different arboviral cycles. For example, little can be done to control the widespread rural populations of Culicine mosquitoes that carry western, St. Louis, and Japanese encephalitis viruses, although campaigns to use nets over cribs of infants in the central valleys of California may have reduced the morbidity from western encephalitis among the age group most severely affected. When St. Louis encephalitis virus enters into the urban cycle, urban spraying and clearing of stagnant-water breeding sites can decrease vector populations. Similarly, the treehole mosquito vector of La Crosse encephalitis virus cannot be cleared from the forests of the central and eastern United States, but in endemic areas campaigns to cement treeholes and to remove old tires (man-made "treeholes") from backyards can reduce exposure of children. Understanding the natural cycle is a prerequisite to control as exemplified in a minor political scuffle in the mid-1960s, when some irate citizens of Republican Ohio accused President Johnson of favoritism for sending military planes to spray a Texas city with an urban epidemic of St. Louis encephalitis and neglecting northeast Ohio, where large numbers of cases of California encephalitis were being reported. The Ohio cases,

however, were acquired in the woods, where spraying would have been imprac-
tical and unacceptable; greater protection would have been afforded by discon-
tinuing the "great society" outdoor summer programs and keeping the children
in the cities.

Dampening the arboviral cycle by immunization of amplifying hosts has been
attempted. Japanese encephalitis vaccine was given to piglets in Japan, which
were important as amplifying hosts of the virus. Immunization of horses can
decrease the spread of the epidemic form of Venezuelan equine encephalitis.

VACCINES

Active Immunization

Vaccines may consist of attenuated or related live viruses or of killed viruses
or of virus components that will induce an immune response and prevent disease
when there is future contact with the natural infection. Rabies is the only virus
infection in which postexposure active immunization is effective (Table 17.2).

Logic dictates that live virus vaccines should be better. They will produce both
humoral and cell-mediated immunity against all components of the virus, they
can be given by the natural route to induce IgA on the appropriate contact sur-

TABLE 17.2. *Available virus vaccines for potentially neuropathic viruses*

Vaccine	Neurologic complications of vaccine
Live virus vaccines	
Vaccinia (no longer in use)	Has effectively eradicated smallpox; formerly caused postvaccinal encephalomyelitis
Yellow fever virus	Very rare potentially fatal encephalitis
Poliovirus	Rare paralytic infections in immunodeficient children and adult contacts; possibly higher rate of Guillain–Barré syndrome
Measles virus	None documented; only anecdotal reports; also reduces incidence of subacute sclerosing panencephalitis
Mumps virus	Aseptic meningitis with Urabe strain (not used in the United States)
Rubella virus	Arthritis; crosses placenta but no evidence of teratogenesis
Varicella–zoster virus	None documented
Inactivated virus vaccines	
Rabies virus	
Neural tissue	High rate of encephalomyelitis with neural tissue, but low
Duck embryo	with duck embryo
Human diploid cells	Few, if any, neurologic complications (Guillain–Barré syndrome and myelopathy reported anecdotally)
Influenza A and B viruses	Guillain–Barré syndrome with swine flu vaccine
Poliovirus	No documented complications
Hepatitis A virus	None
Japanese encephalitis virus	Encephalitis or neuropathy in 1 to 2.3 per million vaccinees
Recombinant protein vaccine	
Hepatitis B virus	None documented; only anecdotal reports of neurologic complications

face, and they have the potential to confer durable lifelong immunity. Indeed, the antibody levels years after live measles, mumps, and rubella virus vaccine are comparable to those after natural infection.

The problems with traditional live virus vaccine lie in their crude methods of development (Table 17.3). To date, attenuated vaccine viruses have been developed by sequential passage of a virulent strain through animals, embryonated eggs or cell cultures, blindly relying on random mutations to attenuate their virulence without the acquisition of new undesirable traits. This procedure can pick up contaminating viruses, as occurred at one time with the inadvertent contamination of yellow fever vaccine with hepatitis virus, as well as with the incorporation of SV40 into early poliovirus vaccines. Alternatively, the attenuated virus can acquire new properties, such as the potential of the rubella virus vaccine to cause arthritis. Greater catastrophes could occur, as exemplified in the development of live virus vaccines in veterinary medicine. The attenuated vaccines for bluetongue virus in sheep, hog cholera in pigs, and feline panleukopenia in cats all proved to be teratogenic. This effect was anticipated with the feline panleukopenia virus, because the wild virus also causes cerebellar hypoplasia in kittens. Similar problems were a concern with the initial introduction rubella virus vaccine. However, wild bluetongue virus was not associated with any natural neurologic disease, and hog cholera was universally fatal; so neural teratogenesis was an unexpected property of the attenuated viruses (see Chapter 13).

The use of killed vaccines is not a panacea for these problems. Contaminating viruses may be present that are more resistant to inactivation than the wild-type virus in the vaccine, such as the live SV40 in the early killed poliovirus vaccine. Furthermore, the immunity usually is of shorter duration and may not be

TABLE 17.3. *Advantages and disadvantages of live and inactivated virus vaccines*

Advantages	Disadvantages
Live virus vaccines	
Durable long-term protection	Possible reversion to virulence
Simulates natural infection	May spread to contacts
Local IgA if given by natural route	May lead to persistent infection or have teratogenic properties
Stimulates cell-mediated immunity	May contain contaminating viruses
One dose amplified in host	Problems of delivery in areas with inadequate refrigeration
Less expense to produce	
Inactivated virus vaccines	
Ease of preparation and storage	Protection usually of shorter duration
Can use virulent strain	May not generate IgA or cell-mediated immunity
Can inactivate contaminating agents	May not generate antibody to some important antigens
No untoward effects of replication	Possible allergic reactions to animal or human proteins or antibiotics
	Incomplete inactivation due to aggregation

IgA, immunoglobulin A.

directed against the appropriate antigens. The inactivated measles vaccine used between 1963 and 1967 gave excellent neutralizing antibody responses in recipients, but after subsequent contact with wild virus, this partial immunity led to a more severe disease called atypical measles. A similar mishap occurred with the killed respiratory syncytial virus vaccine. In addition, unanticipated complications can arise, such as the higher rate of Guillain-Barré syndrome that followed the inactivated swine influenza virus vaccine in 1976 (see Chapter 8).

The control of poliomyelitis with vaccine has been spectacular, first with the use of the killed vaccine and later with the live attenuated virus, which because of its enteric excretion succeeded in immunizing many nonrecipients. With the eradication of wild-type poliomyelitis in the Western Hemisphere only 8 to 10 cases of locally acquired paralytic poliomyelitis occur annually in the United States, and all are related to the vaccine viruses (see Chapter 5). The Advisory Committee on Immunization Practices recently recommended initial immunization of infants with two doses of inactivated poliovirus vaccine followed by two doses of oral poliovirus in childhood (CDC, 1997b). Oral or inactivated vaccine alone are still acceptable, however, and are preferred in some situations including the sole use of inactivated vaccine in the immunosuppressed and the sole use of live vaccine in children who begin vaccination after 6 months of age.

The morbidity and mortality caused by human herpesviruses make vaccine development desirable, but these viruses present unique problems because of their acquisition in early life, their latency, and their oncogenic potential. The oncogenic potential is of concern, even for killed vaccine, because ultraviolet irradiation of cytomegalovirus and herpes simplex virus can convert lytic infection to nonpermissive infection with cell transformation *in vitro* (Albrecht and Rapp, 1973; Rapp and Duff, 1973). The attenuated varicella zoster virus has not been associated with postvaricella encephalomyelitis or ataxia, but no positive or negative effect is available on the incidence of herpes zoster years later. Attenuated viruses or inactivated viruses might prevent primary infection, but they are unlikely to clear latent infections or alter activations.

New technologies promise to provide safer, inexpensive vaccines (Table 17.4). The only current vaccine developed with these technologies is the subunit hepatitis B vaccine, produced by cloning the surface protein gene into yeast. Live attenuated virus vaccines are being developed with focused mutagenesis

TABLE 17.4. *New methods of vaccine development*

Subunit vaccines
Conditional mutants (temperature sensitive)
Deletion mutagenesis
Synthetic polypeptides (with adjuvants)
Antiidiotype antibodies
Recombinant expression vectors
DNA (DNA plasmid carrying antigen-coding gene)

such as temperature sensitive influenza strains that allow replication in the upper but not the lower respiratory tract. Gene reassortment has been added to this strategy to combine the two surface proteins of the circulating epidemic strain of influenza virus with the other 6 genes from a cold-adapted donor virus (Maassab and DeBorde, 1985).

Synthetic peptides also have potential since they can be synthesized quickly and in large amounts (Lerner, 1982). Limitations, however, include the need for a linear epitope and the need to present the peptide with carrier proteins or adjuvants. Antidiotype monoclonal antibodies can similarly serve as vaccines but also may require adjuvants (Gaulton et al., 1986).

Recombinant expression vectors have been of great interest where genes coding for targeted proteins are placed in other viruses, bacteria or yeast (Wilkinson and Borysiewicz, 1995). Vaccinia virus, bacilloviruses, retroviruses, and adenovirus all have been used as virus vectors. For example, the coding sequences for hepatitis B surface antigen, herpes simplex virus glycoprotein D, and influenza virus hemagglutinin were inserted into a single vaccinia virus genome; and intradermally inoculated rabbits developed antibodies to all of the foreign viral antigens (Perkus, et al., 1985). Immunization against multiple agents by a simple scarification that can be done by a nonprofessional aide has obvious advantages in developing countries.

DNA vaccines are the most recent innovation. A DNA plasmid carrying an antigen-coding gene is used to transfect cells *in vivo*, and an immune response to the antigen develops. A variety of DNA vaccines have been tested in animals and preliminary human trials have begun (Whalen, 1996).

Passive Immunization

The administration of preformed antiviral immunoglobulins can lead to short-term protection. After intramuscular or subcutaneous inoculation, maximum titers are found in the blood after 4 to 6 days. Passive immunity of selected hyperimmune serum has been shown to be effective in the postexposure prophylaxis against rabies virus (combined with active immunization) and hepatitis B. Hyperimmune selected immunoglobulins are effective in preventing or modifying varicella in exposed immunocompromised children and in preventing or suppressing cytomegalovirus infections in renal transplant recipients. Pooled immunoglobulins have been useful in providing short-term protection against hepatitis in travelers.

Serum or immunoglobulins of convalescent patients have been employed to treat patients with Lassa and Argentinean hemorrhagic fevers. Administration of antibodies also has had some success in clearing enteroviruses from the CNS and muscle of patients with hypogammaglobulinemia (Misbah et al., 1992). The evanescent protection of passive immunization limits its potential for preventing or treating most infections in the general population.

ANTIVIRAL DRUGS

The intimate relationship of virus replication strategies with normal cellular functions discouraged early searches for antiviral drugs. With knowledge of the molecular biology of virus-cell interactions, however, it became evident that there are multiple sites at which virus-specific functions occur, particularly enzymes coded by the viruses themselves. Furthermore, antimetabolites may be more toxic to rapid replicating cycle of the virus than to normal cell function. The first drug that was championed for the treatment of a CNS infection was idoxuridine for herpes simplex virus encephalitis. In the subsequent controlled study, it was found to have a greater morbidity than placebo and its detrimental myelosuppressive effect outweighed the benefit of inhibition of virus replication. An acceptable drug must be able to reach its target, be capable of acting intracellularly as well as extracellularly and be metabolically stable; they also must do more good than harm (Bean, 1992).

Available Drugs

The drugs with efficacy in the treatment of CNS infections are shown in Table 17.5. The list is limited but promising considering that only one of these had shown efficacy at the time of the first edition of this book. Vidarabine is a purine nucleoside analog. In a double blind controlled trial it had been shown to be a more effective treatment of herpes simplex virus encephalitis than placebo. Acyclovir, aguanosine analog was subsequently shown to be more effective than vidarabine. The two drugs were basically equal in efficacy in the neonatal form of the disease. Gancilovir although structurally similar to acyclovir has greater effectiveness against cytomegalovirus and is more toxic. It is effective in cytomegalovirus retinitis, may be of benefit in cytomegalovirus infections of peripheral nerve, and has not yet been shown to be effective in cytomegalovirus encephalitis and ventriculitis in AIDS patients. There is reasonable data to sup-

TABLE 17.5. *Antiviral drugs in nervous system infections*

Drug	Virus	Efficacy
Vidarabine	Herpes simplex virus	Effective in placebo-controlled trial in herpes simplex virus encephalitis
Acyclovir	Herpes simplex virus	Better than vidarabine in herpes simplex virus encephalitis in controlled trials
Ganciclovir	Cytomegalovirus	Established efficacy in retinitis; anecdotal reports of efficacy in radiculomyelitis and encephalitis
Foscarnet	Cytomegalovirus	Study in progress of ganciclovir plus foscarnet in encephalitis and radiculomyelitis in AIDS patients
Zidovidine (AZT)	HIV	Effective in placebo—controlled trials in AIDS with cognitive abnormalities
Ribavirin	Lassa virus	90% reduction in fatalities vs. controls during first 6 days

port the use of foscarnet in either CMV retinitis or in the case of herpes simplex encephalitis where the virus is thought to have developed resistance to acyclovir.

Zidovidine, a reverse transcriptase inhibitor of HIV, has been documented to delay the onset of dementia, attenuate the neuropathologic findings in AIDS dementia, and actually improve cognition in affected adults and children (see Chapter 12). Similar data are not available for the other reverse transcriptase inhibitors or for the protease inhibitors (Sacktor and McArthur, 1997).

Following the initial description of interferons (Isaacs and Lindenmann, 1957) expectations arose that this group of molecules might be the "broad spectrum antiviral." Although active against a broad range of viruses the interferons are highly species-specific and early studies were constrained by the shortage and expense of preparation of human interferons. In recent years with large volumes of cloned human interferons available efficacy has been shown against hepatitis B active liver disease, hepatitis C chronic liver disease and genital warts. Although used empirically in subacute sclerosing panencephalitis and other chronic CNS infections their efficacy is unproved. Interferon beta reduces the number of exacerbations of multiple sclerosis but this has been accredited to its properties as an immune modulator. Since many multiple sclerosis attacks are precipitated by viruslike illnesses the antiviral properties of interferon beta also may be a factor.

Other immune modulators, drugs that augment immune responses, have been proposed as antiviral agents particularly in persistent and slow infections. Levamisole, isoprinosine and transfer factor have all been advocated, but data of efficacy have never been convincing.

Potential Sites of Drug Actions

Drugs have been described that block replication of viruses in each and every stage of the replicative cycle (Fig. 17.1). Many are of no practical use in the treatment of viral infections of the nervous system because they fail to enter the CNS or are too toxic for human use. However, they do illustrate the potential for drugs to block the early events of adsorption and penetration, to interfere with specific replication events and even to block late events such as assembly and release.

Virus adsorption can be blocked by compounds that react with the positively charged amino acid residues of the viral envelope glycoproteins. Drugs of particular interest in this regard are polyanionic substances including polysulfates, polysulfonates, polycarboxylates and oxometalates. One polyanion that has received wide advocacy for use in HIV infection is dextran sulfate. Dextran sulfate does appear to have the effect of blocking HIV adsorption to cultured T cells but may enhance the infectivity of macrophagetropic virus strains in primary human macrophages (Meylan et al., 1994). Cell fusion can be blocked by some of the same substances but also by negatively charged human serum albumins and by bicyclams.

ATTACHMENT
  Antibody or contructs against receptor
  Heparin
  Polysulfates
  Polysulfonates
  Polycarboxylates
  Oxometalates
  Dextran sulfate

PENETRATION (FUSION)
  Negatively charged serum albumins
  Titerpene derivatives
  Bicyclams

UNCOATING
  Amantadine (influenza)
  Isoxazoles (picornaviruses)
  Aridone (picornaviruses)
  Pyridazinamines (picornaviruses)

NUCLEI ACID REPLICATION
  Reverse transcriptase (retroviruses)
  Dideoxynucleoside analogs
  Acyclic nucleoside phosphonates
  Nonsubstrate analogs
  Integrase inhibition (retroviruses)

DNA polymerase (herpesviruses)
  Pyrimidine nucleotide analogs
  Acyclic nucleoside analogs
  Carbocyclic nucleoside analogs
  Acylic nucleoside phosphonates

MESSAGE TRANSLATION
  Antisence oligonucleotides
  Ribozymes

ASSEMBLY
  Protease inhibitors
  Amantadine
RELEASE
  Neuramidase inhibitors (Influenza)

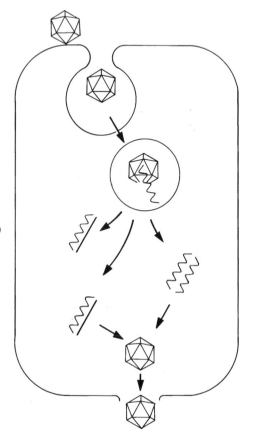

FIG. 17.1. Diagram of the infectious cycle in the host cell. Shown is a naked icosahedral virus that penetrates by endopinocytosis. Nucleic acids are represented by wavy lines and polypeptides by straight lines. The positions of the host-cell nucleus and cytoplasm have been eliminated because different viruses replicate nucleic acids and assemble in different locations. Representative drugs blocking steps of the infectious cycle are listed.

Uncoating is a variable process between different viruses, but drugs have been found that interfere with the uncoating of influenza viruses as well as with picornaviruses. Amantadine is an approved drug for prophylaxis of influenza A virus infections. The drug physically blocks the proton channels formed by a membrane protein; this is critical both for virus uncoating by preventing the disassociation of the matrix protein from the ribonucleoprotein and for virus maturation by altering the hemagglutinin formation and the budding of virus from the cell membrane. Thus amantadine and related drugs affect events in both early and late phases of the infectivity cycle. The picornavirus uncoating can be blocked by a number of agents that bind to the viral capsid and inhibit uncoating (isoxazoles, aridone, pyridazinamines, and others).

Viral polymerases have been the most obvious target for antiviral drugs. The RNA viruses require enzymes to replicate RNA and not simply transcribe RNA from DNA, and these enzymes are not present in normal cells. Some positive-strand RNA viruses direct host cells to manufacture DNA-dependent RNA polymerase, the negative-strand RNA viruses contain their own viral polymerase as do the double-stranded RNA viruses. Retroviruses contain their own unique RNA dependent-DNA polymerase. Among DNA viruses poxviruses have their own DNA polymerase for cytoplasmic replication, and herpesviruses contain a DNA polymerase distinct from cellular DNA polymerase. These enzymes are potential targets and all the drugs except ribavirin on Table 17.5 are directed against these enzymes. A number of nucleoside analogues have been used as antiherpes drugs. Some compete for substrate, some act as chain terminators and some have internal incorporation via internucleotide linkage. Because of these various modes of action the development of resistance does not extend to all drugs. Viruses that have mutations making them resistant to acyclovir or ganciclovir may still remain susceptible to newer drugs like penciclovir or cidofovir.

The antiHIV drugs until recently all represented dideoxynucleotide analogues that targeted the substrate binding site of the reverse transcriptase. The so-called nonnucleoside reverse transcriptase inhibitors interact noncompetitively with an allosteric site distinct from the substrate binding site and are more virus specific in inhibiting reverse transcriptase. HIV integrase also poses an interesting virus specific target for which inhibitors drugs are being sought. The protease inhibitors block maturation. Other agents are being developed that will react with the regulatory proteins that have major roles in the expression of the HIV genome (DeClercq, 1995).

Viral messenger RNA translation also appears to be another ideal site to be targeted with drugs such as antisense oligonucleotides that are complimentary and thus should hybridize to specific sequences of viral messenger RNA. Despite their theoretical appeal, to be effective they must be synthesized easily and in bulk, must be stable *in vivo*, must be able to enter target cells, must be retained by target cells, must be able to interact with their cellular targets and they must not interact in a nonsequence-specific manner with other macromolecules (Stein and Cheng, 1993). There are several proposed variations of antisense antinucleotides. Ribozymes are catalytic antisense molecules that not only bind to but cleave viral RNA; RNA decoys resemble viral RNA for purposes of binding but they do not function after binding (Dropulic and Jeang, 1994).

The protease inhibitors recently have proved to be effective in inhibiting HIV replication. HIV protease is required for cleavage of the HIV gag and gag-pol precursor protein into mature capsid proteins. Therefore blocking this cleavage affects one of the late events in viral maturation. Effective release of virus is blocked by the inhibition of influenza virus neuraminidase. The neuraminidase cleaves the cell surface receptors so that virus released from the cells do not immediately attach to the parent cell.

Ribavirin is a nucleoside analogue that has shown *in vitro* activity against a wide spectrum of RNA and DNA viruses. It does not interfere specifically in the virus cycle but inhibits RNA synthesis and, therefore, affects virus-infected or rapidly growing cells where the need for RNA synthesis is greatest. A variety of similar cytotoxic drugs often developed as antitumor drugs has been tested in viral infections.

The Design of New Drugs

The agents found thus far that interfere with events in virus synthesis have been stumbled upon or uncovered by mass testing of shelf drugs in cell culture systems. Other methods of delivery and design are being actively pursued.

Lioposomes are synthetic phospholipid vesicles that can be used as carriers for biologic molecules including antiviral agents. They are taken up by phagocytic cells and so naturally target themselves to this cell population, but they can be targeted to other cell types by modifying their membranes such as incorporating CD4 to enhance their interaction with HIV-infected lymphocytes.

Fundamental changes in drug design are now taking place. Computer-aided drug design uses X-ray crystallography to determine the three dimensional structure of viral macromolecules and then employs computer simulation and thermodynamic computations to study atomic interactions. These methods can delineate structures with favorable binding characteristics and direct drug synthesis (Bean, 1992). Trial and error will be replaced by logical and systematic drug design.

SUPPLEMENTARY BIBLIOGRAPHY

Galasso GJ, Whitley RJ and Merigan TC (editors): Antiviral Agents and Viral Diseases of Man, 4th Ed. New York: Raven Press, 1997.

Stratton KR, Howe CJ and Johnston RB (editors): Adverse Events Associated with Childhood Vaccines. Washington: National Academy Press, 1994.

18

Postscripts

> At every stage in the past and at every stage in the future, the advancing edge of knowledge in every field has been and will be in a state of confusion. There are phases when the emergence of a new technique or, more rarely, of a fertile generalization allows a swift development of a new area in which ignorance and confusion can be replaced by understanding and the possibility of control and utilization for the satisfaction of human desires. But the edge where ignorance lies beyond the zone of *ad hoc* hypothesis and inadequate experimental technique is always there. Speculation and tentative generalization, as well as the search for and development of new technical approaches, are the legitimate weapons to take us further toward the always receding periphery.
>
> F. Macfarlane Burnet,
> *Enzyme, Antigen and Virus,* 1956

In 1960, Joseph Smadel, then scientific director of the National Institutes of Health, commented to me on new technical approaches as he was committing resources to develop the primate holding facilities for the possible transmission of chronic neurologic diseases. He recalled an earlier time when Webster introduced the white mouse to the Rockefeller Institute as a more susceptible host for "equine" encephalitis; this new host not only aided pathogenesis studies but also led to the isolation of hundreds of arboviruses and later the previously unknown coxsackieviruses. He was convinced that the long-term primate studies would yield answers to human disease, but he said it could be multiple sclerosis, amyotrophic lateral sclerosis, Parkinson's disease, or "maybe even Gajdusek's kuru." Smadel had the instincts to know what would work and the wisdom to not predict the outcome.

Between the white mouse of the 1930s and the chimpanzee of the 1960s, the introduction of cell culture to facilitate studies of polioviruses brought the unanticipated recognition of other enteric viruses. The plaquing of viruses in cell cultures provided a precision in quantitation that not only aided clinical and animal virology but also opened the door for the molecular biologists working with bacteriophage to enter and revolutionize animal virology. The conjugation of antibodies for immunocytochemistry, the development of the ultracentrifuge and differential centrifugation, hybridization, cloning, monoclonal antibodies, rapid sequencing, the ability to detect single fragments of DNA or RNA molecules with polymerase chain reactions (PCR) have all expanded the periphery of knowledge into uncharted zones. At times, the technology has outrun our judgement in interpreting results.

New techniques in molecular biology have recently led to the identification of unculturable bacterial and viral agents in tissues—literally finding organisms without isolating or transmitting them! Representational difference analysis is based on enrichment of DNA fragments present in disease tissue but absent in healthy tissue of the same patient; this method, which combines subtractive hybridization with PCR amplification of "extras" yielded DNA sequences homologous to gamma herpesviruses in Kaposi's sarcoma—the finding of human herpesvirus 8. The same method identified GB hepatitis virus. Consensus sequence-based PCR uses highly conserved DNA sequences of presumed related known organisms to probe infected tissues; this method identified a *Bartonella* bacterium in bacillary angiomatosis and the actinomycete in Whipple disease. Complementary cDNA library screening relies on screening libraries from diseased tissues with hyperimmune serum from patients; this method has been successful in detecting new hepatitis viruses (Gao and Moore, 1996). No new neuropathic viruses have been identified using these new methods, but the time is ripe to apply representational difference analysis, consensus sequence-based PCR and complementary cDNA library screening to inflammatory diseases such as Beçhet disease, uveoencephalitic syndromes, Rasmussen encephalitis, Viluisk encephalitis and multiple sclerosis.

IN DEFENSE OF THE WHITE MOUSE

In this biologic revolution the white mouse is not obsolete. In traditional virology, *in vitro* (in glass) denoted cell cultures and *in vivo* (in the living being) denoted animals. Biochemical studies of virus transcription and translation are now carried out in cell-free systems. In molecular biology these systems are now referred to as *in vitro*, and studies carried out in cell cultures commonly are referred to as *in vivo*. Some investigators have even embraced the antivivisectionists' contention that experimental animals are no longer necessary in research.

While cells in cultures can be lysed or transformed simulating changes in selected cell populations of an organ, these are not models of disease. Incubation periods and clinical remissions or exacerbations and the processes of inflammation, degeneration, and demyelination cannot be faithfully simulated in cell cultures, and the roles of immune responses, so critical in prevention, modulation, or induction of disease, are disregarded. Animal studies provide a crucial bridge between basic virology and application of knowledge to unravel the complexities that separate health from disease.

Observations cannot be wantonly extrapolated from cell culture systems to human disease. In 1949 Enders and his students grew primate kidney cells and fibroblasts in culture and found that these cells that do not replicate polioviruses in the host, develop poliovirus receptors and susceptibility after several days in culture. This work, acknowledged with a Nobel Prize, opened the doors to development of the poliovaccines but also taught an important lesson—cells change in culture. The fact that HIV can replicate in a variety of neural cells in culture does not define which cells are infected in the brain. Conversely, the finding that rabies virus is noncytopathic in cell cultures would lead the naive investigator to believe that the world's most lethal virus has no disease potential. Furthermore, disease and pathologic changes cannot be equated, since rabies virus in animals or humans also can show a paucity of cytopathologic findings in the face of grisly disease.

Studies in animals often prompt new clinical insights. Our serendipitous finding that mumps virus can infect ependymal cells and cause hydrocephalus in hamsters prompted clinical studies of spinal fluid sediments of patients with mumps meningitis. These showed that similar ependymal infection occurs in human mumps and alerted clinicians to seek out the temporal association of mumps and acquired aqueductal stenosis in children.

Animal models provide the basic cornerstone for studies of pathogenesis of varied disease processes applicable to analogous human diseases and for the testing of diagnostic and therapeutic measures prior to human use. In addition, viral infections can induce reproducible lesions for anatomic, physiologic, and pharmacologic studies unrelated to virology. For example, the cerebellar lesion caused by parvoviruses suggests a mechanism whereby a viral infection of the developing nervous system might cause granuloprival cerebellar degeneration in children (Sarnat and Alcala, 1980). Beyond this simulation of human disease, these animals devoid of cellular granular neurons were exploited in neurobiology to provide insights into synaptic development (Herndon et al., 1971), in physiologic studies to investigate the activity of the cerebellum deprived of its sole excitatory cell population (Llinas et al., 1973), and in pharmacologic studies to identify glutamic acid as the transmitter of granular neurons (Young et al., 1974).

Altering the genotype of mice has opened a new approach to studies of nervous system infections. Transgenic mice, commonly produced by microinjection of cloned DNA directly into a pronucleus of a fertilized mouse egg, can express viral genes, which under control of cell-specific promotors, can be targeted to specific cell types. Results such as production of peripheral neuropathy or peripheral nerve tumors with DNA of SV40 and HTLV-I respectively, are of biologic interest but lack apparent clinical relevance (Jaenisch, 1988). On the other hand, selective expression of the early region of JC virus proteins in oligodendrocytes may provide insights into the selective vulnerability of oligodendrocytes to JC virus infection (Small et al., 1986). Different constructs of HIV DNA targeted to different CNS cells have led to an array of findings, some of which do and some of which do not simulate the human neuropathologic changes (see Chapter 12). The most powerful use of transgenic mice in CNS infection has been with prions, where insertion of a mutation in the prion protein gene led to spongiform changes in the mouse (Hsio et al., 1991) and where "knocking out" the prion protein gene abolishes susceptibility of the mice to experimental scrapie (Prusiner et al., 1993) (see Chapter 14). Transgenic and knockout mice will have important roles in studies of viral infections of the nervous system, but the design and interpretation of studies need to be mindful of the true pathogenesis of disease.

KOCH'S POSTULATES REVISITED

The development of microscopic lenses in the seventeenth century revealed a world teeming with microorganisms, but their relationship to disease remained controversial into the late 19th century. Jacob Henle, a teacher of Robert Koch, was skeptical that bacteria caused disease and stressed the need for laboratory investigations to prove their pathogenic potential. As a provocateur and mentor his name is often included in the eponym as Henle-Koch postulates (Evans, 1978). But it was Koch alone who first implemented formal proof by culturing the anthrax bacillus from the blood of sick animals, maintaining the bacteria in an anterior chamber of a bull's eye, and then reproducing clinical disease in experimental animals. He later devised poured-plates from which pure cultures could be obtained (Ford, 1911). On several occasions he described varying proofs of causation (Harden, 1992), but his postulates were put forth most succinctly in a lecture in 1890 where he stated:

> However it can be proved: first that the parasite occurs in every case of disease in question and under circumstances which can account for the pathologic changes in the clinical course of the disease; secondly, that it occurs in no other diseases as fortuitous and nonpathogenic parasite; and thirdly, that it, after being fully isolated from the body and repeatedly grown in pure culture, can induce disease anew; then the occurrence of the parasite in the disease can no longer be accidental, but in this case no other relationship between it and the disease except that of parasite is a cause the disease can be considered (Koch, 1881; translation by Rivers, 1937).

Koch knew the limitations of these criteria and felt they should be applied primarily to animal diseases. At the time he proposed them the postulates had not been fulfilled for typhoid, diphtheria, leprosy, relapsing fever or cholera, yet he believed these diseases were caused by the bacteria isolated from or observed in lesions. Even today his postulates have not been fulfilled for diphtheria and a number of other human bacterial diseases. Koch's postulates were not absolute in their inception even for bacteria, and many modifications have been proposed over the last century.

Viruses

With the 20th century discovery of viruses, Koch's postulates became antiquated. First, because of the limited sensitivity of isolation methods, viruses are almost never isolated from all cases of any disease. Second, pathogenic viruses such as polioviruses or herpesviruses often are recovered from people with no illness. Third, viruses grow in living cells and, therefore, cannot be grown in pure culture, that is poured-plates as defined by Koch. Furthermore, when introduced in experimental animals viruses not infrequently cause different diseases. For example, coxsackie B viruses isolated from patients with pleurodynia or meningitis cause pancreatitis and encephalitis in inoculated mice, and adenoviruses isolated from human respiratory infections or encephalitis cause tumors in hamsters. Other viruses may fail to cause disease in any other species as recently exemplified by HIV and HTLV-1. Rivers addressed this dilemma in his presidential address to the Society of American Bacteriologists in 1936:

> Koch's postulates as proposed by him do not have to be fulfilled in order to prove that a virus is the cause of disease. However, the spirit of his rules of proof still holds in that the worker must demonstrate that a virus is not only associated with disease but it is actually the cause (Rivers, 1937).

Rivers again stressed the importance of regular but not invariable isolation of agents by their transmission to experimental hosts but also the importance of immunologic studies to demonstrate a primary immune response during the infection to be certain that "the virus was neither fortuitously present in the patients nor accidentally picked up in the experimental animals." These immunologic criteria became essential in relating to viruses that only affect humans, such as the association of primary Epstein-Barr virus infection to infectious mononucleosis (Henle et al., 1968). Oddly, it was Jacob Henle's grandson who convinced us of this relation, and he did it without satisfying even one of the original Henle-Koch postulates (Evans, 1978).

Slow Infections

Between 1966 and 1971 viruses or transmissible agents were implicated in four chronic neurologic diseases. Novel methods were employed in the transmission of kuru and Creutzfeldt-Jakob disease to chimpanzees and innovative cell culture methods were devised to recover papillomavirus from multifocal leukoencephalopathy and to rescue measles virus from subacute sclerosing panencephalitis. In the first two diseases no immune response could be detected and in the latter two there was no option to show antibody changes between acute and convalescent sera. A wealth of evidence associated the agents with these diseases, but even River's modifications of Koch's postulates were not satisfied. Because of this dilemma Gibbs and I proposed some alternative criteria for relating viral agents to slow infections:

1. There should be consistency in the transmission of disease to experimental animals or some consistency in the recovery of virus in cell cultures, and this transmission and recovery should be confirmed by more than one laboratory.
2. Either serial transmission of the clinicopathologic process should be accomplished using filtered material and serial dilutions to establish replication of

the agent or the recoverable agent should be demonstrated with consistency in the diseased tissue by electron microscopic, immunofluorescent, or other methods, and should be demonstrated in the appropriate cells to explain the lesions.

3. Parallel studies of normal tissues or tissues of patients with other diseases should be carried out to established that the agent is not an ubiquitous agent or a contaminant (Johnson and Gibbs, 1974).

Human Retrovirus Infections

The recent association of HIV with AIDS and HTLV-1 with chronic myelopathy again raise issues related to Koch's postulates. Indeed, Peter Duesberg and others have stated they do not believe HIV is the cause of AIDS, since the association fails to fulfill Koch's postulates (Duesberg, 1988; Duesberg, 1991). However, the uniform association of each of these viruses with the characteristic clinical disease, transmission of the infections and disease by blood products and transfusions, and the transmission of HIV and AIDS to medical personnel by needle sticks all attest to a causal relationship. HIV is not only transmissible from human to human but the resulting illness is a unique disease complex not seen before. Furthermore, T cells with CD4 receptors are infected and decline in number—an appropriate localization of infection to explain the clinical disease. Evans has added to the criteria for causation "that elimination of the putative cause should decrease the incidence of disease," as demonstrated by the testing of blood and blood products for HIV antibody and the virtual elimination of AIDS in recipients (Evans, 1978).

The issue of causal relationship is more complex in relating the neurologic disease associated with human retrovirus infections to the viruses. First, the arguments for a cause and effect relationship fall short of satisfying the criteria that we previously proposed for slow infections. Second, the variety of very different clinical and pathologic complications does not lend itself to a unified hypothesis of pathogenesis. In terms of the criteria we proposed in 1974, HIV and HTLV-1 associated neurologic diseases have not been transmitted to experimental animals, and although HIV can be detected consistently in the CNS of patients with neurologic disease, HIV can be detected with equal ease in brains of patients without neurologic disease. Finally, neither HIV nor HTLV-1 are detected in the appropriate cells to explain readily the symptoms or the neuropathologic findings (see Chapters 11 and 12).

Over many years studies of the epidemiology of chronic disease have evolved criteria of the causal association quite distinct from Koch's postulates. These are the methods used to associate smoking with lung cancer and dietary factors with coronary artery disease (Yerushalmy and Palmer, 1959; Lilienfeld, 1959). These causal criteria include:

1. the strength of association
2. consistency of association

3. specificity of association
4. temporal sequence of events
5. dose-response relationship
6. biologic plausibility

In the case of HIV dementia, myelopathy, and neuropathy and HTLV-1 associated myelopathy, the strength, consistency and specificity of these associations are good. Yet the long incubation period and middle life onset of HTLV-1 irrespective of whether the virus was acquired peripartum from the mother or as an adult through sexual transmission or blood transfusion does not pose a logical temporal sequence. On the other hand, larger doses of virus may be transmitted by transfusion leading to a shorter incubation period of HTLV-1 myelopathy which may represent a dose-response relationship.

The most difficult issue is biologic plausibility. How HIV infection of macrophages and microglial cells can lead to a wide variety of different clinicopathologic syndromes remains a puzzle. Relating HTLV-1 to spastic paraparesis stretches biologic plausibility even further. Patients with disease do show intrathecal synthesis of antibody to the major polypeptides of the virus, virus can be isolated from the spinal fluid, and morphologically altered lymphocytes are seen within the spinal fluid. Lymphocytes containing antigen have been consistently found in the spinal cord. The rare appearance, the rather uniform middle life onset irrespective of time of infection, and the thoracic cord localization without neural dissemination all defy easy explanation.

There seems little doubt that HIV and HTLV-1 infections are *necessary* to produce the unique neurologic diseases with which they have been associated. The question is whether these infections are *sufficient* or whether some unidentified or even unrelated opportunistic agent or toxin or host factor may be critical in the pathogenesis of the lesions.

To adhere blindly to Koch's postulates would be foolish as both Koch and Rivers acknowledged. The new development of sequence-based identification of microbial pathogens that cannot be cultivated or transmitted will stretch our rules of causation even further (Fredericks and Relman, 1996). As new methods evolve we should still hold to the underlying principle that sufficient evidence needs to be accumulated to make a case beyond reasonable doubt for a cause-and-effect relationship between an infectious agent and a clinical disease. The accumulating data strongly support a cause and effect relationship between HIV and HTLV-1 and their neurologic syndromes, but the documentation of biologic mechanisms leading to lesion induction and confirmation of mechanisms in the analogous animal diseases are needed before we can dispel reasonable doubt.

EMERGING VIRAL INFECTIONS

The global pandemic of AIDS has focused attention on the origins of "new" infectious diseases; and this interest has been more recently intensified by the press coverage of the mysterious outbreaks of Ebola disease and the epidemic of bovine spongiform encephalopathy with possible human transmissions. Such disease outbreaks and pandemics are not unique in history.

Past Epidemics

Some years ago another human virus appeared that was thought to have evolved from an animal virus in Africa. People on the African continent and in the Middle East were the first victims suffering from virus-induced immunodeficiency and dying of pneumonia and diarrhea and less often accompanying demyelinating disease of the brain and spinal cord. When the agent reached the Western world it caused great numbers of deaths; it was said to have been worse than smallpox. The virus was measles; the time was the sixth to eighth century (Johnson et al., 1988b).

Some dispute this scenario positing that measles occurred in ancient China and entered the Middle East along with silk routes. In either case the typical exanthem of measles was not described by the early Greek or Roman physicians. The first convincing description of measles appeared in the Arab world in the sixth century (Mead, 1747). Although the European descriptions of the disease during the middle ages are scanty, it appears the virus spread across the Pyrenees into France with the Saracen invasion of the eighth century (Rolleston, 1937). Measles has no animal host. It is a human morbillivirus that is related to rhinderpest of African cattle. The measles virus must be maintained in human populations, and calculations of incubation period, efficiency of transmission and interval of infectivity indicate that measles virus needs an interactive human population of more than 200,000 people to be sustained. In early millennia a virus such as measles would have caused a brief village outbreak and then disappeared.

Some epidemic diseases in antiquity did disappear such as the great plague of Athens, the English sweating disease and von Economo encephalitis. In the plague of Athens dogs and carrion birds that ate the dead succumbed to the disease, a phenomenon inconsistent with any current known infectious agent (Thucydides, 5th century BC, translated by Warner, 1954). The English sweating disease, which occurred as five distinct epidemics in the 15th and 16th centuries, was characterized by high fever, diffuse sweating, agitation, delirium, and death within 24 hours; furthermore, unlike plague the upper classes such as Oxford students and members of court appeared particularly susceptible (Hunter, 1991). von Economo disease appeared and disappeared within the first half of this century (see Chapter 14). These diseases may have disappeared because of dwindling susceptible populations, microbial mutations, or unappreciated changes in the common human and microbial environment.

During the past two decades a number of new viral infections of the nervous system have been reported. Emerging viral infections include the evolution of genetically new agents, new recognition of agents, or new encounters or accelerated spread of existent viruses. Enteroviruses 70 and 71 with their unusual paralytic disease appear to be newly evolved; whereas parvovirus B19, herpesviruses 6 and 7, snowshoe hare and Jackson Canyon viruses and HTLV-I and II probably have infected human populations for many years but have only recently been isolated and characterized. In contrast, Ebola, Guanarito, and Sabiá viruses and HIV 1 and 2 probably existed in nature but have more recently been disseminated into human populations, while Japanese encephalitis, West Nile and Rift Valley fever viruses, raccoon rabies, herpes simplex virus type 2 and HIV-1 have expanded their habitats because of human activities.

Origins of Emerging Viruses

Previous chapters have addressed the persistence of DNA viruses within individuals by means of latency (Chapter 6) and the persistence of RNA viruses within human and animal populations, in large part, by high mutational rates (Chapter 11) (Table 18.1). Most of the emerging viruses are RNA viruses except where human interactions change such as the recent spread of herpes simplex type 2 with greater sexual license or past epidemics of adenoviruses during military mobilization with crowding of recruits. One of the most intriguing evolutions of new variants is among the influenza viruses. I was assigned to a virologic diagnostic laboratory in 1957 at the peak of the Asian influenza epidemic. A major shift of antigenicity had occurred that allowed infection of the previously immune individuals, and the new influenza virus was also associated with an apparently greater number of neurologic complications. At that time our naivete of molecular genetics led to fanciful hypotheses to explain this antigenic shift and the evolution of new strains of influenza virus. We did not understand that influenza had a multipartite RNA genome, or that when a cell is infected with two different influenza viruses they can reassort genomic segments. Influenza viruses occupy a unique niche between zoonotic and human viruses,

TABLE 18.1. *Mechanisms for viral survival in host populations*

Viruses	Mechanisms
DNA viruses	Latency and activation after new nonimmune hosts born
	Seldom cause fatal disease (host survival)
RNA viruses	
Arboviruses	Mutation/spread in animal populations
Zoonotic viruses	Mutation/spread in animal populations
Human viruses	
Picornaviruses	Mutations that supply new viruses
Influenza	Mutations and reassortment allows reinfection
Measles	"New" virus that requires large human populations
Retroviruses	Latency and high mutation rate
HIV 1 and 2	Low transmissibility, long incubation period, and long infectivity period
HTLV-1	All of above and low disease penetrance

HTLV, human T-cell lymphotropic virus.
Modified from Johnson (1993b).

since some antigenic shifts are due to recombination of human and avian influenza and possibly porcine influenza viruses. Both the major 1957 and 1968 shifts appear to be recombinants of avian and human viruses, and their seemingly mystical origins in China now can be explained by the concentration of humans, ducks and pigs that provide the optimal incubator for reassortment (Kilbourne, 1991). The same, of course, could occur in Iowa, but the population densities of the three species favor the Asian origin.

Population and Travel

Two important factors in this increasing emergence and sustaining of viruses in human populations are the increasing the human population and the remarkable increase and speed of travel (Fig. 18.1). Therefore, exotic viruses are no longer of exotic interest. As mentioned earlier a span of approximately 200 years appears to have passed before the measles virus crossed from the Iberian peninsula to the south of France. Because of the short incubation period and high infectivity the human infection had to cycle during the traverse of the Pyrenees in order to sustain the virus. This transport had to await the massing of the Saracen army. Today a similar virus would cross the Pyrenees in hours.

In 1967 in Yugoslavia and Germany, Marburg virus caused outbreaks of hemorrhagic fever among laboratory workers handling African green monkey cells and serious infections occurred subsequently among medical personnel who

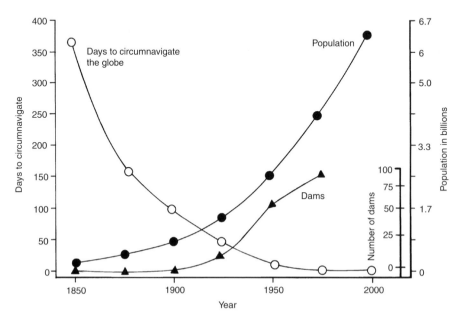

FIG. 18.1. Societal changes that favor emerging viral diseases. (Modified from Nathanson, 1977, with permission.)

cared for them (Kissling et al., 1968). Lassa virus is an arenavirus that causes frequent outbreaks of hemorrhagic fever in Africa. It, too, has a high rate of nosocomial infection and caused major concern when a visitor became ill in London, when a Peace Corps worker brought Lassa to Washington, D.C. and when a young American of Nigerian origin died of the disease in Illinois after a visit to his homeland (Holmes et al., 1990). The increase in human travel and its potential impact on epidemics is enormous; 500 million tourists, immigrants, merchants, students and pilgrims cross national boundaries on commercial airlines each year, 70 million people work outside their home countries, and 50 million are refugees and displaced persons (Wilson, 1995). Travel has become so swift that during a single incubation period of any of these viruses a person from a village in Africa cannot only be in Washington or London but at a grange meeting in Nebraska or a church social in Tennessee (Johnson, 1996a).

The Future

In a world of burgeoning populations we can anticipate that new viruses will emerge with greater frequency, and persistence of these viruses in human populations will be facilitated. Travel will speed the spread and bring a wider population into the equation. Epidemics can be anticipated both in the form of pandemics of new diseases such as AIDS as well as abrupt outbreaks of lethal diseases such as Ebola disease, and these will occur more frequently and over widening geographic areas.

In general these are natural occurrences and new viruses will evolve as mutations and recombination that we have seen in the past. The evolution and spread of new viruses has fascinated biologists and infectious disease specialists for decades. Sensitized by AIDS the lay press has given remarkable coverage to diseases such as "mad cow disease" in Britain and Ebola in Africa. The daily newsprint last year seemed preoccupied with Ebola disease; Hot Zone, a true story of a primate outbreak in Virginia, made a record stay on the best seller list, and Outbreak, a fictitious filovirus flick, was a box office hit. The irony is that at this peak of public interest in emerging infections, funding for basic research was not increased and support for the study of agents that do not currently affect North Americans at home is sparse, despite the fact that we live in a global village where diseases like Ebola and Marburg could be amongst us tomorrow. For many years the Rockefeller Foundation maintained surveillance systems and laboratory facilities in the Caribbean, South America, Africa and India, but funding was curtailed in 1971. The Army closed the research unit in Malaysia in 1989, and the Gorgas Memorial Unit in Panama was relinquished to local control in 1990 (Lederberg et al., 1992). The public seems to have the information and, indeed, a fascination with these microbial threats but lacks the resolve to craft solutions.

Humankind has made remarkable achievements in the control of nature, other species, and, to some extent, its own behavior. Past successes in the development of antimicrobials to control infections and vaccines to eradicate smallpox and to eliminate indigenous wild polio in the Western hemisphere do not prove our invincibility. As Joshua Lederberg wrote, "We have too many illusions that we can, by writ, govern the remaining vital kingdoms, the microbes, that remain our competitors of last resort for domain of the planet. Bacteria and viruses know nothing of human sovereignties. In that natural evolutionary competition there is no guarantee that we will find ourselves the survivor." (Lederberg, 1988).

In this recent concern with emerging viruses there has been the clear implication by some authors that they have arisen from human wickedness. The sexual spread of HIV and type 2 herpes simplex virus has reinforced this judgmental posture as well as the spread of agents resulting from deforestation or the pollution of waterways. Unfortunately this leads to the assumption that emerging diseases might be held in check by political or ecological "correctness," yet many good and generous acts in society can be exploited by microbial adversaries. Provision of day care and schooling for younger children has led to early preimmunization exposure to measles virus and the spread of picornaviruses. Recreational activities have increased the exposure to arboviruses and rabies viruses. Preservation of old trees in suburban housing developments has facilitated the spread of LaCrosse virus to children. Irrigation projects to provide better food and water have led to the spread of Western equine encephalitis in the United States, Japanese encephalitis throughout Asia, and Rift Valley and West Nile viruses in Africa. Development of free international commerce has spread bovine spongiform encephalopathy. Medical advances such as organ transplantation has led to the activation of latent agents, the development of nosocomial infection and the transmission of diseases. Creutzfeldt-Jakob disease, rabies, and HIV have been transmitted within transplanted tissues, and a number of viruses have been transmitted by blood transfusions or blood products (Table 18.2).

Some diseases do emerge because of human foolishness. Allowing hunters to bring raccoons from rabies endemic areas to uninvolved areas and the importation of the Asian tiger mosquito in old automobile tires, an ideal breeding place,

TABLE 18.2. *Societal changes that enhance the evolution and spread of neurotropic viruses*

Providing an adequate pool of susceptibles	Increasing global population Increasing human contacts (travel)
Altering forms of human or animal contact	
Societal mores	Increased sexual contact Day care with early exposure Altering woods for suburbs and recreation Agricultural clearing or irrigation Global movement of animals and animal products
Medical practices	Blood transfusions Immunosuppressive therapy Organ transplants (infected donor) Antiviral drugs (encourage resistance)

Modified from Johnson (1993b).

from Asia to the United States are tragic examples. Last year the translocation of rabies-infected coyotes from Texas to Florida by hunters does not bode well for our ability to learn from past follies. The recognition and sudden appearance of bovine spongiform encephalopathy and the possibility that it has been transmitted to humans represents a scenario that few, if any, could have anticipated; every link in the food chain, including the rendering process has a potential to disseminate disease.

What is needed to face a daunting but exciting future conflict with viruses is greater knowledge of both the molecular biology and the ecology of these microbes. We must anticipate that as we alter our common habitat, the viruses with their facile genetic tactics, can exploit our every move.

SUPPLEMENTARY BIBLIOGRAPHY

Evans AE: Causation and Disease. A chronological journey. New York: Plenum, 1993.

Lederberg J, Shope RE and Oaks SC (editors): Emerging Infections. Microbial Threats to Health in the United States. Washington: National Academy Press, 1992.

References

Abrama F, Bo S, Canese MG, Poli A. Regional distribution of lesions in the central nervous system of cats infected with feline immunodeficiency virus. *AIDS Res Hum Retroviruses* 1995;11:1247–1253.

Abramsky O. Neurological features as presenting manifestations of brucellosis. *Eur Neurol* 1977;15: 281–284.

Abramsky O, Webb C, Teitelbaum D, Aron R. Cell-mediated immunity to neural antigens in idiopathic polyneuritis and myeloradiculitis. *Neurology* 1975;25:1154–1159.

Abzug MJ, Keyserling HL, Lee ML, Levin MJ, Rotbart HA. Neonatal enterovirus infection: virology, serology, and effects of intravenous immune globulin. *Clin Infect Dis* 1995;20:1201–1206.

Achard J-M, Lallement P-Y, Veyssier P. Recurrent aseptic meningitis secondary to intracranial epidermoid cyst and Mollaret's meningitis: two distinct entities or a single disease? A case report and a nosologic discussion. *Am J Med* 1990;89:807–810.

Acheson ED. The clinical syndrome variously called benign myalgic encephalomyelitis Iceland disease, and epidemic neuromyasthenia. *Am J Med* 1959;26:569–595.

Achim CL, Heyes MP, Wiley CA. Quantitation of human immunodeficiency virus, immune activation factors, and quinolinic acid in AIDS brains. *J Clin Invest* 1993;91:2769–2775.

Achim CL, Wang R, Miners DK, Wiley CA. Brain viral burden in HIV infection. *J Neuropathol Exp Neurol* 1994;53:284–294.

Ackermann P, Korver G, Turss R, Wonne R, Hochgesand P. Pranatale Infektion mit dem Virus der lymphocytaren Choriomenigitis. *Dtsch Med Wochenschr* 1974;99:529–632.

Adair JC, Woodley SL, O'Connell JB, Call GK, Baringer JR. Aseptic meningitis following cardiac transplantation: clinical characteristics and relationship to immunosuppressive regimen. *Neurology* 1991; 41:249–252.

Adams JM, Imagawa DT. Measles antibodies in multiple sclerosis. *Proc Soc Exp Biol Med* 1962;111: 562–566.

Adamson DC, Dawson TM, Zink MC, Clements JE, Dawson VL. Neurovirulent simian immunodeficiency virus infection induces neuronal, endothelial, and glial apoptosis. *Mol Med* 1996a;2:417–428.

Adamson DC, Wildemann B, Sasaki M, et al. Immunologic NO synthase: elevation in severe AIDS dementia and induction by HIV-1 gp41. *Science* 1996b;274:1917–1921.

Adjorlolo-Johnson G, DeCock KM, Ekpini E, et al. Prospective comparison of mother-to-child transmission of HIV-1 and HIV-2 in Abidjan, Ivory Coast. *JAMA* 1994;272:462–466.

Adle-Biassette H, Levy Y, Colombel M, et al. Neuronal apoptosis in HIV infection in adults. *Neuropathol Appl Neurobiol* 1995;21:218–227.

Adour JM, Byl FM, Hilsinger RL, Wilcox RD. Meniere's disease as a form of cranial polyganglionitis. *Laryngoscope* 1980;90:392–398.

Adour KK, Bell DN, Hilsinger RL. Herpes simplex virus in idiopathic facial paralysis (Bell's palsy). *JAMA* 1975;233:527–530.

Aguilar MJ, Rasmussen T. Role of encephalitis in pathogenesis of epilepsy. *Arch Neurol* 1960;2:663–676.

Aguzzi A, Wagner EF, Netzer K-O, Bothe K, Anhauser I, Rethwilm A. Human foamy virus proteins accumulate in neurons and induce multinucleated giant cells in the brain of transgenic mice. *Am J Pathol* 1993;142:1061–1071.

Ahlström G, Gunnarsson L-G, Leissner P, Sjödén P-O. Epidemiology of neuromuscular diseases, including the postpolio sequelae, in a Swedish county. *Neuroepidemiology* 1993;12:262–269.

Aicardi J, Goutieres F, Arsenio-Nunes M, Lebon P. Acute measles encephalitis in children with immunosuppression. *Pediatrics* 1977;59:232–239.

Ait-Khaled M, McLaughlin JE, Johnson MA, Emery VC. Distinct HIV-1 long terminal repeat quasispecies present in nervous tissues compared to that in lung, blood and lymphoid tissues of an AIDS patient. *AIDS* 1995;9:675–683.

Aizawa H, Suzutani T, Yahara O, et al. A case of varicella–zoster myelopathy. *Acta Neurol Scand* 1996; 93:470–472

Akizuki S, Setoguchi M, Nakazato O, et al. An autopsy case of human T-lymphotropic virus type I-associated myelopathy. *Hum Pathol* 1988;19:988–990.

Aksamit AJ, Sever JL, Major EO. Progressive multifocal leukoencephalopathy: JC virus detection by in situ hybridization compared with immunohistochemistry. *Neurology* 1986;36:499–504.

Al-Deeb SM, Yaqub BA, Sharif HS, Al-Rajeh SM. Neurobrucellosis. In: Harris AA, ed. *Handbook of clinical neurology,* 8th ed. Amsterdam: Elsevier Science, 1988:581–601.

Albert DM, Lahav ED, Colby JA, Shadduck JA, Sang DN. Retinal neoplasia and dysplasia. I. Introduction by feline leukemia virus. *Invest Ophthalmol* 1977;16:325–337.

Albert DM, Lahav M, Carmichael LE, Percy DH. Canine herpes-induced retinal dysplasia and associated ocular anomalies. *Invest Ophthalmol* 1976;15:267–278.

Albrecht P. Pathogenesis of neurotropic arbovirus infections. *Curr Top Microbiol Immunol* 1968;43:44–91.

Albrecht P, Torrey EF, Boone E, Hicks JT, Daniel N. Raised cytomegalovirus-antibody level in cerebrospinal fluid of schizophrenic patients. *Lancet* 1980;2:769–772.

Albrecht T, Rapp F. Malignant transformation of hamster embryo fibroblasts following exposure to ultraviolet-irradiated human cytomegalovirus. *Virology* 1973;55:53–61.

Aleksic SN, Budzilovich GN, Liberman AN. Herpes zoster oticus and facial paralysis (Ramsay Hunt syndrome). *J Neurol Sci* 1973;20:149–159.

Alford CA, Stagno S, Pass RF, Britt WJ. Congenital and perinatal cytomegalovirus infections. *Rev Infect Dis* 1990;12[Suppl]:S745–S753.

Ali A, Rudge P, Dalgleish AG. Neopterin concentrations in serum and cerebrospinal fluid in HTLV-I infected individuals. *J Neurol* 1992;239:270–272.

Allen IV, McQuaid S, McMahon J, Kirk J, McConnell R. The significance of measles virus antigen and genome distribution in the CNS in SSPE for mechanisms of viral spread and demyelination. *J Neuropathol Exp Neurol* 1996;55:471–480.

Almond JW. The attenuation of poliovirus neurovirulence. *Annu Rev Microbiol* 1987;41:153–180.

Alvarez L, Fajardo R, Lopez E, et al. Partial recovery from rabies in a nine-year-old boy. *Pediatr Infect Dis J* 1994;13:1154–1155.

Ambler M, Stoll J, Tzamaloukas A, Albala MM. Focal encephalomyelitis in infectious mononucleosis. *Ann Intern Med* 1971;75:579–583.

Amirhessami-Aghili N, Spector SA. Human immunodeficiency virus type 1 infection of human placenta: potential route for fetal infection. *J Virol* 1991;65:2231–2236.

Amlie-Lefond C, Kleinschmidt-DeMasters BK, Mahalingam R, Davis LE, Gilden DH. The vasculopathy of varicella–zoster virus encephalitis. *Ann Neurol* 1995;37:784–790.

Amlie-Lefond C, Mackin GA, Ferguson M, Wright RR, Mahalingam R. Another case of virologically confirmed zoster sine herpete, with electrophysiologic correlation. *J Neurovirol* 1996;2:136–138.

Amsterdam JD, Winokur A, Dyson W, et al. Borna disease virus: a possible etiologic factor in human affective disorders? *Arch Gen Psychiatry* 1985;42:1093–1096.

An SF, Giometto B, Scaravilli F. HIV-1 DNA in brains in AIDS and pre-AIDS: correlation with the stage of disease. *Ann Neurol* 1996;40:611–617.

Anand A, Gray ES, Brown T, Clewley JP, Cohen BJ. Human parvovirus infection in pregnancy and hydrops fetalis. *N Engl J Med* 1987;316:183–186.

Andersen O, Lygner P-E, Bergström T, Andersson M, Vahlne A. Viral infections trigger multiple sclerosis relapses: a prospective seroepidemiological study. *J Neurol* 1993;240:417–422.

Anderson AA, Hanson RP. Intrauterine infection of mice with St. Louis encephalitis virus: immunological, physiological, neurological and behavioral effects on progeny. *Infect Immun* 1975;12:1173–1183.

Anderson RM, Donnelly CA, Ferguson NM, et al. Transmission dynamics and epidemiology of BSE in British cattle. *Nature* 1996;382:779–788.

Andrew CG, Drachman DB, Pestronk A, Narayan O. Susceptibility of skeletal muscle to coxsackie A2 virus infection: effects of botulinum toxin and denervation. *Science* 1984;223:714–716.

Andrews JM, Andrews RL. The significance of dense core particles in subacute demyelinating disease in an adult. *Lab Invest* 1973;28:236–243.

Andrews PI, Dichter MA, Berkovic SF, Newton MR, McNamara JO. Plasmapheresis in Rasmussen's encephalitis. *Neurology* 1996;46:242–246.

Angulo JJ, Pimenta-de-Campos E, de Salles-Gomes LF. Postvaccinial meningo-encephalitis. *JAMA* 1964; 187:151–153.

Anlar B, Saatçi I, Köse G, Yalaz K. MRI findings in subacute sclerosing panencephalitis. *Neurology* 1996;47:1278–1283.

Anlar B, Yalaz K, Öktem F, Köse G. Long-term follow-up of patients with subacute sclerosing panencephalitis treated with intraventricular α-interferon. *Neurology* 1997;48:526–528.

Anonymous. The scrapie agent. *Lancet* 1967;2:705–706.

Antoine JC, Michel D, Bertholon P, et al. Creutzfeldt–Jakob disease after extracranial dura mater embolization for a nasopharyngeal angiofibroma. *Neurology* 1997;48:1451–1453.

Appelbaum E, Kreps SI, Sunshine A. Herpes zoster encephalitis. *Am J Med* 1962;32:25–31.

Apstein MD, Koff E, Koff RS. Neuropsychological dysfunction in acute viral hepatitis. *Digestion* 1979; 19:349–358.

Araújo ADQ-C, Leiti ACCB, Dultra SV, Andrada-Serpa MJ. Progression of neurological disability in HTLV-I-associated myelopathy/tropical spastic paraparesis (HAM/TSP). *J Neurol Sci* 1995;129: 147–151.

Arenberg IK, Marovitz WF, Shambaugh GE. The role of the endolymphatic sac in the pathogenesis of endolymphatic hydrops in man. *Acta Otolaryngol (Stockh)* 1970;275:1–49.

Arends MJ, Wyllie AH. Apoptosis: mechanisms and roles in pathology. *Int Rev Exp Pathol* 1991;32: 223–254.

Arey JB. Cytomegalic inclusion disease. *Am J Dis Child* 1954;88:525.

Arlazoroff A, Bleicher Z, Klein C, et al. Vaccine-associated contact paralytic poliomyelitis with atypical neurological presentation. *Acta Neurol Scand* 1987;76:210–214.

Armstrong CL, Miranda AF, Hsu KC, Gamboa ET. Susceptibility of human skeletal muscle culture to influenza virus infection. I. Cytopathology and immunofluorescence. *J Neurol Sci* 1978;35:43–57.

Arnadottir T, Reunanen M, Salmi A. Intrathecal synthesis of virus antibodies in multiple sclerosis patients. *Infect Immun* 1982;38:399–407.

Arnason BGW, Chelmicka-Szorc E. Passive transfer of experimental allergic neuritis in lew rats by direct injection of sensitized lymphocytes into sciatic nerve. *Acta Neuropathol (Berl)* 1972;22:1–6.

Arnason BGW, Soliven B. Acute inflammatory demyelinating polyradiculoneuropathy. In: Dyck PJ, Griffin JW, Low PA, Poduslo JF, eds. *Peripheral neuropathy.* Philadelphia: WB Saunders, 1993: 1437–1497.

Arnason BGW, Winkler GF, Hadler NM. Cell mediated demyelination of peripheral nerve in tissue culture. *Lab Invest* 1969;21:1–10.

Arvin AM. Relationships between maternal immunity to herpes simplex virus and the risk of neonatal herpesvirus infection. *Rev Infect Dis* 1991;13[Suppl 11]:S953–S956.

Asano Y, Yoshikawa T Kajita Y, et al. Fatal encephalitis/encephalopathy in primary human herpesvirus-6 infection. *Arch Dis Child* 1992;67:1484–1485.

Asbury AK, Arnason BGW, Adams RD. The inflammatory lesion in idiopathic polyneuritis. *Medicine (Baltimore)* 1969;48:173–215.

Asher DM. Movement disorders in rhesus monkeys after infection with tick-borne encephalitis virus. *Adv Neurol* 1975;10:277–289.

Assaad F. Measles: summary of worldwide impact. *Rev Infect Dis* 1983;5:452–459.

Assaad F, Cockburn WC. Four-year study of WHO virus reports on enteroviruses other than poliovirus. *Bull WHO* 1972;46:329–339.

Astrom KE, Mancall EL, Richardson EP Jr. Progressive multifocal leukoencephalopathy. *Brain* 1958;81: 93–111.

Aurelius E, Johansson B, Sköldenberg B, Forsgren M. Encephalitis in immunocompetent patients due to herpes simplex virus type 1 or 2 as determined by type-specific polymerase chain reaction and antibody assays of cerebrospinal fluid. *J Med Virol* 1993;39:179–186.

Aylward EH, Henderer JD, McArthur JC, et al. Reduced basal ganglia volume in HIV-1-associated dementia: results from quantitative neuroimaging. *Neurology* 1993;43:2099–2104.

Azimi PH, Cramblett HG, Haynes RE. Mumps meningoencephalitis in children. *JAMA* 1969;207:509–512.

Azzi A, De Santis R, Ciappi S, et al. Human polyomaviruses DNA detection in peripheral blood leukocytes from immunocompetent and immunocompromised individuals. *J Neurovirol* 1996;2:411–416.

Baczko K, Lampe J, Libert UG, et al. Clonal expansion of hypermutated measles virus in a SSPE brain. *Virology* 1993;197:188–195.

Baczko K, Liebert UG, Billeter M, Cattaneo R, Budka H, Ter Meulen V. Expression of defective measles virus genes in brain tissues of patients with subacute sclerosing panencephalitis. *J Virol* 1986;59: 472–478.

Baer GM, Cleary WF. A model in mice for the pathogenesis and treatment of rabies. *J Infect Dis* 1972; 125:520–527.

Bagasra O, Hauptman SP, Lischner HW, Sachs M, Pomerantz RJ. Detection of human immunodeficiency virus type 1 provirus in mononuclear cells by in situ polymerase chain reaction. *N Engl J Med* 1992; 326:1385–1391.

Bagasra O, Lavi E, Bobroski L, et al. Cellular reservoirs of HIV-1 in the central nervous system of infected individuals: identification by the combination of in situ polymerase chain reaction and immunohistochemistry. *AIDS* 1996;10:573–583.

Bahmanyar M, Fayaz A, Nour-Salehi S, Mohammadi M, Koprowski H. Successful protection of human exposed to rabies infection. *JAMA* 1976;235:2751–2754.

Bale JF Jr. Human cytomegalovirus infection and disorders of the nervous system. *Arch Neurol* 1984;41: 310–320.

Balfour HH Jr. Management of cytomegalovirus disease with antiviral drugs. *Rev Infect Dis* 1990; 12[Suppl]:S849–S860.

Balfour HH Jr, Bean B, Laskin OL, et al. Acyclovir halts progression of herpes zoster in immunocompromised patients. *N Engl J Med* 1983;308:1448–1453.

Balfour HH Jr, Siem RA, Bauer H, Quie PG. California arbovirus (LaCrosse) infections. I. Clinical and laboratory findings in 66 children with meningoencephalitis. *Pediatrics* 1973;52:680–691.

Baltazard M, Bahmanyar M. Essai pratique du serum antirabique chez les mordus par loups enrages. *Bull WHO* 1955;13:747–772.

Bang FB, Warwick A. Mouse macrophages as host cells for the mouse hepatitis virus and the genetic basis of their susceptibility. *Proc Natl Acad Sci USA* 1960;46:1065–1075.

Bang HO, Bang J. Involvement of the central nervous system in mumps. *Acta Med Scand* 1943;113: 487–505.

Baratawidjaja RK, Morrissey LP, Labzoffsky NA. Demonstration of vaccinia, lymphocytic choriomeningitis and rabies viruses in the leucocytes of experimentally infected animals. *Arch Ges Virusforsch* 1965;17:273–279.

Barbour AG, Fish D. The biological and social phenomenon of lyme disease. *Science* 1993;260: 1610–1616.

Baringer JR. Recovery of herpes simplex virus from human sacral ganglions. *N Engl J Med* 1974;291: 828–830.

Baringer JR. Herpes simplex virus infection of nervous tissue in animals and man. *Prog Med Virol* 1975; 20:1–26.

Baringer JR, Griffith JF. Experimental herpes simplex encephalitis: early neuropathological changes. *J Neuropathol Exp Neurol* 1970;29:89–104.

Baringer JR, Nathanson N. Parvovirus hemorrhagic encephalopathy of rats: electron microscopic observations of vascular lesions. *Lab Invest* 1972;29:89–104.

Baringer JR, Pisani P. Herpes simplex virus genomes in human nervous system tissue analyzed by polymerase chain reaction. *Ann Neurol* 1994;36:823–829.

Baringer JR, Swoveland P. Recovery from herpes simplex virus from human trigeminal ganglions. *N Engl J Med* 1973;288:648–650.

Barker E, Fujimura SF, Fadem MB, Landay AL, Levy JA. Immunologic abnormalities associated with chronic fatigue syndrome. *Clin Infect Dis* 1994;18[Suppl]:S136–S141.

Barlow RM, Rennie JC, Gardiner AC, Vantsis JT. Infection of pregnant sheep with NADL strain of bovine virus diarrhoea virus and their subsequent challenge with border disease: IIB pool. *J Comp Pathol* 1980;90:67–72.

Barna BP, Estes ML, Jacobs BS, Hudson S, Ransohoff RM. Human astrocytes proliferate in response to tumor necrosis factor alpha. *J Neuroimmunol* 1990;30:239–243.

Barnett EM, Jacobsen G, Evans G, Cassell M, Perlman S. Herpes simplex encephalitis in the temporal cortex and limbic system after trigeminal nerve inoculation. *J Infect Dis* 1994a;169:782–786.

Barnett SW, Murthy KK, Herndier BG, Levy JA. An AIDS-like condition induced in baboons by HIV-2. *Science* 1994b;266:642–646.

Barre-Sinoussi F, Chermann JC, Rey F, et al. Isolation of a T-lymphotropic retrovirus from a patient at risk for AIDS. *Science* 1983;220:868–870.

Barron KD. The microglial cell: a historical review. *J Neurol Sci* 1995;134[Suppl]:S57–S68.

Barry M, Russi M, Armstrong L, Geller D, Tesh R, Dembry L, et al. Brief report: treatment of a laboratory-acquired Sabia virus infection. *N Engl J Med* 1995;333:317–318.

Barthez MA, Billard C, Santini JJ. Relapse of herpes simplex encephalitis. *Neuropediatrics* 1987;18:3–7.

Barton LL, Peters CJ, Ksiazek TG. Lymphocytic choriomeningitis virus: an unrecognized teratogenic pathogen. *Emer Infect Dis* 1995;1:152–153.

Bártová L, Rajcáni J, Pogády J. Herpes simplex virus antibodies in the cerebrospinal fluid of schizophrenic patients. *Acta Virol (Praha)* 1987;31:443–446.

Baskar JF, Peacock J, Sulik KK, Huang E-S. Early-stage developmental abnormalities induced by murine cytomegalovirus. *J Infect Dis* 1987;155:661–666.

Bassili SS, Peyman GA, Gebhardt BM, Daun M, Ganiban GJ, Rifai A. Detection of Epstein–Barr virus DNA by polymerase chain reaction in the vitreous from a patient with Vogt–Koyanagi–Harada syndrome. *Retina* 1996;16:160–161.

Baszler TV, Zachary JF. Murine retroviral-induced spongiform neuronal degeneration parallels resident microglial cell infection: ultrastructural findings. *Lab Invest* 1990;63:612–623.

Bates DW, Buchwald D, Lee J, et al. A comparison of case definitions of chronic fatigue syndrome. *Clin Infect Dis* 1994;18[Suppl]:S11–S15.

Batisse D, Eliaszewicz M, Zazoun L, Baudrimont M, Pialoux G, Dupont B. Acute retinal necrosis in the course of AIDS: study of 26 cases. *AIDS* 1996;10:55–60.

Batra SK, Rasheed BKA, Bigner SH, Bigner DD. Biology of disease: oncogenes and anti-oncogenes in human central nervous system tumors. *Lab Invest* 1994;71:621–637.

Baumgärtner WK, Krakowka S, Koestner A, Evermann J. Ultrastructural evaluation of acute encephalitis and hydrocephalus in dogs caused by canine parainfluenza virus. *Vet Pathol* 1982;19:305–314.

Bean B. Antiviral therapy: current concepts and practices. *Clin Microbiol Rev* 1992;5:146–182.

Bechar M, Davidovich S, Goldhammer G, Machtey I, Gadoth N. Neurological complications following rubella infection. *J Neurol* 1982;226:283–287.

Beck E, Daniel PM, Parry HB. Degeneration of the cerebellar and hypothalamo-neurohypophysial systems in sheep with scrapie, and its relationship to human system degenerations. *Brain* 1964;87:153–176.

Becker LE, Narayan O, Johnson RT. Studies of human papovavirus tumor antigen in experimental and human cerebral neoplasms. *Can J Neurol* 1976;3:105–109.

Beebe GW, Kurtzke JF, Kurland LT, Auth TL, Naglar B. Studies on the natural history of multiple sclerosis. III. Epidemiologic analysis of the Army experience in World War II. *Neurology* 1967;17:1–17.

Beghi E, Nicolosi A, Kurland LT, Mulder DW, Hauser WA, Shuster L. Encephalitis and aseptic meningitis, Olmsted County, Minnesota, 1950–1981. I. Epidemiology. *Ann Neurol* 1984;16:283–294.

Behan PO, Currie S. *Clinical neuroimmunology.* London: WB Saunders, 1978.

Behan PO, Geschwind N, Lamarche JB, Lisak RP, Kies MW. Delayed hypersensitivity to encephalitogenic protein in disseminated encephalomyelitis. *Lancet* 1968;2:1009–1012.

Beilke MA, Riding In D, Hamilton R, et al. HLA-DR expression in macaque neuroendothelial cells in vitro and during SIV encephalitis. *J Neuroimmunol* 1991;33:129–143.

Belec L, Tayot J, Tron P, Mikol J, Scaravilli F, Gray F. Cytomegalovirus encephalopathy in an infant with congenital acquired immuno-deficiency syndrome. *Neuropediatrics* 1990;21:124–129.

Bell EJ, McCartney RA. A study of Coxsackie B virus infections, 1972–1983. *J Hyg* 1984;93:197–203.

Bell EJ, McCartney RA, Riding MH. Coxsackie B viruses and myalgic encephalomyelitis. *J R Soc Med* 1988;81:329–331.

Bell JE, Busuttil A, Ironside JW, et al. Human immunodeficiency virus and the brain: investigation of virus load and neuropathologic changes in pre-AIDS subjects. *J Infect Dis* 1993;168:818–824.

Belloc C, Polack B, Schwartz-Cornil I, Brownlie J, Lèvy D. Bovine immunodeficiency virus: facts and questions. *Vet Res* 1996;27:395–402.

Belman AL, Diamond G, Dickson D, et al. Pediatric acquired immunodeficiency syndrome: neurologic syndromes. *Am J Dis Child* 1988;142:29–35.

Benditt EP, Barrett T, McDougall JK. Viruses in the etiology of atherosclerosis. *Proc Natl Acad Sci USA* 1983;80:6386–6389.

Benirschke K, Mendoza GR, Bazeley PL. Placental and fetal manifestations of cytomegalovirus infection. *Virchows Arch* 1974;16:121–139.

Bennett GJ. Hypotheses on the pathogenesis of herpes zoster-associated pain. *Ann Neurol* 1994;35[Suppl]:S38–S41.

Bennett JL, Gilden DH. The molecular genetics of herpes simplex virus latency and pathogenesis: a puzzle with many pieces still missing. *J Neurovirol* 1996;2:225–229.

Bennett JL, Mahalingam R, Wellish MC, Gilden DH. Epstein–Barr virus-associated acute autonomic neuropathy. *Ann Neurol* 1996;40:453–455.

Bennett M, Hart CA. Feline immunodeficiency virus infection: a model for HIV and AIDS? *J Med Microbiol* 1995;42:233–236.

Bennett NM. Murray Valley encephalitis: 1974 clinical features. *Med J Aust* 1976;2:446–450.

Benveniste EN. Cytokine circuits in brain: implications for AIDS dementia complex. In: Price RW, Perry SW, eds. *HIV, AIDS and the brain.* New York: Raven Press, 1994:71–88.

Berger JR, Mucke L. Prolonged survival and partial recovery in AIDS-associated progressive multifocal leukoencephalopathy. *Neurology* 1988;38:1060–1065.

Bergman I, Painter MJ, Wald ER, Chiponis D, Holland AL, Taylor HG. Outcome in children with enteroviral meningitis during the first year of life. *J Pediatr* 1987;110:705–709.

Bergmans AMC, Groothedde J-W, Schellekens JFP, van Embden JDA, Ossewaarde JM, Schouls LM. Etiology of cat scratch disease: comparison of polymerase chain reaction detection of *Bartonella* (formerly *Rochalimaea*) and *Afipia felis* DNA with serology and skin tests. *J Infect Dis* 1995;171: 916–923.

Bergsagel DJ, Findgold MJ, Butel JS, Kupsky WJ, Garcea RL. DNA sequences similar to those of simian virus 40 in ependymomas and choroid plexus tumors of childhood. *N Engl J Med* 1992;326:988–993.

Bergström T. Polymerase chain reaction for diagnosis of varicella zoster virus central nervous system infections without skin manifestations. *Scand J Infect Dis* 1996;100:41–45.

Bergström T, Andersen O, Vahlne A. Isolation of herpes simplex virus type 1 during first attack of multiple sclerosis. *Ann Neurol* 1989;26:283–285.

Bergström T, Edström S, Tjellström A, Vahlne A. Ménière's disease and antibody reactivity to herpes simplex virus type 1 polypeptides. *Am J Otol* 1992;13:295–300.

Bergström T, Vahlne A, Alestig K, Jeansson S, Forsgren M, Lycke E. Primary and recurrent herpes simplex virus type 2-induced meningitis. *J Infect Dis* 1990;162:322–330.

Bern C, Pallansch MA, Gary HE Jr, et al. Acute hemorrhagic conjunctivitis due to enterovirus 70 in American Samoa: serum-neutralizing antibodies and sex-specific protection. *Am J Epidemiol* 1992; 136:1502–1506.

Bernoulli C, Siegfried J, Baumgartner G, et al. Danger of accidental person-to-person transmission of Creutzfeldt–Jakob disease by surgery. *Lancet* 1977;1:478–479.

Bernton EW, Bryant HU, Decoster MA, et al. No direct neuronotoxicity by HIV-1 virions or culture fluids from HIV-1-infected T cells or monocytes. *AIDS Res Hum Retroviruses* 1992;8:495–503.

Berrada F, Ma D, Michaud J, Doucet G, Giroux L, Kessous-Elbaz A. Neuronal expression of human immunodeficiency virus type 1 env proteins in transgenic mice: distribution in the central nervous system and pathological alterations. *J Virol* 1995;69:6770–6778.

Berry PJ, Nagington J. Fatal infection with echovirus 11. *Arch Dis Child* 1982;57:22–29.

Berti R, Soldan S, Secchiero P, et al. Association of HHV-6 and multiple sclerosis. *J Neurovirol* 1997;3:97.

Bertolli J, Caldwell B, Lindegren ML, Simonds RJ. Epidemiology of HIV disease in children. *Pediatr AIDS* 1995;15:193–204.

Bessen RA, Kocisko DA, Raymond GJ, Nandan S, Lansbury PT, Caughey B. Non-genetic propagation of strain-specific properties of scrapie prion protein. *Nature* 1995;375:698–700.

Bhagavati S, Ehrlich G, Kula RW, et al. Detection of human T-cell lymphoma/leukemia virus type I DNA and antigen in spinal fluid and blood of patients with chronic progressive myelopathy. *N Engl J Med* 1988;318:1141–1147.

Bhamarapravati N, Tuchinda P, Boonyapaknavik V. Pathology of Thailand haemorrhagic fever: a study of 100 autopsy cases. *Ann Trop Med Parasitol* 1967;61:500–510.

Biggs PM. Marek's disease: current state of knowledge. *Curr Top Microbiol Immunol* 1968;43:92–125.

Bigner DD, Kvedar JP, Shaffer TC, Vick NA, Engel WK, Day ED. Factors influencing the cell type of brain tumors induced in dogs by Schmidt–Ruppin Rous sarcoma virus. *J Neuropathol Exp Neurol* 1972;31:583–595.

Bigner DD, Pegram CN. Virus induced experimental brain tumors and putative associations of viruses with human brain tumors, a review. In: Thompson RA, Green JR, eds. *Advances in neurology.* New York: Raven Press, 1976:57–82.

Bilette de Vilemeur T, Deslys J-P, Pradel A, et al. Creutzfeldt–Jakob disease from contaminated growth hormone extracts in France. *Neurology* 1996;47:690–695.

Billeter MA, Cattaneo R, Spielhofer P, Kaelin K, Huber M, Schmid A. Generation and properties of measles virus mutations typically associated with subacute sclerosing panencephalitis. *Ann NY Acad Sci* 1994;724:367–377.

Bistner SI, Rubin LF, Saunders LZ. The ocular lesions of bovine viral diarrhea–mucosal disease. *Pathol Vet* 1970;7:275–286.

Bitzan M. Rubella myelitis and encephalitis in childhood: a report of two cases with magnetic resonance imaging. *Neuropediatrics* 1987;18:84–87.

Blake K, Pillay D, Knowles W, Brown DWG, Griffiths PD, Taylor B. JC virus associated meningoencephalitis in an immunocompetent girl. *Arch Dis Child* 1992;67:956–957.

Blakemore WF, Summers BA, Appel MGJ. Evidence of oligodendrocyte infection and degeneration in canine distemper encephalomyelitis. *Acta Neuropathol (Berl)* 1989;77:550–553.

Blattner WA. HIV epidemiology: past, present, and future. *FASEB J* 1991;5:2340–2348.

Bleier R, Albrecht R. Supendymal macrophages of the third ventricle of hamster: morphological, functional, and histochemical characterization in situ and in culture. *Journal of Comprehensive Neurology* 1980;192:489–504.

Blinzinger K, Muller W. The intercellular gaps of the neuropil as possible pathways for virus spread in viral encephalomyelitis. *Acta Neuropathol (Berl)* 1971;17:37–43.

Bloom DC, Stevens JG. Neuron-specific restriction of a herpes simplex virus recombinant maps to the UL5 gene. *J Virol* 1994;68:3761–3762.

Bloomfield AL. *A bibliography of internal medicine: communicable diseases.* Chicago: University of Chicago Press, 1958.

Bobowick AR, Brody JA, Matthews MR, Roos R, Gajdusek DC. Creutzfeldt–Jakob disease: a case–control study. *Am J Epidemiol* 1973;98:381–394.

Boche D, Hurtrel M, Gray F, et al. Virus load and neuropathology in the FIV model. *J Neurovirol* 1996; 2:377–387.

Bode L, Dürrwald R, Rantam FA, Ferszt R, Ludwig H. First isolates of infectious human Borna disease virus from patients with mood disorders. *Mol Psych* 1996;1:200–212.

Bode L, Ludwig H. Borna disease virus in affective disorders. *Mol Psych* 1996;1:213–214.

Bode L, Riegel S, Lange W, Ludwig H. Human infections with Borna disease virus. *J Med Virol* 1992;36: 309–315.

Bodensteiner JB, Morris HH, Howell JT, Schochet SS. Chronic ECHO type 5 virus meningoencephalitis in x-linked hypogammaglobulinemia: treatment with immune plasma. *Neurology* 1979;29:815–819.

Bodian D. Poliomyelitis: pathologic anatomy. In: *Poliomyelitis: papers and discussion presented at the first international poliomyelitis conference.* Philadelphia: JB Lippincott Co, 1949:62–84.

Bodian D. Viremia in experimental poliomyelitis. I. General aspects of infection after intravascular inoculation with strains of high and of low invasiveness. *Am J Hyg* 1954a;60:339–357.

Bodian D, Howe HA. The rate of progression of poliomyelitis virus in nerves. *Bull Johns Hopkins Hosp* 1941;69:79–85.

Bojinov S. Encephalitis with acute parkinsonian syndrome and bilateral inflammatory necrosis of the substantia nigra. *J Neurol Sci* 1971;12:383–415.

Bolovan CA, Sawtell NM, Thompson RL. ICP34.5 mutants of herpes simplex virus type 1 strain 17syn+ are attenuated for neurovirulence in mice and for replication in confluent primary mouse embryo cell cultures. *J Virol* 1994;68:48–55.

Bondareff W. Distribution of ferritin in the cerebral cortex of the mouse revealed by electron microscopy. *Exp Neurol* 1964;10:377–382.

Bons N, Mestre-Francés N, Charnay Y, Tagliavini F. Spontaneous spongiform encephalopathy in a young adult rhesus monkey. *Lancet* 1996;1:55.

Bordley JE, Brookhauser PE, Worthington EL. Viral infections and hearing: a critical review of the literature. *Laryngoscope* 1972;82:557–577.

Bordley JE, Kapur YP. The histopathological changes in temporal bone resulting from acute smallpox and chickenpox infections. *Laryngoscope* 1972;82:1477–1479.

Borkowsky W, Krasinski K, Cao Y, et al. Correlation of perinatal transmission of human immunodeficiency virus type 1 with maternal viremia and lymphocyte phenotypes. *J Pediatr* 1994;125:345–351.

Bosma TJ, Corbett KM, Eckstein MB, et al. Use of PCR for prenatal and postnatal diagnosis of congenital rubella. *J Clin Microbiol* 1995;33:2881–2887.

Boston Interhospital Virus Study Group. Failure of high dose of 5-iodo-2-deoxyuridine in the therapy of herpes simplex virus encephalitis. *N Engl J Med* 1975;292:600–603.

Bothe K, Aguzzi A, Lassmann H, Rethwilm A, Horak I. Progressive encephalopathy and myopathy in transgenic mice expressing human foamy virus genes. *Science* 1991;253:555–557.

Boufassa F, Bachmeyer C, Carré N, et al. Influence of neurologic manifestations of primary human immunodeficiency virus infection on disease progression. *J Infect Dis* 1995;171:1190–1195.

Bouteille M, Fontaine C, Vedrenne CL, Delarue J. Sur un cas de encéphalite subaiguë à inclusions: étude anatomoclinique et ultrastructurale. *Rev Neurol (Paris)* 1965;118:454–458.

Boycott AE. The transition from live to dead: the nature of filterable viruses. *Annu Rep Smithson Inst* 1929;323–343.

Brady HJM, Pennington DJ, Dzierzak EA. Transgenic mice as models of human immunodeficiency virus expression and related cellular effects. *J Gen Virol* 1994;75:2549–2558.

Brahic M, Smith RA, Gibbs CJ Jr, Garruto RM, Tourtellotte WW, Cash E. Detection of picornavirus sequences in nervous tissue of amyotrophic lateral sclerosis and control patients. *Ann Neurol* 1985; 18:337–343.

Brander S, Raeber A, Sailer A, et al. Normal host prion protein (PrPc) is required for scrapie spread within the central nervous system. *Proc Natl Acad Sci USA* 1996;93:13,148–13,151.

Bray PF, Culp KW, McFarlin DE, Panitch HS, Torkelson RD, Schlight JP. Demyelinating disease after neurologically complicated primary Epstein–Barr virus infection. *Neurology* 1992a;42:278–282.

Bray PF, Luka J, Culp KW, Schlight JP. Antibodies against Epstein–Barr nuclear antigen (EBNA) in multiple sclerosis CSF, and two pentapeptide sequence identities between EBNA and myelin basic protein. *Neurology* 1992b;42:1798–1804.

Bredesen DE. Neural apoptosis. *Ann Neurol* 1995;38:839–851.

Breeden CJ, Hall TC, Tyler HR. Herpes simplex encephalitis treated with systemic 5-iodo-2 deoxyuridine. *Ann Intern Med* 1966;65:1050–1056.

Breningstall GN, Belani KK. Acute transverse myelitis and brainstem encephalitis associated with hepatitis A infection. *Pediatr Neurol* 1995;12:169–171.

Brew BJ, Bhalla RB, Paul M, et al. Cerebrospinal fluid neopterin in human immunodeficiency virus type I infection. *Ann Neurol* 1990;28:556–560.

Brew BJ, Miller J. Human immunodeficiency virus type 1-related transient neurological deficits. *Am J Med* 1996;101:257–261.

Brew BJ, Rosenblum M, Cronin K, Price RW. AIDS dementia complex and HIV-1 brain infection: clinical–virological correlations. *Ann Neurol* 1995;38:563–570.

Brewis EG, Neubauer C, Hurst EW. Another case of louping-ill in man. *Lancet* 1949;1:689–691.

Brierley JB. The penetration of particulate matter from the cerebrospinal fluid into the spinal ganglia, peripheral nerves, and perivascular spaces of the central nervous system. *J Neurol Neurosurg Psychiatry* 1950;13:203–215.

Briese T, Schneemann A, Lewis AJ, et al. Genomic organization of Borna disease virus. *Proc Natl Acad Sci USA* 1994;91:4362–4366.

Briggs NC, Levine PH. A comparative review of systemic and neurological symptomatology in 12 outbreaks collectively described as chronic fatigue syndrome, epidemic neuromyasthenia, and myalgic encephalomyelitis. *Clin Infect Dis* 1994;18[Suppl]:S32–S42.

Brightman MW. The intracerebral movement of proteins injected into blood and cerebrospinal fluid of mice. In: Lajtha A, Ford DH, eds. *Progress in brain research.* Amsterdam: Elsevier Science, 1968:648–677.

Brightman MW, Reese TS. Junctions between intimately apposed cell membranes in the vertebrate brain. *J Cell Biol* 1969;40:648–677.

Brochet B, Henry P, Piquemal-Baluard A, Dupasquier P. Encéphalite herpétique à rechutes. *Rev Neurol (Paris)* 1990;146:6–7 and 450–454.

Brochier B, Kieny MP, Costy F, et al. Large-scale eradication of rabies using recombinant vaccinia–rabies vaccine. *Nature* 1991;354:520–523.

Brody JA, Hadlow WJ, Hotchin J, Johnson RT, Koprowski H, Kurland LT. Soviet search for viruses that cause chronic neurologic diseases in the USSR. *Science* 1965;147:1114–1116.

Brookhauser PE, Bordley JE. Congenital rubella deafness: pathology and pathogenesis. *Arch Otolaryngol* 1973;98:252–257.

Brooks BR. Viral hepatitis type B presenting with seizure. *JAMA* 1977;237:472–473.

Brooks BR. Virus-associated neurological syndromes. In: Lennette D, Spector S, Thompson K, eds. *Diagnosis of Viral Infections: Role of the clinical laboratory.* University Park Press, 1979:183–203.

Brooks BR, Swarz JR, Johnson RT. Spongiform polioencephalopathy caused by a murine retrovirus. I. Pathogenesis of infection in newborn mice. *Lab Invest* 1980;43:480–486.

Brooks BR, Swarz JR, Narayan O, Johnson RT. Murine neurotropic retrovirus spongiform polioencephalomyelopathy: acceleration of disease by virus inoculum concentration. *Infect Immun* 1979;23:540–544.

Brown GC, Karunas RS. Relationship of congenital anomalies and maternal infection with selected enteroviruses. *Am J Epidemiol* 1972;95:207–217.

Brown HR, Goller NL, Rudelli RD, Dymecki J, Wisniewski HM. Postmortem detection of measles virus in non-neural tissues in subacute sclerosing panencephalitis. *Ann Neurol* 1989;26:263–268.

Brown P. The decline and fall of Creutzfeldt–Jakob disease associated with human growth hormone therapy. *Neurology* 1988;38:1135–1137.

Brown P, Cathala F, Raubertas RF, Gajdusek DC, Castaigne P. The epidemiology of Creutzfeldt–Jakob disease: conclusion of a 15-year investigation in France and review of the world literature. *Neurology* 1987a;37:895–904.

Brown P, Cervenáková L, Goldfarb LG, et al. Iatrogenic Creutzfeldt–Jakob disease: an example of the interplay between ancient genes and modern medicine. *Neurology* 1994a;44:291–293.

Brown P, Gajdusek DC. No mouse PMN leukocyte depression after inoculation with brain tissue from multiple sclerosis or spongiform encephalopathies. *Nature* 1974;247:217–218.

Brown P, Gajdusek DC, Gibbs CJ Jr, Asher DM. Potential epidemic of Creutzfeldt–Jakob disease from human growth hormone therapy. *N Engl J Med* 1985;313:728–731.

Brown P, Gibbs CJ Jr, Rodgers-Johnson P, et al. Human spongiform encephalopathy: the National Institutes of Health series of 300 cases of experimentally transmitted disease. *Ann Neurol* 1994b;35:513–529.

Brown RH Jr, Johnson D, Ogonowski M, Weiner HL. Type 1 human poliovirus binds to human synaptosomes. *Ann Neurol* 1987b;21:64–70.

Brown ZA, Vontver LA, Benedetti J, et al. Effects on infants of a first episode of genital herpes during pregnancy. *N Engl J Med* 1987c;317:1246–1251.

Bruce ME, Will RG, Ironside JW, et al. Transmissions to mice indicate that 'new variant' CJD is caused by the BSE agent. *Nature* 1997;389:498–501.

Brunner RL, O'Grady DJ, Partin JC, Partin JS, Schubert WK. Neuropsychologic consequence of Reye syndrome. *J Pediatr* 1979;95:706–711.

Bryson YJ, Pang S, Wei LS, Dickover R, Diagne A, Chen ISY. Clearance of HIV infection in a perinatally infected infant. *N Engl J Med* 1995;332:833–838.

Buchmeier MJ, Lewicki HA, Talbot PJ, Knobler RL. Murine hepatitis virus-4 (strain JHM)-induced neurologic disease is modulated in vivo by monoclonal antibody. *Virology* 1984;132:261–270.

Buchwald D, Cheney PR, Peterson DL, et al. A chronic illness characterized by fatigue, neurologic and immunologic disorders, and active human herpesvirus type 6 infection. *Ann Intern Med* 1992;116:103–113.

Buchwald D, Umali P, Umali J, Kith P, Pearlman T, Komaroff AL. Chronic fatigue and the chronic fatigue syndrome: prevalence in a Pacific Northwest health care system. *Ann Intern Med* 1995;123:81–88.

Budka H. Human immunodeficiency virus (HIV) envelope and core proteins in CNS tissues of patients with the acquired immune deficiency syndrome (AIDS). *Acta Neuropathol (Berl)* 1990;79:611–619.

Budka H, Aguzzi A, Brown P, et al. Neuropathological diagnostic criteria for Creutzfeldt–Jakob disease (CJD) and other human spongiform encephalopathies (prion diseases). *Brain Pathol* 1995;5:459–466.

Buescher EL, Artenstein MS, Olson LC. Central nervous system infections of viral etiology: the changing patterns. *Res Publ Assoc Nerv Ment Dis* 1968;44:147–163.

Bullard DE, Bigner DD. Animal models and virus induction of tumors. In: Thomas DTG, Graham DI, eds. *Brain tumours: scientific basis, clinical investigation and current therapy.* London: Butterworths, 1980;51–84.

Burek JD, Roos RP, Narayan O. Virus induced abortion: studies of equine herpesvirus 1 (abortion virus) in hamsters. *Lab Invest* 1975;33:400–406.

Burgard M, Mayaux M-J, Blanche S, et al. The use of viral culture and p24 antigen testing to diagnose human immunodeficiency virus infection in neonates. *N Engl J Med* 1992;327:1192–1197.

Burgdorfer W, Barbour AG, Hayes SF, Benach JL, Grunwaldt E, Davis JP. Lyme disease: a tick-borne spirochetosis? *Science* 1982;216:1317–1319.

Burke DS. Recombination in HIV: an important viral evolutionary strategy. *Emer Infect Dis* 1997;3:253–271.

Burke DS, Lorsomrudee W, Leake CJ, et al. Fatal outcome in Japanese encephalitis. *Am J Trop Med Hyg* 1985;34:1203–1210.

Burke DS, Nisalak A, Ussery MA. Antibody capture immunoassay detection of Japanese encephalitis virus immunoglobulin M and G antibodies in cerebrospinal fluid. *J Clin Microbiol* 1982;16:1034–1042.

Burks JS, Narayan O, McFarland HF, Johnson RT. Acute encephalopathy caused by defective virus infection. I. Studies of Newcastle disease virus infections in newborn and adult mice. *Neurology* 1976;26:585–588.

Burnet FM. *Enzyme, antigen and virus.* Cambridge: Cambridge University Press, 1956.

Butcher EC, Picker LJ. Lymphocyte homing and homeostasis. *Science* 1996;272:60–66.

Bychkova EN. Viruses isolated from patients with encephalomyelitis and multiple sclerosis. I. Pathogenic and antigenic properties. *Vopr Virusol* 1964;9:173–176.

Byers B. Ribosome crystallization induced in chick embryo tissues by hypothermia. *J Cell Biol* 1966;30: C1–C6.

Byington DP, Johnson KP. Subacute sclerosing panencephalitis virus in immunosuppressed adult hamsters. *Lab Invest* 1975;32:91–97.

Cabrera J, Griffin DE, Johnson RT. Unusual features of the Guillain–Barré syndrome after rabies vaccine prepared in suckling mouse brain. *J Neurol Sci* 1987;81:239–245.

Caekebeke JFV, Peters ACB, Vandvik B, Brouwer OF, de Bakker HM. Cerebral vasculopathy associated with primary varicella infection. *Arch Neurol* 1990;47:1033–1035.

Cairns J. *Cancer: science and society.* San Francisco: WH Freeman, 1978.

Caldemeyer KS, Smith RR, Harris TM, Edwards MK. MRI in acute disseminated encephalomyelitis. *Neuroradiology* 1994;36:216–220.

Calisher CH, Pretzman CI, Muth DJ, Parsons MA, Peterson ED. Serodiagnosis of La Crosse virus infections in humans by detection of immunoglobulin M class antibodies. *J Clin Microbiol* 1986;23:667–671.

Calisher CH, Sever JL. Are North American bunyamwera serogroup viruses etiologic agents of human congenital defects of the central nervous system? *Emer Infect Dis* 1995;1:147–151.

Callis RT, Jahrling PB, DePaoli A. Pathology of Lassa virus infection in the rhesus monkey. *Am J Trop Med Hyg* 1982;31:1038–1045.

Cameron DW, D'Costa LJ, Maitha GM, et al. Female to male transmission of human immunodeficiency virus type 1: risk factors for seroconversion in men. *Lancet* 1989;2:403–407.

Cameron KR, Birchall SM, Moses MA. Isolation of foamy virus from patient with dialysis encephalopathy. *Lancet* 1978;2:796.

Cammer W, Bloom BR, Norton WT, Gordon S. Degradation of basic protein in myelin by neutral proteases secreted by stimulated macrophages: a possible mechanism of inflammatory demyelination. *Proc Natl Acad Sci USA* 1978;75:1554–1558.

Campbell TA, Palmer MS, Will RG, Gibb WRG, Luthert PJ, Collinge J. A prion disease with a novel 96-base pair insertional mutation in the prion protein gene. *Neurology* 1996;46:761–766.

Carbone KM, Park SW, Rubin SA, Waltrip RW II, Vogelsang GB. Borna disease: association with a maturation defect in the cellular immune response. *J Virol* 1991;65:6154–6164.

Carbone KM, Trapp BD, Griffin JW, Duchala CS, Narayan O. Astrocytes and Schwann cells are virus-host cells in the nervous system of rats with Borna disease. *J Neuropathol Exp Neurol* 1989;48:631–644.

Carithers HA, Margileth AM. Cat-scratch disease, acute encephalopathy and other neurologic manifestations. *Am J Dis Child* 1991;145:98–101.

Carp RI, Licursi PC, Merz PA. Multiple sclerosis associated agent. *Lancet* 1977;2:814.

Carrigan DR, Harrington D, Knox KK. Subacute leukoencephalitis caused by CNS infection with human herpesvirus-6 manifesting as acute multiple sclerosis. *Neurology* 1996;47:147–148.

Carrington D, Whittle MJ, Gibson AAM, et al. Maternal serum α-fetoprotein: a marker of fetal aplastic crisis during intrauterine human parvovirus infection. *Lancet* 1987;1:433–435.

Carter GI, Taylor GR, Crow TJ. Search for viral nucleic acid sequences in the post mortem brains of patients with schizophrenia and individuals who have committed suicide. *J Neurol Neurosurg Psychiatry* 1987;50:247–251.

Carter LP, Beggs J, Waggener JD. Ultrastructure of three choroid plexus papillomas. *Cancer* 1972;30: 1130–1136.

Carton CA. Effect of previous sensory loss on the appearance of herpes simplex. *J Neurosurg* 1953;10: 463–468.

Cashman NR, Maselli R, Wollmann RL, Roos R, Simon R, Antel JP. Late denervation in patients with antecedent paralytic poliomyelitis. *N Engl J Med* 1987;317:7–12.

Caspar DLD, Dulbecco R, Klug A, et al. Proposals. *Cold Spring Harb Symp Quant Biol* 1962;27:1–24.

Cassinotti P, Schultze D, Schlageter P, Chevili S, Siegl G. Persistent human parvovirus B19 infection following an acute infection with meningitis in an immunocompetent patient. *Eur J Clin Microbiol Infect Dis* 1993;12:701–704.

Castaigne P, Rondot P, Escourolle R, Ribadeau-Dumas JL, Cathala F, Hauw JJ. Lecoencephalopathie multifocale progressive et "gliomes" multiples. *Rev Neurol (Paris)* 1974;130:379–392.

Cattaneo R, Rebmann G, Baczko K, Ter Meulen V, Billeter MA. Altered ratios of measles virus transcripts in diseased human brains. *Virology* 1987;160:523–526.

Cattaneo R, Rose JK. Cell fusion by the envelope glycoproteins of persistent measles viruses which caused lethal human brain disease. *J Virol* 1993;67:1493–1502.

Cavanagh JB, Greenbaum D, Marshall AHE, Rubinstein LJ. Cerebral demyelination associated with disorders of the reticuloendothelial system. *Lancet* 1959;2:525–529.

Ceccaldi PE, Gillet JP, Tsiang H. Inhibition of the transport of rabies virus in the central nervous system. *J Neuropathol Exp Neurol* 1989;48:620–630.

Centers for Disease Control. Rabies in a laboratory worker: New York. *MMWR* 1977;26:183–184.

Centers for Disease Control. Poliomyelitis: United States, 1978–1979. *MMWR* 1979;28:483.

Centers for Disease Control. Human-to-human transmission of rabies via corneal transplant: France. *MMWR* 1980a;29:25–26.

Centers for Disease Control. Follow-up on Reye's syndrome. *MMWR* 1980b;29:321–322.

Centers for Disease Control. Kaposi's sarcoma and *Pneumocystis* pneumonia among homosexual men: New York City and California. *MMWR* 1981a;30:305–308.

Centers for Disease Control. *Pneumocystis* pneumonia: Los Angeles. *MMWR* 1981b;30:250–252.

Centers for Disease Control. Japanese encephalitis: report of a World Health Organization working group. *MMWR* 1984;33:119–126.

Centers for Disease Control. B-virus infection in humans: Pensacola, Florida. *MMWR* 1987;36:289–295.

Centers for Disease Control. Rubella vaccination during pregnancy: United States, 1971–1988. *MMWR* 1989a;38:289–293.

Centers for Disease Control. Reye syndrome surveillance: United States, 1987 and 1988. *MMWR* 1989b; 38:325–327.

Centers for Disease Control. Aseptic meningitis: New York State and United States, weeks 1–36, 1991a. *MMWR* 1991;40:773–776.

Centers for Disease Control. Rabies prevention: United States, 1991. *MMWR* 1991b;40:1–19.

Centers for Disease Control. St. Louis encephalitis outbreak: Arkansas, 1991. *MMWR* 1991c;40:605–607.

Centers for Disease Control. Inactivated Japanese encephalitis virus vaccine: recommendations of the Advisory Committee on Immunization Practices (ACIP). *MMWR* 1993a;42:1–15.

Centers for Disease Control. Isolation of wild poliovirus type 3 among members of a religious community objecting to vaccination: Alberta, Canada, 1993. *MMWR* 1993b;42:337–340.

Centers for Disease Control. Progress toward global eradication of poliomyelitis, 1988–1991. *MMWR* 1993c;42:486–496.

Centers for Disease Control. Rocky Mountain spotted fever: United States, 1990. *MMWR* 1993d;40:451–460.

Centers for Disease Control. Raccoon rabies epizootic: United States, 1993. *MMWR* 1994a;43:269–274.

Centers for Disease Control. Recommendations of the U.S. Public Health Service Task Force on the use of zidovudine to reduce perinatal transmission of human immunodeficiency virus. *MMWR* 1994b;43:1–20.

Centers for Disease Control. Arboviral disease: United States, 1994. *MMWR* 1995a;44:641–644.

Centers for Disease Control. First 500,000 AIDS cases: United States, 1995. *MMWR* 1995b;44:849–854.

Centers for Disease Control. Human rabies: Alabama, Tennessee, and Texas, 1994. *MMWR* 1995c;44:269–272.

Centers for Disease Control. Translocation of coyote rabies: Florida, 1994. *MMWR* 1995d;44a:580–581.

Centers for Disease Control. Human rabies: Florida, 1996. *MMWR* 1996a;45:719–720.

Centers for Disease Control. Prevention of varicella. *MMWR* 1996b;45:1–36.

Centers for Disease Control. Update: mortality attributable to HIV infection among persons aged 25–44 years—United States, 1994. *MMWR* 1996c;45:121–126.

Centers for Disease Control. World Health Organization consultation on public health issues related to bovine spongiform encephalopathy and the emergence of a new variant of Creutzfeldt–Jakob disease. *MMWR* 1996d;45:295–296.

Centers for Disease Control. Paralytic poliomyelitis: United States, 1980–1994. *MMWR* 1997a;46:79–84.

Centers for Disease Control. Poliomyelitis prevention in the United States: introduction of a sequential vaccination schedule of inactivated poliovirus vaccine followed by oral poliovirus vaccine. *MMWR* 1997b;46:1–25.

Chad DA, Smith TW, Blumenfeld A, Fairchild PG, DeGirolami U. Human immunodeficiency virus (HIV)-associated myopathy: immunocytochemical identification of an HIV antigen (gp 41) in muscle macrophages. *Ann Neurol* 1990;28:579–582.

Chadarevian J-P, Becker WJ. Mollaret's recurrent aseptic meningitis: relationship to epidermoid cysts. *J Neuropathol Exp Neurol* 1980;39:661–669.

Chakrabarti L, Hurtrel M, Maire M-A, et al. Early viral replication in the brain of SIV-infected rhesus monkeys. *Am J Pathol* 1991;139:1273–1280.

Challoner PB, Smith KT, Parker JD, et al. Plaque-associated expression of human herpesvirus 6 in multiple sclerosis. *Proc Natl Acad Sci USA* 1995;92:7440–7444.

Chao CC, Hu S, Peterson PK. Glia: the not so innocent bystanders. *J Neurovirol* 1996;2:234–239.

Chapman BA, Beaven DW. An unusual case of flaccid paralysis of both lower limbs following herpes zoster. *Aust NZ J Med* 1979;9:702–704.

Chaturvedi UC, Mathur A, Chandra A, Das SK, Tandon HO, Singh VK. Transplacental infection with Japanese encephalitis virus. *J Infect Dis* 1980;141:712–714.

Chaves-Carballo E. Epidemiology of Reye's syndrome. In: Schoenberg BS, ed. *Neurological epidemiology: principles and clinical applications.* New York: Raven Press, 1978:231–248.

Chazot G, Broussolle E, Lapras CI, Blättler T, Aguzzi A, Kopp N. New variant of Creutzfeldt–Jakob disease in a 26-year-old French man. *Lancet* 1996;2:1181.

Chen HH, Kong WP, Zhang L, Ward PL, Roos RP. A picornaviral protein synthesized out of frame with the polyprotein plays a key role in a virus-induced immune-mediated demyelinating disease. *Nature Med* 1995;1:927–931.

Chesebro B, Fields BN. Transmissible spongiform encephalopathies: a brief introduction. In: Fields BN, Knipe DM, Howley PM, et al., eds. *Fields virology,* 3rd ed. Philadelphia: Lippincott–Raven Publishers, 1996:2845–2849.

Chesebro B, Wehrly K, Nishio J, Perryman S. Macrophage-tropic human immunodeficiency virus isolates from different patients exhibit unusual V3 envelope sequence homogeneity in comparison with T-cell-tropic isolates: definition of critical amino acids involved in cell tropism. *J Virol* 1992;6:6547–6554.

Chesney PJ, Katcher ML, Nelson DB, Horowitz SD. CSF eosinophilia and chronic lymphocytic choriomeningitis virus meningitis. *J Pediatr* 1979;94:750–752.

Chew-Lim M, Scott T, Webb HE. An ultrastructural study of cerebellar lesions induced in mice by three inoculations of avirulent semliki forest virus. *Acta Neuropathol* 1978;41:55–59.

Child PL, MacKengre RB, Valverde LR, Johnson KM. Bolivian hemorrhagic fever: a pathologic description. *Arch Pathol* 1967;83:434–445.

Childs JE, Glass GE, Korch GW, Ksiazek TG, Leduc JW. Lymphocytic choriomeningitis virus infection and house mouse (*Mus musculus*) distribution in urban Baltimore. *Am J Trop Med Hyg* 1992;47:27–34.

Chin W, Magoffin R, Frierson JG, Lennette EH. Cytomegalovirus infection: a case with meningoencephalitis. *JAMA* 1973;225:740–741.

Chonmaitree T, Menegus MA, Schervish-Swierkosz EM, Schwalenstocker E. Enterovirus 71 infection: report of an outbreak with two cases of paralysis and a review of the literature. *Pediatrics* 1981;67: 489–493.

Chou J, Kern ER, Whitley RJ, Roizman B. Mapping of herpes simplex virus-1 neurovirulence to π1 34.5, a gene nonessential for growth in culture. *Science* 1990;250:1262–1266.

Chou SM. Inclusion body myositis: a chronic persistent mumps myositis? *Hum Pathol* 1986;17:765–777.

Chou SM, Ross R, Burrell R, Gutmann L, Harley JB. Subacute focal adenovirus encephalitis. *J Neuropathol Exp Neurol* 1973;32:34–49.

Chrétien F, Bélec L, Hilton DA, et al. Herpes simplex virus type 1 encephalitis in acquired immunodeficiency syndrome. *Neuropathol Appl Neurobiol* 1996;22:394–404.

Christie AB. *Infectious diseases: epidemiology and clinical practice.* Edinburgh: E & S Livingstone, 1969.

Chumakov M, Voroshilova M, Shindarov L, et al. Enterovirus 71 isolated from cases of epidemic poliomyelitis-like disease in Bulgaria. *Arch Neurol* 1979;60:329–340.

Chusid MJ, Williamson SJ, Murphy JV, Ramey LS. Neuromyelitis optica (Devic disease) following varicella infection. *J Pediatr* 1979;95:737–738.

Cifuentes M, Fernández-Llebrez P, Pérez J, Pérez-Figares JM, Rodriguez EM. Distribution of intraventricularly injected horseradish peroxidase in cerebrospinal fluid compartments of the rat spinal cord. *Cell Tissue Res* 1992;270:485–494.

Cinque P, Baldanti F, Vago L, et al. Ganciclovir therapy for cytomegalovirus (CMV) infection of the central nervous system in AIDS patients: monitoring by CMV DNA detection in cerebrospinal fluid. *J Infect Dis* 1995;171:1603–1606.

Clavel F, Mansinho K, Chamaret S, et al. Human immunodeficiency virus type 2 infection associated with AIDS in West Africa. *N Engl J Med* 1987;316:1180–1185.

Clavel M, Clavel P. Creutzfeldt–Jakob disease transmitted by dura mater graft. *Eur Neurol* 1996;36: 239–240.

Clements JE, Zink MC. Molecular biology and pathogenesis of animal lentivirus infections. *Clin Microbiol Rev* 1996;9:100–117.

Clemis JD, Becker GW. Vestibular neuronitis. *Otolaryngol Clin North Am* 1973;6:139–155.

Cobb WA, Marshall J, Scaravilli F. Long survival in subacute sclerosing panencephalitis. *J Neurol Neurosurg Psychiatry* 1984;47:176–183.

Coetzer JAW, Barnard BJH. Hydrops amnii in sheep associated with hydranencephaly and arthrogryposis with Wesselsbron disease and Rift Valley fever viruses as aetiological agents. *Onderstepoort J Vet Res* 1977;44:119–126.

Coffey VP, Jessop WSE. Maternal influenza and congenital deformities. *Lancet* 1963;1:748–751.

Cogon DG, Kuwabara T, Young GF, Knox DL. Herpes simplex retinopathy in an infant. *Arch Ophthalmol* 1964;72:641–645.

Cohen BA. Prognosis and response to therapy of cytomegalovirus encephalitis and meningomyelitis in AIDS. *Neurology* 1996;46:444–450.

Cohen BA, McArthur JC, Grohman S, Patterson B, Glass JD. Neurologic prognosis of cytomegalovirus polyradiculomyelopathy in AIDS. *Neurology* 1993;43:493–499.

Cohen BA, Rowley AH, Long CM. Herpes simplex type 2 in a patient with Mollaret's meningitis: demonstration by polymerase chain reaction. *Ann Neurol* 1994;35:112–116.

Cohen HA, Ashkenazi A, Nussinovitch M, Amir J, Hart J, Frydman M. Mumps-associated acute cerebellar ataxia. *Am J Dis Child* 1992;146:930–931.

Cohen JI, Corey GR. Cytomegalovirus infection in the normal host. *Medicine (Baltimore)* 1985;64:100–114.

Coimbra TLM, Nassar ES, Burattini MN, et al. New arenavirus isolated in Brazil. *Lancet* 1994;1:391–392.

Cole GA, Gilden DH, Monjan AA, Nathanson N. Lymphocytic choriomeningitis virus: pathogenesis of acute central nervous system disease. *Fed Proc* 1971;30:1821–1841.

Coleman DV, Wolfendale MR, Daniel RA, et al. A prospective of human polyomavirus infection in pregnancy. *J Infect Dis* 1980;142:1–8.

Collee JG, Bradley R. BSE: a decade on—part 1. *Lancet* 1997a;1:636–640.

Collee JG, Bradley R. BSE: a decade on—part 2. *Lancet* 1997b;1:715–721.

Collier AC, Coombs RW, Schoenfeld DA, et al. Treatment of human immunodeficiency virus infection with saquinavir, zidovudine, and zalcitabine. *N Engl J Med* 1996;334:1011–1017.

Connelly KP, DeWitt LD. Neurologic complications of infectious mononucleosis. *Pediatr Neurol* 1994; 10:181–184.

Connolly AM, Dodson WE, Prensky AL, Rust RS. Course and outcome of acute cerebellar ataxia. *Ann Neurol* 1994;35:673–679.

Connolly JH, Allen IV, Hurwitz LJ, Millar JHD. Measles virus antibody and antigen in subacute sclerosing panencephalitis. *Lancet* 1967;1:542–544.

Connolly JH, Hutchinson WM, Allen IV, et al. Carotid artery thrombosis, encephalitis, myelitis, and optic neuritis associated with rubella virus infections. *Brain* 1975;95:583–594.

Constantine DG. Rabies transmission by nonbite route. *Public Health Rep* 1962;77:287–289.

Constantine DG. Bat rabies: current knowledge and future research. In: Nagano Y, Davenport FM, eds. *Rabies.* Tokyo: University of Tokyo Press, 1971:253–262.

Cook ML, Stevens JG. Pathogenesis of herpetic neuritis and ganglionitis in mice: evidence for intraaxonal transport of infection. *Infect Immun* 1973;7:272–288.

Cook SD, Dowling PC. Multiple sclerosis and viruses: an overview. *Neurology* 1980;30:80–91.

Cook SD, Dowling PC. The role of autoantibody and immune complexes in the pathogenesis of Guillain–Barré syndrome. *Ann Neurol* 1981;9[Suppl]:S70–S79.

Cook SD, Dowling PC. Distemper and multiple sclerosis in Sitka, Alaska. *Ann Neurol* 1982;11:192–194.

Cook SD, Dowling PC, Whitaker JN. Serum immunoglobulins in the Guillain–Barré syndrome. *Neurology* 1970;20:403.

Cook SD, MacDonald J, Tapp W, Poskanzer D, Dowling PC. Multiple sclerosis in the Shetland Islands: an update. *Acta Neurol Scand* 1988;77:148–151.

Cook SD, Rohowsky-Kochan C, Bansil S, Dowling PC. Evidence for multiple sclerosis as an infectious disease. *Acta Neurol Scand* 1995;161:34–42.

Cooper JR. Tumor tissue growth: the growth of tumor tissue of the central nervous system in tissue culture. *J Kans Med Soc* 1967;68:340–343.

Copps SC, Giddings LE. Transplacental transmission of western equine encephalitis. *Pediatrics* 1959;24: 31–33.

Corallini A, Pagnani M, Viadana P, et al. Association of BK virus with human brain tumors and tumors of pancreatic islets. *Int J Cancer* 1987;39:60–67.

Corboy JR, Buzy JM, Zink MC, Clements JE. Expression directed from HIV long terminal repeats in central nervous system of transgenic mice. *Science* 1992;258:1804–1808.

Corey L, Adams HG, Brown ZA, Holmes KK. Genital herpes simplex virus infections: clinical manifestations, course, and complications. *Ann Intern Med* 1983;98:958–972.

Corey L, Rubin RJ, Hattwick MAW. Reye's syndrome: clinical progression and evaluation of therapy. *Pediatrics* 1977;60:708–714.

Corey L, Stone EF, Whitley RJ, Mohan K. Difference between herpes simplex virus type 1 and type 2 neonatal encephalitis in neurological outcome. *Lancet* 1988;1:1–4.

Cork LC, Hadlow SJ, Gorham JR, Pyper RC, Crawford TB. Infectious leukoencephalomyelitis of goats (CAEV). *J Infect Dis* 1974;129:134–141.

Corman LC, Dolson DJ. Polyarteritis nodosa and parvovirus B19 infection. *Lancet* 1992;1:491.

Cornblath DE. Electrophysiology in Guillain–Barré syndrome. *Ann Neurol* 1990;27[Suppl]:S17.

Cornblath DR, McArthur JC, Kennedy PGE, Witte AS, Griffin JW. Inflammatory demyelinating peripheral neuropathies associated with human T-cell lymphotropic virus type III infection. *Ann Neurol* 1987;21:32–40.

Cornford ME, McCormick GF. Adult-onset temporal lobe epilepsy associated with smoldering herpes simplex 2 infection. *Neurology* 1997;48:425–430.

Cosby SL, McQuaid S, Taylor MJ, et al. Examination of eight cases of multiple sclerosis and 56 neurological and non-neurological controls for genomic sequences of measles virus, canine distemper virus, simian virus 5 and rubella virus. *J Gen Virol* 1989;70:2027–2036.

Courgnaud V, Laure F, Brossard A, et al. Frequent and early in utero HIV-1 infection. *AIDS Res Hum Retroviruses* 1991;7:337–341.

Cousens SNZ, Esmonde TF, DeSilva R, Wilesmith JW, Smith PG, Will RG. Sporadic Creutzfeldt–Jakob disease in the United Kingdom: analysis of epidemiological surveillance data for 1970–96. *BMJ* 1997;315:389–396.

Coyle PK, Wolinsky JS. Characterization of immune complexes in progressive rubella panencephalitis. *Ann Neurol* 1981;9:557–562.

Coyle PK, Wolinsky JS, Buimovici-Klein E, Moncha R, Cooper LZ. Rubella specific immune complexes following congenital infection and live virus vaccination. *Neurology* 1981;31:126.

Craig CP, Nahmias AJ. Different patterns of neurologic involvement with herpes simplex virus types 1 and 2: isolation of herpes virus type 2 from the buffy coat of two adults with meningitis. *J Infect Dis* 1973;127:365–372.

Creech WB. St. Louis encephalitis in the United States, 1975. *J Infect Dis* 1977;135:1014–1016.

Cremer NE, Johnson KP, Fein G, Likosky WH. Comprehensive viral immunology of multiple sclerosis. II. Analysis of serum and cerebral spinal fluid antibodies by standard serologic methods. *Arch Neurol* 1980;37:610–615.

Cremer NE, Oshiro LS, Norris FJ, Lennette EH. Cultures of tissues from patients with amyotrophic lateral sclerosis. *Arch Neurol* 1973;29:331–333.

Cremer NE, Oshiro LS, Weil ML, Lennette EH, Itabashi HH, Carnay L. Isolation of rubella virus from brain in chronic progressive panencephalitis. *J Gen Virol* 1975;29:331–333.

Crennan JM, Van Scoy RE, McKenna CH, Smith TF. Echovirus polymyositis in patients with hypogammaglobulinemia. *Am J Med* 1986;81:35–42.

Crick F. Central dogma of molecular biology. *Nature* 1970;227:561–563.

Croen KD, Ostrove JM, Dragovic LJ, Smialek JE, Straus SE. Latent herpes simplex virus in human trigeminal ganglia. *N Engl J Med* 1987;317:1427–1432.

Croen KD, Ostrove JM, Dragovic LJ, Straus SE. Patterns of gene expression and sites of latency in human nerve ganglia are different for varicella–zoster and herpes simplex viruses. *Proc Natl Acad Sci USA* 1988;85:9773–9777.

Crow TJ, Johnstone EC, Owens DGC, Ferrier IN, Macmillan JF, Parry RP. Characteristics of patients with schizophrenia or neurological disorder and virus-like agent in cerebrospinal fluid. *Lancet* 1979;1: 842–844.

Cserr HF, Knopf PM. Cervical lymphatics, the blood–brain barrier and the immunoreactivity of the brain: a new view. *Immunol Today* 1992;13:507–512.

Cuatico W, Woldron R Jr, Tyschenko W. Biochemical evidence for viral-like characteristics in cerebrospinal fluids of brain tumor patients. *Cancer* 1977;39:2240–2246.

Cuille J, Chelle PL. Pathologie animale: la maladie dite tremblante du mouton est-elle inoculable. *C R Acad Sci* 1936;201:1552–1554.

Cummins D, McCormick J, Bennett D, et al. Acute sensorineural deafness in Lassa fever. *JAMA* 1990; 264:2093–2096.

Cunningham AJ. Self-tolerance maintained by active suppressor mechanisms. *Transpl Rev* 1976;31:23–43.

Cunningham L, Bowles NE, Lane RJM, Dubowitz V, Archard LC. Persistence of enteroviral RNA in chronic fatigue syndrome is associated with the abnormal production of equal amounts of positive and negative strands of enteroviral RNA. *J Gen Virol* 1990;71:1399–1402.

Cupler EJ, Leon-Monzon M, Miller J, Semino-Mora C, Anderson TL, Dalakas MC. Inclusion body myositis in HIV-1 and HTLV-1 infected patients. *Brain* 1996;119:1887–1893.

Curless RG, Scott GB, Post MJ, Gregorios JB. Progressive cytomegalovirus encephalopathy following congenital infection in an infant with acquired immunodeficiency syndrome. *Childs Nerv Syst* 1987;3: 255–257.

Cushing H. Perineal zoster, with notes upon cutaneous segmentation postaxial to the lower limbs. *Am J Med Sci* 1904;127:375–391.

Cvetkovich TA, Lazar E, Blumberg BM, et al. Human immunodeficiency virus type 1 infection of neural xenografts. *Proc Natl Acad Sci USA* 1992;89:5162–5166.

da Silva EE, Winkler MT, Pallansch MA. Role of enterovirus 71 in acute flaccid paralysis after the eradication of poliovirus in Brazil. *Emer Infect Dis* 1996;2:231–233.

Dal Canto MC, Rabinowitz SG. Murine central nervous system infection by a viral temperature-sensitive mutant. *Am J Pathol* 1981;102:412–426.

Dal Canto MC, Rabinowitz SG, Johnson TC. Virus-induced demyelination: production by a viral temperature-sensitive mutant. *J Neurol Sci* 1979;42:155–168.

Dalakas MC. Polymyositis, dermatomyositis, and inclusion-body myositis. *N Engl J Med* 1991;325: 1487–1498.

Dalakas MC. Pathogenetic mechanisms of post-polio syndrome: morphological, electrophysiological, virological, and immunological correlations. *Ann NY Acad Sci* 1995a;753:167–185.

Dalakas MC. The post-polio syndrome as an evolved clinical entity: definition and clinical description. *Ann NY Acad Sci* 1995b;753:68–80.

Dalakas MC, Illa I, Pezeshkpour GH, Laukaitis JP, Cohen B, Griffin JL. Mitochondrial myopathy caused by long-term zidovudine therapy. *N Engl J Med* 1990;322:1098–1105.

Dalakas MC, London WT, Gravell M, Sever JL. Polymyositis in an immunodeficiency disease in monkeys induced by a type D retrovirus. *Neurology* 1986a;36:569–572.

Dalakas MC, Pezeshkpour GH, Gravell M, Server JL. Polymyositis associated with AIDS retrovirus. *JAMA* 1986b;256:2381–2383.

Dalldorf G. The coxsackie viruses: isolation and properties. In: *Poliomyelitis papers and discussion presented at the second international poliomyelitis conference.* New York: JB Lippincott Co, 1952: 111–137.

DalPan GJ, Glass JD, McArthur JC. Clinicopathologic correlations of HIV-1-associated vacuolar myelopathy: an autopsy-based case–control study. *Neurology* 1994;44:2159–2164.

DalPan GJ, McArthur JH, Aylward E, et al. Patterns of cerebral atrophy in HIV-1-infected individuals: results of a quantitative MRI analysis. *Neurology* 1992;42:2125–2130.

Damjanov I, Moser RL, Moriber Katz S, Lyons P. Immune complex myositis associated with viral hepatitis. *Hum Pathol* 1980;11:478–481.

Daniel MD, Letvin NL, King NW, Kannagi M, Sehgal PK, Hunt RD. Isolation of T-cell tropic HTLV-III-like retrovirus from macaques. *Science* 1985;228:1201–1204.

Daniels R, Shah K, Madden D, Stagno S. Serological investigation of the possibility of congenital transmission of papovavirus JC. *Infect Immun* 1981;33:319–321.

Darling CF, Larsen MB, Byrd SE, Radkowski MA, Palka PS, Allen ED. MR and CT imaging patterns in post-varicella encephalitis. *Pediatr Radiol* 1995;25:241–244.

Darnell RB. The polymerase chain reaction: application to nervous system disease. *Ann Neurol* 1993;34: 513–523.

Davanipour Z, Alter M, Sobel E, Asher DM, Gajdusek DC. A case–control study of Creutzfeldt–Jakob disease. *Am J Epidemiol* 1985b;122:443–451.

Davanipour Z, Alter M, Sobel E, Asher D, Gajdusek DC. Creutzfeldt–Jakob disease: possible medical risk factors. *Neurology* 1985a;35:1483–1486.

Davidson MM, Williams H, Macleod JAJ. Louping ill in man: a forgotten disease. *J Infect* 1991;23: 241–249.

Davidson WL, Hummeler K. B virus infection in man. *Ann NY Acad Sci* 1960;85:970–979.

Davis D, Henslee PJ, Markesbery WR. Fatal adenovirus meningoencephalitis in a bone marrow transplant patient. *Ann Neurol* 1988;23:385–389.

Davis GL, Hawrisiak MM. Experimental cytomegalovirus infection and the developing mouse inner ear: in vivo and in vitro studies. *Otol Rhinol Laryngol* 1977;37:20–29.

Davis GL, Spector GJ, Strauss M, Middlekamp JN. Cytomegalovirus endolabyrinthitis. *Arch Pathol Lab Med* 1977a;101:118–121.

Davis GL, Strauss M. Viral disease of the labyrinth. II. An experimental model using mouse cytomegalovirus. *Otol Rhinol Laryngol* 1973;82:584–594.

Davis LE. Communicating hydrocephalus in newborn hamsters and cats following vaccinia virus infection. *J Neurosurg* 1981;54:767–772.

Davis LE. Influenza B virus model of Reye's syndrome: evidence for a nonpermissive infection of liver and brain. *Lab Invest* 1987;56:32–36.

Davis LE. Reye's syndrome. In: Vinken PJ, Bruyn GW, Klawans HL, eds. Amsterdam: Elsevier Science, 1989a:149–177.

Davis LE. Viruses, vertigo, and deafness. In: McKendall RR, ed. *Handbook of clinical neurology.* Amsterdam: Elsevier Science, 1989b:105–124.

Davis LE, Blisard KS, Kornfeld M. The influenza B virus mouse model of Reye's syndrome: clinical, virologic and morphologic studies of the encephalopathy. *J Neurol Sci* 1990;97:221–231.

Davis LE, Bodian D, Price D, Butler IJ, Vickers JH. Chronic progressive poliomyelitis secondary to vaccination of an immunosuppressed child. *N Engl J Med* 1977b;297:241–245.

Davis LE, Brown JE, Robertson BH, Khanna B, Polish LB. Hepatitis A post-viral encephalitis. *Acta Neurol Scand* 1993;87:67–69.

Davis LE, Harms AC, Chin TDY. Transient cortical blindness and cerebellar ataxia associated with mumps. *Arch Ophthalmol* (a) 1971;85:366–368.

Davis LE, Hjelle BL, Miller VE, et al. Early viral brain invasion in iatrogenic human immunodeficiency virus infection. *Neurology* 1992;42:1736–1739.

Davis LE, Johnson RT. Experimental viral infections of the inner ear. I. Acute infections of the newborn hamster labyrinth. *Lab Invest* 1976;34:349–356.

Davis LE, Johnson RT. An explanation for the localization of herpes simplex encephalitis? *Ann Neurol* 1979;5:2–5.

Davis LE, Johnsson L-G, Kornfeld M. Cytomegalovirus labyrinthitis in an infant: morphological, virological, and immunofluorescent studies. *J Neuropathol Exp Neurol* 1981;40:9–19.

Davis LE, Kornfeld M. Influenza A virus and Reye's syndrome in adults. *J Neurol Neurosurg Psychiatry* 1980;43:516–521.

Davis LE, Shurin S, Johnson RT. Experimental viral labyrinthitis. *Nature* 1975;254:329–331.

Dawson JR Jr. Cellular inclusions in cerebral lesions of lethargic encephalitis. *Am J Pathol* 1933;9:7.

Dawson JR Jr. Cellular inclusions in cerebral lesions of epidemic encephalitis. *Arch Neurol Psychiatry* 1934;31:685–700.

Dawson VL, Dawson TM, Uhl GR, Snyder SH. Human immunodeficiency virus type 1 coat protein neurotoxicity mediated by nitric oxide in primary cortical cultures. *Proc Natl Acad Sci USA* 1993;90:3256–3259.

Day C, Cumming H, Walker J. Enterovirus-specific IgM in the diagnosis of meningitis. *J Infect* 1989;19:219–228.

Dayan AD. Chronic encephalitis in children with severe immunodeficiency. *Acta Neuropathol (Berl)* 1971;19:234–241.

De Clercq E. Antiviral therapy for human immunodeficiency virus infections. *Clin Microbiol Rev* 1995;8:200–239.

De Klippel N, Hautekeete ML, De Keyser J, Ebinger G. Guillain–Barré syndrome as the presenting manifestation of hepatitis C infection. *Neurology* 1993;43:2143.

De La Monte SM, Gabuzda DH, Ho DD, et al. Peripheral neuropathy in the acquired immunodeficiency syndrome. *Ann Neurol* 1988;23:485–492.

De La Monte SM, Ho DD, Schooley RT, Hirsch MS, Richardson EP Jr. Subacute encephalomyelitis of AIDS and its relations to HTLV-III infection. *Neurology* 1987;37:562–569.

De Lorenzo AJD. The olfactory neuron and the blood–brain barrier. In: Wolstenholme GEW, Knight J, eds. *Ciba Foundation symposium on taste and smell in vertebrates.* London: Churchill, 1970:151–176.

de Vries HE, Blom-Roosemalen MCM, van Oosten M, et al. The influence of cytokines on the integrity of the blood–brain barrier in vitro. *J Neuroimmunol* 1996;64:37–43.

Dean DJ, Evans WM, McClure RC. Pathogenesis of rabies. *Bull WHO* 1963;29:803–811.

Dean G. The multiple sclerosis problem. *Sci Am* 1970;223:40–46.

Dean G, Kurtze JF. On the risk of multiple sclerosis according to age at immigration to South Africa. *Brit Med J* 1971;3:725–729.

DeCarli C, Civitello LA, Brouwers P, Pizzo PA. The prevalence of computed tomographic abnormalities of the cerebrum in 100 consecutive children symptomatic with the human immune deficiency virus. *Ann Neurol* 1993;34:198–205.

DeFreitas E, Hilliard B, Cheney PR, et al. Retroviral sequences related to human T-lymphotropic virus type II in patients with chronic fatigue immune dysfunction syndrome. *Proc Natl Acad Sci USA* 1991; 88:2922–2926.

Deibel R, Woodall JP, Decher WJ, Schryver GD. Lymphocytic choriomeningitis virus in man: serological evidence of association with pet hamsters. *JAMA* 1975;232:501–504.

Delsedime M, Mutani R, Giuliani G. Un caso di sindrome tipo sclerosi laterale amiotrofica ad indagine virale positva sul liquor. *Acta Neurol (Napoli)* 1974;29:197–201.

Denning DW, Amos A, Rudge P, Cohen BJ. Neuralgic amyotrophy due to parvovirus infection. *J Neurol Neurosurg Psychiatry* 1987;50:641–642.

Denny-Brown D, Adams RD. Pathologic features of herpes zoster: a note on "geniculate herpes." *Arch Neurol Psychiatry* 1944;51:216–231.

Deresiewicz RL, Thaler SJ, Hsu L, Zamani AA. Clinical and neuroradiographic manifestations of eastern equine encephalitis. *N Engl J Med* 1997;336:1867–1874.

DeSimone PA, Snyder D. Hypoglossal nerve palsy in infectious mononucleosis. *Neurology* 1978;28: 844–847.

Desmond MM, Wilson GS, Melnick JL, et al. Congenital rubella encephalitis. *J Pediatr* 1967;71:311–331.

Desrosiers RC. The simian immunodeficiency viruses. *Annu Rev Immunol* 1990;8:557–578.

Destombes J, Couderc T, Thiesson D, Girard S, Wilt SG, Blondel B. Persistent poliovirus infection in mouse motorneurons. *J Virol* 1997;71:1621–1628.

Detels R, Brody JA, McNew J, Edgar AH. Further epidemiological studies of subacute sclerosing panencephalitis. *Lancet* 1973;2:11–14.

Devinsky O, Cho E-S, Peito CK, Price RW. Herpes zoster myelitis. *Brain* 1991;114:1181–1196.

DeVivo DC, Keating JP. Reye's syndrome. *Adv Pediatr* 1976;22:175–229.

DeVries E. *Postvaccinal perivenous encephalitis.* Amsterdam: Elsevier Science, 1960.

Dhib-Jalbut S, Hoffman PM, Yamabe T, et al. Extracellular human T-cell lymphotropic virus type I tax protein induces cytokine production in adult human microglial cells. *Ann Neurol* 1994;36:787–790.

Di Luca D, Zorzenon M, Mirandola P, Colle R, Batta GA, Cassai E. Human herpesvirus 6 and human herpesvirus 7 in chronic fatigue syndrome. *J Clin Microbiol* 1995;33:1660–1661.

Dick GW, McKeown F, Wilson DC. Virus of acute encephalomyelitis of man and multiple sclerosis. *BMJ* 1958;1:7–9.

Dick GWA, Best AM, Haddow AJ, Smithburn KC. Meningoencephalomyelitis. *Lancet* 1948;2:286–289.

Dickinson AG, Fraser H. Scrapie: pathogenesis in inbred mice: an assessment of host control and response involving many strains of agent. In: Ter Meulen V, Katz M, eds. *Slow virus infections of the central nervous system.* New York: Springer-Verlag, 1977:3–14.

Dickinson AG, Fraser H, Outram GW. Scrapie incubation time can exceed natural lifespan. *Nature* 1975; 256:732–733.

Dietz V, Andrus J, Olivé J-M, Cochi S, de Quadros C. Epidemiology and clinical characteristics of acute flaccid paralysis associated with non-polio enterovirus isolation: the experience in the Americas. *Bull WHO* 1995;73:597–603.

Dietzchold B, Wunner WH, Wiktor TJ, et al. Characterization of an antigenic determinant of the glycoprotein which correlates with pathogenicity. *Proc Natl Acad Sci USA* 1983;80:70.

Dix RD, Waitzman DM, Follansbee S, et al. Herpes simplex virus type 2 encephalitis in two homosexual men with persistent lymphadenopathy. *Ann Neurol* 1985;17:203–206.

Dobler G. Arboviruses causing neurological disorders in the central nervous system. *Arch Virol* 1996;11: 33–40.

Doherty PC, Allan W, Eichelberg M. Roles of αβ and Γσ T cell subsets in viral immunity. *Annu Rev Immunol* 1992;10:123–151.

Dooneief G, Marlink R, Bell K, et al. Neurologic consequences of HTLV-II infection in injection-drug users. *Neurology* 1996;46:1556–1560.

Dorfman LJ. Cytomegalovirus encephalitis in adults. *Neurology* 1973;23:136–144.

Dörries K, Johnson RT, Ter Meulen V. Detection of polyoma virus DNA in PML-brain tissue by in situ hybridization. *J Gen Virol* 1979;42:49–57.

Dörries K, Loeber G, Meixensberger J. Association of polyomaviruses JC, SV40, and BK with human brain tumors. *Virology* 1987;160:268–270.

Douglas JF, Gordon R, Couch RB. A prospective study of chronic herpes simplex virus infections and recurrent herpes labialis in human. *J Immunol* 1970;104:289–295.

Dowling P, Menonna J, Cook S. Cytomegalovirus complement fixation antibody in Guillain–Barré syndrome. *Neurology* 1977;27:1153–1156.

Doyle PW, Gibson G, Dolman CL. Herpes zoster ophthalmicus with contralateral hemiplegia: identification of cause. *Ann Neurol* 1983;14:84–85.

Drachman DA, Adams RD. Herpes simplex and acute inclusion body encephalitis. *Arch Neurol* 1962;7: 61–79.

Drachman DB, Weiner LP, Chase J. Experimental arthrogryposis caused by viral myopathy. *Arch Neurol* 1976;33:362–367.

Dreyer EB, Kaiser PK, Offermann JT, Lipton SA. HIV-1 coat protein neurotoxicity prevented by calcium channel antagonists. *Science* 1990;248:364–367.

Drobyski WR, Knox KK, Majewski D, Carrigan DR. Fatal encephalitis due to variant B human herpesvirus-6 infection in a bone marrow-transplant recipient [Brief report]. *N Engl J Med* 1994;330: 1356–1360.

Dropulic B, Jeang K-T. Gene therapy for human immunodeficiency virus infection: genetic antiviral strategies and targets for intervention. *Hum Gene Ther* 1994;5:927–939.

Dubois V, Lafon M-E, Ragnaud J-M, et al. Detection of JC virus DNA in the peripheral blood leukocytes of HIV-infected patients. *AIDS* 1996;10:353–358.

Dubois-Dalcq M, Barbosa LH, Hamilton R, Sever JL. Comparison between productive and latent subacute sclerosing panencephalitis viral infection in vitro. *Lab Invest* 1974;30:241–250.

Duchowny M, Caplan L, Silber G. Cytomegalovirus infection of the adult nervous system. *Ann Neurol* 1979;5:458–461.

Dudgeon JA. Congenital rubella: pathogenesis and immunology. *Am J Dis Child* 1969;118:35–44.

Dudgeon JW. Virological aspects of Behçet's disease. *Proc R Soc Lond* 1961;54:104–106.

Dueland AN, Devlin M, Martin JR, et al. Fatal varicella–zoster virus meningoradiculitis without skin involvement. *Ann Neurol* 1991;29:569–572.

Duesberg P. HIV is not the cause of AIDS. *Science* 1988;241:514–517.

Duesberg PH. AIDS epidemiology: inconsistencies with human immunodeficiency virus and with infectious disease. *Proc Natl Acad Sci USA* 1991;88:1575–1579.

Duffy J, Lidsky MD, Sharp JT, et al. Polyarthritis, polyarteritis and hepatitis B. *Medicine (Baltimore)* 1976;55:19–37.

Duffy P, Wolf J, Collins G, DeVoe AG, Streeten B, Cowen D. Possible person-to-person transmission of Creutzfeldt–Jakob disease. *N Engl J Med* 1974;290:692.

Duffy PE. Virus induced cerebral sarcoma. *J Neuropathol Exp Neurol* 1970;29:370–391.

Dupont JR, Earle KM. Human rabies encephalitis: a study of forty-nine fatal cases with a review of the literature. *Neurology* 1965;15:1024–1034.

Dykewicz CA, Dato VM, Fisher-Hoch SP, et al. Lymphocytic choriomeningitis outbreak associated with nude mice in a research institute. *JAMA* 1992;267:1349–1353.

Dyson FJ. Unfashionable pursuits. In: Hanle H, ed. *Alexander von Humboldt foundation, bi-national colloquium for Humboldt awardees in cooperation with the Institute for Advanced Study, Princeton, New Jersey, August 23–26, 1981.* Bad Godesberg, Bonn, 1982:29–40.

Earnest MP, Goolishian HA, Calverley JR, Hayes RO, Hill HR. Neurologic, intellectual, and psychologic sequelae following western encephalitis. *Neurology* 1971;21:969–974.

Easton HG. Zoster sine herpete causing acute trigeminal neuralgia. *Lancet* 1970;1:1065–1066.

Ebers GC, Sadovnick AD, Risch NJ. A genetic basis for familial aggregation in multiple sclerosis. *Nature* 1995;377:150–151.

Echevarría JM, Casas I, Tenorio A, de Ory F, Martínez-Martín P. Detection of varicella–zoster virus-specific DNA sequences in cerebrospinal fluid from patients with acute aseptic meningitis and no cutaneous lesions. *J Med Virol* 1994;43:331–335.

Ecker A, Ter Meulen V, Baczko K, Schneider-Schaulies S. Measles virus-specific dsRNAs are targets for unwinding/modifying activity in neural cells in vitro. *J Neurovirol* 1995;1:92–100.

Edelman AS, Zolla-Pazner S. AIDS: a syndrome of immune dysregulation, dysfunction, and deficiency. *FASEB J* 1989;3:22–30.

Edwards JF, Karabatsos N, Collisson EW, De La Concha Bermejillo A. Ovine fetal malformations induced by in utero inoculation with Main Drain, San Angelo, and LaCrosse viruses. *Am J Trop Med Hyg* 1997;56:171–176.

Edwards JF, Livingston CW, Chung SI, Collisson EC. Ovine arthrogryposis and central nervous system malformations associated with in utero Cache Valley virus infection: spontaneous disease. *Vet Pathol* 1989;26:33–39.

Ehrenfeld E, Gebhard JG. Interaction of cellular proteins with the poliovirus 5′ noncoding region. *Arch Virol* 1994;9:269–277.

Ehrenkranz NJ, Ventura AK. Venezuelan equine encephalitis virus infection in man. *Annu Rev Med* 1974; 25:9–14.

Ehrlich GD, Glaser JB, Vryz-Gornia B, et al. Multiple sclerosis, retroviruses, and PCR. *Neurology* 1991; 41:335–343.

Eidelberg D, Sotrel A, Horoupian DS, Neumann PE, Pumarola-Sune T, Price RW. Thrombotic cerebral vasculopathy associated with herpes zoster. *Ann Neurol* 1986;19:7–14.

Eklund CM, Kennedy R, Hadlow WJ. Pathogenesis of scrapie virus infection in the mouse. *J Infect Dis* 1967;117:15–22.

Elfont RM, Griffin DE, Golstein GW. Enhanced endothelial cell adhesion of human cerebrospinal fluid lymphocytes. *Ann Neurol* 1995;38:405–413.

Elizan TS, Ajero-Froehlich L, Fabiyi A, Ley A, Sever JL. Viral infection in pregnancy and congenital CNS malformations in man. *Arch Neurol* 1969;20:115–119.

Ellison PH, Hanson PA. Herpes simplex: a possible cause of brain-stem encephalitis. *Pediatrics* 1977;59: 240–243.

Elsner B, Schwarz E, Mando OG, Maiztegui J, Vilches A. Pathology of 12 fatal cases of Argentine hemorrhagic fever. *Am J Trop Med Hyg* 1973;22:229–236.

Emerson JL, Delez AL. Cerebellar hypoplasia, hypomyelinogenesis and congenital tremors in pigs, associated with prenatal hog cholera vaccination of sows. *J Am Vet Med Assoc* 1967;147:47–54.

Enders G. Varicella–zoster virus infection in pregnancy. *Prog Med Virol* 1984;29:166–196.

Enders G, Miller E, Cradock-Watson J, Bolley I, Ridehalgh M. Consequences of varicella and herpes zoster in pregnancy: prospective study of 1739 cases. *Lancet* 1994;2:1547–1550.

Enders JF, Weller TH, Robbins FC. Cultivation of the Lansing strain of poliomyelitis virus in cultures of various human embryonic tissues. *Science* 1949;109:85–87.

Epstein MA, Achong BG, Barr YM. Virus particle in cultured lymphoblasts from Burkitt's lymphoma. *Lancet* 1964;1:702–703.

Esiri MM, Reading MC, Squier MV, Hughes JT. Immunocytochemical characterization of the macrophage and lymphocyte infiltrate in the brain in six cases of human encephalitis of varied aetiology. *Neuropathol Appl Neurobiol* 1989;15:289–305.

Esmann V, Kroon S, Peterslund NA, et al. Prednisolone does not prevent post-herpetic neuralgia. *Lancet* 1987;2:126–128.

Esolen LM, Takahashi K, Johnson RT, Vaisberg A, Moench TR, Griffin DE. Brain endothelial cell infection in children with acute fatal measles. *J Clin Invest* 1995;96:2478–2481.

Esolen LM, Ward BJ, Moench TR, Griffin DE. Infection of monocytes during measles. *J Infect Dis* 1993; 168:47–52.

Esquilin IO, Hutto C. Mechanisms of HIV transmission and clinical presentation. *Pediatr AIDS* 1995;15: 205–223.

Estes PC, Cheville NF. The ultrastructure of vascular lesions in equine viral arteritis. *Am J Pathol* 1970; 58:235–253.

Estrada R, Mas P, Garlarraga J. Isolation of coxsackie A4 virus in the three cases of acute polyradiculoneuritis of the Landry–Guillain–Barré type. In: *VIIIth International Congress of Neuropathology, Budapest.* Amsterdam: Excerpta Medica, 1975:193–196.

European Collaborative Study. Risk factors for mother-to-child transmission of HIV-1. *Lancet* 1992;1: 1007–1012.

Evans AD, Pallis CA, Spillane JD. Involvement of the nervous system in Behçet's syndrome: report of three cases and isolation of virus. *Lancet* 1957;2:349–353.

Evans AS. Causation and disease: a chronological journey. *Am J Epidemiol* 1978;108:249–257.

Evans CF, Horwitz MS, Hobbs MV, Oldstone MBA. Viral infection of transgenic mice expressing a viral protein in oligodendrocytes leads to chronic central nervous system autoimmune disease. *J Exp Med* 1996;184:2371–2384.

Evans DMA, Dunn G, Minor PD, et al. Increased neurovirulence associated with a single nucleotide change in a noncoding region of the Sabin type 3 poliovaccine genome. *Nature* 1985;314: 548–550.

Everall I, Barnes H, Spargo E, Lantos P. Assessment of neuronal density in the putamen in human immunodeficiency virus (HIV) infection: application of stereology and spatial analysis of quadrants. *J Neurovirol* 1995;1:126–129.

Everberg G. Deafness following mumps. *Acta Otolaryngol (Stockh)* 1957;48:397–403.

Faber DW, Wiley CA, Lynn GB, Gross JG, Freeman WR. Role of HIV and CMV in the pathogenesis of retinitis and retinal vasculopathy in AIDS patients. *Invest Ophthalmol* 1992;33:2345–2353.

Falangola MF, Hanly A, Galvao-Castro B, Petito CK. HIV infection of human choroid plexus: a possible mechanism of viral entry into the CNS. *J Neuropathol Exp Neurol* 1995;54:497–503.

Familusi JB, Osunkoya BO, Moore DL, Kemp GE, Fabiyi A. A fatal human infection with Mokola virus. *Am J Trop Med Hyg* 1972;21:959–963.

Farrell MA, Droogan O, Secor DL, Poukens V, Quinn B, Vinters HV. Chronic encephalitis associated with epilepsy: immunohistochemical and ultrastructural studies. *Acta Neuropathol (Berl)* 1995;89:313–321.

Farrell MK, Partin JC, Bove KE, Jacobs R, Hilton PK. Epidemic influenza myopathy in Cincinnati in 1977. *J Pediatr* 1980;96:545–551.

Farwell JR, Dohrmann GJ, Marrett LD, Meigs JW. Effect of SV40 virus-contaminated polio vaccine on the incidence and type of CNS neoplasms in children: a population based study. *Trans Am Neurol Assoc* 1979;104:261–268.

Fauci AS. Host factors and the pathogenesis of HIV-induced disease. *Nature* 1996;384:529–534.

Fawl RL, Roizman B. The molecular basis of herpes simplex virus pathogenicity. *Semin Virol* 1994;5: 261–271.

Fazakerley JK, Webb HE. Semliki Forest virus induced, immune mediated demyelination: the effect of irradiation. *Br J Exp Pathol* 1987;68:101–113.

Feasby TE, Hahn AF, Gilbert JJ. Passive transfer of demyelinating activity in Guillain–Barré polyneuropathy. *Neurology* 1980;30:363.

Feemster RF. Equine encephalitis in Massachusetts. *N Engl J Med* 1957;257:701–704.

Feinberg WM, Zonis J, Minnich LL. Epstein–Barr virus-associated myelopathy in an adult. *Arch Neurol* 1984;41:454–455.

Fekadu M, Endeshaw T, Alemu W, Bogale Y, Teshager T, Olson JG. Possible human-to-human transmission of rabies in Ethiopia. *Ethiop Med J* 1996;34:123–127.

Feldman W, Larke RPB. Acute cerebellar ataxia associated with the isolation of Coxsackie type A9. *Can Med Assoc J* 1972;106:1104–1107.

Feldmann H, Slenczka W, Klenk H-D. Emerging and reemerging of filoviruses. *Arch Virol* 1996;11:77–100.

Feng Y, Broder CC, Kennedy PE, Berger EA. HIV-1 entry cofactor: functional cDNA cloning of a seven-transmembrane, G protein-coupled receptor. *Science* 1996;272:872–876.

Fenichel GM. Neurological complications of immunization. *Ann Neurol* 1982;12:119–128.

Fenner F. Mouse-pox (infectious ectromelia of mice): a review. *J Immunol* 1949;63:341–373.

Fenner F. Modern trends in animal virology. *Aust J Sci* 1967;30:52–58.

Ferrante MA, Dolan MJ. Q fever meningoencephalitis in a soldier returning from the Persian gulf war. *Clin Infect Dis* 1993;16:489–496.

Field EJ, Cowshall S, Narang HK, Bell TM. Viruses in multiple sclerosis? *Lancet* 1972;2:280–281.

Fields BN. Molecular basis of reovirus virulence. *Arch Virol* 1982;71:95–107.

Fierer J, Bazeley P, Braude AI. Herpes B virus encephalomyelitis presenting as ophthalmic zoster. *Ann Intern Med* 1973;79:225–228.

Figueroa JP, Ashley D, King D, Hull B. An outbreak of acute flaccid paralysis in Jamaica associated with echovirus type 22. *J Med Virol* 1989;29:315–319.

Finkel TH, Török TJ, Ferguson PJ, et al. Chronic parvovirus B19 infection and systemic necrotising vasculitis: opportunistic infection or aetiolgoical agent? *Lancet* 1994;2:1255–1258.

Finley KH, Fitzgerald LH, Richter RW, Riggs N, Shelton JT. Western encephalitis and cerebral ontogenesis. *Arch Neurol* 1967;16:140–164.

Fischer CA, Jones GT. Optic neuritis in dogs. *J Am Vet Assoc* 1972;160:68–79.

Fischl MA, Richman DD, Grieco MH, et al. The efficacy of azidothymidine (AZT) in the treatment of patients with AIDS and AIDS-related complex. *N Engl J Med* 1987;317:185–191.

Fischman HR, Schaeffer M. Pathogenesis of experimental rabies as revealed by immunofluorescence. *Ann NY Acad Sci* 1971;177:78–97.

Fleming JO, Trousdale MD, El-Zaatari FAK, Stohlman SA, Weiner LP. Pathogenicity of antigenic variants of murine coronavirus JHM selected with monoclonal antibodies. *J Virol* 1986;58:869–875.

Flexner S, Lewis PA. Epidemic poliomyelitis in monkeys: a mode of spontaneous infection. *JAMA* 1910; 54:535.

Floeter MK, Civitello LA, Everett CR, Dambrosia J, Luciano CA. Peripheral neuropathy in children with HIV infection. *Neurology* 1997;49:207–212.

Florman AL, Gershon AA, Blackett PR, Nahmias AJ. Intrauterine infection with herpes simplex virus: resultant congenital malformations. *JAMA* 1973;225:129–132.

Folpe A, Lapham LW, Smith HC. Herpes simplex myelitis as a cause of acute necrotizing myelitis syndrome. *Neurology* 1994;44:1955–1957.

Font RL, Jenis EH, Tuck KD. Measles maculopathy associated with subacute sclerosing panencephalitis. *Arch Pathol* 1973;96:168–174.

Forbes SJ, Brumlik J, Harding HB. Acute ascending polyradiculomyelitis associated with ECHO 9 virus. *Dis Nerv Syst* 1967;28:537–540.

Ford WW. The life and work of Robert Koch. *Johns Hopkins Med Bull* 1911;22:1–29.

Foster JD, Fraser H, Bruce ME. Retinopathy in mice with experimental scrapie. *Neuropathol Appl Neurobiol* 1986;12:185–196.

Fox L, Alford M, Achim C, Mallory M, Masliah E. Neurodegeneration of somatostatin-immunoreactive neurons in HIV encephalitis. *J Neuropathol Exp Neurol* 1997;56:360–368.

Fox SA, Finklestone E, Robbins PD, Mastaglia FL, Swanson NR. Search for persistent enterovirus infection of muscle in inflammatory myopathies. *J Neurol Sci* 1994;125:70–76.

Francy DB, Karabatsos N, Wesson DM, et al. A new arbovirus from *Aedes albopictus*, an Asian mosquito established in the United States. *Science* 1990;250:1738–1740.

Frankel SS, Wenig BM, Burke AP, et al. Replication of HIV-1 in dendritic cell-derived syncytia at the mucosal surface of the adenoid. *Science* 1996;272:115–117.

Fredericks DN, Relman DA. Sequence-based identification of microbial pathogens: a reconsideration of Koch's postulates. *Clin Microbiol Rev* 1996;9:18–33.

Frick E, Scheid-Seydel L. Untersuchungen mit J131-markiertem-globulin zur Frage de Abstrammung der Liquorweisskorper. *Klin Wochenschr* 1958;36:857–863.

Friedemann U. Permeability of blood–brain barrier to neurotropic viruses. *Arch Pathol* 1943;35:912–931.

Friedman HM, Gilden DH, Lief FS, Rorke LB, Santoli D, Koprowski H. Hydrocephalus produced by the 6/94 virus. *Arch Neurol* 1975a;32:408–413.

Friedman HM, Gilden DH, Roosa RA, Nathanson N. The effect of neonatal thymectomy on Tamiami virus-induced central nervous system disease. *J Neuropathol Exp Neurol* 1975b;34:159–166.

Frohman EM, van den Noort S, Gupta S. Astrocytes and intracerebral immune responses. *J Clin Immunol* 1989;9:1–9.

Frolova MP, Pogodina VV. Persistence of tick-borne encephalitis virus in monkeys. VI. Pathomorphology of chronic infection in central nervous system. *Acta Virol (Praha)* 1984;28:232–239.

Frumkin LR, Patterson BK, Leverenz JB, et al. Infection of *Macaca nemestrina* brain with human immunodeficiency virus type 1. *J Gen Virol* 1995;76:2467–2476.

Fujinami RS, Oldstone MB. Amino acid homology between the encephalitogenic site of myelin basic protein and virus: mechanism for autoimmunity. *Science* 1985;230:1043–1045.

Fukuda H, Umehara F, Kawahigashi N, Suehara M, Osame M. Acute disseminated myelitis after Japanese B encephalitis vaccination. *J Neurol Sci* 1997;148:113–115.

Fukumoto S, Kinjo M, Hokamura K, Tanaka K. Subarachnoid hemorrhage and granulomatous angiitis of the basilar artery: demonstration of the varicella–zoster virus in the basilar artery lesions. *Stroke* 1986;17:1024–1028.

Fulhorst CF, Hardy JL, Eldridge BF, Presser SB, Reeves WC. Natural vertical transmission of western equine encephalomyelitis virus in mosquitoes. *Science* 1994;263:676–678.

Furuta Y, Takasu T, Fukuda S, et al. Detection of varicella–zoster virus DNA in human geniculate ganglia by polymerase chain reaction. *J Infect Dis* 1992a;166:1157–1159.

Furuta Y, Takasu T, Sato KC, Fukuda S, Inuyama Y, Nagashima K. Latent herpes simplex virus type 1 in human geniculate ganglia. *Acta Neuropathol (Berl)* 1992b;84:39–44.

Furuya T, Nakamura T, Shirabe S, et al. Heightened transmigrating activity of CD4-positive T cells through reconstituted basement membrane in patients with human T-lymphotropic virus type I-associated myelopathy. *Proc Assoc Am Physicians* 1997;109:228–236.

Gabuzda DH, Ho DD, De La Monte SM, Hirsch MS, Rota TR, Sobel RA. Immunohistochemical identification of HTLV-III antigen in brains of patients with AIDS. *Ann Neurol* 1986;20:289–295.

Gadoth N, Weitzman S, Lehmann EE. Acute anterior myelitis complicating West Nile fever. *Arch Neurol* 1979;36:172–173.

Gajdusek DC. Encephalomyocarditis virus infection in childhood [Review article]. *Pediatrics* 1955;16:902–906.

Gajdusek DC. Kuru. *Trans R Soc Trop Med Hyg* 1963;57:151–169.

Gajdusek DC. Slow infections with unconventional viruses. In: *The Harvey lectures.* New York: Academic Press, 1978:283–353.

Gajdusek DC, Gibbs CJ, Alpers M. Experimental transmission of a kuru-like syndrome to chimpanzees. *Nature* 1966;209:794–796.

Gajdusek DC, Gibbs CJ Jr, Rodgers-Johnson P, et al. Infection of chimpanzees by human T-lymphotropic retroviruses in brain and other tissues from AIDS patients. *Lancet* 1985;1:55–56.

Gajdusek DC, Zigas V. Degenerative disease of the central nervous system in New Guinea: the endemic occurrence of "kuru" in the native population. *N Engl J Med* 1957;257:974–978.

Gajdusek DC, Zigas V. Kuru: clinical, pathological and epidemiological study of an acute progressive degenerative disease of the central nervous system among natives of the Eastern Highlands of New Guinea. *Am J Med* 1959;26:442–469.

Galbraith DN, Nairn C, Clements GB. Phylogenetic analysis of short enteroviral sequences from patients with chronic fatigue syndrome. *J Gen Virol* 1995;76:1701–1707.

Gallo RC, Salahuddin SZ, Popovic M, et al. Frequent detection and isolation of cytopathic retroviruses (HTLV-III) from patients with AIDS and at risk for AIDS. *Science* 1984;224:500–504.

Gamboa ET, Eastwood AB, Hays AP, Maxwell J, Penn AS. Isolation of influenza virus from muscle in myoglobinuric polyositis. *Neurology* 1979;29:1323–1335.

Gamboa ET, Wolf A, Yahr MD, et al. Influenza virus antigen in post-encephalitic parkinsonism brain detected by immunofluorescence. *Arch Neurol* 1974;31:228–232.

Gao S-J, Moore PS. Molecular approaches to the identification of unculturable infectious agents. *Emer Infect Dis* 1996;2:159–166.

Gardash'yan AM, Khondkarian OA, Bunina TL, Popova LM, Katkin SG. Experimental data on the study of the etiology of amyotrophic lateral sclerosis. *Vestn Acad Med Sci* 1970;9:80–83.

Gardiner AC, Zakarian B, Barlow RM. Periarteritis in experimental border disease of sheep. III. Immunopathological observations. *J Comp Pathol* 1980;90:469–474.

Gardner SD. Prevalence in England of antibody to human polyomavirus (BK). *BMJ* 1973;1:77–78.

Gardner SD, Field AM, Coleman DV, Hulme B. New human papovavirus (BK) isolated from urine after renal transplantation. *Lancet* 1971;1:1253–1257.

Garruto RM, Yanagihara R. Amyotrophic lateral sclerosis in the Mariana Islands. In: de Jong JMBV, ed. *Handbook of clinical neurology.* New York: Elsevier Science, 1991:253–271.

Gascon G, Yamani S, Crowell J, et al. Combined oral isoprinosine–intraventricular α-interferon therapy for subacute sclerosing panencephalitis. *Brain Dev* 1993;15:346–355.

Gateley A, Gander RM, Johnson PC, Kit S, Otsuka H, Kohl S. Herpes simplex virus type 2 meningoencephalitis resistant to acyclovir in a patient with AIDS. *J Infect Dis* 1990;161:711–715.

Gaulton GN, Sharpe AH, Chang DW, Fields BN, Greene MI. Syngeneic monoclonal internal image anti-idiotopes as prophylactic vaccines. *J Immunol* 1986;137:2930–2936.

Gautier-Smith PC. Neurological complications of glandular fever (infectious mononucleosis). *Brain* 1965;88:323–334.

Gay CL, Armstrong FD, Cohen D, et al. The effects of HIV on cognitive and motor development in children born to HIV-seropositive women with no reported drug use: birth to 24 months. *Pediatrics* 1995; 96:1078–1082.

Geddes JF, Bhattacharjee MB, Savage K, Scaravilli F, McLaughlin JE. Primary cerebral lymphoma: a study of 47 cases probed for Epstein–Barr virus genome. *J Clin Pathol* 1992;45:587–590.

Geissler E. SV40 and human brain tumors. *Prog Med Virol* 1990;37:211–222.

Gelbard HA, James HJ, Sharer LR, et al. Apoptotic neurons in brains from paediatric patients with HIV-1 encephalitis and progressive encephalopathy. *Neuropathol Appl Neurobiol* 1995;21:208–217.

Gelbard HA, Nottet HSLM, Swindells S, et al. Platelet-activating factor: a candidate human immunodeficiency virus type 1-induced neurotoxin. *J Virol* 1994;68:4628–4635.

Gendelman HE, Narayan O, Kennedy-Stoskopf S, et al. Tropism of sheep lentiviruses for monocytes: susceptibility to infection and virus gene expression increase during maturation of monocytes to macrophages. *J Virol* 1986;58:67–74.

Gendelman HE, Narayan O, Molineaux S, Clements JE, Ghotbi Z. Slow, persistent replication of lentiviruses: role of tissue macrophages and macrophage precursors in bone marrow. *Proc Natl Acad Sci USA* 1985a;82:7086–7090.

Gendelman HE, Pezeshkpour GH, Pressman NJ, et al. A quantitation of myelin-associated glycoprotein and myelin basic protein loss in different demyelinating diseases. *Ann Neurol* 1985b;18: 324–328.

Gendelman HE, Wolsinky JS, Johnson RT, Pressman NJ, Pezeshkpour GH, Boisset GF. Measles encephalomyelitis: lack of evidence of viral invasion of the central nervous system and quantitative study of the nature of demyelination. *Ann Neurol* 1984;15:353–360.

Geny C, Gherard R, Boudes P, Lionnet F, Cesaro P, Gray F. Multifocal multinucleated giant cell myelitis in an AIDS patient. *Neuropathol Appl Neurobiol* 1991a;17:157–162.

Geny C, Yulis J, Azoulay A, Brugieres P, Saint-Val C, Degos JD. Thalamic infarction following lingual herpes zoster. *Neurology* 1991b;41:1846.

Georgsson G, Martin JR, Klein J, Pálsson PA, Nathanson N, Pétursson G. Primary demyelination in visna: an ultrastructural study of Icelandic sheep with clinical signs following experimental infection. *Acta Neuropathol (Berl)* 1982;57:171–178.

Gerhard W, Iwasaki Y, Koprowski H. The central nervous system-associated immune response to parainfluenza type I virus in mice. *J Immunol* 1978;120:1256–1260.

Gerhard W, Koprowski H. Persistence of virus-specific memory B cells in mice CNS. *Nature* 1977;266: 360–361.

Gessain A, Barin F, Vernant JC, et al. Antibodies to human T-lymphotropic virus type I in patients with tropical spastic paraparesis. *Lancet* 1985;2:407–409.

Gessain A, Gout O. Chronic myelopathy associated with human T-lymphotropic virus type I (HTLV-I). *Ann Intern Med* 1992;117:933–946.

Ghatak NR, Zimmerman HM. Spinal ganglion in herpes zoster. *Arch Pathol* 1973;95:411–415.

Ghetti B, Tagliavini F, Masters CL, et al. Gerstmann–Sträussler–Scheinker disease. II. Neurofibrillary tangles and plaques with PrP-amyloid coexist in an affected family. *Neurology* 1989;39:1453–1461.

Gibbs AJ, Harrison BD, Watson DH, Wildy P. What's in a virus name? *Nature* 1966;209:450–454.

Gibbs CJ Jr, Asher DM, Brown PW, Fradkin JE, Gajdusek DC. Creutzfeldt–Jakob disease infectivity of growth hormone derived from human pituitary glands. *N Engl J Med* 1993;328:358–359.

Gibbs CJ Jr, Gajdusek DC. Amyotrophic lateral sclerosis, Parkinson's disease, and the amyotrophic lateral sclerosis–parkinsonism–dementia complex on Guam: a review and summary on attempts to demonstrate infection as the etiology. *J Clin Pathol* 1972;25[Suppl]:S132–S140.

Gibbs CJ Jr, Gajdusek DC, Asher DM, et al. Creutzfeldt–Jakob disease (spongiform encephalopathy): transmission to the chimpanzee. *Science* 1968;161:388–389.

Gibbs FA, Gibbs EL, Carpenter PR, Spies HW. Electroencephalographic abnormality in "uncomplicated" childhood diseases. *JAMA* 1959;171:1050–1055.

Gibbs FA, Gibbs EL, Rosenthal IM. Electroencephalographic study of children immunized against measles with live attenuated virus vaccine. *N Engl J Med* 1961;264:800–801.

Giese A, Groschup MH, Hess B, Kretzschmar HA. Neuronal cell death in scrapie-infected mice is due to apoptosis. *Brain Pathol* 1995;5:213–221.

Gilden DH, Beinlich BR, Rubinstien EM, et al. Varicella–zoster virus myelitis: an expanding spectrum. *Neurology* 1995;1994:1818–1823.

Gilden DH, Dueland AN, Cohrs R, Martin JR, Kleinschmidt-DeMasters BK, Mahalingam R. Preherpetic neuralgia. *Neurology* 1991;41:1215–1218.

Gilden DH, Kleinschmidt-DeMasters BK, Wellish M, Hedley-Whyte ET, Rentier B, Mahalingam R. Varicella zoster virus, a cause of waxing and waning vasculitis: the *N Engl J Med* case 5-1995 revisited. *Neurology* 1996;47:1441–1446.

Gilden DH, Murray RS, Wellish M, Kleinschmidt-DeMasters BK, Vafai A. Chronic progressive varicella–zoster virus encephalitis in an AIDS patient. *Neurology* 1988;38:1150–1153.

Gilden DH, Rozenman Y, Murray R, Devlin M, Vafai A. Detection of varicella–zoster virus nucleic acid in neurons of normal human thoracic ganglia. *Ann Neurol* 1987;22:377–380.

Gilden DH, Wright RR, Schneck SA, Gwaltney JM Jr, Mahalingam R. Zoster sine herpete, a clinical variant. *Ann Neurol* 1994;35:530–533.

Giulian D, Vaca K, Noonan CA. Secretion of neurotoxins by mononuclear phagocytes infected with HIV-1. *Science* 1990;250:1593–1596.

Glasgow JFT, Moore R. Reye's syndrome 30 years on. *BMJ* 1993;307:950–951.

Glass JD, Fedor H, Wesselingh SL, McArthur JC. Immunocytochemical quantitation of human immunodeficiency virus in the brain: correlations with dementia. *Ann Neurol* 1995;38:755–762.

Glass JD, Johnson RT. Human immunodeficiency virus and the brain. *Annu Rev Neurosci* 1996;19:1–26.

Glass JD, Wesselingh SL, Selnes OA, McArthur JC. Clinical–neuropathologic correlation in HIV-associated dementia. *Neurology* 1993;43:2230–2237.

Glasse R. Cannibalism in the kuru region of New Guinea. *Trans NY Acad Sci* 1967;29:748–754.

Gledhill AW, Bilbey DLJ, Niven JSF. Effect of certain murine pathogens on phagocytic activity. *Br J Exp Pathol* 1965;46:433–442.

Gocke DJ, Morgan C, Lockshin M, Hsu K, Bombardieri S, Christian CL. Association between polyarteritis and Australia antigen. *Lancet* 1970;2:1149–1153.

Godec MS, Asher DM, Kozachuk WE, et al. Blood buffy coat from Alzheimer's disease patients and their relatives does not transmit spongiform encephalopathy to hamsters. *Neurology* 1994;44:1111–1115.

Godec MS, Asher DM, Murray RS, et al. Absence of measles, mumps, and rubella viral genomic sequences from multiple sclerosis brain tissue by polymerase chain reaction. *Ann Neurol* 1992;32: 401–404.

Goedert JJ, Duliege AM, Amos CI, Felton S, Biggar RJ. High risk of HIV-1 infection for first-born twins: the international registry of HIV-exposed twins. *Lancet* 1991;2:1471–1475.

Gold R, Schmied M, Giegerich G, et al. Differentiation between cellular apoptosis and necrosis by the combined use of in situ tailing and nick translation techniques. *Lab Invest* 1994;71:219–225.

Golden MP, Hammer SM, Wanke CA, Albrecht MA. Cytomegalovirus vasculitis: case reports and review of the literature. *Medicine (Baltimore)* 1994;73:246–255.

Goldfarb LG, Brown P, McCombie WR, et al. Transmissible familial Creutzfeldt–Jakob disease associated with five, seven, and eight extra octapeptide coding repeats in the PRNP gene. *Proc Natl Acad Sci USA* 1991a;88:10,926–10,930.

Goldfarb LG, Brown P, Mitrová E, et al. Creutzfeldt–Jacob disease associated with the PRNP codon 200^{LYS} mutation: an analysis of 45 families. *Eur J Epidemiol* 1991b;7:477–486.

Goldfarb LG, Gajdusek DC. Viliuisk encephalomyelitis in the Iakut people of Siberia. *Brain* 1992;115: 961–978.

Goldfarb LG, Petersen RB, Tabaton M, et al. Fatal familial insomnia and familial Creutzfeldt–Jakob disease: disease phenotype determined by a DNA polymorphism. *Science* 1992;258:806–808.

Gollomp SM, Fahn S. Transient dystonia as a complication of varicella. *J Neurol Neurosurg Psychiatry* 1987;50:1228–1229.

Gómez-Tortosa E, Gadea I, Gegúndez MI, et al. Development of myelopathy before herpes zoster rash in a patient with AIDS. *Clin Infect Dis* 1994;18:810–812.

Gonda MA, Braun MJ, Carter SG, et al. Characterization and molecular cloning of a bovine lentivirus related to human immunodeficiency virus. *Nature* 1987;330:388–391.

Gonda MA, Wong-Staal F, Gallo RC, Clements JE, Narayan O, Gilden RV. Sequence homology and morphologic similarity of HTLV-III and visna virus, a pathogenic lentivirus. *Science* 1985;227:173–177.

Goodman GT, Koprowski H. Study of the mechanism of innate resistance to virus infection. *J Cell Comp Physiol* 1962;59:333–373.

Goodpasture EW, Teague O. Transmission of the virus of herpes febrilis among nerves in experimentally infected rabbits. *J Med Res* 1923;44:139–174.

Goodpasture EW, Woodruff AM, Buddingh GJ. The cultivation of vaccine and other viruses in the chorioallantoic membrane of chick embryos. *Science* 1931;74:371–372.

Goodpasture HC, Poland JD, Francy DB, Bowen GS, Horn KA. Colorado tick fever: clinical, epidemiologic and laboratory aspects of 228 cases in Colorado in 1973–1974. *Ann Intern Med* 1978;88: 303–310.

Gordon B, Selnes OA, Hart J Jr, Hanley DF, Whitley RJ. Long-term cognitive sequelae of acyclovir-treated herpes simplex encephalitis. *Arch Neurol* 1990;47:646–647.

Gordon L, McQuaid S, Cosby SL. Detection of herpes simplex virus (types 1 and 2) and human herpesvirus 6 DNA in human brain tissue by polymerase chain reaction. *Clin Diagn Virol* 1996;6:33–40.

Gorman RJ, Saxon S, Snead OC. Neurologic sequelae of Rocky Mountain spotted fever. *Pediatrics* 1981; 67:354–357.

Goswami KK, Miller RF, Harrison MJ, Hamel DJ, Daniels RS, Tedder RS. Expression of HIV-1 in the cerebrospinal fluid detected by the polymerase chain reaction and its correlation with central nervous system disease. *AIDS* 1991;5:797–803.

Goswami KKA, Randall RE, Lange LS, Russell WC. Antibodies against the paramyxovirus SV5 in the cerebrospinal fluids of some multiple sclerosis patients. *Nature* 1987;327:244–247.

Gosztonyi G, Ludwig H. Borna disease: neuropathology and pathogenesis. In: Koprowski H, Lipkin WI, eds. *Current topics in microbiology and immunology.* Berlin: Springer-Verlag, 1995:39–73.

Goudreau G, Carpenter S, Beaulieu N, Jolicoeur P. Vacuolar myelopathy in transgenic mice expressing human immunodeficiency virus type 1 proteins under the regulation of the myelin basic protein gene promoter. *Nature Med* 1996;2:655–661.

Goudsmit J, Morrow CH, Asher DM, et al. Evidence for and against the transmissibility of Alzheimer disease. *Neurology* 1980;30:945–950.

Gout O, Gessain A, Iba-Zizen M, et al. The effect of zidovudine on chronic myelopathy associated with HTLV-1. *J Neurol* 1991;238:108–110.

Gow JW, Behan WMH, Clements GB, Woodall C, Riding M, Behan PO. Enteroviral RNA sequences detected by polymerase chain reaction in muscle of patients with postviral fatigue syndrome. *BMJ* 1991;302:692–696.

Gow JW, Behan WMH, Simpson K, McGarry F, Keir S, Behan PO. Studies on enterovirus in patients with chronic fatigue syndrome. *Clin Infect Dis* 1994;18[Suppl]:S126–S129.

Gow JW, Simpson K, Schleiphake A, et al. Search for retrovirus in the chronic fatigue syndrome. *J Clin Pathol* 1992;45:1058–1061.

Graman PS. Mollaret's meningitis associated with acute Epstein–Barr virus mononucleosis. *Arch Neurol* 1987;44:1204–1205.

Grau JM, Masanés F, Pedrol E, Casademont J, Fernández-Solá J, Urbano-Márquez A. Human immunodeficiency virus type 1 infection and myopathy: clinical relevance of zidovudine therapy. *Ann Neurol* 1993;34:206–211.

Gravel C, Kay DG, Jolicoeur P. Identification of the infected target cell type in spongiform myeloencephalopathy induced by the neurotropic Cas-Br-E murine leukemia virus. *J Virol* 1993;67:6648–6658.

Graves M, Griffin DE, Johnson RT, et al. Development of antibody to measles virus polypeptides during complicated and uncomplicated measles virus infections. *J Virol* 1984;49:409–412.

Gray F, Bélac L, Keohane C, et al. Zidovudine therapy and HIV encephalitis: a 10-year neuropathological survey. *AIDS* 1994a;8:489–493.

Gray F, Bélec L, Lescs MC, et al. Varicella–zoster virus infection of the central nervous system in the acquired immune deficiency system. *Brain* 1994b;117:987–999.

Gray F, Scaravilli F, Everall I, et al. Neuropathology of early HIV-1 infection. *Brain Pathol* 1996;6:1–15.

Green SH, Wirtschafter JD. Ophthalmoscopic findings in subacute sclerosing panencephalitis. *Br J Ophthalmol* 1973;57:780–787.

Greenberg SJ, Jacobson S, Waldmann TA, McFarlin DE. Molecular analysis of HTLV-I proviral integration and T cell receptor arrangement indicates that T cells in tropical spastic paraparesis are polyclonal. *J Infect Dis* 1989;159:741–744.

Greenfield JG. Encephalitis and encephalomyelitis in England and Wales during the last decade. *Brain* 1950;73:141–166.

Greenlee JE, Becker LE, Narayan O, Johnson RT. Failure to demonstrate papovavirus tumor antigen in human cerebral neoplasms. *Ann Neurol* 1978;3:479–481.

Greenlee JE, Narayan O, Johnson RT, Herndon RM. Induction of brain tumors in hamsters with BK virus, a human papovavirus. *Lab Invest* 1977;36:636–641.

Greenstein JI, McFarland HF, Mingioli ES, McFarlin DE. The lymphoproliferative response to measles virus in twins with multiple sclerosis. *Ann Neurol* 1984;15:79–87.

Gregg NM. Congenital cataract following German measles in mother. *Trans Ophthalmol Soc Aust* 1941;3:35–46.

Gresser I, Lang DJ. Relationships between viruses and leucocytes. *Prog Med Virol* 1966;8:62–130.

Griffin DE. Immunoglobulins in the cerebrospinal fluid: changes during acute viral encephalitis in mice. *J Immunol* 1981;126:27–31.

Griffin DE, Cooper SJ, Hirsch RL, et al. Changes in plasma IgE levels during complicated and uncomplicated measles virus infections. *J Allergy Clin Immunol* 1985;76:206–213.

Griffin DE, Giffels J. Study of protein characteristics that influence entry into the cerebrospinal fluid of normal mice and mice with encephalitis. *J Clin Invest* 1982;70:289–295.

Griffin DE, Hemachudha T, Johnson RT. Postinfectious and postvaccinal encephalomyelitis. In: Gilden DH, Lipton HL, eds. *Clinical and molecular aspects of neurotropic virus infection.* Boston: Kluwer Academic Publishers, 1989a:501–527.

Griffin DE, Hess JL. Cells with natural killer activity in the cerebrospinal fluid of normal mice and athymic nude mice with acute Sindbis virus encephalitis. *J Immunol* 1986;136:1841–1845.

Griffin DE, Hirsch RL, Johnson RT, de Soriano IL, Roedenbeck S, Vaisberg A. Changes in serum C-reactive protein during complicated and uncomplicated measles virus infections. *Infect Immun* 1983;41:861–864.

Griffin DE, Johnson RT. Cellular immune response to viral infection: in vitro studies of lymphocytes from mice infected with Sindbis virus. *Cell Immunol* 1973;9:426–434.

Griffin DE, Levine B, Tyor WR, Irani DN. The immune response in viral encephalitis. *Semin Immunol* 1992a;4:111–119.

Griffin DE, Moench TR, Johnson RT, de Soriano IL, Vaisberg A. Peripheral blood mononuclear cells during natural measles virus infection: cell surface phenotypes and evidence for activation. *Clin Immunol Immunopathol* 1986;40:305–312.

Griffin DE, Mullinix J, Narayan O, Johnson RT. Age-dependence of viral expression: comparative pathogenesis of two rodent-adapted strains of measles virus in mice. *Infect Immun* 1974;9:690–695.

Griffin DE, Narayan O, Adams RJ. Early immune responses in visna, a slow viral disease of sheep. *J Infect Dis* 1978a;138:340–350.

Griffin DE, Narayan O, Bukowski J, Adams RJ, Cohen SR. The cerebrospinal fluid in visna, a slow viral disease of sheep. *Ann Neurol* 1978b;4:212–218.

Griffin DE, Ward BJ, Esolen LM. Pathogenesis of measles virus infection: an hypothesis for altered immune responses. *J Infect Dis* 1994a;170[Suppl]:S24–S31.

Griffin DE, Ward BJ, Jauregui E, Johnson RT, Vaisberg A. Immune activation during measles. *N Engl J Med* 1989b;320:1667–1672

Griffin DE, Wesselingh SL, McArthur JC. Elevated central nervous system prostaglandins in human immunodeficiency virus-associated dementia. *Ann Neurol* 1994b;35:592–597.

Griffin JW, Li CY, Ho TW, et al. Guillain–Barré syndrome in northern China: the spectrum of neuropathological changes in clinically defined cases. *Brain* 1995;118:577–595.

Griffin JW, Watson DF. Axonal transport in neurological disease. *Ann Neurol* 1988;23:3–13.

Griffith JF, Salam MV, Adams RD. The nervous system diseases associated with varicella. *Acta Neurol Scand* 1970;46:279–300.

Grimaldi LME, Murthy KK, Martino G, Furlan R, Franciotta D, Eichberg JW. An immunovirological study of central nervous system involvement during HIV-1 infection of chimpanzees. *J AIDS* 1996; 13:12–17.

Grimstad PR, Ross QE, Craig GB Jr. *Aedes triseriatus* (Diptera: Culicidae) and La Crosse virus. II. Modification of mosquito feeding behavior by virus infection. *J Med Entomol* 1980;17:1–7.

Grimstad PR, Shabino CL, Calisher CH, Waldman RJ. A case of encephalitis in a human associated with a serologic rise to Jamestown Canyon virus. *Am J Trop Med Hyg* 1982;31:1238–1244.

Grinschgl G. Virus meningo-encephalitis in Austria. 2. Clinical features, pathology and diagnosis. *Bull WHO* 1955;12:535–564.

Grist NR, Bell EJ, Assaad F. Enteroviruses in human disease. *Prog Med Virol* 1978;24:114–157.

Gronning M, Riise T, Kvale G, Albrektsen G, Midgard R, Nyland H. Infections in childhood and adolescence in multiple sclerosis. *Neuroepidemiology* 1993;12:61–69.

Grose C, Henle W, Henle G, Feorino PM. Primary Epstein–Barr virus infection in acute neurologic diseases. *N Engl J Med* 1975;292:392–395.

Gsell OR. Leptospiroses and relapsing fever. In: Vinken PJ, Bruyn GW, eds. *Handbook of clinical neurology.* Amsterdam: Elsevier/North-Holland, 1978:395–419.

Gudnadottir M, Helgadottir H, Bjarnason O, Jonsdottir K. Virus isolated from the brain of a patient with multiple sclerosis. *Exp Neurol* 1964;9:85–95.

Guess HA, Broughton DD, Melton LJ III, Kurland LT. Population-based studies of varicella complications. *Pediatrics* 1986;78:723–727.

Guillain G, Barré JA, Strohl A. Sur un syndrome de radiculo-neurite avec hyperalbuminae due liquide cephalomachidien sans reaction cellulaire: remarques sur les caracteres cliniques et graphiques des reflexes tendeneux. *Bull Soc Med Hop Paris* 1916;40:1462.

Gullotta F, Masini T, Scarlato G, Kuchelmesiter K. Progressive multifocal leukoencephalopathy and gliomas in a HIV-negative patient. *Pathol Res Pract* 1992;188:964–972.

Günther G, Haglund M, Lindquist L, Forsgren M, Sköldenberg B. Tick-borne encephalitis in Sweden in relation to aseptic meningo-encephalitis of other etiology: a prospective study of clinical course and outcome. *J Neurol* 1997;244:230–238.

Gurvich EG, Mouseyants AA, Stepanenkova LP. Isolation of vaccinia virus from children with post-vaccinial encephalitis at late intervals after vaccination. *Acta Virol (Praha)* 1975;19:92.

Gutmann DH. Tumor suppressor genes as negative growth regulators in development and differentiation. *Int J Dev Biol* 1995;39:895–907.

Haahr S, Koch-Henriksen N, Moller-Larsen A, Eriksen LS, Andersen HMK. Increased risk of multiple sclerosis after late Epstein–Barr virus infection: a historical prospective study. *Mult Scler* 1995;1: 73–77.

Haahr S, Sommerlund M, Møller-Larsen A, Nielsen R, Hansen HJ. Just another dubious virus in cells from a patient with multiple sclerosis? *Lancet* 1991;2:863–864.

Haase AT. The slow infection caused by visna virus. *Curr Top Microbiol Immunol* 1975;72:101–156.

Haase AT, Ventura P, Gibbs CJ Jr, Tourtellotte WW. Measles virus nucleotide sequences: detection by hybridization in situ. *Science* 1981;212:672–675.

Hackett J Jr, Swanson P, Leahy D, et al. Search for retrovirus in patients with multiple sclerosis. *Ann Neurol* 1996;40:805–809.

Hadlow WJ. Scrapie and kuru. *Lancet* 1959;2:289–290.

Hadlow WJ, Race RE, Kennedy C, Eklund CM. Natural infection of sheep with scrapie virus. In: Prusiner SB, Hadlow WJ, eds. *Slow transmissible diseases of the nervous system,* 2nd ed. New York: Academic Press, 1979:3–12.

Hafer-Macko C, Hsieh S-T, Li CY, et al. Acute motor axonal neuropathy: an antibody-mediated attack on axolemma. *Ann Neurol* 1996a;40:635–644.

Hafer-Macko CE, Sheikh KA, Li CY, et al. Immune attack on the Schwann cell surface in acute inflammatory demyelinating polyneuropathy. *Ann Neurol* 1996b;39:625–635.

Hahn CS, Lustig S, Strauss EG, Strauss JH. Western equine encephalitis virus is a recombinant virus. *Proc Natl Acad Sci USA* 1988;85:5997–6001.

Hainfellner JA, Brantner-Inthaler S, Cervenáková L, et al. The original Gerstmann–Sträussler–Scheinker family of Austria: divergent clinicopathological phenotypes but constant PrP genotype. *Brain Pathol* 1995;5:201–211.

Hainfellner JA, Jellinger K, Budka H. Testing for prion protein does not confirm previously reported conjugal CJD. *Lancet* 1996;2:616–617.

Hainfellner JA, Liberski PP, Guiroy DC, et al. Pathology and immunocytochemistry of a kuru brain. *Brain Pathol* 1997;7:547–553.

Hakosalo J, Saxen L. Influenza epidemic and congenital defects. *Lancet* 1971;2:1346–1347.

Hall CB, Horner FA. Encephalopathy with erythema infectiousum. *Am J Dis Child* 1977;131:65–67.

Hall CB, Long CE, Schnabel KC, et al. Human herpesvirus-6 infection in children: a prospective study of complications and reactivation. *N Engl J Med* 1994;331:432–438.

Hall M, Whaley R, Robertson K, Hamby S, Wilkins J, Hall C. The correlation between neuropsychological and neuroanatomic changes over time in asymptomatic and symptomatic HIV-1-infected individuals. *Neurology* 1996;46:1697–1702.

Hall S, Carlin L, Roach ES, McLean WT Jr. Herpes zoster and central retinal artery occlusion. *Ann Neurol* 1983;13:217–218.

Haltia M, Paetau A, Vaheri A, et al. Fatal measles encephalopathy with retinopathy during cytotoxic chemotherapy. *J Neurol Sci* 1977;9:89–108.

Hamashima Y, Kyogoku M, Hiramatusu S, Nakashima Y, Yamaucki R. Immuno-cytological studies employing labelled active protein. III. Encephalitis Japonica. *Acta Pathol Jpn* 1959;9:89–108.

Hamburger V, Habel K. Teratogenetic and lethal effects of influenza-A and mumps viruses on early chick embryos. *Proc Soc Exp Biol Med* 1947;66:608–617.

Hamilton R. An account of a distemper by the common people of England vulgarly called the mumps. *Trans R Soc Edinb* 1790;2:59–72.

Hanissian AA, Jabbour JT, de Lamerens S, Garcia JH, Horta-Barbosa L. Subacute encephalitis and hypogammaglobulinemia. *Am J Dis Child* 1972;123:151–155.

Hankey GJ, Bucens MR, Chambers JSW. Herpes simplex encephalitis in third trimester of pregnancy: successful outcome for mother and child. *Neurology* 1987;37:1534–1537.

Hanley DF, Johnson RT, Whitley RJ. Yes, brain biopsy should be a prerequisite for herpes simplex encephalitis treatment. *Arch Neurol* 1987;44:1289–1290.

Hanninen P, Arstila P, Lang H, Salmi A, Panelius M. Involvement of the central nervous system in acute, uncomplicated measles virus infection. *J Clin Microbiol* 1980;11:610–613.

Hanshaw JB. Congenital cytomegalovirus infection: a fifteen year perspective. *J Infect Dis* 1971;123: 555–561.

Hanshaw JB, Scheiner AP, Moxley AW, Gaev L, Abel V, Scheiner B. School failure and deafness after "silent" congenital cytomegalovirus infection. *N Engl J Med* 1976;295:468–470.

Hanshaw JB, Scheiner AP, Moxley AW, Gaev L, Abel V. CNS sequelae of congenital cytomegalovirus infection. In: Krugman S, Gershon AA, eds. *Infections of the fetus and newborn infant.* New York: Alan R Liss, 1975:47–54.

Harden VA. Koch's postulates and the etiology of AIDS: an historical perspective. *Hist Philos Life Sci* 1992;14:249–269.

Harding B, Baumer JA. Congenital varicella–zoster. *Acta Neuropathol (Berl)* 1988;76:311–315.

Harding SP, Lipton JR, Wells JCD. Natural history of herpes zoster ophthalmicus: predictors of postherpetic neuralgia and ocular involvement. *Br J Ophthalmol* 1987;71:353–358.

Hardy JB. Clinical and developmental aspects of congenital rubella. *Arch Otolaryngol* 1973a;98:230–236.

Hardy JB. Fetal consequences of maternal viral infections in pregnancy. *Arch Otolaryngol* 1973b;98: 218–227.

Hardy JB, McCracken GH Jr, Gilkeson MR, Sever JL. Adverse fetal outcome following maternal rubella after the first trimester of pregnancy. *JAMA* 1969;207:2141–2142.

Hardy JL. The ecology of western equine encephalomyelitis virus in the central valley of California, 1945–1985. *Am J Trop Med Hyg* 1987;37[Suppl]:18S–32S.

Harjulehto-Mervaala T, Aro T, Hiilesmaa VK, Saxén H, Hovi T, Saxén L. Oral polio vaccination during pregnancy: no increase in the occurrence of congenital malformations. *Am J Epidemiol* 1993;138: 407–414.

Harries-Jones R, Knight R, Will RG, Cousens S, Smith PG, Matthews WB. Creutzfeldt–Jakob disease in England and Wales, 1980–1984: a case–control study of potential risk factors. *J Neurol Neurosurg Psychiatry* 1988;51:1113–1119.

Harrington WJ Jr, Sheremata W, Hjelle B, et al. Spastic ataxia associated with human T-cell lymphotropic virus type II infection. *Ann Neurol* 1993;33:411–414.

Harrison MJG, McArthur JC. *The neurology of AIDS.* Edinburgh: Churchill Livingstone, 1994.

Hart MN, Earle KM. Hemorrhagic and perivenous encephalitis: a clinical–pathological review of 38 cases. *J Neurol Neurosurg Psychiatry* 1975;38:585–591.

Harter DH, Choppin PW. Possible mechanisms in the pathogenesis of "post-infectious" encephalo myelitis. *Res Publ Assoc Nerv Ment Dis* 1971;49:343–355.

Hartley JW, Rowe WP. Naturally occurring murine leukemia viruses in wild mice: characterization of a new "amphotropic" class. *J Virol* 1976;19:19–25.

Hashimoto I, Hagiwara A. Studies on the pathogenesis of and propagation of enterovirus 71 in poliomyelitis-like disease in monkeys. *Acta Neuropathol (Berl)* 1982;58:125–132.

Hattwick MA, Weiss TT, Stechschulte J, Baer GM, Gregg MB. Recovery from rabies: a case report. *Ann Intern Med* 1972;76:931–942.

Hattwick MAW, Sayetta RB. Time trends of Reye's syndrome based on national statistics. In: Crocker JFS, ed. *Reye's syndrome.* New York: Grune & Stratton, 1979:13–32.

Hawkins SA, Lyttle JA, Connolly JH. Two cases of influenza B encephalitis. *J Neurol Neurosurg Psychiatry* 1987;50:1236–1237.

Hayashi K, Iwasaki Y, Yanagi K. Herpes simplex virus type 1-induced hydrocephalus in mice. *J Virol* 1986;57:942–951.

Hayes K, Gibas H. Placental cytomegalovirus infection without fetal involvement following primary infection in pregnancy. *J Pediatr* 1978;62:965–969.

Haynes BF, Pantaleo G, Fauci AS. Toward an understanding of the correlates of protective immunity to HIV infection. *Science* 1996;271:324–328.

He JL, Chen YZ, Farzan M, et al. CCR3 and CCR5 are co-receptors for HIV-1 infection of microglia. *Nature* 1997;385:645–649.

Head H, Campbell AW. Pathology of herpes zoster and its bearing on sensory localization. *Brain* 1900; 23:353–523.

Heath CW, Alexander AD, Galton MM. Leptospirosis in the United States. *N Engl J Med* 1965;273: 857–864 and 915–922.

Heathfield KWG, Pilsworth R, Wall J, Corsellis JAN. Coxsackie B5 infections in Essex, 1965, with particular reference to the nervous system. *Q J Med* 1967;36:579–595.

Heinonen OP, Shapiro S, Monson RR, Hartz SC, Rosenberg L, Slone D. Immunization during pregnancy against poliomyelitis and influenza in relation to childhood malignancy. *Int J Epidemiol* 1973;2: 229–235.

Held JR, Adaros HL. Neurological disease in man following administration of suckling mouse brain antirabies vaccine. *Bull WHO* 1972;46:321–327.

Hemachudha T. Rabies. In: Vinken PJ, Bruyn GW, Klawans HL, eds. *Handbook of clinical neurology.* Amsterdam: Elsevier Science, 1989:383–404.

Hemachudha T. Human rabies: clinical aspects, pathogenesis, and potential therapy. *Curr Top Microbiol Immunol* 1994;187:121–143.

Hemachudha T, Griffin DE, Chen WW, Johnson RT. Immunologic studies of rabies vaccination-induced Guillain–Barré syndrome. *Neurology* 1988a;38:375–378.

Hemachudha T, Griffin DE, Giffels JJ, Johnson RT, Moser AB, Phanuphak P. Myelin basic protein as an encephalitogen in encephalomyelitis and polyneuritis following rabies vaccination. *N Engl J Med* 1987a;316:369–374.

Hemachudha T, Griffin DE, Johnson RT, Giffels JJ. Immunologic studies of patients with chronic encephalitis induced by post-exposure Semple rabies vaccine. *Neurology* 1988b;38:42–44.

Hemachudha T, Panpanich P, Phanuphak P, Manatsathit S, Wilde H. Immune activation in human rabies. *Trans R Soc Trop Med Hyg* 1993;87:106–108.

Hemachudha T, Phanuphak P, Johnson RT, Griffin DE, Ratanavongsiri J, Siriprasomsup W. Neurologic complications of Semple-type rabies vaccine: clinical and immunologic studies. *Neurology* 1987b; 37:550–556.

Hemachudha T, Phanuphak P, Sriwanthana B, et al. Immunologic study of human encephalitic and paralytic rabies, preliminary report of 16 patients. *Am J Med* 1988c;84:673–677.

Hemachudha T, Phuapradit P. Rabies. *Curr Opin Neurol* 1997;10:260–267.

Henderson DA, Shelokov A. Epidemic neuromyasthenia: clinical syndrome? *N Engl J Med* 1959;260: 757–818.

Heneine W, Woods TC, Sinha SD, et al. Lack of evidence for infection with known human and animal retroviruses in patients with chronic fatigue syndrome. *Clin Infect Dis* 1994;18[Suppl]:S121–S125.

Henle G, Henle W, Diehl V. Relation of Burkitt's tumor-associated herpes type virus to infectious mononucleosis. *Proc Natl Acad Sci USA* 1968;59:94–101.

Hermans PE, Goldstein NP, Wellman WE. Mollaret's meningitis and differential diagnosis of recurrent meningitis. *Am J Med* 1972;52:128–140.

Herndon RM, Griffin DE, McCormick U, Weiner LP. Mouse hepatitis virus-induced recurrent demyelination: a preliminary report. *Arch Neurol* 1975a;32:32–35.

Herndon RM, Johnson RT, Davis LE, Descalzi LR. Ependymitis in mumps virus meningitis: electron microscopical studies of cerebrospinal fluid. *Arch Neurol* 1974;30:475–479.

Herndon RM, Margolis G, Kilham L. The synaptic organization of the malformed cerebellum induced by perinatal infection with feline panleukopenia virus (PLV). I. Elements forming the cerebella glomeruli. *J Neuropathol Exp Neurol* 1971;30:196–205.

Herndon RM, Rena-Descalzi L, Griffin DE, Coyle PK. Age dependence of viral expression: electron microscopic and immunoperoxidase studies of measles virus replication in mice. *Lab Invest* 1975b; 33:544–553.

Hickey WF. Trafficking of hematogenous cells into the CNS. *J Neurovirol* 1997;3[Suppl]:S66–S67.

Hickey WF, Kimura H. Perivascular microglial cells of the CNS are bone marrow-derived and present antigen in vivo. *Science* 1988;239:290–292.

Hickey WF, Vass K, Lassmann H. Bone marrow-derived elements in the central nervous system: an immunohistochemical and ultrastructural survey of rat chimeras. *J Neuropathol Exp Neurol* 1992;51: 246–256.

Hierholzer JC. Adenoviruses in the immunocompromised host. *Clin Microbiol Rev* 1992;5:262–274.

Hill AF, Desbruslais M, Joiner S, et al. The same prion strain causes CJD and BSE. *Nature* 1997;389: 448–450.

Hiller F. Heinrich Irenaeus Quinke. In: Haymaker W, ed. *The founders of neurology.* Springfield, IL: Charles C Thomas, 1953:356–359.

Hilt DC, Buchholz D, Krumholz A, Weiss H, Wolinsky JS. Herpes zoster ophthalmicus and delayed contralateral hemiparesis due to cerebral angiitis: diagnosis and management approaches. *Ann Neurol* 1983;14:543–553.

Hilton DA, Love S, Fletcher A, Pringle JH. Absence of Epstein–Barr virus RNA in multiple sclerosis as assessed by in situ hybridisation. *J Neurol Neurosurg Psychiatry* 1994;57:975–976.

Hinman AR, Fraser DW, Douglas RG, et al. Outbreak of lymphocytic choriomeningitis virus infections in medical center personnel. *Am J Epidemiol* 1975;101:103–110.

Hirsch RL, Griffin DE, Johnson RT, et al. Cellular immune responses during complicated and uncomplicated measles virus infections of man. *Clin Immunol Immunopathol* 1984;31:1–12.

Hirsch RL, Griffin DE, Winkelstein JA. The effect of complement depletion on the course of Sindbis virus infection in mice. *J Immunol* 1978;121:1276–1278.

Hirsch RL, Winkelstein JA, Griffin DE. The role of complement in viral infections. III. Activation of the classical and alternative complement pathways by Sindbis virus. *J Immunol* 1980;124: 2507–2510.

Hjelle B, Appenzeller O, Mills R, et al. Chronic neurodegenerative disease associated with HTLV-II infection. *Lancet* 1992;1:645–646.

Ho DD, Rota TR, Schooley RT, et al. Isolation of HTLV-III from cerebrospinal fluid and neural tissues of patients with neurologic syndromes related to the acquired immunodeficiency syndrome. *N Engl J Med* 1985;313:1493–1497.

Ho TW, Mishu B, Li CY, et al. Guillain–Barré syndrome in northern China: relationship to *Campylobacter jejuni* infection and anti-glycolipid antibodies. *Brain* 1995;118:597–605.

Hoagland RJ. *Infectious mononucleosis.* New York: Grune & Stratton, 1969.

Hochberg FH, Miller G, Schooley RT, Hirsch MS, Feorino P, Henle W. Central-nervous-system lymphoma related to Epstein–Barr virus. *N Engl J Med* 1983;309:748.

Hogan EL, Krigman MR. Herpes zoster myelitis: evidence for viral invasion of spinal cord. *Arch Neurol* 1973;29:309–313.

Hogan RN, Baringer JR, Prusiner SB. Progressive retinal degeneration in scrapie-infected hamsters: a light and electron microscopic analysis. *Lab Invest* 1981;44:34–42.

Hogan RN, Kingsbury DT, Baringer JR, Prusiner SB. Retinal degeneration in experimental Creutzfeldt–Jakob disease. *Lab Invest* 1983;49:708–715.

Hoke CH, Nisalak A, Sangawhipa N, et al. Protection against Japanese encephalitis by inactivated vaccines. *N Engl J Med* 1988;319:608–614.

Hoke CH, Vaughn DW, Nisalak A, et al. Effect of high-dose dexamethasone on the outcome of acute encephalitis due to Japanese encephalitis virus. *J Infect Dis* 1992;165:631–637.

Holden H, Schuknecht H. Distribution pattern of blood in the inner ear following spontaneous subarachnoid hemorrhage. *J Laryngol Otol* 1968;82:321–329.

Holland NR, Power C, Mathews VP, Glass JD, Forman M, McArthur JC. Cytomegalovirus encephalitis in acquired immunodeficiency syndrome (AIDS). *Neurology* 1994;44:507–514.

Hollander H, Stringari S. Human immunodeficiency virus-associated meningitis. *Am J Med* 1987;83: 813–816.

Holman RC, Khan AS, Belay ED, Schonberger LB. Creutzfeldt–Jakob disease in the Untied States, 1979–1994: using national mortality data to assess the possible occurrence of variant cases. *Emer Infect Dis* 1996;2:333–337.

Holman RC, Khan AS, Kent J, Strine TW, Schonberger LB. Epidemiology of Creutzfeldt–Jakob disease in the United States, 1979–1990: analysis of national mortality data. *Neuroepidemiology* 1995;14: 174–181.

Holmberg CA, Gribble DH, Takemoto KK, Howley PM, Espana C, Osburn BI. Isolation of simian virus 40 from rhesus monkeys (*Macaca mulatta*) with spontaneous progressive multifocal leukoencephalopathy. *J Infect Dis* 1977;136:593–596.

Holmes GP, Kaplan JE, Gantz NM, et al. Chronic fatigue syndrome: a working case definition. *Ann Intern Med* 1988;108:387–389.

Holmes GP, McCormick JB, Trock SC, et al. Lassa fever in the United States. *N Engl J Med* 1990;323: 1120–1123.

Holmes KV. Localization of viral infections. In: Nathanson N, ed. *Viral pathogenesis*. Philadelphia: Lippincott–Raven Publishers, 1997:35–53.

Holmgren EB, Forsgren M. Epidemiology of tick-borne encephalitis in Sweden 1956–1989: a study of 1116 cases. *Scand J Infect Dis* 1990;22:287–295.

Holt S, Hudgins D, Krishnan KR, Critchley EMR. Diffuse myelitis associated with rubella vaccination. *BMJ* 1976;2:1037–1038.

Hook EW, Luttrell CN, Slaten K, Wagner RR. Hemorrhagic encephalopathy in chicken embryos infected with influenza virus. IV. Endothelial localization of viral antigens determined by immunofluorescence. *Am J Pathol* 1962;41:593–602.

Hooks JJ, Percopo C, Wang Y, Detrick B. Retina and retinal pigment epithelial cell autoantibodies are produced during murine coronavirus retinopathy. *J Immunol* 1993;151:3381–3389.

Hope-Simpson RE. The nature of herpes zoster: a long-term study and a new hypothesis. *Proc R Soc Lond* 1965;58:9–20.

Hopkins SJ, Rothwell NJ. Cytokines and the nervous system. I. Expression and recognition. *Trends Neurosci* 1995;18:83–88.

Horie H, Koike S, Kurata T, et al. Transgenic mice carrying the human poliovirus receptor: new animal model for study of poliovirus neurovirulence. *J Virol* 1994;68:681–688.

Hornabrook RW. Kuru: a subacute cerebellar degeneration. *Brain* 1968;91:53–74.

Horner FA. Neurologic disorders after Asian influenza. *N Engl J Med* 1958;258:983–985.

Horta-Barbosa L, Fuccillo DA, Sever JL, Zeman W. Isolation of measles virus from a brain biopsy. *Nature* 1969;221:974.

Horten B, Price RW, Jimenez D. Multifocal varicella–zoster virus leukoencephalitis temporally remote from herpes zoster. *Ann Neurol* 1981;9:251–266.

Houff SA, Burton RC, Wilson RW, et al. Human-to-human transmission of rabies virus by a corneal transplant. *N Engl J Med* 1979;300:603–604.

Hoult JG, Flewett TH. Influenza encephalopathy and post-influenzal encephalitis: histological and other observations. *BMJ* 1960;1:1847–1850.

Houtman JJ, Fleming JO. Dissociation of demyelination and viral clearance in congenitally immunodeficient mice infected with murine coronavirus JHM. *J Neurovirol* 1996a;2:101–110.

Houtman JJ, Fleming JO. Pathogenesis of mouse hepatitis virus-induced demyelination. *J Neurovirol* 1996b;2:361–376.

Howard RS, Lees AJ. Encephalitis lethargica, a report of four recent cases. *Brain* 1987;110:19–33.

Howard RS, Wiles CM, Spencer GT. The late sequelae of poliomyelitis. *Q J Med* 1988;66:219–232.

Howell PG, Verwoerd DW. Bluetongue virus. *Virol Monogr* 1971;9:35–74.

Hrdy DB, Rubin DH, Fields BN. Molecular basis of reovirus neurovirulence: role of the M2 gene in avirulence. *Proc Natl Acad Sci USA* 1982;79:1298–1302.

Hsiao K, Baker HF, Crow TJ, et al. Linkage of a prion protein missense variant to Gerstmann–Sträussler syndrome. *Nature* 1989;338:342–345.

Hsiao K, Dlouhy SR, Farlow MR, et al. Mutant prion proteins in Gerstmann–Sträussler–Scheinker disease with neurofibrillary tangles. *Nature Gen* 1992;1:68–71.

Hsiao K, Meiner Z, Kahana E, et al. Mutation of the prion protein in Libyan Jews with Creutzfeldt–Jakob disease. *N Engl J Med* 1991;324:1091–1097.

Hsich G, Kenney K, Gibbs CJ Jr, Lee KH, Harrington MG. The 14-3-3 brain protein in cerebrospinal fluid as a marker for transmissible spongiform encephalopathies. *N Engl J Med* 1996;335:924–930.

Huang AS. Defective interfering viruses. *Annu Rev Microbiol* 1973;27:101–117.

Huang CH, Wong C. Relation of the peripheral multiplication of Japanese B encephalitis virus to the pathogenesis of the infection in mice. *Acta Virol (Praha)* 1963;7:322–330.

Huang E-S, Alford CA, Reynolds DW, Stagno S, Pass RF. Molecular epidemiology of cytomegalovirus infections in women and their infants. *N Engl J Med* 1980;303:958–962.

Hubert C, Brahic M. Early infection of the central nervous system by the GDVII and DA strains of Theiler's virus. *J Virol* 1995;69:3197–3200.

Huet P-M, Layrargues GP, Lebrun L-H, Richer G. Hepatitis B surface antigen in the cerebrospinal fluid in a case of Guillain–Barré syndrome. *CMA J* 1980;122:1157–1159.

Huet T, Cheynier R, Meyerhans A, Roelants G, Wain-Hobson S. Genetic organization of a chimpanzee lentivirus related to HIV-1. *Nature* 1990;345:356–359.

Huff JC, Drucker JL, Clemmer A, et al. Effect of oral acyclovir on pain resolution in herpes zoster: a reanalysis. *J Med Virol* 1993;1[Suppl]:S93–S96.

Hughes RAC, Newsom-Davis JM, Perkins GD, Pierce JM. Controlled trial of prednisolone in acute polyneuropathy. *Lancet* 1978;1:750–753.

Hull HF, Birmingham ME, Melgaard B, Lee JW. Progress toward global polio eradication. *J Infect Dis* 1997;175:4–9.

Hung TP, Kono R. Neurological complications of acute haemorrhagic conjunctivitis. In: Vinken PJ, Bruyn GW, eds. *Handbook of clinical neurology.* Amsterdam: North-Holland, 1979:595–623.

Hunter PR. The English sweating sickness, with particular reference to the 1551 outbreak in Chester. *Rev Infect Dis* 1991;13:303–306.

Hurst EW, Pawan JL. A further account of the Trinidad outbreak of acute rabic myelitis: histology of the experimental disease. *J Pathol Bacteriol* 1932;35:301–321.

Hurtrel B, Chakrabarti L, Hurtrel M, Montagnier L. Target cells during early SIV encephalopathy. *Res Virol* 1993;144:41–46.

Hurwitz ES. Reye's syndrome. *Epidemiol Rev* 1989;11:249–253.

Hurwitz ES, Barrett MJ, Bregman D, et al. Public health service study of Reye's syndrome and medications: report of the main study. *JAMA* 1987;257:1905–1911.

Hutto C, Arvin A, Jacobs R, et al. Intrauterine herpes simplex virus infections. *J Pediatr* 1987;110:97–101.

Hwang YM, Lee MC, Suh DC, Lee WY. *Coxiella* (Q fever)-associated myelopathy. *Neurology* 1993;43:338–342.

Hyman RW, Ecker JR, Tenser RB. Varicella–zoster virus RNA in human trigeminal ganglia. *Lancet* 1983;2:814–816.

Hypiä T, Hovi T, Knowles NJ, Stanway G. Classification of enteroviruses based on molecular and biological properties. *J Gen Virol* 1997;78:1–11.

Ichiyama T, Houdou S, Kisa T, Ohno K, Takeshita K. Varicella with delayed hemiplegia. *Pediatr Neurol* 1990;6:279–281.

Iida T, Kitamura T, Guo J, et al. Origin of JC polyomavirus variants associated with progressive multifocal leukoencephalopathy. *Proc Natl Acad Sci USA* 1993;90:5062–5065.

Ilienko VI, Komandenko NI, Platonov BG, Prozorova IN, Panov AG. Pathogenetic study on chronic forms of tick-borne encephalitis. *Acta Virol (Praha)* 1974;18:341–346.

Illa I, Ortiz N, Gallard E, Juarez C, Grau JM, Dalakas MC. Acute axonal Guillain–Barré syndrome with IgG antibodies against motor axons following parenteral gangliosides. *Ann Neurol* 1995;38:218–224.

Inaba G. Behçet's disease. In: Vinken PJ, Bruyn GW, Klawans HL, eds. *Handbook of clinical neurology.* Amsterdam: Elsevier Science, 1989:593–610.

Innes JRM, Kurland LT. Is multiple sclerosis caused by a virus? *Am J Med* 1952;12:574–585.

Inomata H, Kato M. Vogt–Koyanagi–Harada disease. In: Vinken PJ, Bruyn GW, Klawans HL, eds. *Handbook of clinical neurology.* Amsterdam: Elsevier Science, 1989:611–626.

Inoue A, Tsukada N, Koh C-S, Yanagisawa N. Chronic relapsing demyelinating polyneuropathy associated with hepatitis B infection. *Neurology* 1987;37:1663–1666.

Iorio RM. Mechanisms of neutralization of animal viruses: monoclonal antibodies provide a new perspective. *Microb Pathog* 1988;5:1–7.

Iqbal A, Orger JJ-F, Arnason BGW. Cell-mediated immunity in idiopathic polyneuritis. *Ann Neurol* 1981; 9[Suppl]:S65–S69.

Irani DN, Griffin DE. Regulation of lymphocyte homing into the brain during viral encephalitis at various stages of infection. *J Immunol* 1996;156:3850–3857.

Irani DN, Johnson RT. New approaches to the treatment of herpes zoster. *Infect Med* 1996;13:897–902.

Isaacs A, Lindenmann J. Virus interference. I. The interferon. *Proc R Soc Lond* 1957;147:258–267.

Ito H, Sayama S, Irie S, et al. Antineuronal antibodies in acute cerebellar ataxia following Epstein–Barr virus infection. *Neurology* 1994;44:1506–1507.

Ito M, Go T, Okuno T, Mikawa H. Chronic mumps virus encephalitis. *Pediatr Neurol* 1991;7:467–470.

Itoyama Y, Webster HF, Sternberger NH, et al. Distribution of papovavirus, myelin-associated glycoprotein, and myelin basic protein in progressive multifocal leukoencephalopathy lesions. *Ann Neurol* 1982;11:396–407.

Iwasaki Y, Clark HF. Cell to cell transmission of virus in the central nervous system. II. Experimental rabies in mouse. *Lab Invest* 1975;33:391–399.

Izumi KM, Stevens JG. Molecular and biological characterization of a herpes simplex virus type 1 (HSV-1) neuroinvasiveness gene. *J Exp Med* 1990;172:487–496.

Izumo S, Goto I, Itoyama Y, et al. Interferon-alpha is effective in HTLV-I-associated myelopathy: a multicenter, randomized, double-blind, controlled trial. *Neurology* 1996;46:1016–1021.

Jabs DA. Controversies in the treatment of cytomegalovirus retinitis: foscarnet versus ganciclovir. *Infect Agents Dis* 1995;4:131–142.

Jackson AC. Biological basis of rabies virus neurovirulence in mice: comparative pathogenesis study using the immunoperoxidase technique. *J Virol* 1991;65:537–540.

Jackson AC, Johnson RT. Aseptic meningitis and acute viral encephalitis. In: Vinken PJ, Bruyn GW, Klawans HL, eds. *Handbook of clinical neurology.* Amsterdam: Elsevier Science, 1989:125–148.

Jackson AC, Moench TR, Griffin DE, Johnson RT. The pathogenesis of spinal cord involvement in the encephalomyelitis of mice caused by neuroadapted Sindbis virus infection. *Lab Invest* 1987;56: 418–423.

Jacob H. The neuropathology of the Marburg disease in man. In: Martini GA, Siegert R, eds. *Marburg virus disease.* New York: Springer-Verlag, 1971:54–61.

Jacobs BC, van Doorn PA, Schmitz PIM, et al. *Campylobacter jejuni* infections and anti-GM1 antibodies in Guillain–Barré syndrome. *Ann Neurol* 1996;40:181–187.

Jacobson LP, Kirby AJ, Polk S, et al. Changes in survival after acquired immunodeficiency syndrome (AIDS): 1984–1991. *Am J Epidemiol* 1993a;138:952–964.

Jacobson S, Flerlage ML, McFarland HF. Impaired measles virus-specific cytotoxic T cell responses in multiple sclerosis. *J Exp Med* 1985;162:839–850.

Jacobson S, Lehky T, Nishimura M, Robinson S, McFarlin DE, Dhib-Jalbut S. Isolation of HTLV-II from a patient with chronic, progressive neurological disease clinically indistinguishable from HTLV-I-associated myelopathy/tropical spastic paraparesis. *Ann Neurol* 1993b;33:392–396.

Jacobson S, Shida H, McFarlin DE, Fauci AS, Koenig S. Circulating CD8 cytotoxic T lymphocytes specific for HTLV-1 pX in patients with HTLV-1 associated neurological disease. *Nature* 1990;348:245–248.

Jaenisch R. Transgenic animals. *Science* 1988;240:1468–1474.

Jagelman S, Suckling AJ, Webb HE. The pathogenesis of avirulent Semliki Forest virus infections in athymic nude mice. *J Gen Virol* 1978;41:599–607.

Jakob J, Roos RP. Molecular determinants of Theiler's murine encephalomyelitis-induced disease. *J Neurovirol* 1996;2:70–77.

Jamieson BD, Ahmed R. T cell memory. *J Exp Med* 1989;169:1993–2005.

Jamieson GA, Maitland NJ, Wilcock GK, Craske J, Itzhaki RF. Latent herpes simplex virus type 1 in normal and Alzheimer's disease brains. *J Med Virol* 1991;33:224–227.

Jay V, Becker LE, Otsubo H, et al. Chronic encephalitis and epilepsy (Rasmussen's encephalitis): detection of cytomegalovirus and herpes simplex virus 1 by the polymerase chain reaction and in situ hybridization. *Neurology* 1995;45:108–117.

Jefferson M, Riddoch D, Smith WT. Fatal encephalopathy complicating lymphoid interstitial pneumonia. *J Neurol Neurosurg Psychiatry* 1971;34:341–347.

Jeffery DR, Mandler RN, Davis LE. Transverse myelitis. *Arch Neurol* 1993;50:532–535.

Jellinek EH, Tulloch WS. Herpes zoster with dysfunction of bladder and anus. *Lancet* 1976;1:1219–1222.

Jenner E. *The origin of the vaccine inoculation.* London: DN Shury, 1801.

Joachims HZ, Eliacher I. Cochlear hearing loss following rubella in an adult. *Scand Audiol* 1982;11:89–90.

Joag SV, Stephens EB, Galbreath D, et al. Simian immunodeficiency virus SIV$_{mac}$ chimeric virus whose *env* gene was derived from SIV-encephalitis brain is macrophage-tropic but not neurovirulent. *J Virol* 1995;69:1367–1369.

Johansson PJH, Sveger T, Ahlfors K, Ekstrand J, Svensson L. Reovirus type 1 associated with meningitis. *Scand J Infect Dis* 1996;28:117–120.

John GC, Kreiss J. Mother-to-child transmission of human immunodeficiency virus type 1. *Epidemiol Rev* 1996;18:149–157.

Johnson BK, Stone GA, Godec MS, Asher DM, Gajdusek DC, Gibbs CJ, Jr. Long-term observations of human immunodeficiency virus-infected chimpanzees. *AIDS Res Hum Retroviruses* 1993;9:375–378.

Johnson BL, Wisotzkey HM. Neuroretinitis associated with herpes simplex encephalitis in an adult. *Am J Ophthalmol* 1977;83:481–489.

Johnson KP. Mouse cytomegalovirus: placenta infection. *J Infect Dis* 1969;120:445–450.

Johnson KP, Ferguson LC, Byington DP, Redman D. Multiple fetal malformations due to persistent viral infection. I. Abortion, intrauterine death, and gross abnormalities in fetal swine infected with hog cholera vaccine virus. *Lab Invest* 1974a;30:608–617.

Johnson KP, Johnson RT. California encephalitis. II. Studies of experimental infection in the mouse. *J Neuropathol Exp Neurol* 1968a;27:390–400.

Johnson KP, Johnson RT. Granular ependymitis: occurrence in myxovirus infected rodents and prevalence in man. *Am J Pathol* 1972;67:511–526.

Johnson KP, Klasnja R, Johnson RT. Neural tube defects of chick embryos: an indirect result of influenza A virus infection. *J Neuropathol Exp Neurol* 1971;30:68–74.

Johnson KP, Lepow ML, Johnson RT. California encephalitis. I. Clinical and epidemiological studies. *Neurology* 1968a;18:250–254.

Johnson KP, Wolinsky JS, Swoveland P. Central nervous system infections (chronic). In: Huang GD, Green RH, eds. CRC Handbook Series in Clinical Laboratory Science. Section H. *Virology and Rickettsiology* vol. 1, part 2; CRC Press, West Palm Beach; 1978.

Johnson R, Milbourn PE. Central nervous system manifestations of chickenpox. *Can Med Assoc J* 1970; 102:831–834.

Johnson RT. The pathogenesis of herpes virus encephalitis. I. Virus pathways to the nervous system of suckling mice demonstrated by fluorescent antibody staining. *J Exp Med* 1964a;119:343–356.

Johnson RT. The pathogenesis of herpes virus encephalitis. II. A cellular basis for the development of resistance with age. *J Exp Med* 1964b;120:359–374.

Johnson RT. Experimental rabies: studies of cellular vulnerability and pathogenesis using fluorescent antibody staining. *J Neuropathol Exp Neurol* 1965a;24:662–674.

Johnson RT. Virus invasion of the central nervous system: a study of Sindbis virus infection in the mouse using fluorescent antibody. *Am J Pathol* 1965b;46:929–943.

Johnson RT. Mumps virus encephalitis in the hamster: studies of the inflammatory response and noncytopathic infection of neurons. *J Neuropathol Exp Neurol* 1968;27:80–95.

Johnson RT. The pathogenesis of experimental rabies. In: Nagano Y, Davenport FM, eds. *Rabies.* Tokyo: University of Tokyo Press, 1970a:59–75.

Johnson RT. Subacute sclerosing panencephalitis. *J Infect Dis* 1970b;121:227–230.

Johnson RT. Inflammatory response to viral infection. *Res Publ Assoc Nerv Ment Dis* 1971;49:305–312.

Johnson RT. Effects of viral infections on the developing nervous system. *N Engl J Med* 1972a;287:599–604.

Johnson RT. Treatment of herpes simplex encephalitis. *Arch Neurol* 1972b;27:97–98.

Johnson RT. Pathophysiology and epidemiology of acute viral infections of the nervous system. *Adv Neurol* 1974;6:27–40.

Johnson RT. Hydrocephalus and viral infections. *Dev Med Child Neurol* 1975a;17:807–816.

Johnson RT. Progressive rubella encephalitis. *N Engl J Med* 1975b;292:1020–1021.

Johnson RT. Problems in relating viral infections to malformations in man. *Contr Epidem Biostat* 1979;1: 138–146.

Johnson RT. Selective vulnerability of neural cells to viral infection. *Brain* 1980;103:447–472.

Johnson RT. *Viral infections of the nervous system.* New York: Raven Press, 1982.

Johnson RT. Late progression of poliomyelitis paralysis: discussion of pathogenesis. *Rev Infect Dis* 1984; 6[Suppl]:S568–S570.

Johnson RT. Nononcogenic retrovirus infections as models for chronic and relapsing human diseases: introduction. *Rev Infect Dis* 1985a;7:66–67.

Johnson RT. Viral aspects of multiple sclerosis. In: Vinken PJ, Bruyn GW, Klawans HL, eds. *Handbook of clinical neurology.* Amsterdam: Elsevier Science, 1985b:319–336.

Johnson RT. The pathogenesis of acute viral encephalitis and postinfectious encephalomyelitis. *J Infect Dis* 1987;155:359–364.

Johnson RT. The viral infections of the developing nervous system: an overview. In: Johnson RT, Lyon G, eds. *Viruses and the developing nervous system.* Lancaster, UK: Kluwer Academic Publishers, 1988: 1–19.

Johnson RT. Arboviral encephalitis. In: Warren KS, Mahmoud AAF, eds. *Tropical and geographical medicine.* New York: McGraw-Hill, 1990:691–699.

Johnson RT. "Herpetic infection, with especial reference to involvement of the nervous system": an appraisal. *Medicine (Baltimore)* 1993a;72:133–135.

Johnson RT. Neurovirology: the evolution of new challenges. In: Gandevia SC, Burke D, Anthony M, eds. *Science and practice in clinical neurology.* Cambridge: Cambridge University Press, 1993b:363–373.

Johnson RT. Emerging infections of the nervous system. *J Neurol Sci* 1994a:124:3–14.

Johnson RT. The virology of demyelinating diseases. *Ann Neurol* 1994b:36[Suppl]:S54–S60.

Johnson RT. Pathogenesis of poliovirus infections. *Ann NY Acad Sci* 1995;753:361–365.

Johnson RT. Acute encephalitis. *Clin Infect Dis* 1996a;23:219–226.

Johnson RT. Emerging viral infections. *Arch Neurol* 1996b;53:18–22.

Johnson RT. Real and theoretical threats to human health posed by the epidemic of bovine spongiform encephalopathy. In: Gibbs CJ Jr, ed. *Bovine spongiform encephalopathy: the BSE dilemma.* New York: Springer-Verlag, 1996c:359–363.

Johnson RT, Brooks BR. The possible viral etiology of amyotrophic lateral sclerosis. In: Serratrice G, Crus D, Desnuelle C, eds. *Neuromuscular diseases.* New York: Raven Press, 1984:353–359.

Johnson RT, Buescher EL, Rogers NG, Funkenbusch MJ, Oliu WE. Epidemic central nervous system disease of mixed enterovirus etiology. II. Analysis of laboratory investigations. *Am J Hyg* 1960a;71: 331–341.

Johnson RT, Burke DS, Elwell M, et al. Japanese encephalitis: immunocytochemical studies of viral antigen and inflammatory cells in fatal cases. *Ann Neurol* 1985a;18:567–573.

Johnson RT, Gibbs CJ Jr. Koch's postulates and slow infections of the nervous system. *Arch Neurol* 1974; 30:36–38.

Johnson RT, Glass JD, McArthur JC, Chesebro BW. Quantitation of human immunodeficiency virus in brains of demented and nondemented patients with acquired immunodeficiency syndrome. *Ann Neurol* 1996;39:392–395.

Johnson RT, Griffin DE. Pathogenesis of viral infections. In: Vinken PJ, Bruyn GW, eds. *Handbook of clinical neurology.* Amsterdam: North-Holland, 1978:15–37.

Johnson RT, Griffin DE. Postinfectious encephalomyelitis. In: Kennedy PGE, Johnson RT, eds. *Infections of the nervous system.* London: Butterworths, 1987:209–226.

Johnson RT, Griffin DE, Arregui A, et al. Spastic paraparesis and HTLV-1 infection in Peru. *Ann Neurol* 1988a;23[Suppl]:S151–S155.

Johnson RT, Griffin DE, Gendelman HE. Postinfectious encephalomyelitis. *Semin Neurol* 1985b;5: 180–190.

Johnson RT, Griffin DE, Hirsch RL. Escape from immune surveillance within the central nervous system. In: Miescher PA, Bolis L, Gorini S, Lambo TA, Nossal GJV, Torrigiani G, eds. *Immunopathology of the central and peripheral nervous system.* Basel: Schwabe, 1979:113–121.

Johnson RT, Griffin DE, Hirsch RL, et al. Measles encephalomyelitis: clinical and immunological studies. *N Engl J Med* 1984;310:137–141.

Johnson RT, Griffin DE, Moench TR. Pathogenesis of measles immunodeficiency and encephalomyelitis: parallels to AIDS. *Microb Pathog* 1988b;4:169–174.

Johnson RT, Herndon RM. Virological studies of multiple sclerosis and other chronic and relapsing neurological diseases. *Prog Med Virol* 1974;18:214–228.

Johnson RT, Intralawan P, Puapanwatton S. Japanese encephalitis: identification of inflammatory cells in cerebrospinal fluid. *Ann Neurol* 1986;20:691–695.

Johnson RT, Johnson KP. Hydrocephalus following viral infection: the pathology of aqueductal stenosis developing after experimental mumps virus infection. *J Neuropathol Exp Neurol* 1968b;27:591–606.

Johnson RT, Johnson KP. Slow and chronic virus infections of the nervous system. In: Plum F, ed. *Recent advances in neurology.* Philadelphia: FA Davis, 1969:33–78.

Johnson RT, Johnson KP, Edmonds CJ. Virus-induced hydrocephalus: development of aqueductal stenosis in hamsters after mumps infection. *Science* 1967;157:1066–1067.

Johnson RT, Lazzarini RA, Waksman BH. Mechanisms of virus persistence. *Ann Neurol* 1981;9:616–617.

Johnson RT, McArthur JC. AIDS and the brain. *Trends Neurosci* 1986;9:91–94.

Johnson RT, McArthur JC, Narayan O. The neurobiology of human immunodeficiency virus infections. *FASEB J* 1988c;2:2970–2981.

Johnson RT, McFarland HF, Levy SE. Age-dependent resistance to viral encephalitis: studies of infections due to Sindbis virus in mice. *J Infect Dis* 1972;125:257–262.

Johnson RT, Mercer EH. The development of fixed rabies virus in mouse brain. *Aust J Exp Biol* 1964;42: 449–456.

Johnson RT, Mims CA. Medical progress, pathogenesis of viral infections of the nervous system. *N Engl J Med* 1968;278:23–30 and 84–92.

Johnson RT, Narayan O. Experimental neurological diseases of animals caused by viruses. In: Klawans HL, ed. *Models of human neurological diseases.* Amsterdam: Excerpta Medica, 1974:40–82.

Johnson RT, Narayan O, Weiner LP. The relationship of SV40 related viruses to progressive multifocal leukoencephalopathy. In: Robinson WS, Fox CF, eds. *Mechanisms of virus disease.* Menlo Park, NJ: WA Benjamin, 1974b:187–197.

Johnson RT, Olson LC, Buescher EL. Herpes simplex virus infections in the nervous system: problems in laboratory diagnosis. *Arch Neurol* 1968b;18:260–264.

Johnson RT, Portnoy B, Rogers NG, Buescher EL. Acute benign pericarditis: virologic study of 34 patients. *Arch Intern Med* 1961;108:823–932.

Johnson RT, Shuey HE, Buescher EL. Epidemic central nervous system disease of mixed enterovirus etiology. I. Clinical and epidemiological description. *Am J Hyg* 1960b;71:321–330.

Johnstone JA, Ross CAC, Dunn M. Meningitis and encephalitis associated with mumps infection: a 10-year survey. *Arch Dis Child* 1972;47:647–651.

Jolicoeur P, Massé G, Kay DG. The prion protein gene is dispensable for the development of spongiform myeloencephalopathy induced by the neurovirulent Cas-Br-E murine leukemia virus. *J Virol* 1996;70: 9031–9034.

Joly E, Mucke L, Oldstone MBA. Viral persistence in neurons explained by lack of major histocompatibility class I expression. *Science* 1991;253:1283–1285.

Jones HR Jr, Ho DD, Forgacs P, et al. Acute fulminating fatal leukoencephalopathy as the only manifestation of human immunodeficiency virus infection. *Ann Neurol* 1988;23:519–522.

Jones JF, Ray CG, Minnich LL, Hicks MJ, Kibler R, Lucas DO. Evidence for active Epstein–Barr virus infection in patients with persistent, unexplained illnesses: elevated anti-early antigen antibodies. *Ann Intern Med* 1985;102:1–7.

Jones TC, Doll ER, Bryans JT. The lesions of equine viral arteritis. *Cornell Vet* 1957;47:52–68.

Jordan EK, Sever JL. Fetal damage caused by parvoviral infections. *Reprod Toxicol* 1994;8:161–189.

Joseph BS, Oldstone MBA. Immunological injury in measles virus infection. II. Suppression of immune injury through antigenic modulation. *J Exp Med* 1975;142:864–876.

Joy JL, Carlo JR, Vélez-Borrás JR. Cerebral infarction following herpes zoster: the enlarging clinical spectrum. *Neurology* 1989;39:1640.

Joyce J, Hotopf M, Wessely S. The prognosis of chronic fatigue and chronic fatigue syndrome: a systematic review. *Q J Med* 1997;90:223–233.

Jubelt B, Cashman NR. Neurological manifestations of the post-polio syndrome. *Crit Rev Neurobiol* 1987;3:199–220.

Jubelt B, Drucker J. Post-polio syndrome: an update. *Semin Neurol* 1993;13:283–290.

Jubelt B, Gallez-Hawkins G, Narayan O, Johnson RT. Pathogenesis of human poliovirus infection in mice. I. Clinical and pathological studies. *J Neuropathol Exp Neurol* 1980a;39:138–148.

Jubelt B, Narayan O, Johnson RT. Pathogenesis of human poliovirus infection in mice. II. Age-dependency of paralysis. *J Neuropathol Exp Neurol* 1980b;39:149–159.

Jubelt B, Salazar-Grueso EF, Roos RP, Cashman NR. Antibody titer to the poliovirus in blood and cerebrospinal fluid of patients with post-polio syndrome. *Ann NY Acad Sci* 1995;753:201–207.

Juel-Jensen BE. The national history of shingles: events associated with reactivation of varicella–zoster virus. *J R Coll Gen Pract* 1970;20:323–327.

Juel-Jensen BE, MacCallum FO. *Herpes simplex, varicella and zoster.* Philadelphia: JB Lippincott Co, 1972.

Julkunen I, Koskiniemi M, Lehtokoski-Lehtiniemi E, Sainio K, Vaheri A. Chronic mumps virus encephalitis. *J Neuroimmunol* 1985;8:167–175.

Kabat EA, Wolfe A, Bezer AE. The rapid production of acute disseminated encephalomyelitis in rhesus monkey by injection of heterologous and homologous brain tissue with adjuvants. *J Exp Med* 1947; 85:117–130.

Kai K, Furuta T. Isolation of paralysis-inducing murine leukemia viruses from Friend virus passaged in rats. *J Virol* 1984;50:970–973.

Kalayjian RC, Cohen ML, Bonomo RA, Flanigan TP. Cytomegalovirus ventriculoencephalitis in AIDS. *Medicine (Baltimore)* 1993;72:67–77.

Kalman CM, Laskin OL. Herpes zoster and zosteriform herpes simplex virus infections in immunocompetent adults. *Am J Med* 1986;81:775–778.

Kaluza G, Lell G, Reinacher M, Stitz L, Willems WR. Neurogenic spread of Semliki Forest virus in mice. *Arch Virol* 1987;93:97–110.

Kamei S, Hersch SM, Kurata T, Takei Y. Coxsackie B antigen in the central nervous system of a patient with fatal acute encephalitis: immunohistochemical studies of formalin-fixed paraffin-embedded tissue. *Acta Neuropathol (Berl)* 1990;80:216–221.

Kamei S, Tetsuka T, Takasu T, Shimizu K. New non-invasive rapid diagnosis of herpes simplex virus encephalitis by quantitative detection of intrathecal antigen with a chemiluminescence assay. *J Neurol Neurosurg Psychiatry* 1994;57:1112–1114.

Kanamitsu M, Kasamaki A, Ogawa M, Kasahara S, Imamura M. Immunofluorescent study on the pathogenesis of oral infection of poliovirus in monkey. *Jpn J Med Sci Biol* 1967;20:175–194.

Kanki PJ, Alroy J, Essex M. Isolation of T-lymphotropic retrovirus related to HTLV-III/LAV from wild-caught African green monkeys. *Science* 1985;230:951–954.

Kannagi M, Matsushita S, Shida H, Harada S. Cytotoxic T cell response and expression of the target antigen in HTLV-1 infection. *Leukemia* 1994;8[Suppl]:S54–S59.

Kaplan AM, Koveleski JT. St. Louis encephalitis with particular involvement of the brain stem. *Arch Neurol* 1968;35:45–46.

Karmody CS. Asymptomatic maternal rubella and congenital deafness. *Arch Otolaryngol* 1969;89: 720–726.

Karp CL, Wysocka M, Wahl LM, et al. Mechanism of suppression of cell-mediated immunity by measles virus. *Science* 1996;273:228–231.

Karpas A. Origin and spread of AIDS [Letter]. *Nature* 1990;348:578.

Kascsak RJ, Carp RI, Vilcek JT, Donnenfeld H, Bartfeld H. Virological studies in amyotrophic lateral sclerosis. *Muscle Nerve* 1982;5:93–101.

Katz M, Koprowski H. The significance of failure to isolate infectious viruses in cases of subacute sclerosing panencephalitis. *Arch Ges Virusforsch* 1973;41:390–393.

Katz M, Rorke LB, Masland WS, Broadano GB, Koprowski H. Subacute sclerosing panencephalitis: isolation of a virus encephalitogenic for ferrets. *J Infect Dis* 1970;121:188–195.

Kaufmann CA, Weinberger DR, Stevens JR, et al. Intracerebral inoculation of experimental animals with brain tissue from patients with schizophrenia. *Arch Gen Psychiatry* 1988;45:648–652.

Kawahara H, Tohyama J, Ingaki M, Ohno K. Congenital hydrocephalus due to intrauterine HTLV-1 infection. *Lancet* 1990;2:1442.

Kay DG, Gravel C, Pothier F, Lapperière A, Robitaille Y. Neurological disease induced in transgenic mice expressing the env gene of the Cas-Br-E murine retrovirus. *Proc Natl Acad Sci USA* 1993;90: 4538–4542.

Kay DG, Gravel C, Robitaille Y, Jolicoeur P. Retrovirus-induced spongiform myeloencephalopathy in mice: regional distribution of infected target cells and neuronal loss occurring in the absence of viral expression in neurons. *Proc Natl Acad Sci USA* 1991;88:1281–1285.

Keenlyside RA, Schoenberger LB, Bregman DJ, Sullivan-Bolyai JZ. Fatal Guillain–Barré syndrome after the national influenza immunization program. *Neurology* 1980;39:929–933.

Kennedy PGE. Neurological complications of varicella–zoster virus. In: Kennedy PGE, Johnson RT, eds. *Infections of the nervous system.* London: Butterworths, 1987:177–208.

Kennedy PGE. On the possible role of viruses in the aetiology of motor neurone disease: a review. *J R Soc Med* 1990;83:784–787.

Kennedy PGE, Narayan O, Ghotbi Z, Hopkins J, Gendelman HE, Clements JE. Persistent expression of

Ia antigen and viral genome in visna–maedi virus-induced inflammatory cells: possible role of lentivirus-induced interferon. *J Exp Med* 1985;162:1970–1982.

Kennedy PGE, Newsome DA, Hess J, et al. Cytomegalovirus but not human T lymphotropic virus type III/lymphadenopathy associated virus detected by in situ hybridisation in retinal lesions in patients with the acquired immune deficiency syndrome. *BMJ* 1986;293:162–164.

Kennedy PGE, Steiner I. A molecular and cellular model to explain the differences in reactivation from latency by herpes simplex and varicella–zoster viruses. *Neuropathol Appl Neurobiol* 1994;20: 368–374.

Kennedy RH, Danielson MA, Mulder DM, Kurland LT. Guillain–Barré syndrome: a 42-year-old epidemiologic and clinical study. *Mayo Clin Proc* 1978;53:93–99.

Kenyon RH, Green DE, Eddy GA, Peters CJ. Treatment of Junin virus-infected guinea pigs with immune serum: development of late neurological disease. *J Med Virol* 1986;20:207–218.

Kernéis S, Bogdanova A, Kraehenbuhl J-P, Pringault E. Conversion by Peyer's patch lymphocytes of human enterocytes into M cells that transport bacteria. *Science* 1997;277:949–952.

Kerr DA, Chang CF, Gordon J, Bjornsti MA, Khalili K. Inhibition of human neurotropic virus (JCV) DNA replication in glial cells by camptothecin. *Virology* 1993;196:612–618.

Kesselring J, Miller DH, Robb SA, et al. Acute disseminated encephalomyelitis: MRI findings and the distinction from multiple sclerosis. *Brain* 1990;113:291–302.

Kessler HA, Trenholme GM, Harris AA, Levin S. Acute myopathy associated with influenza A/Texas/1/77 infection. *JAMA* 1980;243:461–462.

Ketzler S, Weis S, Haug H, Budka H. Loss of neurons in the frontal cortex in AIDS brains. *Acta Neuropathol (Berl)* 1990;80:92–94.

Khabbaz RF, Hartel D, Lairmore M, et al. Human T lymphotropic virus type II (HTLV-II) infection in a cohort of New York intravenous drug users: an old infection? *J Infect Dis* 1991;163:252–256.

Khabbaz RF, Heneine W, George JR, et al. Infection of a laboratory worker with simian immunodeficiency virus [Brief report]. *N Engl J Med* 1994;330:172–177.

Khalifa MA, Rodrigues MM, Rajagopalan S, Swoveland P. Eye pathology associated with measles encephalitis in hamsters. *Arch Virol* 1991;119:165–173.

Khan AS, Heneine WM, Chapman LE, et al. Assessment of a retrovirus sequence and other possible risk factors for the chronic fatigue syndrome in adults. *Ann Intern Med* 1993;118:241–245.

Khanna R, Burrows SR, Moss DJ. Immune regulation in Epstein–Barr virus-associated diseases. *Microbiol Rev* 1995;59:387–405.

Kibayashi K, Mastri AR, Hirsch CS. Neuropathology of human immunodeficiency virus infection at different disease stages. *Hum Pathol* 1996;27:637–642.

Kibrick S. Current status of Coxsackie and ECHO viruses in human disease. *Prog Med Virol* 1964;6:27–70.

Kidd D, Howard RS, Williams AJ, Heatley FW, Panayiotiopoulos CP, Spencer GT. Late functional deterioration following paralytic poliomyelitis. *Q J Med* 1997;90:189–196.

Kilbourne ED. New viruses and new disease: mutation, evolution and ecology. *Curr Opin Immunol* 1991; 3:518–524.

Kilham L, Margolis G. Cerebellar ataxia in hamsters inoculated with rat virus. *Science* 1964;143: 1047–1048.

Kilham L, Margolis G. Viral etiology of spontaneous ataxia of cats. *Am J Pathol* 1966;48:991–1011.

Kimberlin RH, Walker CA. Pathogenesis of mouse scrapie: evidence for neural spread of infection to the CNS. *J Gen Virol* 1980;51:183–187.

Kimura H, Aso K, Kuzushima K, Hanada N, Shibata M, Morishima T. Relapse of herpes simplex encephalitis in children. *Pediatrics* 1992;89:891–894.

Kinnunen E, Valle M, Piirainen L, et al. Viral antibodies in multiple sclerosis, a nationwide co-twin study. *Arch Neurol* 1990;47:743–746.

Kira J-i, Koyanagi Y, Yamada T, et al. Increased HTLV-I proviral DNA in HTLV-I-associated myelopathy: a quantitative polymerase chain reaction study. *Ann Neurol* 1991;29:194–201.

Kira J, Minato S, Itoyama Y, Goto I, Kato M, Hasuo K. Leukoencephalopathy in HTLV-I-associated myelopathy: MRI and EEG data. *J Neurol Sci* 1988;87:221–232.

Kirk J. Pseudoviral hollow-cored vesicles in multiple sclerosis brain. *Acta Neuropathol (Berl)* 1979;48: 63–66.

Kirk J, Hutchinson WM. The fine structure of the CNS in multiple sclerosis. I. Interpretation of cytoplasmic papovavirus-like and paramyxovirus-like inclusions. *Neuropathol Appl Neurobiol* 1978;4: 343–356.

Kirk JL, Fine DP, Sexton DJ, Muchmore HG. Rocky Mountain spotted fever, a clinical review based on 48 confirmed cases, 1943–1986. *Medicine (Baltimore)* 1990;69:35–45.

Kissling RE, Robinson RQ, Murphy FA, Whitfield SG. Agent of disease contracted from green monkeys. *Science* 1968;160:888–890.

Kitano Y, Ohzono H, Yasuda N, Shimizu T. Hydranencephaly, cerebellar hypoplasia, and myopathy in chick embryos infected with aino virus. *Vet Pathol* 1996;33:672–681.

Kittur SD, Hoh JH, Kawas CH, Hayward GS, Endo H, Adler WH. A molecular hybridization study for the presence of herpes simplex, cytomegalovirus and Epstein–Barr virus in brain and blood of Alzheimer's disease patients. *Arch Gerontol Geriatr* 1992;15:35–41.

Klatzo I, Gajdusek DC, Zigas V. Pathology of kuru. *Lab Invest* 1959;8:799–847.

Kleinschmidt-DeMasters BK, Amlie-Lefond C, Gilden DH. The patterns of varicella zoster virus encephalitis. *Hum Pathol* 1996;27:927–938.

Klemola E, Weckman N, Haltia K, Kaariainen L. The Guillain–Barre syndrome associated with acquired cytomegalovirus infection. *Acta Med Scand* 1967;181:603–607.

Kliks SC, Wara DW, Landers DV, Levy JA. Features of HIV-1 that could influence maternal–child transmission. *JAMA* 1994;272:467–474.

Knipe DM. Virus–host cell interactions. In: Fields BN, Knipe DM, Howley PM, et al., eds. *Fields virology,* 3rd ed. New York. Lippincott–Raven Publishers, 1996:273–300.

Knopf PM, Cserr HF, Nolan SC, Wu T-Y, Harling-Berg CJ. Physiology and immunology of lymphatic drainage of interstitial and cerebrospinal fluid from the brain. *Neuropathol Appl Neurobiol* 1995;21: 175–180.

Knox KK, Harrington DP, Carrigan DR. Fulminant human herpesvirus six encephalitis in a human immunodeficiency virus-infected infant. *J Med Virol* 1995;45:288–292.

Koduri PR, Naides SJ. Aseptic meningitis caused by parvovirus B19. *Clin Infect Dis* 1995;21:1053.

Koeda T, Inagaki M, Kawahara H, et al. Progressive encephalopathy associated with cytomegalovirus infection without immune deficiency. *J Child Neurol* 1993;8:373–377.

Kogon A, Spigland I, Frothingham TE, et al. The Virus Watch Program: a continuing surveillance of viral infections in metropolitan New York families. *Am J Epidemiol* 1969;89:51–61.

Komori S, Ludwig J, Okazaki H, Komori T, Kurland LT. Reye's syndrome in Olmsted County, Minnesota: did it exist before 1963? *Mayo Clin Proc* 1992;67:871–875.

Komurasaki Y, Nagineni CN, Wang Y, Hooks JJ. Virus RNA persists within the retina in coronavirus-induced retinopathy. *Virology* 1996;222:446–450.

Kondo K, Kuroiwa Y. A case control study of Creutzfeldt–Jakob disease: association with physical injuries. *Ann Neurol* 1982;11:377–381.

Konno S, Koeda T, Madarame H, et al. Myopathy and encephalopathy in chick embryos experimentally infected with Akabane virus. *Vet Pathol* 1988;25:1–8.

Konno S, Moriwaki M, Nakagawa M. Akabane disease in cattle: congenital abnormalities caused by viral infection: spontaneous disease. *Vet Pathol* 1982;19:246–266.

Kono R, Uchida N, Sasagawa A, et al. Neurovirulence of acute haemorrhagic conjunctivitis virus in monkeys. *Lancet* 1973;1:61–63.

Koprowski H, DeFreitas EC, Harper ME, et al. Multiple sclerosis and human T-cell lymphotropic retroviruses. *Nature* 1985;318:154–160.

Kosaka H, Sano Y, Matsukado Y, Sairenji T, Hinuma Y. Failure to detect papovavirus-associated T antigens in human brain tumor cells by anticomplement immunofluorescence. *J Neurosurg* 1980;52:367–370.

Koschel K, Halbach M. Rabies virus infection selectively impairs membrane receptor functions in neuronal model cells. *J Gen Virol* 1979;42:627–632.

Koschel K, Muenzel P. Persistent paramyxovirus infections and behavior of β-adrenergic receptors in C-6 rat glioma cells. *J Gen Virol* 1980;47:513–517.

Koski CL, Chou DKH, Jungalwala FB. Anti-peripheral nerve myelin antibodies in Guillain–Barré syndrome bind a neutral glycolipid of peripheral myelin and cross-react with Forssman antigen. *J Clin Invest* 1989;84:280–287.

Koskiniemi M. CNS manifestations associated with *Mycoplasma pneumoniae* infections: summary of cases at the University of Helsinki and review. *Clin Infect Dis* 1993;17[Suppl 1]:S52–S57.

Koskiniemi M, Rautonen J, Lehtokoski-Lehtiniemi E, Vaheri A. Epidemiology of encephalitis in children: a 20-year survey. *Ann Neurol* 1991;29:492–497.

Koyanagi Y, Tanaka Y, Kira J-i, et al. Primary human immunodeficiency virus type 1 viremia and central nervous system invasion in a novel hu-PBL-immunodeficient mouse strain. *J Virol* 1997;71: 2417–2424.

Krakowka S, Miele JA, Mathes LE, Metzler AE. Antibody responses to measles virus and canine distemper virus in multiple sclerosis. *Ann Neurol* 1983;14:533–538.

Krauss GL, Campbell ML, Roche KW, Huganir RL, Neidermeyer E. Chronic steroid-responsive encephalitis without autoantibodies to glutamate receptor GluR3. *Neurology* 1996;46:247–249.

Krebs JW, Strine TW, Smith JS, Rupprecht CE, Childs JE. Rabies surveillance in the United States during 1994. *J Am Vet Med Assoc* 1995;207:1562–1575.

Kreutzberg GW. Microglia: a sensor for pathological events in the CNS. *Trends Neurosci* 1996;19: 312–318.

Krey HF, Ludwig H, Boschek CB. Multifocal retinopathy in Borna disease virus infected rabbits. *Am J Ophthalmol* 1979a;87:157–164.

Krey HF, Ludwig H, Rott P. Spread of infectious virus along the optic nerve into the retina in Borna disease virus-infected rabbits. *Arch Virol* 1979b;61:283–288.

Kristensson K, Ghetti B, Wisniewski HM. Study on the propagation of herpes simplex virus (type 2) into brain after intraocular injection. *Brain Res* 1974;69:189–201.

Kristensson K, Lycke E, Sjostrand J. Spread of herpes simplex virus in peripheral nerves. *Acta Neuropathol (Berl)* 1971;17:44–53.

Kuban KC, Ephros MA, Freeman RL, Laffell LB, Bresnan MJ. Syndrome of opsoclonus–myoclonus caused by coxsackie B3 infection. *Ann Neurol* 1983;13:69–71.

Kucera P, Dolivo M, Coulon P, Flamand A. Pathways of the early propagation of virulent and avirulent rabies strains from the eye to the brain. *J Virol* 1985;55:158–162.

Kulhanjian JA, Soroush V, Au DS, et al. Identification of women at unsuspected risk of primary infection with herpes simplex virus type 2 during pregnancy. *N Engl J Med* 1992;326:916–920.

Kumagami H. Experimental facial nerve paralysis. *Arch Otolaryngol* 1972;95:305–312.

Kumar M, Resnick L, Loewenstein DA, Berger J, Eisdorfer C. Brain-reactive antibodies and the AIDS dementia complex. *J AIDS* 1989;2:469–471.

Kumar ML, Nankervis GA, Gold E. Inapparent congenital cytomegalovirus infection: a follow-up study. *N Engl J Med* 1973;288:1370–1372.

Kure K, Lyman WD, Weidenheim KM, Dickson DW. Cellular localization of an HIV-1 antigen in subacute AIDS encephalitis using an improved double-labeling immunohistochemical method. *Am J Pathol* 1990;136:1085–1091.

Kurent JE, Brooks BR, Madden DL, Sever JL, Engel WK. CSF viral antibodies: evaluation in amyotrophic lateral sclerosis and late onset post-poliomyelitis progressive muscular atrophy. *Arch Neurol* 1979;36:269–273.

Kurland LT, Wiederholt WC, Kirkpatrick JW, Potter G, Armstrong P. Swine influenza vaccine and Guillain–Barré syndrome. *Arch Neurol* 1985;42:1089–1090.

Kuroda Y, Matsui M. Cerebrospinal fluid interferon-gamma is increased in HTLV-I-associated myelopathy. *J Neuroimmunol* 1993;42:223–226.

Kuroda Y, Takashima H, Ideda A, et al. Treatment of HTLV-I-associated myelopathy with high-dose intravenous gammaglobulin. *J Neurol* 1991;238:309–314.

Kuroda Y, Yukitake M, Kurohara K, Takashima H, Matsui M. A follow-up study on spastic paraparesis in Japanese HAM/TSP. *J Neurol Sci* 1995;132:174–176.

Kurogi H, Inaba Y, Goto Y, et al. Serologic evidence for etiologic role of Akabane virus in epizootic abortion–arthrogryposis–hydranencephaly in cattle in Japan, 1972–1974. *Arch Virol* 1975;47:71–83.

Kurtzke JF. Epidemiologic evidence for multiple sclerosis as an infection. *Clin Microbiol Rev* 1993;6: 382–427.

Kurtzke JF, Gudmundsson KR, Bergmann S. Multiple sclerosis Iceland. I. Evidence of a post-war epidemic. *Neurology* 1982;32:143–150.

Kurtzke JF, Hyllested K. Multiple sclerosis in the Faroe Islands. I. Clinical and epidemiological features. *Ann Neurol* 1979;5:6–21.

Kurtzke JF, Hyllested K, Arbuckle JD, et al. Multiple sclerosis in the Faroe Islands. IV. The lack of a relationship between canine distemper and the epidemics of MS. *Acta Neurol Scand* 1988;78:484–500.

La Monica N, Almond JW, Racaniello VR. A mouse model for poliovirus neurovirulence identifies mutations that attenuate the virus for humans. *J Virol* 1987;61:2917–2920.

Lackner AA, Dandekar S, Gardner MB. Neurobiology of simian and feline immunodeficiency virus infections. *Brain Pathol* 1991;1:201–212.

Lackritz EM, Satten GA, Aberle-Grasse J, et al. Estimated risk of transmission of the human immunodeficiency virus by screened blood in the United States. *N Engl J Med* 1995;333:1721–1725.

Lafaille JJ, Nagashima K, Katsuki M, Tonegawa S. High incidence of spontaneous autoimmune encephalomyelitis in immunodeficient anti-myelin basic protein T cell receptor transgenic mice. *Cell* 1994;78:399–408.

Lafferty WE, Coombs RW, Bennedetti J, Critchlow C, Corey L. Recurrences after oral and genital herpes simplex virus infection, influence of site of infection and viral type. *N Engl J Med* 1987;316: 1444–1449.

Lagacé-Simard J, Descôteaux J-P, Lussier G. Experimental pneumovirus infections. *Am J Pathol* 1980; 101:31–40.

Lagacé-Simard J, Descôteaux J-P, Lussier G. Experimental pneumovirus infections. 2. Hydrocephalus of hamsters and mice due to infection with human respiratory syncytial virus (RS). *Am J Pathol* 1982; 107:36–40.

Lai D-W, Gragasin ME. Electroencephalography in herpes simplex encephalitis. *J Clin Neurophysiol* 1988;5:87–103.

Lakeman FD, Koga J, Whitley RJ. Detection of antigen to herpes simplex virus in cerebrospinal fluid from patients with herpes simplex encephalitis. *J Infect Dis* 1987;155:1172–1178.

Lakeman FD, Whitley RJ. Diagnosis of herpes simplex encephalitis: application of polymerase chain reaction to cerebrospinal fluid from brain-biopsied patients and correlation with disease. *J Infect Dis* 1995;171:857–863.

Lampert F, Lampert P. Multiple sclerosis. *Arch Neurol* 1975;32:425–427.

Lampert PW. Autoimmune and virus-induced demyelinating diseases. *Am J Pathol* 1978;91:175–208.

Lampert PW, Gajdusek DC, Gibbs CJ Jr. Subacute spongiform virus encephalopathies. *Am J Pathol* 1972; 40:103–110.

Lampert PW, Sims JK, Kniazeff AJ. Mechanism of demyelination in JHM virus encephalomyelitis: electron microscopic studies. *Acta Neuropathol (Berl)* 1973;24:76–85.

Landesman SH, Kalish LA, Burns DN, et al. Obstetrical factors and the transmission of human immunodeficiency virus type 1 from mother to child. *N Engl J Med* 1996;334:1617–1623.

Landgren M, Kyllerman M, Bergström T, Dotevall L, Ljungström L, Ricksten A. Diagnosis of Epstein–Barr virus-induced central nervous system infections by DNA amplification from cerebrospinal fluid. *Ann Neurol* 1994;35:631–635.

Landrigan PJ, Witte JJ. Neurologic disorders following live measles virus vaccination. *JAMA* 1973;223: 1459–1462.

Landry O. Note sur la paralysie ascendante aique. *Gaz Hebd Med Paris* 1859;6:472–486.

Lane TE, Buchmeier MJ, Watry DD, Fox HS. Expression of inflammatory cytokines and inducible nitric oxide synthase in brains of SIV-infected rhesus monkeys: applications to HIV-induced central nervous system disease. *Mol Med* 1996;2:27–37.

Langston C, Lewis DE, Hammill HA, et al. Excess intrauterine fetal demise associated with maternal human immunodeficiency virus infection. *J Infect Dis* 1995;172:1451–1460.

Lapinleimu K, Koskimies O, Cantell K, Saxen L. Viral antibodies in mothers of defective children. *Teratology* 1972;5:345–352.

Larder BA, Darby G, Richman DD. HIV with reduced sensitivity to zidovudine (AZT) isolated during prolonged therapy. *Science* 1989;243:1731–1734.

Lascelles RG, Jonson PJ, Longso M, Chiang A. Infectious mononucleosis presenting as acute cerebellar syndrome. *Lancet* 1973;2:707–709.

Laver WG, Webster RG. Ecology of influenza viruses in lower mammals and birds. *Br Med Bull* 1979; 35:29–33.

Lavi E, Fishman PS, Highkin MK, Weiss SR. Limbic encephalitis after inhalation of a murine coronavirus. *Lab Invest* 1988;58:31–36.

Lawton AH, Seaburg C, Branch LC, Azar GJ, Bond JO. Follow-up studies of St. Louis encephalitis in Florida: comparison of 1964 and 1965 health question findings. *South Med J* 1966;59:1409–1414.

Leake CJ, Johnson RT. The pathogenesis of Japanese encephalitis virus in *Culex tritaemiorhynchus* mosquitoes. *Trans R Soc Trop Med Hyg* 1987;81:681–687.

Lebon P, Lyon G. Non-congenital rubella encephalitis. *Lancet* 1974;2:468.

Lederberg J. Medical science, infectious disease, and the unity of humankind. *JAMA* 1988;260:684–685.

Lederberg J, Shope RE, Oaks SC Jr. *Emerging infections, microbial threats to health in the United States.* Washington, DC: National Academy Press, 1992.

Lednicky JA, Garcea RL, Bergsagel DJ, Butel JS. Natural simian virus 40 strains are present in human choroid plexus and ependymoma tumors. *Virology* 1995;212:710–717.

Leduc, JW. Epidemiology and ecology of the California serogroup viruses. *Am J Trop Med Hyg* 1987; 37[Suppl]:60S–68S.

Lee MR, Ho DD, Gurney ME. Functional interaction and partial homology between human immunodeficiency virus and neuroleukin. *Science* 1987;237:1047–1052.

Lefebvre S, Hubert B, Tekaia F, Brahic M, Bureau JF. Isolation from human brain of six previously unreported cDNAs related to the reverse transcriptase of human endogenous retroviruses. *AIDS Res Hum Retroviruses* 1995;11:231–237.

Leff RL, Love LA, Miller FW, et al. Viruses in idiopathic inflammatory myopathies: absence of candidate viral genomes in muscle. *Lancet* 1992;2:1192–1195.

Lehky TJ, Flerlage N, Katz D, et al. Human T-cell lymphotropic virus type II-associated myelopathy: clinical and immunologic profiles. *Ann Neurol* 1996;40:714–723.

Lehky TJ, Fox CH, Koenig S, et al. Detection of human T-lymphotropic virus type I (HTLV-I) tax RNA in the central nervous system of HTLV-I-associated myelopathy/tropical spastic paraparesis patients by in situ hybridization. *Ann Neurol* 1995;37:167–175.

Lehmann-Grube F. Lymphocytic choriomeningitis virus. *Virol Monogr* 1971;10:1–173.

Leib DA, Bogard CL, Kosz-Vnenchak M, et al. A deletion mutant of the latency-associated transcript of herpes simplex virus type 1 reactivates from the latent state with reduced frequency. *J Virol* 1989;63: 2893–2900.

Leis AA, Butler IJ. Infantile herpes zoster ophthalmicus and acute hemiparesis following intrauterine chickenpox. *Neurology* 1987;37:1537–1538.

Lelong M, Lépine P, Alison F, Le-Tan-Vinh, Satgé P, Chany C. La pneumonie à virus de groupe A.P.C. chez de nourrison isolement du virus: les lésions anatomohistologiques. *Arch Fr Pediatr* 1956;13: 1091–1096.

LeNaour R, Clayette P, Henin Y, et al. Infection of human macrophages with an endogenous tumour necrosis factor-alpha (TNF-alpha)-independent human immunodeficiency virus type 1 isolate is unresponsive to the TNF-alpha synthesis inhibitor RP 55778. *J Gen Virol* 1994;75:1379–1388.

Leneman F. The Guillain–Barré syndrome. *Arch Intern Med* 1966;118:139–144.

Lennette EH, Caplan GE, Magoffin RL. Mumps virus infections simulating paralytic poliomyelitis. *Pediatrics* 1960;25:788–797.

Lentz TL, Burrage TG, Smith AL, Crick J, Tignor GH. Is the acetylcholine receptor a rabies virus receptor? *Science* 1982;215:182–184.

Leon-Monzon M, Dalakas MC. Absence of persistent infection with enteroviruses in muscles of patients with inflammatory myopathies. *Ann Neurol* 1992;32:219–222.

Leon-Monzon ME, Dalakas MC. Detection of poliovirus antibodies and poliovirus genome in patients with the post-polio syndrome. *Ann NY Acad Sci* 1995;753:208–218.

Leonard JC, Tobin OH. Polyneuritis associated with cytomegalovirus infections. *Q J Med* 1971;40: 435–442.

Leparc I, Kopecka H, Fuchs F, Janatova I, Aymard M, Julien J. Search for poliovirus in specimens from patients with the post-polio syndrome. *Ann NY Acad Sci* 1995;753:233–236.

Lepow ML, Coyne N, Thompson LB, Carver DH, Robbins FC. A clinical, epidemiological and laboratory investigation of aseptic meningitis during the four-year period 1955–1958. II. The clinical disease and its sequelae. *N Engl J Med* 1962;266:1188–1193.

Lerner RA. Tapping the immunological repertoire to produce antibodies of predetermined specificity. *Nature* 1982;299:592–596.

Letson GW, Bailey RE, Pearson J, Tsai TF. Eastern equine encephalitis (EEE): a description of the 1989 outbreak, recent epidemiologic trends, and the association of rainfall with EEE occurrence. *Am J Trop Med Hyg* 1993;49:677–685.

Letvin NL, King NW. Immunologic and pathologic manifestations of the infection of rhesus monkeys with simian immunodeficiency virus of macaques. *J AIDS* 1990;3:1023–1040.

Levin MC, Jacobson S. HTLV-I associated myelopathy/tropical spastic paraparesis (HAM/TSP): a chronic progressive neurologic disease associated with immunologically mediated damage to the central nervous system. *J Neurovirol* 1997;3:126–140.

Levin MC, Lehky TJ, Flerlage AN, et al. Immunologic analysis of a spinal cord-biopsy specimen from a patient with human T-cell lymphotropic virus type I-associated neurologic disease. *N Engl J Med* 1997;336:839–845.

Levine B, Hardwick JM, Trapp BD, Crawford TO, Bollinger RC, Griffin DE. Antibody-mediated clearance of alphavirus infection from neurons. *Science* 1991;254:856–860.

Levine B, Huang Q, Isaacs JT, Reed JC, Griffin DE, Hardwick JM. Conversion of lytic to persistent alphavirus infection by the bcl-2 cellular oncogene. *Nature* 1993;361:739–742.

Levine S, Wenk EJ. A hyperacute form of allergic encephalomyelitis. *Am J Pathol* 1965;47:61–88.

Levitt LP, Rich TA, Kinde SW, Lewis AL, Gates EH, Bond JO. Central nervous system mumps: a review of 64 cases. *Neurology* 1970;20:829–834.

Levy JA. *HIV and the pathogenesis of AIDS.* Washington, DC: ASM Press, 1994:1–359.

Levy JA, Shimabukuro J, Hollander H, Mills J, Kaminsky L. Isolation of AIDS-associated retroviruses from cerebrospinal fluid and brain of patients with neurological symptoms. *Lancet* 1985;2:586–588.

Lewis J, Wesselingh SL, Griffin DE, Hardwick JM. Alphavirus-induced apoptosis in mouse brains correlates with neurovirulence. *J Virol* 1996;70:1828–1835.

Lewis JM, Utz JP. Orchitis, parotitis, and meningoencephalitis due to lymphocytic choriomeningitis virus. *N Engl J Med* 1961;265:776–780.

Li J, Zhang LB, Yoneyama T, et al. Genetic basis of the neurovirulence of type 1 polioviruses isolated from vaccine-associated paralytic patients. *Arch Virol* 1996;141:1047–1054.

Liberski PP, Yanagihara R, Gibbs CJ Jr, Gajdusek DC. Spread of Creutzfeldt-Jakob disease virus along visual pathways after intraocular inoculation. *Arch Virol* 1990;111:141–147.

Libíková H, Pogády J, Stancek D, Mucha V. Hepatitis B and herpes viral components in the cerebrospinal fluid of chronic schizophrenic and senile demented patients. *Acta Virol (Praha)* 1981;25:182–190.

Libman MD, Dascal A, Kramer MS, Mendelson J. Strategies for the prevention of neonatal infection with herpes simplex virus: a decision analysis. *Rev Infect Dis* 1991;13:1093–1104.

Liebert UG, Schneider-Schaulies S, Baczko K, Ter Meulen V. Antibody-induced restriction of viral gene expression in measles encephalitis in rats. *J Virol* 1990;64:706–713.

Liedtke W, Malessa R, Faustmann PM, Eis-Hübinger A-M. Human herpesvirus 6 polymerase chain reaction findings in human immunodeficiency virus associated neurological disease and multiple sclerosis. *J Neurovirol* 1995;1:253–258.

Likar M, Dane DW. An illness resembling acute poliomyelitis caused by a virus of the Russian spring–summer encephalitis/louping ill group of Northern Ireland. *Lancet* 1958;1:456–458.

Lilienfeld AM. On the methodology of investigations of etiologic factors in chronic diseases: some comments. *J Chronic Dis* 1959;10:41–46.

Lin S-M, Ryu S-J, Liaw Y-F. Guillain–Barré syndrome associated with acute delta hepatitis virus superinfection. *J Med Virol* 1989;28:144–145.

Lindegren ML, Fehrs LJ, Hadler SC, Hinman AR. Update: rubella and congenital rubella syndrome, 1980–1990. *Epidemiol Rev* 1991;13:341–348.

Lindsay JR. Histopathology of deafness due to postnatal viral disease. *Arch Otolaryngol* 1973;98:258–264.

Linneman CC, Alvira MM. Pathogenesis of varicella–zoster angiitis in the CNS. *Arch Neurol* 1980;37:239–240.

Linssen WHJP, Fabreëls FJM, Wevers RA. Infective acute transverse myelopathy: report of two cases. *Neuropediatrics* 1991;22:107–109.

Lionnet F, Pulik M, Genet P, et al. Myelitis due to varicella–zoster virus in two patients with AIDS: successful treatment with acyclovir. *Clin Infect Dis* 1996;22:138–140.

Lipton HL. Theiler's virus infection in mice: an unusual biphasic disease process leading to demyelination. *Infect Immun* 1975;11:1147–1155.

Lipton HL. Is JC virus latent in brain? *Ann Neurol* 1991a;29:433–434.

Lipton HL, Friedmann A, Sethi P, Crowther JR. Characterization of Vilyuisk virus as a picornavirus. *J Med Virol* 1983;12:195–203.

Lipton HL, Gonzalez-Scarano F. Central nervous system immunity in mice infected with Theiler's virus. I. Local neutralizing antibody response. *J Infect Dis* 1978;137:145–151.

Lipton HL, Johnson RT. The pathogenesis of rat virus infections in the newborn hamster. *Lab Invest* 1972;27:508–513.

Lipton HL, Melvold R, Miller SD, DalCanto MC. Mutation of a major histocompatibility class I locus, H-2D, leads to an increased virus burden and disease susceptibility in Theiler's virus-induced demyelinating disease. *J Neurovirol* 1995;1:138–144.

Lipton SA. Calcium channel antagonists and human immunodeficiency virus coat protein-mediated neuronal injury. *Ann Neurol* 1991b;30:110–114.

Lisak RP, Mitchell M, Zweiman B, Orrechio E, Asbury AK. Guillain–Barre syndrome and Hodgkin's disease: three cases with immunological studies. *Ann Neurol* 1977;1:72–78.

Liu C, Yoth DW, Rodina P, Shauf LR, Gonzalez G. A comparative study of the pathogenesis of western equine and eastern equine encephalomyelitis viral infections in mice by intracerebral and subcutaneous inoculations. *J Infect Dis* 1970;122:53–63.

Liu GT, Holmes GL. Varicella with delayed contralateral hemiparesis detected by MRI. *Pediatr Neurol* 1990;6:131–134.

Llinas R, Hillman DE, Precht W. Neuronal circuit reorganization in mammalian agranular cerebellar cortex. *J Neurobiol* 1973;4:69–94.

Lodmell DL, Ewalt LC. Pathogenesis of street rabies virus infections in resistant and susceptible strains of mice. *J Virol* 1985;55:788–795.

Loffel NB, Rossi LN, Mumenthaler M, Lutschg J, Ludin HP. The Landry–Guillain–Barré syndrome: complications, prognosis, and natural history in 123 cases. *J Neurol Sci* 1977;33:71–79.

Logigian EL, Kaplan RF, Steere AC. Chronic neurologic manifestations of Lyme disease. *N Engl J Med* 1990;323:1438–1444.

London WT, Fuccillo DA, Sever JL, Kent SG. Influenza virus as a teratogen in rhesus monkeys. *Nature* 1975;255:483–484.

Louis J-C, Magal E, Takayama S, Varon S. CNTF protection of oligodendrocytes against natural and tumor necrosis factor-induced death. *Science* 1993;259:689–692.

Love S, Hill TJ, Maitland NJ. MS strain of type 2 herpes simplex virus produces necrotizing retinitis in mice. *J Neurol Sci* 1993;115:144–152.

Lum LCS, Lam SK, Choy YS, George R, Harun F. Dengue encephalitis: a true entity? *Am J Trop Med Hyg* 1996;54:256–259.

Lunch B, Kristensson K, Norrby E. Selective infections of olfactory and respiratory epithelium by vesicular stomatitis and Sendai viruses. *Neuropathol Appl Neurobiol* 1987;13:111–122.

Lundstrom R. Rubella during pregnancy. *Acta Paediatr Scand* 1962;51[Suppl]:S1–S110.

Luppi M, Barozzi P, Maiorana A, Marasca R, Torelli G. Human herpesvirus 6 infection in normal human brain tissue. *J Infect Dis* 1994;169:943–944.

Luria SE, Darnell JE, Baltimore D, Campbell A. *General virology,* 3rd ed. New York: John Wiley & Sons, 1978.

Lusher JM, Operskalski EA, Aledort LM, et al. Risk of human immunodeficiency virus type 1 infection among sexual and nonsexual household contacts of persons with congenital clotting disorders. *Pediatrics* 1991;88:242–249.

Lwoff A. The concept of virus. *J Gen Microbiol* 1957;17:239–253.

Lyman WD, Kress Y, Kure K, Rashbaum WK, Rubinstein A, Soeiro R. Detection of HIV in fetal central nervous system tissue. *AIDS* 1990;4:917–920.

Lynberg MC, Khoury MJ, Lu X, Cocian T. Maternal flu, fever, and the risk of neural tube defects: a population-based case–control study. *Am J Epidemiol* 1994;140:244–255.

Lynch WP, Czub S, McAtee FJ, Hayes SF, Portis JL. Murine retrovirus-induced spongiform encephalopathy: productive infection of microglia and cerebellar neurons in accelerated CNS disease. *Neuron* 1991;7:365–379.

Lynch WP, Portis JL. Murine retrovirus-induced spongiform encephalopathy: disease expression is dependent on postnatal development of the central nervous system. *J Virol* 1993;67:2601–2610.

Lynch WP, Robertson SJ, Portis JL. Induction of focal spongiform neurodegeneration in developmentally resistant mice by implantation of murine retrovirus-infected microglia. *J Virol* 1995;69:1408–1419.

Lyon G, Dodge PR, Adams RD. The acute encephalopathies of obscure origin in infants and children. *Brain* 1961;84:680–708.

Maas JJ, Beersma MFC, Haan J, Jonkers GJPM, Kroes ACM. Bilateral brachial plexus neuritis following parvovirus B19 and cytomegalovirus infection. *Ann Neurol* 1996;40:928–932.

Maassab HF, DeBorde DC. Development and characterization of cold-adapted viruses for use as live virus vaccines. *Vaccine* 1985;3:355–369.

Maassab JF. The role of viruses in sudden deafness. *Adv Otorhinolaryngol* 1973;20:229–235.

Mabruk MJEMF, Glasgow GM, Flack AM, et al. Effect of infection with the ts22 mutant of Semliki Forest virus on development of the central nervous system in the fetal mouse. *J Virol* 1989;63:4027–4033.

MacDonald H, Tobin JOH. Congenital cytomegalovirus infection: a collaborative study on epidemiological, clinical, and laboratory findings. *Dev Med Child Neurol* 1978;20:471–482.

MacDonald MG, Ginzburg HM, Bolan JC. HIV infection in pregnancy: epidemiology and clinical management. *J AIDS* 1991;4:100–108.

MacDonald ST, Sutherland K, Ironside JW. Prion protein genotype and pathological phenotype studies in sporadic Creutzfeldt–Jakob disease. *Neuropathol Appl Neurobiol* 1996;22:285–292.

MacFarlane DW, Boyd RD, Dodrill CB, Tufts E. Intrauterine rubella, head size, and intellect. *Pediatrics* 1975;55:797–801.

Mackenzie IRA, Carrigan DR, Wiley CA. Chronic myelopathy associated with human herpesvirus-6. *Neurology* 1995;45:2015–2017.

Mackenzie JS, Lindsay MD, Coelen RJ, Broom AK, Hall RA, Smith DW. Arboviruses causing human disease in the Australasian zoogeographic region. *Arch Virol* 1994;136:447–467.

MacMahon EME, Glass JD, Hayward SD, et al. Epstein–Barr virus in AIDS-related primary central nervous system lymphoma. *Lancet* 1991;2:969–973.

Magliocco AM, Demetrick DJ, Sarnat HB, Hwang WS. Varicella embryopathy. *Arch Pathol Lab Med* 1992;116:181–186.

Magliulo E, Torre D, Dietz A, Portelli V, Armignacco O. Post-varicella acute transverse myelitis. *Infection* 1979;7:260–261.

Mahalingam R, Wellish M, Brucklier J, Gilden DH. Persistence of varicella–zoster virus DNA in elderly patients with postherpetic neuralgia. *J Neurovirol* 1995;1:130–133.

Mahalingam R, Wellish M, Wolf W, et al. Latent varicella–zoster viral DNA in human trigeminal and thoracic ganglia. *N Engl J Med* 1990;323:627–631.

Mahalingam R, Wellish MC, Dueland AN, Cohrs RJ, Gilden DH. Localization of herpes simplex virus and varicella zoster virus DNA in human ganglia. *Ann Neurol* 1992;31:444–448.

Maiztegui JI, Fernandez NJ, de Damilano A. Efficacy of immune plasma in treatment of Argentine haemorrhagic fever and association between treatment and a late neurological syndrome. *Lancet* 1979;2: 1216–1217.

Manco-Johnson MJ, Nuss R, Key N, et al. Lupus anticoagulant and protein S deficiency in children with postvaricella purpura fulminans or thrombosis. *Pediatrics* 1996;128:319–323.

Manian FA, Kindred M, Fulling KH. Chronic varicella–zoster virus myelitis without cutaneous eruption in a patient with AIDS: report of a fatal case. *Clin Infect Dis* 1995;21:986–988.

Mankowski JL, Spelman JP, Ressetar HG, et al. Neurovirulent simian immunodeficiency virus replicates productively in endothelial cells of the central nervous system in vivo and in vitro. *J Virol* 1994;68: 8202–8208.

Mann JM. AIDS in the 1990s: a global analysis. *Pharos* 1993;56:2–11.

Manuelidis EE, de Figueiredo JM, Kim JH, Fritch WW, Manuelidis L. Transmission studies from blood of Alzheimer disease patients and healthy relatives. *Proc Natl Acad Sci USA* 1988;85:4898–4901.

Manuelides EE, Thomas L. Occlusion of brain capillaries by endothelial swelling in *Mycoplasma* infections. *Proc Natl Acad Sci USA* 1973;70:706–709.

Manuelidis L, Sklaviadis T, Akowitz A, Fritch W. Viral particles are required for infection in neurodegenerative Creutzfeldt–Jakob disease. *Proc Natl Acad Sci USA* 1995;92:5124–5128.

Marberg K, Goldblum N, Sterk VV, Jasinska-Klingberg W, Klingberg MA. The natural history of West Nile fever. I. Clinical observations during an epidemic in Israel. *Am J Hyg* 1956;64:259–269.

Marés-Segura R, Solá-Lomaglia R, Soler-Singla L, Pou-Serradell A. Guillain–Barré syndrome associated with hepatitis A. *Ann Neurol* 1986;19:100.

Margolis G, Kilham L. In pursuit of an ataxic hamster, or virus-induced cerebellar hypoplasia. In: *International Academy of Pathology Monograph 9: Central nervous system*. Baltimore: Williams & Wilkins, 1968:157–183.

Margolis G, Kilham L. Hydrocephalus in hamsters, ferrets, rats and mice following inoculations with reovirus type 1. II. Pathologic studies. *Lab Invest* 1969;21:189–198.

Margolis TP, Sedarati F, Dobson AT, Feldman LT, Stevens JG. Pathways of viral gene expression during acute neuronal infection with HSV-1. *Virology* 1992;189:150–160.

Margulis MS, Soloviev VD, Schubladze AK. Aetiology and pathogenesis of acute sporadic disseminated encephalomyelitis and multiple sclerosis. *J Neurol Neurosurg Psychiatry* 1946;9:63–74.

Marie P. Scléroe en plaques et maladies infectieuses. *Prog Med* 1884;12:287–289.

Marinesco G, Draganesco S. Recherches experimentales sur la neurotropisme du virus herpetique. *Ann Inst Pasteur* 1923;37:753–783.

Marion RW, Wiznia AA, Hutcheon RG, Rubinstein A. Fetal AIDS syndrome score: correlation between severity of dysmorphism and age at diagnosis of immunodeficiency. *Am J Dis Child* 1987;141:429–431.

Marra CM. Neurologic complications of *Bartonella henselae* infection. *Curr Opin Neurol* 1995;8:164–169.

Marsden JP, Hurst EW. Acute perivascular myelinoclasis ("acute dissemination encephalomyelitis") in smallpox. *Brain* 1932;55:181–225.

Marsh RF, Bessen RA, Lehmann S, Hartsough GR. Epidemiological and experimental studies on a new incident of transmissible mink encephalopathy. *J Gen Virol* 1991;72:589–594.

Martin JR, Goudswaard J, Palsson PA, et al. Cerebrospinal fluid immunoglobulins in sheep with visna, a slow virus infection of the central nervous system. *J Neuroimmunol* 1982;3:139–148.

Martin JR, Holt RK, Webster HF. Herpes-simplex-related antigen in human demyelinative disease and encephalitis. *Acta Neuropathol (Berl)* 1988;76:325–337.

Martin R, McFarland HF. Immunological aspects of experimental allergic encephalomyelitis and multiple sclerosis. *Crit Rev Clin Lab Sci* 1995;32:121–182.

Martone WJ, Kaufmann AF. Leptospirosis in humans in the United States, 1974–1978. *J Infect Dis* 1979; 140:1020–1022.

Marttila RJ, Rinne UK, Tiilikainen A. Virus antibodies in Parkinson's disease. *J Neurol Sci* 1982;54:227–238.

Martyn CN, Cruddas M, Compston DAS. Symptomatic Epstein–Barr virus infection and multiple sclerosis. *J Neurol Neurosurg Psychiatry* 1993;56:167–168.

Masliah E, Ge N, Morey M, Deteresa R, Terry RD, Wiley CA. Cortical dendritic pathology in human immunodeficiency virus encephalitis. *Lab Invest* 1992;66:285–291.

Masters CL, Gajdusek DC. The spectrum of Creutzfeldt–Jakob disease and the virus-induced subacute spongiform encephalopathies. In: Smith WT, Cavanagh JB, eds. *Recent advances in neuropathology,* 2nd ed. Edinburgh: Churchill Livingstone, 1982:139–163.

Masters CL, Gajdusek DC, Gibbs CJ Jr. Creutzfeldt–Jakob disease virus isolations from the Gerstmann–Sträussler syndrome with an analysis of the various forms of amyloid plaque deposition in the virus-induced spongiform encephalopathies. *Brain* 1981;104:559–588.

Masters CL, Richardson EP Jr. Subacute spongiform encephalopathy (Creutzfeldt–Jakob disease): the nature and progression of spongiform change. *Brain* 1978;101:333–344.

Mastrianni JA, Iannicola C, Myers RM, DeArmond S, Prusiner SB. Mutation of the prion protein gene at codon 208 in familial Creutzfeldt–Jakob disease. *Neurology* 1996;47:1305–1312.

Masuda M, Hoffman PM, Ruscetti SK. Viral determinants that control the neuropathogenicity of PVC-211 murine leukemia virus in vivo determine brain capillary endothelial cell tropism of the virus in vitro. *J Virol* 1993;67:4580–4587.

Matsui M, Kakigi R, Watanabe S, Kuroda Y. Recurrent demyelinating transverse myelitis in a high titer HBs-antigen carrier. *J Neurol Sci* 1996;139:235–237.

Matsuo H, Tsujihata M, Satoh A, et al. Plasmapheresis in treatment of human T-lymphotropic virus type-I associated myelopathy. *Lancet* 1988;2:1109–1114.

Matthews WB. Epidemiology of Creutzfeldt–Jakob disease in England and Wales. *J Neurol Neurosurg Psychiatry* 1975;38:210–213.

Mawle AC, Nisenbaum R, Dobbins JB, et al. Immune responses associated with chronic fatigue syndrome: a case–control study. *J Infect Dis* 1997;175:136–141.

Mawle AC, Nisenbaum R, Dobbins JG, et al. Seroepidemiology of chronic fatigue syndrome: a case–control study. *Clin Infect Dis* 1995;21:1386–1389.

Max MB. Treatment of post-herpetic neuralgia: antidepressants. *Ann Neurol* 1994;35[Suppl]:S50–S53.

Mayer JLR, Beardsley DS. Varicella-associated thrombocytopenia: autoantibodies against platelet surface glycoprotein V. *Pediatr Res* 1996;40:615–619.

McArthur JC. Neurologic manifestations of AIDS. *Medicine (Baltimore)* 1987;66:407–437.

McArthur JC, Cohen BA, Farzedegan H, et al. Cerebrospinal fluid abnormalities in homosexual men with and without neuropsychiatric findings. *Ann Neurol* 1988;23[Suppl]:S34–S37.

McArthur JC, Cohen BA, Selnes OA, et al. Low prevalence of neurological and neuropsychological abnormalities in otherwise healthy HIV-1-infected individuals: results from the multicenter AIDS cohort study. *Ann Neurol* 1989;26:601–611.

McArthur JC, Hoover DR, Bacellar H, et al. Dementia in AIDS patients: incidence and risk factors. *Neurology* 1993;43:2245–2252.

McArthur JC, Nance-Sproson TE, Griffin DE, et al. The diagnostic utility of elevation in cerebrospinal fluid β-microglobulin in HIV-1 dementia. *Neurology* 1992;42:1707–1712.

McArthur JC, Sipos E, Cornblath DR, et al. Identification of mononuclear cells in CSF of patients with HIV infection. *Neurology* 1989;39:66–70.

McArthur JC, Sipos E, Cornblath DR, et al. Identification of mononuclear cells in cerebrospinal fluid of patients with HIV infection. *Neurology* 1992 (*in press*).

McCance DJ, Sebesteny A, Griffin BE, Balkwill F, Tilly R, Gregson NA. A paralytic disease in nude mice associated with polyoma virus infection. *J Gen Virol* 1983;64:57–67.

McCarthy JT, Amer J. Post-varicella acute transverse myelitis: a case presentation and review of the literature. *Pediatrics* 1978;62:202–204.

McCarthy M, Fay DB, Jubelt B, Johnson RT. Comparative studies of five strains of mumps virus *in vitro* as in neonatal hamsters: evaluation of growth, cytopathogenicity and neurovirulence. *J Med Virol* 1980;5:1–15.

McCarthy VP, Zimmerman AW, Miller CA. Central nervous system manifestations of parainfluenza virus type 3 infections in childhood. *Pediatr Neurol* 1990;6:197–201.

McClure JJ, Lindsay WA, Taylor W, Ochoa R, Issel CJ, Coulter SJ. Ataxia in four horses with equine infectious anemia. *J Am Vet Med Assoc* 1982;180:279–283.

McComas AJ, Upton AR, Sica RE. Motoneurone disease and ageing. *Lancet* 1973;2:1477–1480.

McCormick WF, Rodnitzky RL, Schochet SS, McKee AP. Varicella–zoster encephalomyelitis. *Arch Neurol* 1969;21:559–570.

McCullers JA, Lakeman FD, Whitley RJ. Human herpesvirus 6 is associated with focal encephalitis. *Clin Infect Dis* 1995;21:571–576.

McCutchan JA. Cytomegalovirus infections of the nervous system in patients with AIDS. *Clin Infect Dis* 1995;20:747–754.

McFarland HF, Griffin DE, Johnson RT. Specificity of the inflammatory response in viral encephalitis. I. Adoptive immunization of immunosuppressed mice infected with Sindbis virus. *J Exp Med* 1972; 136:216–226.

McGrath NM, Anderson NE, Hope JKA, Croxson MC, Powell KF. Anterior opercular syndrome, caused by herpes simplex encephalitis. *Neurology* 1997;49:494–497.

McGuire D, Barhite S, Hollander H, Miles M. JC virus DNA in cerebrospinal fluid of human immunodeficiency virus-infected patients: predictive value for progressive multifocal leukoencephalopathy. *Ann Neurol* 1995;37:395–399.

McGuire TC, Crawford TB, Henson JB. Immunofluorescent localization of equine infectious anemia virus in tissue. *Am J Pathol* 1971;62:283–292.

McKeating JA. Biological consequences of human immunodeficiency virus type 1 envelope polymorphism: does variation matter? *J Gen Virol* 1996;77:2905–2919.

McKenna MJ, Mills BG. Immunohistochemical evidence of measles virus antigens in active osteosclerosis. *Otolaryngol Head Neck Surg* 1989;101:415–421.

McKhann GM, Cornblath DR, Griffin JW, et al. Acute motor axonal neuropathy: a frequent cause of acute flaccid paralysis in China. *Ann Neurol* 1993;33:333–342.

McKinney RE Jr, Katz SL, Wilfert CM. Chronic enteroviral meningoencephalitis in agammaglobulinemic patients. *Rev Infect Dis* 1987;9:886–887.

McLean CA, Masters CL, Vladimirtsev VA, et al. Viliuisk encephalomyelitis: review of the spectrum of pathological changes. *Neuropathol Appl Neurobiol* 1997;23:212–217.

McLean DM, Donohue WL. Powassan virus: isolation of virus from a fatal case of encephalitis. *Can Med Assoc J* 1959;80:708–711.

McVoy MA, Adler SP. Immunologic evidence for frequent age-related cytomegalovirus reactivation in seropositive immunocompetent individuals. *J Infect Dis* 1989;160:1–10.

Mead R. *A discourse on the small pox and measles.* London: A Dodd, 1747.

Meade RH, Chang TW. Zoster-like eruption due to echovirus 6. *Am J Dis Child* 1979;133:283–284.

Medori R, Tritschler H-J, LeBlanc A, et al. Fatal familial insomnia: a prion disease with a mutation at codon 178 of the prion protein gene. *N Engl J Med* 1992;326:444–449.

Mehta PD, Kulczycki J, Mehta SP, et al. Increased levels of β2-microglobulin, soluble interleukin-2 receptor, and soluble CD8 in patients with subacute sclerosing panencephalitis. *Clin Immunol Immunopathol* 1992;65:53–59.

Meier JL, Holman RP, Croen KD, Smialek JE, Straus SE. Varicella–zoster virus transcription in human trigeminal ganglia. *Virology* 1993;193:193–200.

Melanson M, Chalk C, Georgevich L, et al. Varicella–zoster virus DNA in CSF and arteries in delayed contralateral hemiplegia: evidence for viral invasion of cerebral arteries. *Neurology* 1996;47:569–570.

Melchers W, de Villser M, Jongen P, et al. The postpolio syndrome: no evidence for poliovirus persistence. *Ann Neurol* 1992;32:728–732.

Melnick JL, Dressman GR, McCollum CH, Petrie BL, Purek J, DeBakey ME. Cytomegalovirus antigen within human arterial smooth muscle cells. *Lancet* 1983;2:644–647.

Melnick SC, Flewett TH. Role of infection in the Guillain–Barré syndrome. *J Neurol Neurosurg Psychiatry* 1964;27:397–407.

Menninger KA. Influenza and schizophrenia. *Am J Psychiatry* 1926;5:469–479.

Menser MA, Dods L, Harley JD. A twenty-five year follow-up of congenital rubella. *Lancet* 1967;2: 1347–1350.

Menser MA, Forrest JM. Rubella: high incidence of defects in children considered normal at birth. *Med J Aust* 1974;1:123–126.

Meredith TA, Aaberg TM, Reeser FH. Rhegmatogenous retinal detachment complicating cytomegalovirus retinitis. *Am J Ophthalmol* 1979;87:793–796.

Merelli E, Sola P, Faglioni P, Poggi M, Montorsi M, Torelli G. Newest human herpesvirus (HHV-6) in the Guillain–Barré syndrome and other neurological diseases. *Acta Neurol Scand* 1992;85:334–336.

Merigan TC, Baer GM, Winkler WG, et al. Human leukocyte interferon administration to patients with symptomatic and suspected rabies. *Ann Neurol* 1984;16:82–87.

Merrill JE, Chen ISY. HIV-1, macrophages, glial cells, and cytokines in AIDS nervous system disease. *FASEB J* 1991;5:2391–2397.

Mertens G, Ieven M, Ursi D, Pattyn SR, Martin JJ, Parizel PM. Detection of herpes simplex virus in the cerebrospinal fluid of patients with encephalitis using the polymerase chain reaction. *J Neurol Sci* 1993;118:213–216.

Meyer HM Jr, Johnson RT, Crawford IP, Dascomb HE, Rogers NG. Central nervous system syndromes of "viral" etiology: a study of 713 cases. *Am J Med* 1960;29:334–347.

Meylan PR, Kornbluth RS, Zbinden I, Richman DD. Influence of host cell type and V3 loop of the surface glycoprotein on susceptibility of human immunodeficiency virus type 1 to polyanion compounds. *Antimicrob Agents Chemother* 1994;38:2910–2916.

Michaud J, Helle TL. Acute haemorrhagic leucoencephalitis localised to the brainstem and cerebellum: a report of two cases. *J Neurol Neurosurg Psychiatry* 1982;45:151–157.

Mihas A, Kirby JD, Kent SP. Hepatitis B antigen and polymyositis. *JAMA* 1978;239:221–222.

Mikol J, Felten-Papaiconomou A, Ferchal F, et al. Inclusion-body myositis: clinicopathological studies and isolation of an adenovirus type 2 from muscle biopsy specimen. *Ann Neurol* 1982;11:576–581.

Miller A. Selective decline in cellular immune response to varicella zoster in the elderly. *Neurology* 1980;30:582–587.

Miller E, Cradock-Watson JE, Pollock TM. Consequences of confirmed maternal rubella at successive stages of pregnancy. *Lancet* 1982;2:781–784.

Miller E, Goldacre M, Pugh S, et al. Risk of aseptic meningitis after measles, mumps, and rubella vaccine in UK children. *Lancet* 1993;1:979–982.

Miller HG. Prognosis of neurologic illness following vaccination against smallpox. *Arch Neurol* 1953;69:695–706.

Miller HG, Stanton JB. Neurological sequelae of prophylactic inoculation. *Q J Med* 1954;23:1–27.

Miller HG, Stanton JB, Gibbons JL. Parainfectious encephalomyelitis and related syndromes. *Q J Med* 1956;25:427–505.

Miller JR. Prolonged intracerebral infection with poliovirus in asymptomatic mice. *Ann Neurol* 1981;9:590–596.

Miller JR, Ramareddy VG, Myers JC. Amyotrophic lateral sclerosis: search for poliovirus by nucleic acid hybridization. *Neurology* 1980;30:884–886.

Miller SD, McRae BL, Vanderlugt CL, et al. Evolution of the T-cell repertoire during the course of experimental immune-mediated demyelinating diseases. *Immunol Rev* 1995;144:225–244.

Mims CA. Intracerebral injections and the growth of viruses in the mouse brain. *Br J Exp Pathol* 1960;41:52–59.

Mims CA. Aspects of the pathogenesis of virus diseases. *Bacteriol Rev* 1964;28:30–71.

Mims CA. Immunofluorescence study of the carrier state and mechanism of vertical transmission of lymphocytic choriomeningitis virus infection in mice. *J Pathol Bacteriol* 1966;91:395–402.

Mims CA. Pathogenesis of viral infections of the fetus. *Prog Med Virol* 1968;10:194–237.

Mims CA. Viral aetiology of diseases of obscure origin. *Br Med Bull* 1985;41:63–69.

Mims CA, Murphy FA, Taylor WP, Marshall ID. The pathogenesis of Ross River virus infections in mice. I. Ependymal infection, cortical thinning and hydrocephalus. *J Infect Dis* 1973;127:121–128.

Minckler DS, McLean EB, Shaw CM, Hendrickson A. Herpesvirus hominis encephalitis and retinitis. *Arch Ophthalmol* 1976;94:89–95.

Misbah SA, Spickett GP, Ryba PCJ, et al. Chronic enteroviral meningoencephalitis in agammaglobulinemia: case report and literature review. *J Clin Immunol* 1992;12:266–270.

Mitchell CJ, Niebylski ML, Smith GC, et al. Isolation of eastern equine encephalitis virus from *Aedes albopictus* in Florida. *Science* 1992;257:526–527.

Mitchell DN, Goswami KKA, Taylor P, et al. Failure to isolate a transmissible agent from the bone-marrow of patients with multiple sclerosis. *Lancet* 1979;2:415–416.

Mizrahi EM, Tharp BR. A characteristic EEG pattern in neonatal herpes simplex encephalitis. *Neurology* 1982;32:1215–1220.

Modlin JF. Perinatal echovirus infection: insights from a literature review of 61 cases of serious infection and 16 outbreaks in nurseries. *Rev Infect Dis* 1986;8:918–926.

Modlin JF, Jabbour JT, Witte JJ, Halsey NA. Epidemiologic studies of measles, measles vaccine, and subacute sclerosing panencephalitis. *Pediatrics* 1977;59:505–512.

Moench TR, Griffin DE. Immunocytochemical identification and quantitation of the mononuclear cells in the cerebrospinal fluid, meninges, and brain during acute viral meningoencephalitis. *J Exp Med* 1984;159:77–88.

Moench TR, Griffin DE, Obriecht CR, Vaisberg AJ, Johnson RT. Acute measles in patients with and without neurological involvement: distribution of measles virus antigen and RNA. *J Infect Dis* 1988;158: 433–442.

Mollaret P. La menigite endothelio-leucocytaire multi-recurrent benigne. *Rev Neurol (Paris)* 1977;133: 225–244.

Monath TP, Cropp DB, Harrison AK. Mode of entry of a neurotropic arbovirus into the central nervous system. *Lab Invest* 1983;48:399–410.

Monath TP, Nystrom RR, Bailey RE, Calisher CH, Muth DJ. Immunoglobulin M antibody capture enzyme-linked immunosorbent assay for diagnosis of St. Louis encephalitis. *J Clin Microbiol* 1984; 20:784–790.

Monath TP, Tsai TF. St. Louis encephalitis: lessons from the last decade. *Am J Trop Med Hyg* 1987; 37[Suppl]:40S–59S.

Monif GRG, Dische RM. Viral placentitis in congenital cytomegalovirus infection. *Am J Clin Pathol* 1972;58:445–449.

Monjan AA, Gilden DH, Cole GA, Nathanson N. Cerebellar hypoplasia in neonatal rats caused by lymphocytic choriomeningitis virus. *Science* 1970;171:194–196.

Monjan AA, Silverstein AM, Cole G.A. Lymphocytic choriomeningitis virus-induced retinopathy in newborn rats. *Invest Ophthalmol* 1972;11:850–856.

Monteyne P, Sindic CJM, Laterre EC. Recurrent meningitis and encephalitis associated with herpes simplex type 2: demonstration by polymerase chain reaction. *Eur Neurol* 1996;36:176–177.

Montgomery JR, Flanders RW, Yow MD. Congenital anomalies and herpesvirus infection. *Am J Dis Child* 1973;126:364–366.

Montgomery RD. The epidemiology of myelopathy associated with human T-lymphotropic virus 1. *Trans R Soc Trop Med Hyg* 1993;87:154–159.

Moore M, Baron RC, Filstein MR, et al. Aseptic meningitis and high school football players, 1978 and 1980. *JAMA* 1983;249:2039–2042.

Mora CA, Garruto RM, Brown P, et al. Seroprevalence of antibodies to HTLV-I in patients with chronic neurological disorders other than tropical spastic paraparesis. *Ann Neurol* 1988;23[Suppl]: S192–S195.

Morgan M, Nathwani D. Facial palsy and infection: the unfolding story. *Clin Infect Dis* 1992;14:263–271.

Morgani JB. *The seats and causes of disease investigated by anatomy, 1769.* London: Millar and Cadell, 1769.

Mori M, Kurata H, Tajima M, Shimada H. JC virus detection by in situ hybridization in brain tissue from elderly patients. *Ann Neurol* 1991;29:428–432.

Morimoto K, Patel M, Corisdeo S, et al. Characterization of a unique variant of bat rabies virus responsible for newly emerging human cases in North America. *Proc Natl Acad Sci USA* 1996;93: 5653–5658.

Moritoyo T, Reinhart TA, Moritoyo H, et al. Human T-lymphotropic virus type I-associated myelopathy and tax gene expression in CD4+ T lymphocytes. *Ann Neurol* 1996;40:84–90.

Morrison RE, Shatsky SA, Holmes GE, Top FH, Martins AN. Herpes simplex virus type 1 from a patient with radiculoneuropathy. *JAMA* 1979;241:393–394.

Mortimer EA Jr, Lepow M, Gold E, Robbins FC, Burton GJ, Fraumeni JF Jr. Long-term follow-up of persons inadvertently inoculated with SV40 as neonates. *N Engl J Med* 1981;3056:1517–1518.

Moulignier A, Mikol J, Gonzalez-Canali G, et al. AIDS-associated cytomegalovirus infection mimicking central nervous system tumors: a diagnostic challenge. *Clin Infect Dis* 1996;22:626–631.

Moulignier A, Pialoux G, Dega H, Dupont B, Huerre M, Baudrimont M. Brain stem encephalitis due to varicella–zoster virus in a patient with AIDS. *Clin Infect Dis* 1995;20:1378–1380.

Mucke L, Eddleston M. Astrocytes in infectious and immune-mediated diseases of the central nervous system. *FASEB J* 1993;7:1226–1232.

Mucke L, Oldstone MBA. The expression of major histocompatibility complex (MHC) class I antigens in the brain differs markedly in acute and persistent infections with lymphocytic choriomeningitis virus (LCMV). *J Neuroimmunol* 1992;36:193–198.

Mühlemann K, Miller RK, Metlay L, Menegus MA. Cytomegalovirus infection of the human placenta: an immunocytochemical study. *Hum Pathol* 1992;23:1234–1237.

Muir P, Nicholson F, Sharief MK, et al. Evidence for persistent enterovirus infection of the central nervous system in patients with previous paralytic poliomyelitis. *Ann NY Acad Sci* 1995;753:219–232.

Muir P, Nicholson F, Spencer GT, et al. Enterovirus infection of the central nervous system of humans: lack of association with chronic neurological disease. *J Gen Virol* 1996;77:1469–1476.

Mukai N, Kobayashi S. Primary brain and spinal cord tumors induced by human adenovirus type 12 in hamsters. *J Neuropathol Exp Neurol* 1973;32:523–541.

Mulder DW, Rosenbaum RA, Layton DD. Late progression of poliomyelitis or forme fruste amyotrophic lateral sclerosis. *Mayo Clin Proc* 1972;47:756–761.

Müller CF, Fatzer RS, Beck K, Vandevelde M, Zurbriggen A. Studies on canine distemper virus persistence in the central nervous system. *Acta Neuropathol (Berl)* 1995;89:438–445.

Muller WK, Schaltenbrand G. Attempts to reproduce amyotrophic lateral sclerosis in laboratory animals by inoculation of Schu virus isolated from a patient with apparent amyotrophic lateral sclerosis. *J Neurol* 1979;220:1–19.

Murakami S, Mizobuchi M, Nakashiro Y, Doi T, Hato N, Yanagihara N. Bell palsy and herpes simplex virus: identification of viral DNA in endoneurial fluid and muscle. *Ann Intern Med* 1996;124:27–30.

Murao T. Induction of intracranial tumors in mice by human adenovirus type 12. I. Immunofluorescent studies on T antigen and the predilection sites for tumor development in the brain. *Acta Pathol Jap* 1972;22:41–51.

Murphy EL, Fridey J, Smith JW, et al. HTLV-associated myelopathy in a cohort of HTLV-I and HTLV-II-infected blood donors. *Neurology* 1997;48:315–320.

Murphy FA. Rabies pathogenesis [Brief review]. *Arch Virol* 1977;54:279–297.

Murphy FA. Virus taxonomy. In: Fields BN, Knipe DM, Howley PM, et al., eds. *Fields virology,* 3rd ed. New York: Lippincott–Raven Publishers, 1996:15–58.

Murphy FA, Fauqet CM, Bishop DHL, et al. *Virus taxonomy: sixth report of the International Committee on Taxonomy of Viruses.* Vienna: Springer-Verlag, 1994.

Murphy FA, Harrison AK, Winn WC, Bauer SP. Comparative pathogenesis of rabies and rabies-like viruses: infection of the central nervous system and centrifugal spread of virus to peripheral tissues. *Lab Invest* 1973a;29:1–16.

Murphy FA, Taylor WP, Mims CA, Marshall ID. Pathogenesis of Ross River virus infection in mice. II. Muscle, heart, and brown fat lesions. *J Infect Dis* 1973b;127:129–138.

Murphy FA, Whitfield SG. Eastern equine encephalitis virus infection: electron microscopic studies of mouse central nervous system. *Exp Mol Pathol* 1970;13:131–146.

Murray EA, Rausch DM, Lendvay J, Sharer LR, Eiden LE. Cognitive and motor impairments associated with SIV infection in rhesus monkeys. *Science* 1992a;255:1246–1249.

Murray HW, Knox DL, Green WR, Susel RM. Cytomegalovirus retinitis in adults. *Am J Med* 1977;63:574–584.

Murray HW, Masur H, Senterfit LB, Roberts RB. The protean manifestations of *Mycoplasma pneumoniae* infection in adults. *Am J Med* 1975;58:229–242.

Murray RS, Brown B, Brian D, Cabirac GF. Detection of coronavirus RNA and antigen in multiple sclerosis brain. *Ann Neurol* 1992d;31:525–533.

Mustafa MM, Weitman SD, Winick NJ, Bellini WJ, Timmons CF, Siegel JD. Subacute measles encephalitis in the young immunocompromised host: report of two cases diagnosed by polymerase chain reaction and treated with ribavirin and review of the literature. *Clin Infect Dis* 1993;16:654–660.

Myers EN, Stool S. Cytomegalic inclusion disease of the inner ear. *Laryngoscope* 1968;78:1904–1914.

Naeye RL, Blanc W. Pathogenesis of congenital rubella. *JAMA* 1965;194:1277–1283.

Nagano I, Nakamura S, Yoshioka M, Onodera J, Kogure K, Itoyama Y. Expression of cytokines in brain lesions in subacute sclerosing panencephalitis. *Neurology* 1994;44:710–715.

Nahmias AJ, Alford CA, Korones SB. Infection of the newborn with herpesvirus hominis. *Adv Pediatr* 1970;17:185–226.

Nahmias AJ, Hirsch MS, Kramer JH, Murphy FA. Effect of antithymocyte serum on herpesvirus hominis (type 1) infection in adult mice. *Proc Natl Acad Sci USA* 1969;132:696–698.

Nakagawa M, Izumo S, Ijichi S, et al. HTLV-I-associated myelopathy: analysis of 213 patients based on clinical features and laboratory findings. *J Neurovirol* 1995;1:50–61.

Nakagawa M, Nakahara K, Maruyama Y, et al. Therapeutic trials in 200 patients with HTLV-I-associated myelopathy/tropical spastic paraparesis. *J Neurovirol* 1996;2:345–355.

Narayan O, Clements JE. Biology and pathogenesis of lentiviruses. *J Gen Virol* 1989;70:1617–1639.

Narayan O, Herzog S, Frese K, Scheefers H, Rott R. Behavioral disease in rats caused by immunopathological responses to persistent Borna virus in the brain. *Science* 1983a;220:1401–1403.

Narayan O, Herzog S, Frese K, Scheefers H, Rott R. Pathogenesis of Borna disease in rats: immune-mediated viral ophthalmoencephalopathy causing blindness and behavioral abnormalities. *J Infect Dis* 1983b;148:305–315.

Narayan O, Johnson RT. Effects of viral infection on nervous system development. I. Pathogenesis of bluetongue virus infection in mice. *Am J Pathol* 1972;68:1–14.

Narayan O, Kennedy-Stoskopf S, Sheffer D, Griffin DE, Clements JE. Activation of caprine arthritis–encephalitis virus expression during maturation of monocytes to macrophages. *Infect Immun* 1983c;41:67–73.

Narayan O, McFarland HF, Johnson RT. Effects of viral infection on nervous system development. II. Attempts to modify bluetongue virus-induced malformations with cyclophosphamide and anti-thymocyte serum. *Am J Pathol* 1972;68:15–22.

Narayan O, Penney JB Jr, Johnson RT, Herndon RM, Weiner LP. Etiology of progressive multifocal leukoencephalopathy: identification of papovavirus. *N Engl J Med* 1973;289:1278–1282.

Narayan O, Sheffer D, Clements JE, Tennekoon G. Restricted replication of lentiviruses: visna viruses induce a unique interferon during interaction between lymphocytes and infected macrophages. *J Exp Med* 1985;162:1954–1969.

Narayan O, Silverstein AM, Price D, Johnson RT. Visna virus infection of American lambs. *Science* 1974; 183:1202–1203.

Nath A, Psooy K, Martin C, et al. Identification of a human immunodeficiency virus type 1 tat epitope that is neuroexcitatory and neurotoxic. *J Virol* 1996;70:1475–1480.

Nath A, Wolinsky JS. Antibody response to rubella virus structural proteins in multiple sclerosis. *Ann Neurol* 1990;27:533–536.

Nathanson JA, Chun LLY. Immunological function of the blood–cerebrospinal fluid barrier. *Proc Natl Acad Sci USA* 1989;86:1684–1688.

Nathanson N. The emergence of infectious diseases: societal causes and consequences. *ASM News* 1997; Amer Soc Microbiol;63:83–88.

Nathanson N, Cole GA, Santos GW, Squire RA, Smith KO. Viral hemorrhagic encephalopathy or rats. I. Isolation, identification, and properties of the HER strains of rat virus. *Am J Epidemiol* 1970;91: 328–338.

Nathanson N, Martin JR. The epidemiology of poliomyelitis: enigmas surrounding its appearance, epidemicity, and disappearance. *Am J Epidemiol* 1979;110:672–691.

Nathanson N, McGann KA, Wilesmith J, Desrosiers R, Brookmeyer R. The evolution of virus diseases: their emergence, epidemicity, and control. *Virus Res* 1993;29:3–20.

National Institutes of Health. Current understanding of persistent viral infections and their implication in human disease: summary of a workshop. *J Infect Dis* 1976;133:707–714.

Navia BA, Cho E-S, Petito CK, Price RW. The AIDS dementia complex. II. Neuropathology. *Ann Neurol* 1986a;19:525–535.

Navia BA, Jordan BD, Price RW. The AIDS dementia complex. I. clinical features. *Ann Neurol* 1986b;19: 517–524.

Navia BA, Price RW. The acquired immunodeficiency syndrome dementia complex as the presenting or sole manifestation of human immunodeficiency virus infection. *Arch Neurol* 1987;44:65–69.

Navin JJ, Angevine JM. Congenital cytomegalic inclusion disease with porencephaly. *Neurology* 1968;18: 470–472.

Negrini M, Rimessi P, Mantovani C, et al. Characterization of BK virus variants rescued from human tumours and tumour cell lines. *J Gen Virol* 1990;71:2731–2736.

Neumann H, Cavalié DE, Wekerle H. Induction of MHC class I genes in neurons. *Science* 1995;269: 549–552.

Neumann-Haefelin D, Fleps U, Renne R, Schweizer M. Foamy viruses. *Intervirology* 1993;35:196–207.

Nevin S, McMenemey WH, Behrman S, Jones DP. Subacute spongiform encephalopathy: a subacute form of encephalopathy attributable to vascular dysfunction (spongiform cerebral atrophy). *Brain* 1960;83: 519–564.

Newton L, Hall SM. Reye's syndrome in the British Isles: report for 1990/91 and the first decade of surveillance. *Community Dis Rep* 1993;3:R11–R16.

Nichols WW. Virus-induced chromosome abnormalities. *Annu Rev Microbiol* 1970;24:479–500.

Nicholson DH. Cytomegalovirus infection of the retina. *Int Ophthalmol Clin* 1975;15:151–162.

Nicola L, Hanshaw S. Congenital and neonatal varicella. *J Pediatr* 1979;94:175–176.

Nicolau S, Meteiesco E. Septinevrites a virus rabique des rue: preuves de la marche centrifuge du virus dans les nerfs peripheriques des lapins. *C R Acad Sci* 1928;186:1072–1074.

Nicoll JAR, Kinrade E, Love S. PCR-mediated search for herpes simplex virus DNA in sections of brain from patients with multiple sclerosis and other neurological disorders. *J Neurol Sci* 1992;113: 144–151.

Nicoll JAR, Maitland NJ, Love S. Autopsy neuropathological findings in 'burnt out' herpes simplex encephalitis and use of the polymerase chain reaction to detect viral DNA. *Neuropathol Appl Neurobiol* 1991;17:375–382.

Nicolosi A, Hauser WA, Beghi E, Kurland LT. Epidemiology of central nervous system infections in Olmsted County, Minnesota, 1950–1981. *J Infect Dis* 1986;154:399–408.

Niedermeyer HP, Arnold W. Otosclerosis: a measles virus associated inflammatory disease. *Acta Otolaryngol (Stockh)* 1995;115:300–303.

Nielsen SL, Petito CK, Urmacher CD, Posner JB. Subacute encephalitis in acquired immune deficiency syndrome: a postmortem study. *Am J Clin Pathol* 1984;82:678–682.

Nir Y, Beemer A, Goldwasser RA. West Nile virus infection in mice following exposure to a viral aerosol. *Br J Exp Pathol* 1965;46:443–449.

Nishimura M, McFarlin DE, Jacobson S. Sequence comparisons of HTLV-I from HAM/TSP patients and their asymptomatic spouses. *Neurology* 1993;43:2621–2624.

Nishimura M, Saida T, Kuroki S, et al. Post-infectious encephalitis with anti-galactocerebroside antibody subsequent to *Mycoplasma pneumoniae* infection. *J Neurol Sci* 1996;140:91–95.

Nishino H, Engel AG, Rima BK. Inclusion body myositis: the mumps virus hypothesis. *Ann Neurol* 1989; 25:260–264.

Niu MT, Stein DS, Schnittman SM. Primary human immunodeficiency virus type 1 infection: review of pathogenesis and early treatment intervention in humans and animal retrovirus infections. *J Infect Dis* 1993;168:1490–1501.

Noah DL, Smith MG, Gotthardt JC, Krebs JW, Green D, Childs JE. Mass human exposure to rabies in New Hampshire: exposures, treatment, and cost. *Am J Public Health* 1996;86:1149–1151.

Noorbehesht B, Enzmann DR, Sullender W, Bradley JS. Neonatal herpes simplex encephalitis: correlation of clinical and CT findings. *Radiology* 1987;162:813–819.

Norkin LC. Virus receptors: implications for pathogenesis and the design of antiviral agents. *Clin Microbiol Rev* 1995;8:293–315.

Norman S, Smith MC. Caprine arthritis–encephalitis: review of the neurologic form in 30 cases. *J Am Vet Med Assoc* 1983;182:1342–1345.

Norrby E. Viral antibodies in multiple sclerosis. *Prog Med Virol* 1978;24:1–39.

Norrby E, Link H, Olsson J-E, Panelius M, Salmi A, Vandvik B. Comparison of antibodies against different viruses in cerebrospinal fluid and serum samples from patients with multiple sclerosis. *Infect Immun* 1974;10:688–694.

Norris FJ Jr, Leonards R, Calanchini PR, Calder CD. Herpes zoster meningoencephalitis. *J Infect Dis* 1970;122:335–338.

Nzilambi N, De Cock KM, Forthal DN, et al. The prevalence of infection with human immunodeficiency virus over a 10-year period in rural Zaire. *N Engl J Med* 1988;318:276–279.

O'Brien WA, Hartigan PM, Martin D, et al. Changes in plasma HIV-1 RNA and CD4+ lymphocyte counts and the risk of progression to AIDS. *N Engl J Med* 1996;334:426–431.

Oesch B, Westaway D, Wälchli M, et al. A cellular gene encodes scrapie PrP 27-30 protein. *Cell* 1985;40: 735–746.

Ogata A, Nagashima K, Tashiro K, Miyakawa A, Mikuni C. MRI-pathological correlate of brain lesions in a necropsy case of HTLV-I associated myelopathy. *J Neurol Neurosurg Psychiatry* 1993;56: 194–196.

Ojala A. On changes in the cerebrospinal fluid during measles. *Ann Med Intern Fenn* 1947;36:321–331.

Ojeda VJ. Fatal herpes simplex encephalitis with demonstration of virus in the olfactory pathway. *Pathology* 1980;12:429–437.

Okuno T. An epidemiological review of Japanese encephalitis. *WHO Stat Rep* 1978;31:120–133.

Okuno T, Oya A, Ito T. The identification of Negishi virus: a presumably new member of Russian spring–summer encephalitis virus family isolated in Japan. *Jpn J Med Sci Biol* 1961;14:51–59.

Olding LB, Jensen FC, Oldstone MBA. Pathogenesis of cytomegalovirus infection. I. Activation of virus from bone marrow-derived lymphocytes by in vitro allogenic reaction. *J Exp Med* 1975;141:561–572.

Oldstone MBA, Dixon FJ. Pathogenesis of chronic disease associated with persistent lymphocytic choriomeningitis viral infection. II. Relationship of the antilymphocytic choriomeningitis immune response to tissue injury in chronic lymphocytic choriomeningitis disease. *J Exp Med* 1970;131:1–19.

Oldstone MBA, Dixon FJ. Acute viral infection: tissue injury mediated by antiviral antibody through a complement effector system. *J Immunol* 1971;107:1274–1280.

Oldstone MBA, Homstoen J, Welsh RM Jr. Alterations of acetylcholine enzymes in neuroblastoma cells persistently infected with lymphocytic choriomeningitis virus. *J Cell Physiol* 1977;91:459–472.

Oldstone MBA, Rall GF. Mechanism and consequence of viral persistence in cells of the immune system and neurons. *Intervirology* 1993;35:116–121.

Oldstone MBA, Schwimmbeck P, Dyrberg T, Fujinami R. Mimicry by virus of host molecules: implications for autoimmune disease. In: *Progress in immunology VI,* 6th ed. New York: Academic Press, 1986:787–795.

Oldstone MBA, Sinha YN, Blount P, et al. Virus-induced alterations in homeostasis: alterations in differentiated functions of infected cells in vivo. *Science* 1982;218:1125–1127.

Olson LC, Buescher EL, Artenstein MS, Parkman PD. Herpesvirus infections of the human central nervous system. *N Engl J Med* 1967;277:1271–1277.

Oomes PG, Jacobs BC, Hazenberg MP, Banffer JR, van der Meche FG. Anti-GM1 IgG antibodies and *Campylobacter* bacteria in Guillain–Barre syndrome: evidence of molecular mimicry. *Ann Neurol* 1995;38:170–175.

Orgel LE. The maintenance of the accuracy of protein synthesis and its relevance to ageing. *Proc Natl Acad Sci USA* 1963;49:517–521.

Orlowski JP, Gillis J, Kilham HA. A catch in the Reye. *Pediatrics* 1987;80:638–642.

Osame M, Janssen R, Kubota H, et al. Nationwide survey of HTLV-I-associated myelopathy in Japan: association with blood transfusion. *Ann Neurol* 1990;28:50–56.

Osame M, Nakagawa M, Umehara F, et al. Recent studies on the epidemiology, clinical features and pathogenic mechanisms of HTLV-I associated myelopathy (HAM/TSP) and other diseases associated to HTLV. *J Neurovirol* 1997;3[Suppl]:S50–S51.

Osame M, Usuku K, Izumo S, et al. HTLV-I associated myelopathy, a new clinical entity. *Lancet* 1986;1: 1031–1032.

Osburn BI, Johnson RT, Silverstein AM, Prendergast RA, Jochim MM, Levy SE. Experimental viral-induced congenital encephalopathies. II. The pathogenesis of bluetongue vaccine virus infection in fetal lambs. *Lab Invest* 1971a;25:206–210.

Osburn BI, Silverstein AM, Prendergast RA, Johnson RT, Parshall CJ. Experimental viral-induced congenital encephalopathies. I. Pathology of hydranencephaly and porencephaly caused by bluetongue vaccine virus. *Lab Invest* 1971b;25:197–205.

Osler W. *The principles and practice of medicine.* New York: Appleton and Company, 1892:777–778.

Oster-Granite ML, Herndon RM. Studies of cultured human and simian fetal brain cells. I. Characterization of the cell types. *Neuropathol Appl Neurobiol* 1978;4:429–442.

Oster-Granite ML, Narayan O, Johnson RT, Herndon RM. Studies of cultured human and simian fetal brain cells. II. Infections with human (BK) and simian (SV40) papovaviruses. *Neuropathol Appl Neurobiol* 1978;4:443–455.

Owen F, Lofthouse R, Crow TJ, et al. Insertion in prion protein gene in familial Creutzfeldt–Jakob disease. *Lancet* 1989;1:51–52.

Özel M, Xi Y-G, Baldauf E, Diringer H, Pocchiari M. Small virus-like structure in brains from cases of sporadic and familial Creutzfeldt–Jakob disease. *Lancet* 1994;2:923–924.

Padgett BL, Walker DL. Prevalence of antibodies in human sera against JC virus, an isolate from a case of progressive multifocal leukoencephalopathy. *Prog Med Virol* 1976;22:1–35.

Padgett BL, Walker DL, ZuRhein GM, Varakis JN. Differential neurooncogenicity of strains of JC virus, a human polyoma virus, in newborn Syrian hamsters. *Cancer Res* 1977;37:718–720.

Padgett BL, Walker DL, ZuRhein GM, Eckroade RJ, Dessel BH. Cultivation of papova-like virus from human brain with progressive multifocal leucoencephalopathy. *Lancet* 1971;1:1257.

Page LK, Tyler HR, Shillito J. Neurosurgical experiences with herpes simplex encephalitis. *J Neurosurg* 1967;27:346–352.

Paisley JW, Bruhn FW, Lauer BA, McIntosh K. Type A2 influenza viral infections in children. *Am J Dis Child* 1978;132:34–36.

Palmer MS, Dryden AJ, Hughes JT, Collinge J. Homozygous prion protein genotype predisposes to sporadic Creutzfeldt–Jakob disease. *Nature* 1991;352:340–342.

Pan K-M, Baldwin M, Nguyen J, et al. Conversion of α helices into β-sheets features in the formation of scrapie prion proteins. *Proc Natl Acad Sci USA* 1993;90:10,962–10,966.

Panitch HS. Influence of infection on exacerbations of multiple sclerosis. *Ann Neurol* 1994;36[Suppl]: S25–S28.

Panum PL. *Observations made during the epidemic of measles on the Faroe Islands in the year 1846.* New York: American Public Health Association, Delta Omega Society, 1940.

Paquette Y, Hanna Z, Savard P, Brousseau R, Robitaille Y, Jolicoeur P. Retrovirus-induced murine motor neuron disease: mapping the determinant of spongiform degeneration within the envelope gene. *Proc Natl Acad Sci USA* 1989;86:3896–3900.

Parchi P, Castellani R, Capellari S, et al. Molecular basis of phenotypic variability in sporadic Creutzfeldt–Jakob disease. *Ann Neurol* 1996;36:767–778.

Parhad IM, Johnson KP, Wolinsky JS, Swoveland P. Measles retinopathy: a hamster model of acute and chronic lesions. *Lab Invest* 1980;43:52–60.

Parkman PD, Buescher EL, Artenstein MS. Recovery of rubella virus from army recruits. *Proc Soc Exp Biol Med* 1962;111:225–230.

Parks WP, Queiroga LT, Melnick JL. Studies of infantile diarrhea in Karachi, Parkistan. II. Multiple virus isolations from rectal swabs. *Am J Epidemiol* 1967;85:469–478.

Parry HB. Scrapie: a transmissible and hereditary disease of sheep. *Heredity* 1962;17:75–105.

Partin JC, Partin JS, Schubert WK, McLaurin RL. Brain ultrastructure in Reye's syndrome. *J Neuropathol Exp Neurol* 1975;34:425–444.

Partridge JW, Flewett TH, Whitehead JEM. Congenital rubella affecting an infant whose mother had rubella antibodies before conception. *BMJ* 1981;282:187–188.

Paryani SG, Arvin AM. Intrauterine infection with varicella–zoster virus after maternal varicella. *N Engl J Med* 1986;314:1542–1546.

Paskavitz JF, Anderson CA, Filley CM, Kleinschmidt-DeMasters BK, Tyler KL. Acute arcuate fiber demyelinating encephalopathy following Epstein–Barr virus infection. *Ann Neurol* 1995;38:127–131.

Pastuszak AL, Levy M, Schick B, et al. Outcome after maternal varicella infection in the first 20 weeks of pregnancy. *N Engl J Med* 1994;330:901–905.

Paterson PY. Transfer of allergic encephalomyelitis in rats by means of lymph node cells. *J Exp Med* 1960; 111:119–136.

Paterson PY. Neuroimmunologic diseases of animals and humans. *Rev Infect Dis* 1979;1:468–482.

Paton P, Poly H, Gonnaud P-M, et al. Acute meningoradiculitis concomitant with seroconversion to human immunodeficiency virus type 1. *Res Virol* 1990;141:427–433.

Patterson WJ, Dealler S, Bovine spongiform encephalopathy and the public health. *J Public Health Med* 1995;17:261–268.

Paul JR. *The history of poliomyelitis.* New Haven: Yale University Press, 1971.

Pavesi G, Gemignani F, Macaluso GM, et al. Acute sensory and autonomic neuropathy: possible association with Coxsackie B virus infection. *J Neurol Neurosurg Psychiatry* 1992;55:613–615.

Payne FE, Baublis JV, Habashi HH. Isolation of measles virus from cell cultures of brain from a patient with subacute sclerosing panencephalitis. *N Engl J Med* 1969;281:585–589.

Payne SL, Salinovich O, Nauman SM, Issel CJ, Montelaro RC. Course and extent of variation of equine infectious anemia virus during parallel persistent infections. *J Virol* 1987;61:1266–1270.

Pearl PL, Hussam A-F, Starke JR, Dreyer Z, Louis PT, Kirkpatrick JB. Neuropathology of two fatal cases of measles in the 1988–1989 Houston epidemic. *Pediatr Neurol* 1990;6:126–130.

Pedersen NC, Ho EW, Brown ML, Yamamoto JK. Isolation of a T-lymphotropic virus from domestic cats with an immunodeficiency-like syndrome. *Science* 1987;235:790–793.

Pedneault L, Katz BZ, Miller G. Detection of Epstein–Barr virus in the brain by the polymerase chain reaction. *Ann Neurol* 1992;32:184–192.

Pellegrini M, O'Brien TJ, Hoy J, Sedal L. *Mycoplasma pneumoniae* infection associated with an acute brainstem syndrome. *Acta Neurol Scand* 1996;93:203–206.

Pena Rossi C, Delcroix M, Huitinga I, et al. Role of macrophages during Theiler's virus infection. *J Virol* 1997;71:3336–3340.

Penman HG. Fatal infectious mononucleosis: a critical review. *J Clin Pathol* 1970;2:765–771.

Penney JB Jr, Weiner LP, Herndon RM, Narayan O, Johnson RT. Virions from progressive multifocal leukoencephalopathy: rapid serological identification by electron microscopy. *Science* 1972;178: 60–62.

Pepose JS, Stevens JG, Cook ML, Lampert PW. Marek's disease as a model for the Landry–Guillain–Barré syndrome: latent viral infection in non-neural cells accompanied by specific immune responses to peripheral nerve and myelin. *Am J Pathol* 1981;103:309–320.

Perelson AS, Neumann AU, Markowitz M, Leonard JM, Ho DD. HIV-1 dynamics in vivo: virion clearance rate, infected cell life-span, and viral generation time. *Science* 1996;271:1582–1586.

Perkus ME, Piccini A, Lipinskas B, Paoletti E. Recombinant vaccinia virus: immunization against multiple pathogens. *Science* 1985;229:981–984.

Perlman HB, Lindsay JR. Relation of inner ear spaces to the meninges. *Arch Otolaryngol* 1939;29:12–23.

Perlman JM, Argyle C. Lethal cytomegalovirus infection in preterm infants: clinical, radiological, and neuropathological findings. *Ann Neurol* 1992;31:64–68.

Perron H, Lalande B, Gratacap B, et al. Isolation of retrovirus from patients with multiple sclerosis. *Lancet* 1991;2:862–863.

Perry VH, Gordon S. Macrophages and microglia in the nervous system. *Trends Neurosci* 1988;11: 273–277.

Persidsky Y, Limoges J, McComb R, et al. Human immunodeficiency virus encephalitis in SCID mice. *Am J Pathol* 1996;149:1027–1053.

Petereit H-F, Bamborschke S, Lanfermann H. Acute transverse myelitis caused by herpes simplex virus. *Eur Neurol* 1996;36:52–53.

Peters ACB, Versteeg J, Lindeman J, Bots GTAM. Varicella and acute cerebellar ataxia. *Arch Neurol* 1978; 35:769–771.

Peters ACB, Vielvoye GJ, Versteeg J, Bots GTAM, Lindeman J. Echo 25 focal encephalitis and subacute hemichorea. *Neurology* 1979;29:767–681.

Petersen RB, Tabaton M, Berg L, et al. Analysis of the prion protein gene in thalamic dementia. *Neurology* 1992;42:1859–1863.

Peterslund NA. Herpes zoster associated encephalitis: clinical findings and acyclovir treatment. *Scand J Infect Dis* 1988;20:583–592.

Petito CK, Navia BA, Cho E-S, Jordan BD, George DC, Price RW. Vacuolar myelopathy pathologically resembling subacute combined degeneration in patients with the acquired immunodeficiency syndrome. *N Engl J Med* 1985;312:874–879.

Petito CK, Vecchio D, Chen Y-T. HIV antigen and DNA in AIDS spinal cords correlate with macrophage infiltration but not with vacuolar myelopathy. *J Neuropathol Exp Neurol* 1994;53:86–94.

Pette H, Doring G. Uber einheimische Panencephalomyelitis vom Charakter der Encephalitis Japonica. *Dtsch Z Nervenheilkd* 1939;149:7–44.

Petursson G, Nathanson N, Georgsson G, Panitch H, Palsson PA. Pathogenesis of visna. I. Sequential virologic, serologic, and pathologic studies. *Lab Invest* 1976;35:402–412.

Philip RN, Reinhard KR, Lackmar DB. Observations on a mumps epidemic in a "virgin" population. *Am J Hyg* 1959;69:91–111.

Phillips CA, Fanning WL, Gump DW, Phillips CF. Cytomegalovirus encephalitis in immunologically normal adults: successful treatment with vidarabine. *JAMA* 1977;21:2299–2300.

Picard FJ, Dekaban GA, Silva J, Rice GPA. Mollaret's meningitis associated with herpes simplex type 2 infection. *Neurology* 1993;43:1722–1727.

Piot P. AIDS: a global response. *Science* 1996;272:1855.

Pizzo PA, Eddy J, Falloon J, et al. Effect of continuous intravenous infusion of zidovudine (AZT) in children with symptomatic HIV infection. *N Engl J Med* 1988;319:889–896.

Plesner A-M, Arlien-Soborg P, Herning M. Neurological complications and Japanese encephalitis vaccination. *Lancet* 1996;1:202–203.

Plum F. Sensory loss with poliomyelitis. *Neurology* 1956;6:166–173.

Pogo BGT, Casals J, Elizan TS. A study of viral genomes and antigens in brains of patients with Alzheimer's disease. *Brain* 1987;110:907–915.

Pohl-Koppe A, Kaiser R, Ter Meulen V, Liebert UG. Antibody reactivity to individual structural proteins of measles virus in the CSF of SSPE and MS patients. *Clin Diagn Virol* 1995;4:135–147.

Poiesz BJ, Ruscetti FW, Gazdar AF, Bunn PA, Minna JD, Gallo RC. Detection and isolation of type C retrovirus particles from fresh and cultured lymphocytes of a patient with cutaneous T-cell lymphoma. *Proc Natl Acad Sci USA* 1980;77:7415–7419.

Pomerantz RJ, Kuritzkes DR, De La Monte SM, et al. Infection of the retina by human immunodeficiency virus type I. *N Engl J Med* 1987;317:1643–1647..

Ponka A. Central nervous system manifestations associated with serologically verified *Mycoplasma pneumoniae* infection. *Scand J Infect Dis* 1980;12:175–184.

Pönkä A, Pettersson T. The incidence and aetiology of central nervous system infections in Helsinki in 1980. *Acta Neurol Scand* 1982;66:529–535.

Porras C, Barboza JJ, Fuenzalida E, Adaros HL, Oviedo de Diaz AM, Furst J. Recovery from rabies in man. *Ann Intern Med* 1976;85:44–48.

Portegies P, de Gans J, Lange JMA, et al. Declining incidence of AIDS dementia complex after introduction of zidovudine treatment. *BMJ* 1989;299:819–821.

Portenoy RK, Duma C, Foley KM. Acute herpetic and postherpetic neuralgia: clinical review and current management. *Ann Neurol* 1986;20:651–664.

Porter DD. Aleutian disease: a persistent parvovirus infection of mink with a maximal but ineffective host humoral immune response. *Prog Med Virol* 1986;33:42–60.

Porter DD, Larsen AE, Porter HG. The pathogenesis of Aleutian disease of mink. III. Immune complex arteritis. *Am J Pathol* 1973;71:331–344.

Portis JL, Czub S, Garon CF, McAtee FJ. Neurodegenerative disease induced by the wild mouse ecotropic retrovirus is markedly accelerated by long terminal repeat and gag–pol sequences from nondefective Friend murine leukemia virus. *J Virol* 1990;64:1648–1656.

Poskanzer DC, Schapira K, Miller H. Epidemiology of multiple sclerosis in the counties of Northumberland and Durham. *J Neurol Neurosurg Psychiatry* 1963;26:368–376.

Potts BJ, Berry LJ, Osburn BI, Johnson KP. Viral persistence and abnormalities of the central nervous system after congenital infection of sheep with border disease virus. *J Infect Dis* 1985;151: 337–341.

Potts BJ, Sever JL, Tzan NR, Huddleston D, Elder GA. Possible role of pestiviruses in microcephaly [Letter]. *Lancet* 1987;1:972–973.

Power C, Johnson RT. HIV-1 associated dementia: clinical features and pathogenesis. *Can J Neurol Sci* 1995;22:92–100.

Power C, Kong P-A, Crawford TO, et al. Cerebral white matter changes in acquired immunodeficiency syndrome dementia: alterations of the blood–brain barrier. *Ann Neurol* 1993;34:339–350.

Power C, McArthur JC, Johnson RT, et al. Demented and nondemented patients with AIDS differ in brain-derived human immunodeficiency virus type 1 envelope sequences. *J Virol* 1994;68:4643–4649.

Power C, Poland SD, Blume WT, Girvin JP, Rice GPA. Cytomegalovirus and Rasmussen's encephalitis. *Lancet* 1990;2:1282–1284.

Pranzatelli MR. The neurobiology of the opsoclonus–myoclonus syndrome. *Clin Neuropharmacol* 1992; 15:186–228.

Price RA, Garcia JH, Rightsel WA. Choriomeningitis and myocarditis in an adolescent with isolation of Coxsackie B5 virus. *Am J Clin Pathol* 1970;53:825–831.

Price RW, Nielsen S, Horten B, Rubino M, Padgett B, Walker D. Progressive multifocal leukoencephalopathy: a burnt-out case. *Ann Neurol* 1983;13:485–490.

Pritchard AE, Jensen K, Lipton HL. Assembly of Theiler's virus recombinants used in mapping determinants of neurovirulence. *J Virol* 1993;67:3901–3907.

Proctor L, Lindsay J, Perlman H, Matz G. Acute vestibular paralysis in herpes zoster oticus. *Ann Otol Rhinol Laryngol* 1979;88:303–310.

Provisor AJ, Iacuone JJ, Chilcote RR, Neiburger RG, Crussi FG, Baehner RL. Acquired agammaglobulinemia after a life threatening illness with clinical and laboratory features of infectious mononucleosis in three related male children. *N Engl J Med* 1975;293:62–65.

Prusiner S. Novel proteinaceous infectious particles cause scrapie. *Science* 1982;216:136–144.

Prusiner SB. Prions and neurodegenerative diseases. *N Engl J Med* 1987;317:1571–1581.

Prusiner SB. Molecular biology of prion diseases. *Science* 1991;252:1515–1522.

Prusiner SB. Human prion diseases and neurodegeneration. *Curr Top Microbiol Immunol* 1996;207:1–17.

Prusiner SB, Groth D, Serban A, et al. Ablation of the prion protein (PrP) gene in mice prevents scrapie and facilitates production of anti-PrP antibodies. *Proc Natl Acad Sci USA* 1993;90:10,608–10,612.

Prusiner SB, Telling G, Cohen FE, DeArmond SJ. Prion diseases of humans and animals. *Semin Virol* 1996;7:159–173.

Pryce G, Male D, Sedgwick J. Antigen presentation in brain: brain endothelial cells are poor stimulators of T-cell proliferation. *Immunology* 1989;66:207–212.

Pulec JL. Meniere's disease: results of a two and one-half year study of etiology, natural history and results of treatment. *Laryngoscope* 1972;82:1703–1715.

Purdham DR, Batty PF. A case of acute measles meningoencephalitis with virus isolation. *J Clin Pathol* 1974;27:994–996.

Pyykkö I, Vesanen M, Asikainen K, Koskiniemi M, Airaksinen L, Vaheri A. Human spumaretrovirus in the etiology of sudden hearing loss. *Acta Otolaryngol (Stockh)* 1993;113:109–112.

Quagliarello V. The acquired immunodeficiency syndrome: current status. *Yale J Biol Med* 1982;55: 443–452.

Querfurth H, Swanson PD. Vaccine-associated paralytic poliomyelitis. *Arch Neurol* 1990;47:541–544.

Quinke H. Ueber Hydrocephalus. *Veehandl Cong Innere Med* 1891;10:321–331.

Quinn TC. Global burden of the HIV pandemic. *Lancet* 1996;1:99–106.

Quinn TC, Kline RL, Halsey N, et al. Early diagnosis of perinatal HIV infection by detection of viral-specific IgA antibodies. *JAMA* 1991;266:3439–3442.

Raff MC, Barres BA, Burne JF, Coles HS, Ishizaki Y, Jacobson MD. Programmed cell death and the control of cell survival: lessons from the nervous system. *Science* 1993;262:695–700.

Raghavan R, Stephens EB, Joag SV, et al. Neuropathogenesis of chimeric simian/human immunodeficiency virus infection in pig-tailed and rhesus macaques. *Brain Pathol* 1997;7:851–861.

Ragozzino MW, Melton LJ III, Kurland LT, Chu CP, Perry HO. Population-based study of herpes zoster and its sequelae. *Medicine (Baltimore)* 1982;61:310–316.

Ramlow J, Alexander M, LaPorte R, Kaufmann C, Kuller L. Epidemiology of the post-polio syndrome. *Am J Epidemiol* 1992;136:769–786.

Rammohan KW, McFarland HF, McFarlin DE. Subacute sclerosing panencephalitis after passive immunization and natural measles infection: role of antibody in persistence of measles virus. *Neurology* 1982;32:390–394.

Rance NE, McArthur JC, Cornblath DR, Landstrom DL, Griffin JW, Price DL. Gracile tract degeneration in patients with sensory neuropathy and AIDS. *Neurology* 1988;38:265–271.

Rapoport SI. *Blood–brain barrier in physiology and medicine.* New York: Raven Press, 1976.

Rapp F, Duff R. Transformation of hamster embryo fibroblasts by herpes simplex viruses type 1 and 2. *Cancer Res* 1973;33:1527–1534.

Rasmussen HB, Clausen J. Possible involvement of endogenous retroviruses in the development of autoimmune disorders, especially multiple sclerosis. *Acta Neurol Scand* 1997;169:32–37.

Raubertas RF, Brown P, Cathala F, Brown I. The question of clustering of Creutzfeldt–Jakob disease. *Am J Epidemiol* 1989;129:146–154.

Ravenholt RT, Foege WH. 1918 influenza, encephalitis lethargica, parkinsonism. *Lancet* 1982;2:860–864.

Ravi V, Desai AS, Shenoy PK, Satishchandra P, Chandramuki A, Gourie-Devie M. Persistence of Japanese encephalitis virus in the human nervous system. *J Med Virol* 1993;40:326–329.

Rawls WE. Viral persistence in congenital rubella. *Prog Med Virol* 1974;18:273–288.

Rawls WE, Melnick JL. Rubella virus carrier cultures derived from congenitally infected infants. *J Exp Med* 1966;123:795–816.

Rebiere I, Galy-Eyraud C. Estimation of the risk of aseptic meningitis associated with mumps vaccination, France, 1991–1993. *Int J Epidemiol* 1995;24:1223–1227.

Redford EJ, Hall SM, Smith KJ. Vascular changes and demyelination induced by the intraneural injection of tumour necrosis factor. *Brain* 1995;118:869–878.

Reed W. Recent researches concerning the etiology, propagation and prevention of yellow fever by the United States Army commission. *J Hyg* 1902;2:101–119.

Rees JH, Gregson NA, Griffith PL, Hughes RAC. *Campylobacter jejuni* and Guillain–Barré syndrome. *Q J Med* 1993;86:623–634.

Rees JH, Gregson NA, Hughes RAC. Anti-ganglioside GM1 antibodies in Guillain–Barré syndrome and their relationship to *Campylobacter jejuni* infection. *Ann Neurol* 1995;38:809–816.

Reik L Jr. Spirochaetal infections of the nervous system. In: Kennedy PGE, Johnson RT, eds. *Infections of the nervous system.* London: Butterworths, 1987:43–75.

Reimann HA. Infectious diseases: review of current literature. *Arch Intern Med* 1937;60:337–384.

Ren R, Racaniello VR. Poliovirus spreads from muscle to the central nervous system by neural pathways. *J Infect Dis* 1992;166:747–752.

Resnick L, DiMarzo-Veronese F, Schüpbach J, et al. Intra–blood-brain-barrier synthesis of HTLV-III-specific IgG in patients with neurologic symptoms associated with AIDS or AIDS-related complex. *N Engl J Med* 1985;313:1498–1504.

Reux I, Fillet A-M, Fourneri J-G, et al. In situ hybridization of HIV-1 RNA in retinal vascular wall. *Am J Pathol* 1993;143:1275–1279.

Revol A, Vighetto A, Jouvet A, Aimard G, Trillet M. Encephalitis in cat scratch disease with persistent dementia. *J Neurol Neurosurg Psychiatry* 1992;55:133–135.

Reye RDK, Morgan G, Baral J. Encephalopathy and fatty degeneration of viscera: a disease entity in childhood. *Lancet* 1963;2:749–752.

Reyes M, Gary HE Jr, Dobbins JG, et al. Surveillance for chronic fatigue syndrome: four U.S. cities, September 1989 through August 1993. *MMWR* 1997;46:1–13.

Reyes MG, Fresco R, Chokroverty S, Salud EQ. Virus-like particles in granulomatous angiitis of the central nervous system. *Neurology* 1976;26:797–799.

Reynolds DW, Stagno S, Stubbs KG, et al. Inapparent congenital cytomegalovirus infection with elevated cord IgM levels: causal relation with auditory and mental deficiency. *N Engl J Med* 1974;290:291–296.

Rhodes RH. Evidence of serum-protein leakage across the blood–brain barrier in the acquired immunodeficiency syndrome. *J Neuropathol Exp Neurol* 1991;50:171–183.

Richards WPC, Cordy DR. Bluetongue virus infection: pathologic responses of nervous systems in sheep and mice. *Science* 1967;156:530–531.

Richardson EP Jr. Progressive multifocal leukoencephalopathy. *N Engl J Med* 1961;265:815–823.

Richert JR, Potolicchio S Jr, Garagusi VF, et al. Cytomegalovirus encephalitis associated with episodic neurologic deficits and OKT-8+ pleocytosis. *Neurology* 1987;37:149–152.

Ricker W, Blumberg A, Peters CH, Widerman A. The association of the Guillain–Barre syndrome with infectious mononucleosis with a report of two fatal cases. *Blood* 1947;2:217–226.

Rinaldo CR Jr. Modulation of major histocompatibility complex antigen expression by viral infection. *Am J Pathol* 1994;144:637–650.

Rivers TM. Viruses and Koch's postulates. *J Bacteriol* 1937;33:1–12.

Rivers TM. *Tom Rivers: reflections on a life in medicine and science—an oral history memoir.* Cambridge: MIT Press, 1967.

Rivers TM, Schwentker FF. Encephalomyelitis accompanied by myelin destruction experimentally produced in monkeys. *J Exp Med* 1935;61:689–702.

Rizzuto N, Cavallaro T, Monaco S, et al. Role of HIV in the pathogenesis of distal symmetrical peripheral neuropathy. *Acta Neuropathol (Berl)* 1995;90:244–250.

Robbins SG, Hamel CP, Detrick B, Hooks JJ. Murine coronavirus induces an acute and long-lasting disease of the retina. *Lab Invest* 1990;62:417–426.

Robertson GG, Williamson AP, Blattner RJ. A study of abnormalities in early chick embryos inoculated with Newcastle disease virus. *J Exp Zool* 1955;129:5–43.

Robertson GG, Williamson AP, Blattner RJ. Origin of myeloschisis in chick embryos infected with influenza-A virus. *Yale J Biol Med* 1960;32:449–463.

Rocklin RE, Sheremata WA, Feldman RG, Kies MW, David JR. The Guillain–Barré syndrome and multiple sclerosis: in vitro cellular responses to nervous tissue antigens. *N Engl J Med* 1971;284: 803–808.

Rodden VJ, Canton HE, O'Connor DM, Schmidt RR, Cherry JD. Acute hemiplegia of childhood associated with Coxsackie A9 viral infection. *J Pediatr* 1975;86:56–58.

Rodgers SE, Barton ES, Oberhaus SM, et al. Reovirus-induced apoptosis of MDCK cells is not linked to viral yield and is blocked by Bcl-2. *J Virol* 1997;71:2540–2546.

Rodgers-Johnson P, Gajdusek DC, Morgan OSC, Zaninovic V, Sarin PS, Graham DS. HTLV-I and HTLV-III antibodies and tropical spastic paraparesis. *Lancet* 1985;2:1247–1248.

Rodriguez M, Oleszak E, Leibowitz J. Theiler's murine encephalomyelitis: a model of demyelination and persistence of virus. *Crit Rev Immunol* 1987;7:325–365.

Rodriguez M, Rivera-Quinones C, Murray PD, Kariuki Njenga M, Wettstein PJ, Mak T. The role of CD4 and CD8 T cells in demyelinating disease following Theiler's virus infection: a model for multiple sclerosis. *J Neurovirol* 1997;3:543–545.

Rogers SW, Andrew PI, Gahring LC, et al. Autoantibodies to glutamate receptor GluR3 in Rasmussen's encephalitis. *Science* 1994;265:648–651.

Rohwer RG. Alzheimer's disease transmission: possible artifact due to intercurrent illness. *Neurology* 1992;42:287–288.

Roizman B. An inquiry into the mechanisms of recurrent herpes infections of man. *Perspect Virol* 1965; 4:283–304.

Roizman B, Palese P. Multiplication of viruses: an overview. In: Fields BN, Knipe DM, Howley PM, et al., eds. *Fields virology,* 3rd ed. New York: Lippincott–Raven Publishers, 1996:101–112.

Rolleston JD. *History of the acute exanthemata.* London: William Heinemann, 1937.

Roman GC, Schoenberg BS, Madden DL, et al. Human T-lymphotropic virus type I antibodies in the serum of patients with tropical spastic paraparesis in the Seychelles. *Arch Neurol* 1987;44:605–607.

Román GC, Spencer PS, Schoenberg BS, et al. Tropical spastic paraparesis in the Seychelles Islands: a clinical and case–control neuroepidemiologic study. *Neurology* 1987;37:1323–1328.

Roman-Campos G, Toro G. Herpetic brainstem encephalitis. *Neurology* 1980;30:981–985.

Roos R, Chou SM, Rogers NG, Basnight M, Gajdusek DC. Isolation of an adenovirus 32 strain from human brain in a case of subacute encephalitis. *Proc Soc Exp Biol Med* 1972;139:636–640.

Roos R, Gajdusek DC, Gibbs CJ Jr. The clinical characteristics of transmissible Creutzfeldt–Jakob disease. *Brain* 1973;96:1–20.

Roos RP. Adenovirus. In: Vinken PJ, Bruyn GW, Klawans HL, eds. *Handbook of clinical neurology.* Amsterdam: Elsevier Science, 1989:281–293.

Roos RP, Viola MV, Wollmann R, Hatch MH, Antel JP. Amyotrophic lateral sclerosis with antecedent poliomyelitis. *Arch Neurol* 1980;37:312–313.

Roos RP, Wollmann R. DA strain of Theiler's murine encephalomyelitis virus induces demyelination in nude mice. *Ann Neurol* 1984;15:494–499.

Roques P, Marce D, Courpotin C, et al. Correlation between HIV provirus burden and in utero transmission. *AIDS* 1993;7[Suppl]:S39–S43.

Rorabaugh ML, Berlin LE, Heldrich F, et al. Aseptic meningitis in infants younger than 2 years of age: acute illness and neurologic complications. *Pediatrics* 1993;92:206–211.

Rorke LB, Spiro AJ. Cerebral lesions in congenital rubella syndrome. *J Pediatr* 1967;70:243–255.

Roscelli JD, Bass JW, Pang L. Guillain–Barré syndrome and influenza vaccination in the US army, 1980–1988. *Am J Epidemiol* 1991;133:952–955.

Rose JW, Stroop WG, Matsuo F, Henkel J. Atypical herpes simplex encephalitis: clinical virologic and neuropathologic evaluation. *Neurology* 1992;42:1809–1812.

Rosen L. Overwintering mechanisms of mosquito-borne arboviruses in temperate climates. *Am J Trop Med Hyg* 1987;37[Suppl]:69S–76S.

Rosenberg NL, Rotbart HA, Abzug MJ, Ringel SP, Levin MJ. Evidence for a novel picornavirus in human dermatomyositis. *Ann Neurol* 1989;26:204–209.

Rosenberg RN, Neuwelt EA, Kirkpatrick J, Kohler P. Encephalopathy associated with cryoprecipitable Australia antigen. *Ann Neurol* 1977;1:298–300.

Rosenblum M, Scheck AC, Cronin K, et al. Dissociation of AIDS-related vacuolar myelopathy and productive HIV-1 infection of the spinal cord. *Neurology* 1989;39:892–896.

Rosenblum MK, Brew BJ, Hahn B, et al. Human T-lymphotropic virus type I-associated myelopathy in patients with the acquired immunodeficiency syndrome. *Hum Pathol* 1992;23:513–519.

Rosenblum WI. Biology of disease, aspects of endothelial malfunction and function in cerebral microvessels. *Lab Invest* 1986;55:252–268.

Rosenblum WI, Hadfield MG. Granulomatous angiitis of the nervous system in cases of herpes zoster and lymphosarcoma. *Neurology* 1972;22:348–354.

Rösener M, Hahn H, Kranz M, Heeney J, Rethwilm A. Absence of serological evidence for foamy virus infection in patients with amyotrophic lateral sclerosis. *J Med Virol* 1996;48:222–226.

Rosenfeld J, Taylor CL, Atlas SW. Myelitis following chickenpox: a case report. *Neurology* 1993;43: 1834–1836.

Ross MH, Abend WK, Schwartz RB, Samuels MA. A case of C2 herpes zoster with delayed bilateral pontine infarction. *Neurology* 1991;41:1685–1686.

Ross RT, Cheang M. Geographic similarities between varicella and multiple sclerosis: an hypothesis on the environmental factor of multiple sclerosis. *J Clin Epidemiol* 1995;48:731–737.

Rotbart HA. Human parvovirus infections. *Annu Rev Med* 1990;41:25–34.

Roth AM, Purcell TW. Ocular findings associated with encephalomyelitis caused by herpesvirus simiae. *Am J Ophthalmol* 1977;85:345–348.

Rous P. A sarcoma of the foul transmissible by an agent separable from the tumor cells. *J Exp Med* 1911; 13:397–411.

Rowe WP. Studies of genetic transmission of murine leukemia virus by AKR mice. I. Crosses with Fr-1n strains of mice. *J Exp Med* 1972;136:1272–1285.

Rowe WP, Hartley JW, Waterman S, Turner HC, Huebner RL. Cytopathogenic agent resembling human salivary gland virus recovered from tissue cultures of human adenoids. *Proc Soc Exp Biol Med* 1956; 92:418–424.

Rowson KE, Hinchcliffe R, Gamble DR. A virological and epidemiological study of patients with acute hearing loss. *Lancet* 1975;1:471–473.

Royal W III, Selnes OA, Concha M, Nance-Sproson TE, McArthur JC. Cerebrospinal fluid human immunodeficiency virus type 1 (HIV-1) p24 antigen levels in HIV-1-related dementia. *Ann Neurol* 1994;36:32–39.

Royal W III, Updike M, Selnes OA, et al. HIV-1 infection and nervous system abnormalities among a cohort of intravenous drug users. *Neurology* 1991;41:1905–1910.

Rubin RH, Gregg MB, Sikes RK. Rabies in citizens of the United States, 1963–1968: epidemiology, treatment, and complications of treatment. *J Infect Dis* 1969;120:168–173.

Ruff RL, Secrist D. Viral studies in benign acute childhood myositis. *Arch Neurol* 1982;39:261–263.

Rupprecht CE, Smith JS, Fekadu M, Childs JE. The ascension of wildlife rabies: a cause for public health concern or intervention? *Emer Infect Dis* 1995;1:107–114.

Russell DS. *Observations on the pathology of hydrocephalus.* London: Her Majesty's Stationery Office, 1949.

Ryder JW, Croen K, Kleinschmidt-DeMasters BK, Ostrove JM, Straus SE, Cohn DL. Progressive encephalitis three months after resolution of cutaneous zoster in a patient with AIDS. *Ann Neurol* 1986;19:182–188.

Rziha H-J, Belohradsky BH, Schneider U, Schwenk HU, Bornkamm GW, zur Hausen H. BK virus II. Serological studies in children with congenital disease and patients with malignant tumors and immunodeficiencies. *Med Microbiol Immunol* 1978;165:83–92.

Sabin AB. The nature and rate of centripetal progression of certain neurotropic viruses along peripheral nerves. *Am J Pathol* 1937;13:615–617.

Sabin AB. Pathogenesis of poliomyelitis, reappraisal in the light of new data. *Science* 1956;123: 1151–1157.

Sabin AB. Pathologic and virologic studies on three cases of so-called post-influenza encephalitis. In: Van Bogaert L, Radermecker J, Hozay J, Lowenthal A, eds. *Encephalitides*. Amsterdam: Elsevier, 1959: 79–83.

Sabin AB. Comments on paper by ZuRhein and Chou. *Res Publ Assoc Nerv Ment Dis* 1968;44:110–111.

Sabin AB, Wright AM. Acute ascending myelitis following a monkey bite, with isolation of a virus capable of reproducing the disease. *J Exp Med* 1934;59:115–135.

Sabin AG, Krumbiegel ER, Wigand R. ECHO type 9 virus disease. *AMA J Dis Child* 1958;96:197–219.

Sacktor N, McArthur J. Prospects for therapy of HIV-associated neurologic diseases. *J Neurovirol* 1997; 3:89–101.

Sadovnick AD, Armstrong H, Rice GPA, et al. A population-based study of multiple sclerosis in twins: update. *Ann Neurol* 1993;33:281–285.

Safranek TJ, Lawrence DN, Kurland LT, et al. Reassessment of the association between Guillain–Barré syndrome and receipt of swine influenza vaccine in 1976–1977: results of a two-state study. *Am J Epidemiol* 1991;133:940–951.

Safrit JT, Koup RA. The immunology of primary HIV infection: which immune responses control HIV replication? *Curr Opin Immunol* 1995;7:456–461.

Sagawa K, Mochizuki M, Masuoka K, et al. Immunopathological mechanisms of human T cell lymphotropic virus type 1 (HTLV-I) uveitis. *J Clin Invest* 1995;95:852–858.

Said G, Lacroix C, Chemouilli P, et al. Cytomegalovirus neuropathy in acquired immunodeficiency syndrome: a clinical and pathological study. *Ann Neurol* 1991;29:139–146.

Saida T, Saida K, Lisak RP, Brown MJ, Silberberg DH, Asbury AK. In vivo demyelinating activity of sera from patients with Guillain–Barré syndrome. *Ann Neurol* 1982;11:69–75.

Saito H, Takahashi Y, Harata S, et al. Isolation and characterization of mumps virus strains in a mumps outbreak with a high incidence of aseptic meningitis. *Microbiol Immunol* 1996;40:271–275.

Saito Y, Sharer LR, Epstein LG, et al. Overexpression of *nef* as a marker for restricted HIV-1 infection of astrocytes in postmortem pediatric central nervous tissues. *Neurology* 1994;44:474–481.

Salas R, De Manzione N, Tesh RB, et al. Venezuelan haemorrhagic fever. *Lancet* 1991;2:1033–1036.

Salazar A, Podzamczer D, Reñe R, et al. Cytomegalovirus ventriculoencephalitis in AIDS patients. *Scand J Infect Dis* 1995;27:165–169.

Salazar-Grueso EF, Grimaldi LME, Roos RP, Variakojis R, Jubelt B, Cashman NR. Isoelectric focusing studies of serum and cerebrospinal fluid in patients with antecedent poliomyelitis. *Ann Neurol* 1989; 26:709–713.

Salmi A, Reunanen M, Ilonen J, Panelius M. Intrathecal antibody synthesis to virus antigens in multiple sclerosis. *Clin Exp Immunol* 1983;52:241–249.

Salonen R. Cerebrospinal fluid and serum interferon in multiple sclerosis: longitudinal study. *Neurology* 1983;33:1604–1606.

Salonen O, Koshkiniemi M, Saari A, Myllylä V, Pyhälä R, Airaksinen L. Myelitis associated with influenza A virus infection. *J Neurovirol* 1997;3:83–85.

Sanchez A, Ksiazek TG, Rollin PE, et al. Reemergence of Ebola virus in Africa. *Emer Infect Dis* 1995;1: 96–97.

Sanders VJ, Waddell AE, Felisan SL, Li X, Conrad AJ, Tourtellotte WW. Herpes simplex virus in postmortem multiple sclerosis brain tissue. *Arch Neurol* 1996;53:125–133.

Sankalé J-L, Sallier de la Tour R, Marlink RG, et al. Distinct quasi-species in the blood and the brain of an HIV-2-infected individual. *Virology* 1996;226:418–423.

Sarnat HB, Alcala H. Human cerebellar hypoplasia: a syndrome of diverse causes. *Arch Neurol* 1980;37: 300–305.

Sarradet PM. Un cas de tremblante sur un boeuf. *Rev Vet* 1883;3:310–312.

Sasaki A, Nakazato Y. The identity of cells expressing MHC class II antigens in normal and pathological human brain. *Neuropathol Appl Neurobiol* 1992;18:13–26.

Sasaki K, Morooka I, Inomata H, Kashio N, Akamine T, Osame M. Retinal vasculitis in human T-lymphotropic virus type I associated myelopathy. *Br J Ophthalmol* 1989;73:812–815.

Sasseville VG, Lackner AA. Neuropathogenesis of simian immunodeficiency virus infection in macaque monkeys. *J Neurovirol* 1997;3:1–9.

Sasseville VG, Newman W, Brodie SJ, Hesterberg P, Pauley D, Ringler DJ. Monocyte adhesion to endothelium in simian immunodeficiency virus-induced AIDS encephalitis is mediated by vascular cell adhesion molecule-1/α4β1 integrin interactions. *Am J Pathol* 1994;144:27–40.

Sasseville VG, Smith MM, Mackay CR, et al. Chemokine expression in simian immunodeficiency virus-induced AIDS encephalitis. *Am J Pathol* 1996;149:1459–1467.

Sauder C, Müller A, Cubitt B, et al. Detection of Borna disease virus (BDV) antibodies and BDV RNA in psychiatric patients: evidence for high sequence conservation of human blood-derived BDV RNA. *J Virol* 1996;70:7713–7724.

Scheid W. Mumps virus and the central nervous system. *World Neurol* 1961;2:117–118.

Schiff JA, Schaefer JA, Robinson JE. Epstein–Barr virus in cerebrospinal fluid during infectious mononucleosis encephalitis. *Yale J Biol Med* 1982;55:59–63.

Schlesinger Y, Tebas P, Gaudreault-Keener M, Buller RS, Storch GA. Herpes simplex virus type 2 meningitis in the absence of genital lesions: improved recognition with use of the polymerase chain reaction. *Clin Infect Dis* 1995;20:842–848.

Schmidbauer M, Budka H, Ambros P. Herpes simplex virus (HSV) DNA in microglial nodular brainstem encephalitis. *J Neuropathol Exp Neurol* 1989;48:645–652.

Schmidbauer M, Budka H, Pilz P, Kurata T, Hondo R. Presence, distribution and spread of productive varicella zoster virus infection in nervous tissues. *Brain* 1992;115:383–398.

Schmidtmayerova H, Nottet HSLM, Nuovo G, et al. Human immunodeficiency virus type 1 infection alters chemokine β peptide expression in human monocytes: implications for recruitment of leukocytes into brain and lymph nodes. *Proc Natl Acad Sci USA* 1996;93:700–704.

Schmitt B, Seeger J, Kreuz W, Enenkel S, Jacobi G. Central nervous system involvement of children with HIV infection. *Dev Med Child Neurol* 1991;33:535–540.

Schmitt FA, Bigley JW, McKinnis R, et al. Neuropsychological outcome of zidovudine (AZT) treatment of patients with AIDS and AIDS-related complex. *N Engl J Med* 1988;319:1573–1578.

Schmitz H, Enders G. Cytomegalovirus as a frequent cause of Guillain–Barre syndrome. *J Med Virol* 1977;1:21–27.

Schmitz H, Kampa D, Doerr HW, Luthardt T, Hillemanns HG, Wurtele A. IgM antibodies to cytomegalovirus during pregnancy. *Arch Virol* 1977;53:177–184.

Schneck SA. Neuropathological features of human organ transplantation. I. Possible cytomegalovirus infection. *J Neuropathol Exp Neurol* 1965;24:415–429.

Schneemann A, Schneider PA, Lamb RA, Lipkin WI. The remarkable coding strategy of Borna disease virus: a new member of the nonsegmented negative strand RNA viruses. *Virology* 1995;210:1–8.

Schober R, Herman MM. Neuropathology of cardiac transplantation. *Lancet* 1973;1:962–967.

Schonberger LB, Bregman DJ, Sullivan-Bolyai JZ, et al. Guillain–Barré syndrome following vaccination in the national influenza immunization program, United States, 1976–1977. *Am J Epidemiol* 1979; 110:105–123.

Schroth G, Gawehn J, Thron A, Vallbracht A, Voigt K. Early diagnosis of herpes simplex encephalitis by MRI. *Neurology* 1987;37:179–183.

Schuknecht HF, Kitamura K. Vestibular neuritis. *Ann Otol Rhinol Laryngol* 1981;90:1–19.

Schultz G, DeLay PD. Losses in newborn lambs associated with bluetongue vaccination of pregnant ewes. *J Am Vet Assoc* 1955;127:224–226.

Schwartz J, Elizan TS. Herpes simplex virus encephalitis in suckling mice: ultrastructural studies of virus replication. *J Neuropathol Exp Neurol* 1975;34:359–368.

Schwartz J, Elizan TS. Search for viral particles and virus-specific products in idiopathic Parkinson disease brain material. *Ann Neurol* 1979;6:261–263.

Schwartz JN, Cashwell F, Hawkins HK, Klintworth GK. Necrotizing retinopathy with herpes zoster ophthalmicus. *Arch Pathol* 1976;100:386–391.

Schwarz GA, Yang DC, Noone EL. Meningoencephalomyelitis with epidemic parotitis. *Arch Neurol* 1964;11:453–462.

Schwarz TF, Nerlich A, Hottenträger B, et al. Parvovirus B19 infection of the fetus: histology and in situ hybridization. *Am J Clin Pathol* 1996;96:121–126.

Scott JR, Davies D, Fraser H. Scrapie in the central nervous system: neuroanatomical spread of infection and Sinc control of pathogenesis. *J Gen Virol* 1992;73:1637–1644.

Scott TW, Hildreth SW, Beaty BJ. The distribution and development of eastern equine encephalitis virus in its enzootic mosquito vector, *Culiseta melanura*. *Am J Trop Med Hyg* 1984;33:300–310.

Scott TW, Weaver SC. Eastern equine encephalomyelitis virus: epidemiology and evolution of mosquito transmission. *Adv Virus Res* 1989;37:277–328.

Seay AR, Griffin DE, Johnson RT. Experimental viral polymyositis: age-dependency and immune responses to Ross River virus infection in mice. *Neurology* 1981;31:656–661.

Seay AR, Wolinsky JS. Ross river virus-induced demyelination. I. Pathogenesis and histopathology. *Ann Neurol* 1982;12:380–389.

Seay AR, Wolinsky JS. Ross River virus-induced demyelination. II. Ultrastructural studies. *Ann Neurol* 1983;14:559–568.

Sedarati F, Izumi KM, Wagner EK, Stevens JG. Herpes simplex virus type 1 latency-associated transcription plays no role in establishment or maintenance of a latent infection in murine sensory neurons. *J Virol* 1989;63:4455–4458.

Sei S, Saito K, Stewart SK, et al. Increased human immunodeficiency virus (HIV) type 1 DNA content and quinolinic acid concentration in brain tissues from patients with HIV encephalopathy. *J Infect Dis* 1995;172:638–647.

Seif I, Coulon P, Rollin PE, Flamand A. Rabies virulence: effect on pathogenicity and sequence characterization of rabies virus mutations affecting antigenic site III of the glycoprotein. *J Virol* 1985;53:926–934.

Seilhean D, Dzia-Lepfoundzou A, Sazdovitch V, et al. Astrocytic adhesion molecules are increased in HIV-1-associated cognitive/motor complex. *Neuropathol Appl Neurobiol* 1997;23:83–92.

Selbst RG, Selhorst JB, Harbison JW, Myer EC. Parainfectious optic neuritis. *Arch Neurol* 1983;40:347–350.

Selby G, Walker GL. Cerebral arteritis in cat-scratch disease. *Neurology* 1979;29:1413–1418.

Selinka H-C, Zibert A, Wimmer E. Poliovirus can enter and infect mammalian cells by way of an intercellular adhesion molecule 1 pathway. *Proc Natl Acad Sci USA* 1991;88:3598–3602.

Selmaj K, Raine CS, Farooq M, Norton WT, Brosnan CF. Cytokine cytotoxicity against oligodendrocytes, apoptosis induced by lymphotoxin. *J Immunol* 1991;147:1522–1529.

Selnes OA, Galai N, McArthur JC, et al. HIV infection and cognition in intravenous drug users: long-term follow-up. *Neurology* 1997;48:223–230.

Selnes OA, Miller E, McArthur JC, et al. HIV-1 infection: no evidence of cognitive decline during the asymptomatic stages. *Neurology* 1990;40:204–208.

Sempere AP, Elizaga J, Duarte J, et al. Q fever mimicking herpetic encephalitis. *Neurology* 1993;43:2713–2714.

Senkowski A, Shim B, Roos RP. The effect of Theiler's murine encephalomyelitis virus (TMEV) VP1 carboxyl region on the virus-induced central nervous system disease. *J Neurovirol* 1995;1:101–110.

Sergent JS, Lockshin MD, Christian CL, Cocke DJ. Vasculitis with hepatitis B antigenemia. *Medicine (Baltimore)* 1976;55:1–18.

Server AC, Johnson RT. Guillain–Barré syndrome. *Curr Clin Top Infect Dis* 1982;3:74–96.

Sexton DJ, Rollin PE, Breitschwerdt EB, et al. Life-threatening Cache Valley virus infection. *N Engl J Med* 1997;336:547–549.

Sezer N. Further investigations on virus of Behçet's disease. *Am J Ophthalmol* 1956;41:41–55.

Shaffer MF, Rake G, Hodes HL. Isolation of virus from a patient with fatal encephalitis complicating measles. *Am J Dis Child* 1942;64:815–819.

Shafran SD. The chronic fatigue syndrome. *Am J Med* 1991;90:730–739.

Shah KV, Daniel RW, Warszawski R. High prevalence of antibodies to BK, an SV40 related papovavirus, in residents of Maryland. *J Infect Dis* 1973;128:784–787.

Shah KV, Nathanson N. Human exposure to SV40: review and comment. *Am J Epidemiol* 1976;103:1–12.

Shaked Y. Rickettsial infection of the central nervous system: the role of prompt antimicrobial therapy. *Q J Med* 1991;79:301–306.

Sharer LR. Pathology of HIV-1 infection of the central nervous system: a review. *J Neuropathol Exp Neurol* 1992;51:3–11.

Sharer LR, Dowling PC, Michaels J, et al. Spinal cord disease in children with HIV-1 infection: a combined molecular biological and neuropathological study. *Neuropathol Appl Neurobiol* 1990;16:317–331.

Sharief MK, Hentges R, Ciardi M. Intrathecal immune response in patients with the post-polio syndrome. *N Engl J Med* 1991;325:749–755.

Sharma DP, Zink MC, Anderson M, et al. Derivation of neurotropic SIV from exclusively lymphotropic parental virus: pathogenesis of infection in macaques. *J Virol* 1992;66:3550–3556.

Sharma KR, Sriram S, Fries T, Bevan HJ, Bradley WG. Lumbosacral radiculoplexopathy as a manifestation of Epstein–Barr virus infection. *Neurology* 1993;43:2550–2554.

Sharma S, Mathur A, Prakash V, Kulshreshtha R, Kumar R, Chaturvedi UC. Japanese encephalitis virus latency in peripheral blood lymphocytes and recurrence of infection in children. *Clin Exp Immunol* 1991;85:85–89.

Sharpe M, Hawton K, Seagroatt V, Pasvol G. Follow up of patients presenting with fatigue to an infectious diseases clinic. *BMJ* 1992;305:147–152.

Shaw C-M, Alvord EC. Multiple sclerosis beginning in infancy. *J Child Neurol* 1987;2:252–256.

Shaw GM, Harper ME, Hahn BH, et al. HTLV-III infection in brains of children and adults with AIDS encephalopathy. *Science* 1985;227:177–182.

Shearer GM, Clerici M, Lucey DR. Cytokines and HIV infection. *Semin Virol* 1994;5:449–455.

Shein HM. Transformation of astrocytes and destruction of spongioblasts induced by a simian tumor virus SV40 in cultures of human fetal neuroglia. *J Neuropathol Exp Neurol* 1967;26:60–76.

Shein HM. Neoplastic transformation of hamster astrocytes in vitro by simian virus 40 and polyoma virus. *Science* 1968;159:1476–1477.

Sheinberg MM. Antibody to lymphocytic choriomeningitis virus in children with congenital hydrocephalus. *Acta Virol (Praha)* 1975;19:165–166.

Sherman MP, Amin RM, Rodgers-Johnson PEB, et al. Identification of human T cell leukemia/lymphoma virus type I antibodies, DNA and protein in patients with polymyositis. *Arthritis Rheum* 1995;38:690–698.

Shi B, DeGirolami U, He J, et al. Apoptosis induced by HIV-1 infection of the central nervous system. *J Clin Invest* 1996;98:1979–1990.

Shill M, Baynes RD, Miller SD. Fatal rabies encephalitis despite appropriate post-exposure prophylaxis. *N Engl J Med* 1987;316:1257–1258.

Shimeld C, Whiteland JL, Williams NA, Easty DL, Hill TJ. Reactivation of herpes simplex virus type 1 in the mouse trigeminal ganglion: an in vivo study of virus antigen and immune cell infiltration. *J Gen Virol* 1996;77:2583–2590.

Shimizu T, Kawakami Y, Fukuhara S, Matumoto M. Experimental stillbirth in pregnant swine infected with Japanese encephalitis virus. *Jpn J Exp Med* 1954;24:363–375.

Shoji H, Honda Y, Murai I, Sato Y, Oizumi K, Hondo R. Detection of varicella–zoster virus DNA by polymerase chain reaction in cerebrospinal fluid of patients with herpes zoster meningitis. *J Neurol* 1992;239:69–70.

Shope RE. Arbovirus-related encephalitis. *Yale J Biol Med* 1980;53:93–99.

Shyu W-C, Lin J-C, Chang B-C, Harn H-J, Lee C-C, Tsao W-L. Recurrent ascending myelitis: an unusual presentation of herpes simplex virus type 1 infection. *Ann Neurol* 1993;34:625–627.

Sibley WA, Bamford CR, Clark K. Clinical viral infections and multiple sclerosis. *Lancet* 1985;2:1313–1315.

Sidhu MS, Crowley J, Lowenthal A, et al. Defective measles virus in human subacute sclerosing panencephalitis brain. *Virology* 1994;202:631–641.

Sidtis JJ, Gatsonis C, Price RW, et al. Zidovudine treatment of the AIDS dementia complex: results of a placebo-controlled trial. *Ann Neurol* 1993;33:343–349.

Siegel M. Congenital malformations following chickenpox, measles, mumps and hepatitis: results of a cohort study. *JAMA* 1973;226:1521–1524.

Sierra-Honigmann AM, Carbone KM, Yolken RH. Polymerase chain reaction (PCR) search for viral nucleic acid sequences in schizophrenia. *Br J Psychiatry* 1995;166:55–60.

Sigerist HE. *A history of medicine: primitive and archaic medicine.* New York: Oxford University Press, 1951.

Sigurdsson B. Rida; a chronic encephalitis of sheep: with general remarks on infections which develop slowly and some of their special characteristics. *Br Vet J* 1954;110:341–354.

Sigurdsson B, Palsson PA, Grimsson H. Visna, a demyelinating transmissible disease of sheep. *J Neuropathol Exp Neurol* 1957;15:389–403.

Silver B, McAvoy K, Mikesell S, Smith TW. Fulminating encephalopathy with perivenular demyelination and vacuolar myelopathy as the initial presentation of human immunodeficiency virus infection. *Arch Neurol* 1997;54:647–650.

Silverstein A, Steinberg G, Nathanson M. Nervous system involvement in infectious mononucleosis. *Arch Neurol* 1972;26:353–358.

Silverstein AM, Parshall CJ, Osburn BI, Prendergast RA. An experimental virus induced retinal dysplasia in the fetal lamb. *Am J Ophthalmol* 1971;72:22–34.

Sima AAF, Finkelstein SD, McLachlan DR. Multiple malignant astrocytomas in a patient with spontaneous progressive multifocal leukoencephalopathy. *Ann Neurol* 1983;14:183–188.

Simas JP, Dyson H, Fazakerley JK. The neurovirulent GDVII strain of Theiler's virus can replicate in glial cells. *J Virol* 1995;69:5599–5606.

Simila S, Jouppila R, Salmi A, Pohjonen R. Encephalomeningitis in children associated with an adenovirus type 7 epidemic. *Acta Paediatr Scand* 1970;59:310–316.

Simonon A, Lepage P, Karita E, et al. An assessment of the timing of mother-to-child transmission of human immunodeficiency virus type 1 by means of polymerase chain reaction. *J AIDS* 1994;7:952–957.

Simonsen JN, Cameron DW, Gakinya MN, et al. Human immunodeficiency virus infection among men with sexually transmitted diseases. *N Engl J Med* 1988;319:274–278.

Simpson DM, Wolfe DE. Neuromuscular complications of HIV infection and its treatment. *AIDS* 1991;5:917–926.

Singer DB, Rudolph AJ, Rosenberg HS, Rawls WE, Boniuk M. Pathology of the congenital rubella syndrome. *J Pediatr* 1967;71:667–675.

Singh U, Scheld WM. Infectious etiologies of rhabdomyolysis: three case reports and review. *Clin Infect Dis* 1996;22:642–649.

Siwasontiwat D, Lumlertdacha B, Polsuwan C, Hemachudha T, Chutvongse S, Wilde H. Rabies: is provocation of the biting dog relevant for risk assessment? *Trans R Soc Trop Med Hyg* 1992;86:443.

Sköldenberg B. Herpes simplex encephalitis. *Scand J Infect Dis* 1991;78:40–46.

Sköldenberg B. Herpes simplex encephalitis. *Scand J Infect Dis* 1996;100:8–13.

Sköldenberg B, Alestig K, Burman L, et al. Acyclovir versus vidarabine in herpes simplex encephalitis. *Lancet* 1984;2:707–711.

Sköldenberg B, Kalimo K, Carlstrom A, Forsgren M, Halonen P. Herpes simplex encephalitis: a serological follow-up study. *Acta Neurol Scand* 1981;63:273–285.

Small JA, Khoury G, Jay G, Howley PM, Scangos GA. Early regions of JC virus and BK virus induce distinct and tissue-specific tumors in transgenic mice. *Proc Natl Acad Sci USA* 1986;83:8288–8292.

Smith JS, Fishbein DB, Rupprecht CE, Clark K. Unexplained rabies in three immigrants in the United States. *N Engl J Med* 1991;324:205–211.

Smith MD, Scott GM, Rom S, Patou G. Herpes simplex virus and facial palsy. *J Infect* 1987;15:259–261.

Smith MG. Propagation in tissue cultures of a cytopathogenic virus from human salivary gland virus (SGV) disease. *Proc Soc Exp Biol Med* 1956;94:424–430.

Smith MW, Dean M, Carrington M, et al. Contrasting genetic influence of CCR2 and CCR5 variants on HIV-1 infection and disease progression. *Science* 1997;277:959–965.

Sobel RA, Collins AB, Colvin RB, Bhan AK. The in situ cellular immune response in acute herpes simplex encephalitis. *Am J Pathol* 1986;125:332–338.

Sorensen O, Collins A, Flintoff W, Ebers G, Dales S. Probing for the human coronavirus OC43 in multiple sclerosis. *Neurology* 1986;36:1604–1606.

Sorice M, Griggi T, Circella A, et al. Cerebrospinal fluid antiganglioside antibodies in patients with AIDS. *Infection* 1995;23:288–291.

Soto-Ramirez LE, Renjifo B, McLane MF, et al. HIV-1 Langerhans' cell tropism associated with heterosexual transmission of HIV. *Science* 1996;271:1291–1292.

Sotrel A, Rosen S, Ronthal M, Ross DB. Subacute sclerosing panencephalitis: an immune complex disease? *Neurology* 1983;33:885–890.

South MA, Tompkins WAF, Morris CR, Rawls WE. Congenital malformation of the central nervous system associated with genital (type 2) herpesvirus. *J Pediatr* 1969;75:13–18.

Southern PM, Smith JW, Luby JP, Barnett JA, Sanford JP. Clinical and laboratory features of epidemic St. Louis encephalitis. *Ann Intern Med* 1969;71:681–689.

Spataro RF, Lin S-R, Horner FA, Hall CB, McDonald JV. Aqueductal stenosis and hydrocephalus: rare sequelae of mumps virus infection. *Neuroradiology* 1976;12:11–13.

Speck PG, Simmons A. Divergent molecular pathways of productive and latent infection with a virulent strain of herpes simplex virus type 1. *J Virol* 1991;65:4001–4005.

Spehar T, Strand M. Molecular mimicry between HIV-1 gp41 and an astrocyte isoform of alpha-actinin. *J Neurovirol* 1995;1:381–390.

Sperling RS, Shapiro DE, Coombs RW, et al. Maternal viral load, zidovudine treatment, and the risk of transmission of human immunodeficiency virus type 1 from mother to infant. *N Engl J Med* 1996;335:1621–1629.

Sperling RS, Stratton P, O'Sullivan JJ, et al. A survey of zidovudine use in pregnant women with human immunodeficiency virus infection. *N Engl J Med* 1992;326:857–861.

Spiegelberg HL. Biological activities of immunoglobulins of different classes and subclasses. *Adv Immunol* 1974;19:259.

Spillane JD, Wells CEC. The neurology of Jennerian vaccination: a clinical account of the neurological complications which occurred during the smallpox epidemic in South Wales in 1962. *Brain* 1964;87: 1–44.

Sprent J, Tough DF. Lymphocyte life-span and memory. *Science* 1994;265:1395–1400.

Spriggs DR, Bronson RT, Fields BN. Hemagglutinin variants of reovirus type 3 have altered central nervous system tropism. *Science* 1983;220:505–507.

Spruance L, Bailey A. Colorado tick fever: a review of 115 laboratory confirmed cases. *Arch Intern Med* 1973;131:288–310.

Srabstein JC, Morris N, Larke R, de Sa DJ, Castelino BB, Sum E. Is there a congenital varicella syndrome? *J Pediatr* 1974;84:239–243.

Stagno S, Huang ES, Thames SD. Congenital cytomegalovirus infection: occurrence in an immune population. *N Engl J Med* 1977;296:1254–1258.

Stagno S, Pass RF, Cloud G, et al. Primary cytomegalovirus infection in pregnancy. *JAMA* 1986;256: 1904–1908.

Stagno S, Reynolds DW, Tsiantos A, Fuccillo DA, Long W, Alford CA. Comparative serial virologic and serologic studies of symptomatic and subclinical congenitally and naturally acquired cytomegalovirus infection. *J Infect Dis* 1975;132:568–577.

Starr JG, Bart RD, Gold E. Inapparent congenital cytomegalovirus infection: clinical and epidemiologic characteristics in early infancy. *N Engl J Med* 1970;282:1075–1078.

Staud R, Corman LC. Association of parvovirus B19 infection with giant cell arteritis. *Clin Infect Dis* 1996;22:1123.

Steck AJ, Siegrist P, Herschkowitz N, Schaefer R. Phosphorylation of myelin basic protein by vaccinia virus cores. *Nature* 1976;263:436–438.

Steel JG, Dix RD, Baringer JR. Isolation of herpes simplex virus type 1 in recurrent (Mollaret) meningitis. *Ann Neurol* 1982;11:17–21.

Steeper TA, Horwitz CA, Ablashi DV, et al. The spectrum of clinical and laboratory findings resulting from human herpesvirus-6 (HHV-6) in patients with mononucleosis-like illnesses not resulting from Epstein–Barr virus or cytomegalovirus. *Am J Clin Pathol* 1990;93:776–783.

Steere AC, Grodzicki RL, Arnold MS, et al. The spirochetal etiology of Lyme disease. *N Engl J Med* 1983;308:733–740.

Stein CA, Cheng Y-C. Antisense oligonucleotides as therapeutic agents: is the bullet really magical? *Science* 1993;261:1004–1012.

Steiner I, Kennedy PGE. Molecular biology of herpes simplex virus type 1 latency in the nervous system. *Mol Neurobiol* 1993;7:137–159.

Steiner I, Kennedy PGE. Herpes simplex virus latent infection in the nervous system. *J Neurovirol* 1995; 1:19–29.

Steinhardt E, Israeli C, Lambert RA. Studies on the cultivation of the virus of vaccinia. *J Infect Dis* 1913; 13:294–300.

Steinhauer DA, Holland JJ. Rapid evolution of RNA viruses. *Annu Rev Microbiol* 1987;41:409–433.

Steller H. Mechanisms and genes of cellular suicide. *Science* 1995;267:1445–1462.

Stevens DA, Ferrington RA, Jordan GW, Merigan TC. Cellular events in zoster vesicles: relation to clinical course and immune parameters. *J Infect Dis* 1975;131:509–515.

Stevens JG. Latent characteristics of selected herpesviruses. *Adv Cancer Res* 1978;26:227–256.

Stevens JG. Human herpesviruses: a consideration of the latent state. *Microbiol Rev* 1989;53:318–332.

Stevens JG. HSV-1 neuroinvasiveness. *Intervirology* 1993;35:152–163.

Stevens JG. Overview of herpesvirus latency. *Semin Virol* 1994;5:196.

Stevens JG, Wagner EK, Devi-Rao GB, Cook ML, Feldman LT. RNA complementary to a herpesvirus alpha gene mRNA is prominent in latently infected neurons. *Science* 1987;235:1056–1059.

Stevenson PG, Hawke S, Sloan DJ, Bangham CRM. The immunogenicity of intracerebral virus infection depends on anatomical site. *J Virol* 1997;71:145–151.

Stohlman SA, Lin M, Parra B, Bergmann CC, Hinton DR. Immune regulation of coronavirus-induced demyelinating encephalomyelitis. *J Neurovirol* 1997;3[Suppl]:S56–S57.

Stover SL, Wanglee P, Kennedy C. Acute hemorrhagic pancreatitis and other visceral changes associated with acute encephalopathy. *J Pediatr* 1968;73:235–241.

Straus SE. The chronic mononucleosis syndrome. *J Infect Dis* 1988;157:405–412.

Straus SE. History of chronic fatigue syndrome. *Rev Infect Dis* 1991;13[Suppl]:S2–S7.

Straus SE, Cohen JI, Tosato G, Meier J. NIH conference: Epstein–Barr virus infections—biology, pathogenesis, and management. *Ann Intern Med* 1993;118:45–58.

Straus SE, Dale JK, Tobi M, et al. Acyclovir treatment of the chronic fatigue syndrome: lack of efficacy in a placebo-controlled trial. *N Engl J Med* 1988;319:1692–1698.

Straus SE, Tosato G, Armstrong G, et al. Persisting illness and fatigue in adults with evidence of Epstein–Barr virus infection. *Ann Intern Med* 1985;102:7–16.

Strebel PM, Sutter RW, Cochi SL, et al. Epidemiology of poliomyelitis in the United States one decade after the last reported case of indigenous wild virus-associated disease. *Clin Infect Dis* 1992;14: 568–579.

Strizki JM, Albright AV, Sheng H, O'Connor M, Perrin L, Gonzalez-Scarano F. Infection of primary human microglia and monocyte-derived macrophages with human immunodeficiency virus type 1 isolates: evidence of differential tropism. *J Virol* 1996;70:7654–7662.

Studahl M, Ricksten A, Sandberg T, et al. Cytomegalovirus infection of the CNS in non-compromised patients. *Acta Neurol Scand* 1994;89:451–457.

Suarez GA, Giannini C, Bosch EP, et al. Immune brachial plexus neuropathy: suggestive evidence for an inflammatory-immune pathogenesis. *Neurology* 1996;46:559–561.

Subak-Sharpe I, Dyson H, Fazakerley J. In vivo depletion of CD8+ T cells prevents lesions of demyelination in Semliki Forest virus infection. *J Virol* 1993;67:7629–7633.

Suga S, Yoshikawa T, Asano Y, et al. Clinical and virological analyses of 21 infants with exanthem subitum (roseola infantum) and central nervous system complications. *Ann Neurol* 1993;33:597–603.

Sugamata M, Miyazawa M, Mori S, Spangrude GJ, Ewalt LC, Lodmell DL. Paralysis of street rabies virus-infected mice is dependent on T lymphocytes. *J Virol* 1992;66:1252–1260.

Sugihara H, Mutoh Y, Tsuchiyama H. Neuro-Beçhet's syndrome: report of two autopsy cases. *Acta Pathol Jpn* 1969;19:95–101.

Sulkava R, Rissanen A, Phyala R. Post-influenzal encephalitis during the influenza A outbreak in 1979/1980. *J Neurol Neurosurg Psychiatry* 1981;44:161–163.

Suter C, Westmoreland BF, Sharbrough FW, Hermann RC Jr. Electroencephalographic abnormalities in interferon encephalopathy: a preliminary report. *Mayo Clin Proc* 1984;59:847–850.

Sutton AL, Smithwick EM, Seligman SJ, Kim D-S. Fatal disseminated herpesvirus hominis type 2 infection in an adult with associated thymic dysplasia. *Am J Med* 1974;56:545–553.

Swan C, Tostevin AL. Congenital abnormalities in infants following infectious diseases during pregnancy, with special reference to rubella: third series of cases. *Med J Aust* 1946;1:645–659.

Swan C, Tostevin AL, Moore B, Mayo H, Black GHB. Congenital defects in infants following infectious disease during pregnancy. *Med J Aust* 1943;2:201–210.

Swanink CMA, van der Meer JWM, Vercoulen JHMM, Bleijenberg G, Fennis JFM, Galama JMD. Epstein–Barr virus (EBV) and the chronic fatigue syndrome: normal virus load in blood and normal immunologic reactivity in the EBV regression assay. *Clin Infect Dis* 1995;20:1390–1392.

Swanink CMA, Vercoulen JHMM, Galama JMD, et al. Lymphocyte subsets, apoptosis and cytokines in patients with chronic fatigue syndrome. *J Infect Dis* 1996;173:460–463.

Swarz JR, Brooks BR, Johnson RT. Spongiform polioencephalomyelopathy caused by a murine retrovirus. II. Ultrastructural localization of virus replication and spongiform changes in the central nervous system. *Neuropathol Appl Neurobiol* 1981;7:365–380.

Syrjänen J, Valtonen VV, Iivanainen M, Kaste M, Huttunen JK. Preceding infection as an important risk factor for ischaemic brain infarction in young and middle aged patients. *BMJ* 1988;296:1156–1160.

Tada H, Rappaport J, Lashgari M, Amini S, Wong-Staal F, Khalili K. Trans-activation of the JC virus late promoter by the tat protein of type 1 human immunodeficiency virus in glial cells. *Proc Natl Acad Sci USA* 1990;87:3479–3483.

Takahashi K, Wesselingh SL, Griffin DE, McArthur JC, Johnson RT, Glass JD. Localization of HIV-1 in human brain using polymerase chain reaction/in situ hybridization and immunocytochemistry. *Ann Neurol* 1996;39:705–711.

Takashima S, Becker LE. Neuropathology of fatal varicella. *Arch Pathol Lab Med* 1979;103:209–213.

Takemoto KK, Rabson AS, Mullarkey MF, Blaese RM, Garon CF, Nelson D. Isolation of papovaviruses from brain tumor and urine of a patient with Wiskott–Aldrich syndrome. *J Natl Cancer Inst* 1974;53: 1205–1207.

Tamashiro VG, Perez HH, Griffin DE. Prospective study of the magnitude and duration of changes in tuberculin reactivity during complicated and uncomplicated measles. *Pediatr Infect Dis J* 1987;6:451–454.

Tan SV, Guiloff RJ, Henderson DC, Gazzard BG, Miller R. AIDS-associated vacuolar myelopathy and tumor necrosis factor-alpha (TNFα). *J Neurol Sci* 1996;138:134–144.

Tan SV, Guiloff RJ, Scaravilli F. AIDS-associated vacuolar myelopathy, a morphometric study. *Brain* 1995;118:1247–1261.

Tan SV, Guiloff RJ, Scaravilli F, Klapper PE, Cleator GM, Gazzard BG. Herpes simplex type 1 encephalitis in acquired immunodeficiency syndrome. *Ann Neurol* 1993;34:619–622.

Tang TT, Sedmak GV, Siegesmund KA, McCreadie SR. Chronic myopathy associated with coxsackie virus type A9. *N Engl J Med* 1975;292:608–611.

Tardieu M, Grospiere B, Durandy A. Circulating immune complexes containing rubella antigens in late onset rubella syndrome. *J Pediatr* 1980;97:370–373.

Taskinen E, Koskiniemi M-L, Vaheri A. Herpes simplex virus encephalitis. *J Neurol Sci* 1984;63:331–338.

Taylor GR, Crow TJ, Markakis DA, Lofthouse R, Neeley S, Carter GI. Herpes simplex virus and Alzheimer's disease: a search for virus DNA by spot hybridisation. *J Neurol Neurosurg Psychiatry* 1987;47:1061–1065.

Taylor-Wiedeman J, Sissons JGP, Borysiewicz LK, Sinclair JH. Monocytes are a major site of persistence of human cytomegalovirus in peripheral blood mononuclear cells. *J Gen Virol* 1991;72:2059–2064.

Tedder DG, Ashley R, Tyler KL, Levin MJ. Herpes simplex virus infection as a cause of benign recurrent lymphocytic meningitis. *Ann Intern Med* 1994;121:334–338.

Tellez-Nagel I, Harter DH. Subacute sclerosing leukoencephalitis: ultrastructure of intranuclear and intracytoplasmic inclusions. *Science* 1966;154:899.

Telling GC, Parchi P, DeArmond SJ, et al. Evidence for the conformation of the pathologic isoform of the prion protein enciphering and propagating prion diversity. *Science* 1996;274:2079–2082.

Telling GC, Scott M, Hsiao KK, et al. Transmission of Creutzfeldt–Jakob disease from humans to transgenic mice expressing chimeric human–mouse prion protein. *Proc Natl Acad Sci USA* 1994;91:9936–9940.

Templer DI, Trent NH, Spencer DA, et al. Season of birth in multiple sclerosis. *Acta Neurol Scand* 1992;85:107–109.

Tenser RB. Role of herpes simplex virus thymidine kinase expression in viral pathogenesis and latency. *Intervirology* 1991;32:76–92.

Tenser RB, Hay KA, Edris WA. Latency-associated transcript but not reactivatable virus is present in sensory ganglion neurons after inoculation of thymidine kinase-negative mutants of herpes simplex virus type 1. *J Virol* 1989;63:2861–2865.

Tentsov YY, Zuev VA, Rzhaninova AA, Schevchenko AM, Bukrinskaya AG. Influenza virus genetic sequences in the blood of children with congenital pathology of the CNS. *Arch Virol* 1989;108:301–306.

Teodora JG, Branton PE. Regulation of apoptosis by viral gene products. *J Virol* 1997;71:1739–1746.

Thaler M. Pathogenesis of Reye's syndrome: a working hypothesis. *Pediatrics* 1975;56:1081–1084.

Thomas FP, Chalk C, Lalonde R, Robitaille Y, Jolicoeur P. Expression of human immunodeficiency virus type 1 in the nervous system of transgenic mice leads to neurological disease. *J Virol* 1994;68:7099–7107.

Thomas NH, Collins JE, Robb SA, Robinson RO. *Mycoplasma pneumoniae* infection and neurological disease. *Arch Dis Child* 1993;69:573–576.

Thompson CB. Apoptosis in the pathogenesis and treatment of disease. *Science* 1995;267:1456–1462.

Thompson JA. Mumps: a cause of acquired aqueductal stenosis. *J Pediatr* 1979;94:923–924.

Thompson JA, Glasgow LA. Intrauterine viral infection and the cell-mediated immune response. *Neurology* 1980;30:212–215.

Thompson RL, Devi-Rao GV, Stevens JG, Wagner EK. Rescue of a herpes simplex virus type 1 neurovirulence function with a cloned DNA fragment. *J Virol* 1985;55:504–508.

Thompson WH, Beaty BJ. Venereal transmission of LaCrosse (California encephalitis) arbovirus in *Aedes triseriatus* mosquitoes. *Science* 1977;196:530–531.

Thompson WH, Kalfayan B, Anslow RO. Isolation of California encephalitis virus from a fatal human illness. *Am J Epidemiol* 1965;81:245–253.

Thucydides. *History of the Peloponnesian War.* Baltimore: Penguin Books, 1954.

Tillack TW. The transport of ferritin across the placenta of the rat. *Lab Invest* 1966;15:896–909.

Tirawatnpong S, Hemachudha T, Manutsathit S, Shuangshoti S, Phanthumchinda K, Phanuphak P. Regional distribution of rabies viral antigen in central nervous system of human encephalitic and paralytic rabies. *J Neurol Sci* 1989;92:91–99.

Tobin JD, ten Bensel RW. Varicella with thrombocytopenia causing fatal intracerebral hemorrhage. *Am J Dis Child* 1972;124:577–578.

Toerner JG, Kumar PN, Garagusi VF. Guillain–Barré syndrome associated with Rocky Mountain spotted fever: case report and review. *Clin Infect Dis* 1996;22:1090–1091.

Toggas SM, Masliah E, Rockenstein EM, Rall GF, Abraham CR, Mucke L. Central nervous system damage produced by expression of the HIV-1 coat protein gp 120 in transgenic mice. *Nature* 1994;367: 188–193.

Tohyama J, Kawahara H, Inagaki M, Ohno K, Takeshita K, Egi T. Clinical and neuroradiologic findings of congenital hydrocephalus in infant born to mother with HTLV-I associated myelopathy. *Neurology* 1992;42:1406–1408.

Tomaru U, Ikeda H, Ohya O, et al. Human T lymphocyte virus type I-induced myeloneuropathy in rats: implication of local activation of the pX and tumor necrosis factor-α genes in pathogenesis. *J Infect Dis* 1996;174:318–323.

Tomlinson BE, Irving D. The numbers of limb motor neurons in the human lumbosacral cord throughout life. *J Neurol Sci* 1977;34:213–219.

Tondury G, Smith DW. Fetal rubella pathology. *J Pediatr* 1966;68:867–879.

Tooze J. *The molecular biology of tumour viruses.* Cold Spring Harbor, NY: Cold Spring Harbor Press, 1973.

Torigoe S, Kumamoto T, Koide W, Taya K, Yamanishi K. Clinical manifestations associated with human herpesvirus 7 infection. *Arch Dis Child* 1995;72:518–519.

Tornatore C, Berger JR, Houff SA, et al. Detection of JC virus DNA in peripheral lymphocytes from patients with and without progressive multifocal leukoencephalopathy. *Ann Neurol* 1992;31:454–462.

Tornatore C, Chandra R, Berger JR, Major EO. HIV-1 infection of subcortical astrocytes in the pediatric central nervous system. *Neurology* 1994;44:481–487.

Torrey EF, Torrey BB, Peterson MR. Seasonality of schizophrenic births in the United States. *Arch Gen Psychiatry* 1977;34:1065–1070.

Torrey EF, Yolken RH, Winfrey CJ. Cytomegalovirus antibody in cerebrospinal fluid of schizophrenic patients detected by enzyme immunoassay. *Science* 1982;216:892–894.

Townsend JJ, Baringer JR, Wolinsky JS, et al. Progressive rubella encephalitis: late onset after congenital rubella. *N Engl J Med* 1975;292:990–993.

Townsend JJ, Stroop WG, Baringer JR, Wolinsky JS, McKerrow JH, Berg BO. Neuropathology of progressive rubella panencephalitis after childhood rubella. *Neurology* 1982;32:185–190.

Townsend JJ, Wolinsky JS, Baringer JR. The neuropathology of progressive rubella panencephalitis of late onset. *Brain* 1976;99:81–90.

Trapp BD, Small JA, Pulley M, Khoury G, Scangos GA. Dysmyelination in transgenic mice containing JC virus early region. *Ann Neurol* 1988;23:38–48.

Travers RL, Hughes GRV, Cambridge G, Sewell JR. Coxsackie B neutralisation titres in polymyositis/dermatomyositis. *Lancet* 1977;1:1268.

Troendle-Atkins J, Demmier GJ, Buffone GJ. Rapid diagnosis of herpes simplex virus encephalitis by using the polymerase chain reaction. *J Pediatr* 1993;123:376–380.

Troost D, Van Den Oord JJ, Vianney De Jong JMB. Immunohistochemical characterization of the inflammatory infiltrate in amyotrophic lateral sclerosis. *Neuropathol Appl Neurobiol* 1990;16:401–410.

Trujillo JR, Navia BA, Worth J, et al. High levels of anti-HIV-1 envelope antibodies in cerebrospinal fluid as compared to serum from patients with AIDS dementia complex. *J AIDS* 1996;12:19–25.

Tsai TF, Canfield MA, Reed CM, et al. Epidemiological aspects of a St. Louis encephalitis outbreak in Harris County, Texas, 1986. *J Infect Dis* 1988;157:351–356.

Tselis A, Duman R, Storch GA, Lisak RP. Epstein–Barr virus encephalomyelitis diagnosed by polymerase chain reaction: detection of the genome in the CSF. *Neurology* 1997;48:1351–1355.

Tsiang H. Pathophysiology of rabies virus infection of the nervous system. *Adv Virus Res* 1993;42: 375–412.

Tsukada N, Koh C-S, Inoue A, Yanagisawa N. Demyelinating neuropathy associated with hepatitis B virus infection: detection of immune complexes composed of hepatitis B virus surface antigen. *J Neurol Sci* 1987;77:203–216.

Tsukamoto T, Hirano N, Iwasaki Y, Haga S, Terunuma H, Yamamoto T. Vacuolar degeneration in mice infected with a coronavirus JHM-CC strain. *Neurology* 1990;40:904–910.

Tsunoda I, Kurtz CIB, Fujinami RS. Apoptosis in acute and chronic central nervous system disease induced by Theiler's murine encephalomyelitis virus. *Virology* 1997;228:388–393.

Tucker PC, Strauss EG, Kuhn RJ, Strauss JH, Griffin DE. Viral determinants of age-dependent virulence of Sindbis virus for mice. *J Virol* 1993;67:4605–4610.

Tyler HR. Neurological complications of rubeola (measles). *Medicine (Baltimore)* 1957;36:147–167.

Tyler KL, Gross RA, Cascino GD. Unusual viral causes of transverse myelitis: hepatitis A virus and cytomegalovirus. *Neurology* 1986a;36:855–858.

Tyler KL, Mcphee DA, Fields BN. Distinct pathways of viral spread in the host determined by reovirus S1 gene segment. *Science* 1986b;233:770–774.

Tyler KL, Tedder DG, Yamamoto LJ, et al. Recurrent brainstem encephalitis associated with herpes simplex virus type 1 DNA in cerebrospinal fluid. *Neurology* 1995;45:2246–2250.

Tyor WR, Glass JD, Baumrind N, et al. Cytokine expression of macrophages in HIV-1-associated vacuolar myelopathy. *Neurology* 1993a;43:1002–1009.

Tyor WR, Glass JD, Griffin JW, et al. Cytokine expression in the brain during the acquired immunodeficiency syndrome. *Ann Neurol* 1992a;31:349–360.

Tyor WR, Moench TR, Griffin DE. Characterization of the local and systemic B cell response of normal and athymic nude mice with Sindbis virus encephalitis. *J Neuroimmunol* 1989;24:207–215.

Tyor WR, Power C, Gendelman HE, Markham R. A model of human immunodeficiency virus encpehalitis in SCID mice. *Proc Natl Acad Sci USA* 1993b;90:8658–8662.

Tyor WR, Stoll G, Griffin DE. The characterization of Ia expression during Sindbis virus encephalitis in normal and athymic nude mice. *J Neuropathol Exp Neurol* 1990;49:21–30.

Tyor WR, Wesselingh S, Levine B, Griffin DE. Long term intraparenchymal Ig secretion after acute viral encephalitis in mice. *J Immunol* 1992b;149:4016–4020.

Tyrrell DAJ, Crow TJ, Parry RP, Johnstone E, Ferrier IN. Possible virus in schizophrenia and some neurological disorders. *Lancet* 1979;1:839–844.

Ubol S, Tucker PC, Griffin DE, Hardwick JM. Neurovirulent strains of alphavirus induce apoptosis in bcl-2-expressing cells: role of a single amino acid change in the E2 glycoprotein. *Proc Natl Acad Sci USA* 1994;91:5202–5206.

Uchiyama T, Yodoi J, Sagawa K, Takatsuki K, Uchino H. Adult T-cell leukemia: clinical and hematologic features of 16 cases. *Blood* 1977;50:481–492.

Umehara F, Izumo S, Takeya M, Takahashi K, Sato E, Osame M. Expression of adhesion molecules and monocyte chemoattractant protein-1 (MCP-1) in the spinal cord lesions in HTLV-1-associated myelopathy. *Acta Neuropathol (Berl)* 1996;91:343–350.

Underwood M. *A treatise on the diseases of children.* London: J Mathews, 1787.

Vafai A, Wellish M, Gilden DH. Expression of varicella–zoster virus in blood mononuclear cells of patients with postherpetic neuralgia. *Proc Natl Acad Sci USA* 1988;85:2767–2770.

Vago L, Cinque P, Sala E, et al. JCV-DNA and BKV-DNA in the CNS tissue and CSF of AIDS patients and normal subjects: study of 41 cases and review of the literature. *J AIDS* 1996;12:139–146.

Vaheri A, Julkunen I, Koskiniemi M-L. Chronic encephalomyelitis with specific increase in intrathecal mumps antibodies. *Lancet* 1982;2:685–688.

Vahlne A, Nystrom B, Sandberg M, Hamberger A, Lycke E. Attachment of herpes simplex virus to neurons and glial cells. *J Gen Virol* 1978;40:359–371.

Vallee H, Carre H. Sur la nature infectieuse de l'anémie du cheval. *C R Acad Sci* 1904;139:331–333.

van Bogaert L. Une leuco-encéphalite sclérosante subaigü. *J Neurol Neurosurg Psychiatry* 1945;8:101.

Vanderlugt CJ, Miller SD. Epitope spreading. *Curr Opin Immunol* 1996;8:831–836.

Vandvik B. Oligoclonal IgG and free light chains in the cerebrospinal fluid of patients with multiple sclerosis and infectious diseases of the central nervous system. *Scand J Immunol* 1977;6:913–922.

Vandvik B, Nilsen RE, Vartdal F, Norrby E. Mumps meningitis: specific and non-specific antibody responses in the central nervous system. *Acta Neurol Scand* 1982;65:468–487.

Vandvik B, Norrby E, Steen-Johnsen J, Stensvold K. Mumps meningitis: prolonged pleocytosis and occurrence of mumps virus-specific oligoclonal IgG in the cerebrospinal fluid. *Eur Neurol* 1978;17:13–22.

Vandvik B, Sköldenberg B, Forsgren M, Stiernstedt G, Jeansson S, Norrby E. Long-term persistence of intrathecal virus-specific antibody responses after herpes simplex virus encephalitis. *J Neurol* 1985;231:307–312.

VanLandingham KE, Marsteller HB, Ross GW, Hayden FG. Relapse of herpes simplex encephalitis after conventional acyclovir therapy. *JAMA* 1988;259:1051–1053.

Varmus H. Retroviruses. *Science* 1988;240:1427–1435.

Vazeux R, Lacroix-Ciaudo C, Blanche S, et al. Low levels of human immunodeficiency virus replication in the brain tissue of children with severe acquired immunodeficiency syndrome encephalopathy. *Am J Pathol* 1991;140:137–144.

Vazquez-Lopez E. On the growth of Rous sarcoma inoculated into the brain. *Am J Cancer* 1936;26:29–55.

Vinters HV, Wang R, Wiley CA. Herpesviruses in chronic encephalitis associated with intractable childhood epilepsy. *Hum Pathol* 1993;24:871–879.

Viola MV, Frazier M, White L, Brody J, Spiegelman S. RNA-instructed DNA polymerase activity in a cytoplasmic particulate fraction in brains from Guamanian patients. *J Exp Med* 1975;142:483–494.

Viola MV, Myers JC, Gann KL, Gibbs CJ Jr, Roos RP. Failure to detect poliovirus genetic information in amyotrophic lateral sclerosis. *Ann Neurol* 1979;5:402–403.

Visser LH, van der Meché FGA, van Doorn PA, et al. Guillain–Barré syndrome without sensory loss (acute motor neuropathy): a subgroup with specific clinical, electrodiagnostic and laboratory features. *Brain* 1995;118:841–847.

Visudhiphan P, Chiemchanya S, Sirinavin S. Internal carotid artery occlusion associated with *Mycoplasma pneumoniae* infection. *Pediatr Neurol* 1992;8:237–239.

von Bokay J. Uber den atiologischen Zusammenhang der Varizellen mit gewissen Fallen von Herpes Zoster. *Wien Klin Wochenschr* 1909;22:1323.

von Pirquet C. Das Verhalten der kutanen Tuberkulin-reaktion wahrend der Masern. *Dtsch Med Wochenschr* 1908;34:1297–1300.

Wadia NH. Neurological manifestations of enterovirus 70: a 15-year review from India. In: Ishii K, Uchida Y, Miyamura K, Yamazaki S, eds. *Acute hemorrhagic conjunctivitis: etiology, epidemiology and clinical manifestations.* Tokyo: University of Tokyo Press, 1989:251–266.

Wain-Hobson S, Szathmary E, Szamado S, Meyerhans A. An antigenic demise of the immune system, or AIDS. *Dixieme Colloque Des Cent Gardes* 1995;17–24.

Waksman BH, Adams RD. Allergic neuritis. An experimental disease of rabbits induced by the injection of peripheral nervous tissue and adjuvants. *J Exp Med* 1955;102:213–235.

Walker DH, McCormick JB, Johnson KM, et al. Pathologic and virologic study of fatal Lassa fever in man. *Am J Pathol* 1982;107:349–356.

Walker DL. Progressive multifocal leukoencephalopathy: an opportunistic viral infection of the central nervous system. In: *Handbook of clinical neurology.* Amsterdam: Elsevier North-Holland, 1978: 307–329.

Walker DL, Padgett BL, ZuRhein GM, Albert AE, Marsh RF. Human papovavirus (JC): induction of brain tumors in hamsters. *Science* 1973;181:674–676.

Wallgren A. Une nouvelle maladie dur systeme nerveux central? *Acta Paediatr* 1925;4:158–182.

Walsh KJ, Armstrong RD, Turner AM. Brachial plexus neuropathy associated with human parvovirus infection. *BMJ* 1988;296:896.

Walter GF, Renella RR. Epstein–Barr virus in brain and Rasmussen's encephalitis. *Lancet* 1989;1: 279–280.

Walters JH. Postencephalitic Parkinson syndrome after meningoencephalitis due to Coxsackie virus group B, type 2. *N Engl J Med* 1960;263:744–746.

Waltrip RW II, Buchanan RW, Summerfelt A, Breier A, Carpenter WT Jr. Borna disease virus and schizophrenia. *Psychiatry Res* 1995;56:33–44.

Wang F-I, Stohlman SA, Fleming JO. Demyelination induced by murine hepatitis virus JHM strain (MHV-4) is immunologically mediated. *J Neuroimmunol* 1990;30:31–41.

Wang L, Robb CW, Cloyd MW. HIV induces homing of resting T lymphocytes to lymph nodes. *Virology* 1997;228:141–152.

Ward AC. Changes in the neuraminidase of neurovirulent influenza virus strains. *Virus Genes* 1995;10: 253–260.

Ward AC. Neurovirulence of influenza A virus. *J Neurovirol* 1996;2:139–151.

Ward BJ, Johnson RT, Vaisberg A, Jauregui E, Griffin DE. Spontaneous proliferation of peripheral mononuclear cells in natural measles virus infection: identification of dividing cells and correlation with mitogen responsiveness. *Clin Immunol Immunopathol* 1990;55:315–326.

Ward BJ, Johnson RT, Vaisberg A, Jauregui E, Griffin DE. Cytokine production in vitro and the lymphoproliferative defect of natural measles virus infection. *Clin Immunol Immunopathol* 1991;61: 236–248.

Ward JM, O'Leary TJ, Baskin GB, et al. Immunohistochemical localization of human and simian immunodeficiency viral antigens in fixed tissue sections. *Am J Pathol* 1987;127:199–205.

Warrell DA, Davidson NM, Pope HM, et al. Pathophysiologic studies in human rabies. *Am J Med* 1976; 60:180–190.

Warrell MJ, Looareesuwan S, Manatsathit S, et al. Rapid diagnosis of rabies and post-vaccinal encephalitides. *Clin Exp Immunol* 1988;71:229–234.

Warren KG, Brown SM, Wroblewska Z, Gilden D, Koprowski H, Subak-Sharpe J. Isolation of latent herpes simplex virus from the superior cervical and vagus ganglions of human beings. *N Engl J Med* 1978;287:1068–1069.

Watanabe R, Wege H, Ter Meulen V. Adoptive transfer of EAE-like lesions from rats with coronavirus-induced demyelinating encephalomyelitis. *Nature* 1983;305:150–153.

Watanabe T, Satoh M, Oda Y. Human parvovirus B19 encephalopathy. *Arch Dis Child* 1994;70:71.

Watson HD, Tignor GH, Smith AL. Entry of rabies virus into the peripheral nerves of mice. *J Gen Virol* 1981;56:372–382.

Wear DJ, Rapp F. Latent measles virus infection of the hamster central nervous system. *J Immunol* 1971; 107:1593–1598.

Weaver SC, Salas R, Rico-Hesse R, et al. Re-emergence of epidemic Venezuelan equine encephalo-myelitis in South America. *Lancet* 1996;1:436–440.

Webb HE, Rao RL. Kyasanur Forest disease: a general clinical study in which some cases with neuro-logical complications were observed. *Trans R Soc Trop Med Hyg* 1961;55:284–298.

Weber T, Turner RW, Frye S, et al. Specific diagnosis of progressive multifocal leukoencephalopathy by polymerase chain reaction. *J Infect Dis* 1994;169:1138–1141.

Wechsler B, Dell'Isola B, Vidailhet M, et al. MRI in 31 patients with Behçet's disease and neurological involvement: prospective study with clinical correlation. *J Neurol Neurosurg Psychiatry* 1993;56: 793–798.

Weigler BJ. Biology of B virus in macaque and human hosts: a review. *Clin Infect Dis* 1992;14:555–567.

Weil ML, Itabashi HH, Cremer NE, Oshiro LS, Lennette EH, Carnay L. Chronic progressive panen-cephalitis due to rubella virus simulating subacute sclerosing panencephalitis. *N Engl J Med* 1975; 292:994–998.

Weiland F, Cox JH, Meyer S, Dahme E, Reddehase MJ. Rabies virus neuritic paralysis: immunopatho-genesis of nonfatal paralytic rabies. *J Virol* 1992;66:5096–5099.

Weiland HT, Vermey-Keers C, Salimans MMM, Fleuren GJ, Verwey RA, Anderson MJ. Parvovirus B19 associated with fetal abnormality. *Lancet* 1987;1:682–683.

Weiner LP. Pathogenesis of demyelination induced by mouse hepatitis virus (JHM virus). *Arch Neurol* 1973;28:298–303.

Weiner LP, Herndon RM, Johnson RT. Viral infections and demyelinating diseases. *N Engl J Med* 1973; 288:1103–1110.

Weiner LP, Herndon RM, Narayan O, et al. Isolation of virus related to SV40 from patients with pro-gressive multifocal leukoencephalopathy. *N Engl J Med* 1972;286:385–390.

Weiner LP, Narayan O. Virologic studies of progressive multifocal leukoencephalopathy. *Prog Med Virol* 1974;18:229–240.

Weiner LP, Stohlman SA, Davis RL. Attempts to demonstrate virus in amyotrophic lateral sclerosis. *Neu-rology* 1980;30:1319–1322.

Weinstein L. Influence of age and sex on susceptibility and clinical manifestations in poliomyelitis. *N Engl J Med* 1957;257:47–52.

Weiser B, Nachman S, Tropper P, et al. Quantitation of human immunodeficiency virus type 1 during pregnancy: relationship of viral titer to mother-to-child transmission and stability of viral load. *Proc Natl Acad Sci USA* 1994;91:8037–8041.

Weiss AF, Portmann R, Fischer H, Simon J, Zang KD. Simian virus 40-related antigens in three human meningiomas with defined chromosome loss. *Proc Natl Acad Sci USA* 1975a;72:609–613.

Weiss RA. HIV receptors and the pathogenesis of AIDS. *Science* 1996;272:1885–1888.

Weiss S, Streifler M, Weiser HJ. Motor lesions in herpes zoster: incidence and special features. *Eur Neu-rol* 1975b;13:332–338.

Weiss SR. Coronaviruses SD and SK share extensive nucleotide homology with murine coronavirus MHV-A59, more than that shared between human and murine coronaviruses. *Virology* 1983;126: 669–677.

Weller TH, Neva FA. Propagation in tissue culture of cytopathic agents from patients with rubella-like ill-ness. *Proc Soc Exp Biol Med* 1962;111:215–225.

Weller TH, Witton HM. The etiologic agents of varicella and herpes zoster. *J Exp Med* 1958;108:869–890.

Wells CEC. Neurological complications of so-called "influenza": A winter study in Southeast Wales. *BMJ* 1971;1:369–373.

Wells GAH, Scott AC, Johnson CT, et al. A novel progressive spongiform encephalopathy in cattle. *Vet Res* 1987;121:419–420.

Welsh RM. Host cell modification of lymphocytic choriomeningitis virus and Newcastle disease virus altering viral inactivation by human complement. *J Immunol* 1977;118:348–354.

Wenger F. Necrosis cerebral masiva del feto en casos de encefalitis equine Venezolana. *Invest Clin* 1967; 21:13–31.

Wenner HA, Abel D, Barrick S, Seshumurty P. Clinical and pathogenetic studies of Medical Lake macaque virus infections in cynomolgus monkeys (simian varicella). *J Infect Dis* 1977;135:611–622.

Wesselingh SL, Power C, Glass JD, et al. Intracerebral cytokine messenger RNA expression in acquired immunodeficiency syndrome dementia. *Ann Neurol* 1993;33:576–582.

Wessely S, Powell R. Fatigue syndromes: a comparison of chronic "postviral" fatigue with neuromuscular and affective disorders. *J Neurol Neurosurg Psychiatry* 1989;52:940–948.

Westarp ME, Kornhuber HH, Rössler J, Flügel RM. Human spuma retrovirus antibodies in amyotrophic lateral sclerosis. *Neurol Psychiatry Brain Res* 1992;1:1–4.

Westmore GA, Pickard BH, Stern H. Isolation of mumps virus from the inner ear after sudden deafness. *BMJ* 1979;1:14–15.

Wetmur JG, Schwartz J, Elizan TS. Nucleic acid homology studies of viral nucleic acids in idiopathic Parkinson's disease. *Arch Neurol* 1979;36:462–464.

Whalen RG. DNA vaccines for emerging infectious diseases: what if? *Emer Infect Dis* 1996;2: 168–175.

White DO, Fenner FJ. Medical Virology. 4th ed. Academic Press. 1994.

White FA III, Ishaq M, Stoner GL, Frisque RJ. JC virus DNA is present in many human brain samples from patients without progressive multifocal leukoencephalopathy. *J Virol* 1992;66:5726–5734.

White HH, Kepes JH, Kirkpatrick CH, Schimke RN. Subacute encephalitis and congenital hypogenital hypogammaglobulinemia. *Arch Neurol* 1972;36:462–464.

Whitley R, Arvin A, Prober C, et al. A controlled trial comparing vidarabine with acyclovir in neonatal herpes simplex virus infection. *N Engl J Med* 1991a;324:444–449.

Whitley R, Arvin A, Prober C, et al. Predictors of morbidity and mortality in neonates with herpes simplex virus infections. *N Engl J Med* 1991b;324:450–454.

Whitley R, Lakeman AD, Nahmias A, Roizman B. DNA restriction-enzyme analysis of herpes simplex virus isolates obtained from patients with encephalitis. *N Engl J Med* 1982;307:1060–1062.

Whitley RJ. Neonatal herpes simplex virus infections. *J Med Virol* 1993;S1:13–21.

Whitley RJ, Alford CA, Hirsch MS, et al. Vidarabine versus acyclovir therapy in herpes simplex encephalitis. *N Engl J Med* 1986;314:144–149.

Whitley RJ, Cobbs CG, Alford CA, et al. Diseases that mimic herpes simplex encephalitis. *JAMA* 1989; 262:234–239.

Whitley RJ, Gnann JW Jr, Hinthorn D, et al. Disseminated herpes zoster in the immunocompromised host: a comparative trial of acyclovir and vidarabine. *J Infect Dis* 1992;165:450–455.

Whitley RJ, Lakeman F. Herpes simplex virus infections of the central nervous system: therapeutic and diagnostic considerations. *Clin Infect Dis* 1995;20:414–420.

Whitley RJ, Soong S-J, Dolin R, Galasso GJ, Ch'ien LT, Alford CA. Adenine arabinoside therapy of biopsy-proved herpes simplex encephalitis. *N Engl J Med* 1977;297:289–294.

Whitley RJ, Soong S-J, Hirsch MS, et al. Herpes simplex encephalitis: vidarabine therapy and diagnostic problems. *N Engl J Med* 1981;304:313–318.

Whittle HC, Dossetor J, Oduloju A, Bryceson ADM, Greenwood BM. Cell-mediated immunity during natural measles infection. *J Clin Invest* 1978;62:678–684.

Wientjens DPWM, Davanipour Z, Hofman A, et al. Risk factors for Creutzfeldt–Jakob disease: a reanalysis of case–control studies. *Neurology* 1996;46:1287–1291.

Wigdahl B, Brady JN. Molecular aspects of HTLV-I: relationship to neurological diseases. *J Neurovirol* 1996;2:307–322.

Wikstrand CJ, Bigner DD. Immunobiologic aspects of the brain and human gliomas. *Am J Pathol* 1980; 98:517–567.

Wilborn F, Schmidt CA, Brinkmann V, Jendroska K, Oettle H, Siegert W. A potential role for human herpesvirus type 6 in nervous system disease. *J Neuroimmunol* 1994;49:213–214.

Wild NJ, Sheppard S, Smithells RW, Holzel H, Jones G. Onset and severity of hearing loss due to congenital rubella infection. *Arch Dis Child* 1989;64:1280–1283.

Wildy P. The progression of herpes simplex virus to the central nervous system of the mouse. *J Hyg* 1967; 65:173–192.

Wilesmith JW. Bovine spongiform encephalopathy: epidemiological factors associated with the emergence of an important new animal pathogen in Great Britain. *Semin Virol* 1994;5:179–187.

Wiley CA, Achim C. Human immunodeficiency virus encephalitis is the pathological correlate of dementia in acquired immunodeficiency syndrome. *Ann Neurol* 1994;36:673–676.

Wiley CA, Gardner M. The pathogenesis of murine retroviral infection of the central nervous system. *Brain Pathol* 1993;3:128.

Wiley CA, Grafe M, Kennedy C, Nelson JA. Human immunodeficiency virus (HIV) and JC virus in acquired immune deficiency syndrome (AIDS) patients with progressive multifocal leukoencephalopathy. *Acta Neuropathol (Berl)* 1988;76:338–346.

Wiley CA, Masliah E, Morey M, et al. Neocortical damage during HIV infection. *Ann Neurol* 1991;29: 651–657.

Wiley CA, Schrier RD, Denaro FJ, Nelson JA, Lampert PW, Oldstone MBA. Localization of cytomegalovirus proteins and genome during fulminant central nervous system infection in an AID patient. *J Neuropathol Exp Neurol* 1986;45:127–139.

Wilfert CM, Buckley RH, Mokanakumar T, et al. Persistent and fatal central nervous system echovirus infections in patients with agammaglobulinemia. *N Engl J Med* 1977;296:1485–1489.

Wilfong RF, Bigner DD, Self DJ, Wechsler W. Brain tumor types induced by the Schmidt–Ruppin strain of Rous sarcoma virus in inbred Fischer rats. *Acta Neuropathol (Berl)* 1973;25:196–206.

Wilkinson GWG, Borysiewicz LK. Gene therapy and viral vaccination: the interface. *Br Med Bull* 1995; 51:205–216.

Wilkinson L. The development of the virus concept as reflected in corpora of studies on individual pathogens. 1. Beginnings at the turn of the century. *Med Hist* 1974;18:211–221.

Will RG, Ironside JW, Zeidler M, et al. A new variant of Creutzfeldt–Jakob disease in the UK. *Lancet* 1996;2:921–925.

Will RG, Knight RSG, Zeidler M, et al. Reporting of suspect new variant Creutzfeldt–Jakob disease. *Lancet* 1997;2:847.

Will RG, Matthews WB. A retrospective study of Creutzfeldt–Jakob disease in England and Wales 1970–79. I. Clinical features. *J Neurol Neurosurg Psychiatry* 1984;47:134–140.

Williamson AP, Blattner RJ, Robertson GG. The relationship of viral antigen to virus-induced defects in chick embryos: Newcastle disease virus. *Dev Biol* 1965;12:498–519.

Wilson ME. Travel and the emergence of infectious diseases. *Emer Infect Dis* 1995;1:39–46.

Wilson MG, Stein AM. Teratogenic effects of Asian influenza. *JAMA* 1969;210:336–337.

Wimalaratna HSK, Capildeo R, Lee HY. Herpes zoster of second and third segments causing ipsilateral Horner's syndrome. *BMJ* 1987;294:1463.

Windebank AJ, Litchy WJ, Daube JR, Iverson RA. Lack of progression of neurologic deficit in survivors of paralytic polio: a 5-year prospective population-based study. *Neurology* 1996;46:80–84.

Winkler WG, Fashinell TR, Leffingwell L, Howard P, Conomy JP. Airborne rabies transmission in a laboratory worker. *JAMA* 1973;226:1219–1221.

Wisniewski HM, Bloom BR. Primary demyelination as a non-specific consequence of a cell-mediated immune reaction. *J Exp Med* 1975;141:346.

Wisniewski HM, Keith AB. Chronic relapsing experimental allergic encephalomyelitis: an experimental model of multiple sclerosis. *Ann Neurol* 1977;1:144–148.

Wolf A, Cowen D. Perinatal infections of the central nervous system. In: Minckler J, ed. *Pathology of the nervous system.* New York: McGraw-Hill, 1972:2565–2611.

Wolf JL, Rubin DH, Finberg R, et al. Intestinal M cells: a pathway for entry of reovirus into the host. *Science* 1981;212:471–472.

Wolf SM, Schotland DL, Phillips LL. Involvement of nervous system in Behçet's syndrome. *Arch Neurol* 1965;12:315–325.

Wolfe L, Denhardt F. Induction of gliomas in marmosets by simian sarcoma virus–type 1 (SSV-1). *Proc Am Assoc Cancer Res* 1975;16:119.

Wolinsky JS. Progressive rubella panencephalitis. In: Vinken PJ, Bruyn GW, eds. *Handbook of clinical neurology.* Amsterdam: Elsevier North-Holland, 1978:331–341.

Wolinsky JS. Herpes simplex encephalitis. *Johns Hopkins Med Bull* 1980;147:157–163.

Wolinsky JS, Baringer JR, Margolis G, Kilham L. Ultrastructure of mumps virus replication in newborn hamster central nervous system. *Lab Invest* 1974;31:403–412.

Wolinsky JS, Berg BO, Maitland CJ. Progressive rubella panencephalitis. *Arch Neurol* 1976;33:722–723.

Wolinsky JS, Dau PC, Buimovici-Klein E, et al. Progressive rubella panencephalitis: immunological studies and results of isoprinosine therapy. *Clin Exp Immunol* 1979;35:397–404.

Wolinsky JS, Johnson RT. Role of viruses in chronic neurological diseases. In: Fraenkel-Conrat H, Wagner RR, eds. *Comprehensive virology.* New York: Plenum Press, 1980:257–296.

Wolinsky JS, Jubelt B, Burke S, Narayan O. Hematogenous origin of the inflammatory response in acute poliomyelitis. *Ann Neurol* 1982a;11:59–68.

Wolinsky JS, Swoveland P, Johnson KP, Baringer JR. Subacute measles encephalitis complicating Hodgkin's disease in an adult. *Ann Neurol* 1977;1:452–457.

Wolinsky JS, Waxham MN, Hess JL, Townsend JJ, Baringer JR. Immunochemical features of a case of progressive rubella panencephalitis. *Clin Exp Immunol* 1982b;48:359–366.

Wood MJ. Herpes zoster and pain. *Scand J Infect Dis* 1991;78[Suppl]:S53–S61.

Wood MJ. Current experience with antiviral therapy for acute herpes zoster. *Ann Neurol* 1994;35[Suppl]: S65–S68.

Woodall CJ, Riding MH, Graham DI, Clements GB. Sequences specific for enterovirus detected in spinal cord from patients with motor neurone disease. *BMJ* 1994;308:1541–1543.

Woodfin BM, Davis LE. Displacement of hepatic ornithine carbamoyltransferase from mitochondria to cytosol in Reye's syndrome. *Biochem Med Metab Biol* 1991;46:255–262.

Woods WA, Johnson RT, Hostetler DD, Lepow ML, Robbins FC. Immunofluorescent studies on rubella-infected tissue cultures and human tissues. *J Immunol* 1966;96:253–260.

Woolf NK, Koehrn FJ, Harris JP, Richman DD. Congenital cytomegalovirus labyrinthitis and sensorineural hearing loss in guinea pigs. *J Infect Dis* 1989;160:929–937.

Wright GP. Nerve trunks as pathways in infection. *Proc R Soc Lond* 1953;46:319–330.

Wrobleska Z, Gilden D, Devlin M, et al. Cytomegalovirus isolation from a chimpanzee with acute demyelinating disease after inoculation of multiple sclerosis brain cells. *Infect Immun* 1979;25: 1008–1015.

Wu E, Dickson DW, Jacobson S, Raine CS. Neuroaxonal dystrophy in HTLV-1-associated myelopathy/tropical spastic paraparesis: neuropathologic and neuroimmunologic correlations. *Acta Neuropathol (Berl)* 1993;86:224–235.

Wucherpfenning KW, Strominger JL. Molecular mimicry in T cell-mediated autoimmunity: viral peptides activate human T cell clones specific for myelin basic protein. *Cell* 1995;80:695–705.

Wynn DR, Rodriguea M, O'Fallon M, Kurland LT. A reappraisal of the epidemiology of multiple sclerosis in Olmsted County, Minnesota. *Neurology* 1990;40:780–786.

Xu X, Heidenreich O, Nerenberg M. HAM/TSP and ATL: persistent paradoxes and new hypotheses. *J Neurovirol* 1996;2:60–69.

Yahr MD. Encephalitis lethargica (von Economo's disease, epidemic encephalitis). In: *Handbook of clinical neurology.* Amsterdam: North-Holland, 1978:451–457.

Yamada M, Zurbriggen A, Oldstone MBA, Fujinami RS. Common immunologic determinant between human immunodeficiency virus type 1 gp41 and astrocytes. *J Virol* 1991;65:1370–1376.

Yamamoto LJ, Tedder DG, Ashley R, Levin MJ. Herpes simplex virus type 1 DNA in cerebrospinal fluid of a patient with Mollaret's meningitis. *N Engl J Med* 1991;325:1082–1085.

Yamanishi K, Shiraki K, Kondo T, et al. Identification of human herpesvirus-6 as a causal agent for exanthem subitum. *Lancet* 1988;1:1065–1067.

Yawn DH, Pyeatte JC, Joseph JM, Eichler SL, Garcia-Bunuel R. Transplacental transfer of influenza virus. *JAMA* 1971;216:1022–1023.

Yerushalmy J, Palmer CE. On the methodology of investigations of etiologic factors in chronic diseases. *J Chronic Dis* 1959;10:27–40.

Yokomori K, Asanaka M, Stohlman SA, et al. Neuropathogenicity of mouse hepatitis virus JHM isolates differing in hemagglutinin-esterase protein expression. *J Neurovirol* 1995;1:330–339.

Yolken RH. Summary of meeting. *J Neurovirol* 1996;2:196–197.

Yoneda T, Urade M, Sakuda M, Miyazaki T. Altered growth, differentiation, and responsiveness to epidermal growth factor of human embryonic mesenchymal cells of palate by persistent rubella virus infection. *J Clin Invest* 1986;77:1613–1621.

Yoshiki T. Chronic progressive myeloneuropathy in WKAH rats induced by HTLV-I infection as an animal model for HAM/TSP in humans. *Intervirology* 1995;38:229–237.

Young AB, Oster-Granite ML, Herndon RM, Snyder SH. Glutamic acid: selective depletion by viral induced granule cell loss in hamster cerebellum. *Brain Res* 1974;73:1–13.

Yow MD, White NH, Taber LH, et al. Acquisition of cytomegalovirus infection from birth to 10 years: a longitudinal serologic study. *J Pediatr* 1986;109:35–37.

Yuki N, Taki T, Takahashi M, et al. Molecular mimicry between GQ1b ganglioside and lipopolysaccharides of *Campylobacter jejuni* isolated from patients with Fisher's syndrome. *Ann Neurol* 1994;36:791–793.

Zakarian B, Barlow RM, Rennie JC. Periarteritis in experimental border disease of sheep. *J Comp Pathol* 1975;23:635–659.

Zerr I, Bodemer M, Otto M, et al. Diagnosis of Creutzfeldt–Jakob disease by two-dimensional gel electrophoresis of cerebrospinal fluid. *Lancet* 1996;2:846–849.

Zhdanov VM. Integration of viral genomes. *Nature* 1975;256:471–473.

Zhu T, Mo H, Wang N, et al. Genotypic and phenotypic characterization of HIV-1 patients with primary infection. *Science* 1993;261:1179–1181.

Zil'ber LA, Bajdakova ZL, Gardas'jan AN, Konovalov NV, Bunina TL, Barabadze EM. Study of the etiology of amyotrophic lateral sclerosis. *Bull WHO* 1963;29:449–456.

Zimmerman LE. Histopathologic basis for ocular manifestations of congenital rubella syndrome. *Am J Ophthalmol* 1968;65:837–862.

Zisman B, Wheelock EF, Allison AC. Role of macrophages and antibody in resistance of mice against yellow fever virus. *J Immunol* 1971;107:236–243.

Zoll J, Jongen P, Galama J, van Kuppeveld F, Melchers W. Coxsackievirus B1-induced murine myositis: no evidence for viral persistence. *J Gen Virol* 1993;74:2071–2076.

zur Hausen H. The role of viruses in human tumors. *Adv Cancer Res* 1980;33:77–107.

zur Hausen H. Viruses in human cancers. *Science* 1991;254:1167–1173.

ZuRhein GM. Association of papova-virions with a human demyelinating disease (progressive multifocal leukoencephalopathy). *Prog Med Virol* 1969;11:185–247.

ZuRhein GM, Chou S-M. Papova virus in progressive multifocal leukoencephalopathy. In: Zimmerman HM, ed. *Infections of the nervous system.* Baltimore: Williams & Wilkins, 1968:307–362.

ZuRhein GM, Chou SM. Particles resembling papovavirus in human cerebral demyelinating disease. *Science* 1965;148:1477–1479.

Subject Index

A

Acquired immunodeficiency syndrome. *See also*
    Human immunodeficiency virus
clinical syndromes of congenital infection,
    331–332
dementia in, 297–299
encephalopathy in, 296–297
lamivudine therapy, 312
meningitis in, 296–297
opportunistic neurologic processes, 294–295
pathogenesis, 292–293, 313
peripheral neuropathies, 300–301
prevalence of, 290–291
progression, rate and factors affecting,
    293–294
protease inhibitor therapy, 312–313, 421–422
vacuolar myelopathy in, 299–300
zidovidine therapy, 294, 311–312
Acute disseminated encephalomyelitis. *See*
    Postinfectious encephalomyelitis
Acute hemorrhagic leukoencephalitis
diagnosis of, 201
time of onset, 201
viruses associated with, 201–202
Acute neurologic disease. *See also* Encephalitis,
    Menigitis, Poliomyelitis
herpesviruses in, 133–168
postviral syndromes, 181–224
rabies virus in, 169–179
Acyclovir
herpetic encephalitis treatment, 147–149, 418
immunocompromised patient treatment, 160
Adenoviruses
cerebral tumor, association with, 381–383
characteristics of, 102–103
CNS infections, 103–104
distinguishing features in, 16
epidemiology, 103
immunodeficiency, association with, 83–84

morphology of, 15, 20
Reye's syndrome, association with, 215
specimens for isolation and diagnosis, 125
Adsorption. *See* Attachment
Aino virus, 344
Akabane virus, 344
Aleutian mink disease virus, cerebrovascular dis-
    ease, 407–409
Alphavirus. *See* Eastern encephalitis virus,
    Venezuelan equine encephalitis virus,
    Western encephalitis virus
Alzheimer's disease
histologic findings of, 368
prion, possible roles in, 369–370
virus, possible roles in, 368–369
Amantadine, prophylaxis of influenza A,
    420–421
Amitryptyline, postherpetic neuralgia treatment,
    160
Amyotrophic lateral sclerosis
epidemiology, 370
virus, possible roles in, 7–8, 370–372
Animal studies of viruses
deafness, 400–402
cerebral malformations, 340–345
human immunodeficiency virus models,
    309–311
hydrocephalus, 345–347
retinitis, 392–394
vasculitis, cerebrovascular disease, 407–409
Antibody. *See* Immunoglobulin
Antisense oligonucleotide, viral therapy, 421
Apoptosis
central nervous system development role, 32
comparison to necrosis, 32–33
HIV dementia association, 299
viral mechanisms of induction, 32–33
Arboviruses
agents causing encephalitis, 110–112

Arboviruses (*contd.*)
  alphavirus. *See* Alphavirus
  arthropod infection, 112–114
  bunyaviridae. *See* Bunyaviridae
  California encephalitis virus. *See* California
    encephalitis virus
  Colorado tick fever virus. *See* Colorado tick
    fever virus
  Eastern encephalitis virus. *See* Eastern
    encephalitis virus
  environmental control of, 413–414
  epidemiology of encephalitis, 112
  flavivirus. *See* Flaviviridae
  Japanese encephalitis virus. *See* Japanese
    encephalitis virus
  portals of entry, 39
  Ross River virus. *See* Ross River virus
  St. Louis encephalitis virus. *See* St. Louis
    encephalitis virus
  specimens for isolation and diagnosis, 125
  Semliki Forest virus. *See* Semliki Forest virus
  Sindbis virus. *See* Sindbis virus
  tick-borne encephalitis viruses. *See* Tick-borne
    encephalitis viruses
  transmission, 109
  Venezuelan equine encephalitis virus. *See*
    Venezuelan equine encephalitis virus
  West Nile virus. *See* West Nile virus
  Western encephalitis virus. *See* Western
    encephalitis virus
Arenaviridae
  distinguishing features in, 18
  hemorrhagic fever from, 105, 107–108
  Junin virus. *See* Junin virus
  Lassa fever, 107, 399
  Lymphocytic choriomeningitis virus. *See* Lym-
    phocytic choriomeningitis virus
  Machupo virus. *See* Machupo virus
  morphology of, 15, 20
Arteritis. *See* Vasculitis
Arthropod-borne viruses. *See* Arboviruses
Aseptic meningitis. *See* Meningitis
Assembly, overview of viral mechanisms, 27
Attachment, virus infection
  blocking by drugs, 419
  efficiency, 24
  receptors, 24–26
Avian sarcoma virus
  cerebral tumor, association with, 381–382
  discovery of, 265
Axonal transport of viruses, 42–43
Azidothymidine. *See* Zidovidine

B

B cell
  activation of, 64–65
  differentiation and maturation of, 62–64
  surface markers, 63, 65
  viral antigens, 69
B virus
  encephalitis with, 151
  myelitis with, 151
Beçet's disease
  features of, 260
  virus involvement in, 260–261
Biopsy of brain, 148
BK virus
  cerebral tumor, association with, 381–383,
    385–386
  fetal infection, 339
  progressive multifocal leukoencephalopathy,
    association with, 245–248
Blood–brain barrier
  attenuation in inflammation, 80, 82
  changes in HIV dementia, 302, 309
  structure, 49
  virus permeability, 46–47, 49–50
Blood–cerebrospinal fluid barrier
  immunoglobulin permeability, 76–77
  structure of, 50
Bluetongue virus, fetal cerebral effects of vac-
    cine, 342–343
Border disease virus
  cerebrovascular disease, 407–408
  teratogenesis, 344
Borna disease
  features of, 262
  human disease, 262–263
Bornavirus, retinitis, 392–393
Bovine immunodeficiency virus, features of dis-
    ease, 283
Bovine papilloma virus, cerebral tumor induction,
    381
Bovine spongiform encephalopathy
  history of, 364–365, 367–368
  human variant of, 366–367
  incubation period, 365
  prevention, 365
  transmission, 364–366
Bovine viral diarrhea virus
  retinitis with, 392
  teratogenesis, 344
Brachial neuritis, postinfection, 209
Budding, overview of viral mechanisms, 27
Bunyaviridae

California encephalitis virus. *See* California
  encephalitis virus
  distinguishing features in, 17
  La Crosse virus. *See* La Crosse virus
  morphology of, 15, 20
Burkitt's lymphoma, Epstein–Barr virus, isolation
  from, 160, 378

C

California encephalitis virus
  clinical features of infection, 120
  epidemiology, 118
  La Crosse strain, 118
  life cycle of, 119–120
Campylobacter, Guillain–Barré syndrome association, 208–209
Cancer. *See also* Burkitt's lymphoma, Cerebral
  tumor, Transformation
  multistep oncogenesis, 377
  tumor suppressor genes, 378
  viral oncogenes, 378
Canine distemper
  demyelination in, 187, 189
  retinitis with, 392
Cannibalism, and kuru, 356
Caprine arthritis–encephalitis virus
  demyelination in infection, 187
  features of disease, 282
Capsomer, structure in viruses, 13
Cardiovirus. *See* Encephalomyocarditis virus
Cat-scratch disease
  clinical features, 132
  differential diagnosis from acute viral CNS
    infections, 132
  pathogens, 132
Cell cultures of viruses, 15, 21
Cell-mediated immune response. *See* T cell
Cercopithecine herpesvirus 1. *See* B virus
Cerebellar hypoplasia, virus-induced in animals,
  342
Cerebral tumor
  adenoviruses in, 381–383
  epidemiologic studies, 386
  Epstein–Barr virus in, 383–384
  laboratory induction by viruses, 378–383
  papovaviruses in, 381–386
  retroviruses in, 381–383
  virus recovery from, 383–386
Cerebrospinal fluid
  antigen efflux to, 78
  herpetic encephalitis diagnosis, 144–146
  history of examination, 4

immunoglobulins in, 76–77
  lymphocytes in, 77
Chandipura virus, demyelination in infection,
  187, 189
Chemokines, synthesis and effects, 66
Chemotherapy of virus infections, 418–422
Chickenpox
  epidemiology, 152
  fetal effects of, 335–336
  neurological complications of, 153, 157–158
  postinfectious encephalomyelitis, 193, 197
  vaccination against, 159
  virus. *See* Varicella–zoster virus
Chronic fatigue syndrome
  definition of, 223–224
  and epidemic neuromyasthenia, 221
  epidemiology, 224
  history of, 211, 220
  prognosis of, 224
  types of, 220
  viruses in sporadic cases, 221–223
Chronic infection, differentiation from chronic
  disease, 225–226
Chronic neurologic diseases
  Alzheimer's disease, 368–370
  amyotrophic lateral sclerosis, 370–372
  Borna disease, 262–263
  bovine immunodeficiency virus, 283
  bovine spongiform encephalopathy, 364–368
  caprine arthritis–encephalitis virus, 282
  Creutzfeldt–Jakob disease, 349, 356–364
  equine infectious anemia virus, 282–283
  feline immunodeficiency virus, 283–284
  human immunodeficiency virus, 265, 267,
    287–315
  human T–cell lymphotropic viruses, 268–277
  Kozhevnikov's disease, 258–259
  kuru, 349, 353–356
  lentiviruses, 279–280
  mechanism of viral persistence, 228–231
  multiple sclerosis, 248–258
  murine leukemia virus, 277–279
  Parkinson's disease, 372–373
  progressive multifocal leukoencephalopathy,
    241–243, 245–248
  progressive rubella panencephalitis, 239–241
  Rasmussen's disease, 258–259
  recurrent inflammatory diseases, 259–261
  schizophrenia, 373–374
  scrapie, 227–228, 349–353
  simian immunodeficiency virus, 284–286
  subacute sclerosing panencephalitis, 231–239

Chronic neurologic diseases (*contd.*)
  Viliusk encephalomyelitis, 261–262
  visna, 227–228, 281–282
Classification of viruses, 14–15
Colony-stimulating factors, synthesis and effects, 66
Colorado tick fever virus
  clinical features of infection, 122
  epidemiology, 122
Complement
  activation, 73–74
  components, 73
  depletion in viral infection, 74
Complementation, 29
Continuous focal epilepsy. *See* Kozhevnikov's epilepsy
Coronaviridae
  distinguishing features in, 18
  morphology of, 15, 20
  mouse hepatitis virus. *See* Mouse hepatitis virus
  recovery in multiple sclerosis, 255, 257
Coxsackie virus
  chronic fatigue syndrome, association with, 221–223
  and encephalitis, 98–99
  epidemics, 99
  fetal infection, 337–338
  meningitis with, 97–98
  myositis with, 403–404
  nonpolio manifestations, 96–97
  Reye's syndrome, association with, 215
  seasonal distribution of infection, 96–97
  serotypes, 93
  specimens for isolation and diagnosis, 125
Creutzfeldt–Jakob disease
  bovine spongiform encephalopathy in cause, 366–367
  diagnosis, 357–358
  disease description, 357–358
  incidence, 357
  nosology, 356–357
  transmission
    familial cases, 359–362
    iatrogenic transmission, 362–363
    laboratory transmission, 358–359
    sporadic cases, 363–364
Cultivation, viruses
  animal cultures, 15
  cell cultures, 15, 21
  egg cultures, 15
  explant cultures, 21
Cytokines

  cells of origin, 66–68
  classification of, 66
  neural response to, 68
  neurotoxicity of, 307–309
  overview of effects, 66–68
  viral defense mechanisms, 68
Cytomegalovirus, 16
  cytomegalic inclusion disease, 326–327
  deafness with, 398, 400–401
  diagnosis of infection, 167
    mothers and infants, 326, 328–329
    specimens for isolation, 125
  diseases in immunocompromised patients, 165–167
  encephalitis with, 166
  foscarnet therapy, 329
  ganciclovir therapy, 329
  Guillain–Barré syndrome, association with, 205–206
  humoral immunity, 164
  latency, 164
  portals of entry, 39
  prevalence of infection
    fetal, 325–326
    maternal, 326
  receptor, 25
  retinitis with, 389–390
  silent fetal infection, 328

D

Dawson's encephalitis. *See* Subacute sclerosing panencephalitis
Deafness. *See also* Labyrinthitis
  animal studies of viral effects, 400–402
  cytomegalovirus in, 398, 400–401
  pathogenesis, 396–397
  rubella virus in, 397–398
  sudden acquired deafness, viral induction, 398–400
  virus types and lesions, 395
Degenerative diseases
Alzheimer's disease, 368–370
  amyotrophic lateral sclerosis, 7–8, 370–372
  Creutzfeldt–Jakob disease, 356–364, 366–367
  kuru, 353–356, 364
  Parkinson's disease, 372–373
  scrapie, 7, 215, 227–228, 255, 257, 349–353, 364, 394, 426
Dementia
  AIDS, 297–299, 302
  Alzheimer's disease, 368–370
Demyelination
  mechanisms in viral demyelination, 189–192

rabies vaccine induction, 183–185
viruses in, 186–189
Dengue viruses, clinical features of infection, 124–125
Diagnosis
acute hemorrhagic leukoencephalitis, 201
adenoviruses, 125
arboviruses, 125
cat-scratch disease, 132
coxsackie virus, 125
Creutzfeldt–Jakob disease, 357–358
cytomegalovirus, 125, 167, 326, 328–329
echovirus, 125
enteroviruses, 125
Guillain–Barré syndrome, 203
herpes encephalitis, 125, 144–146, 148
human immunodeficiency virus, 333
infectious mononucleosis, 125
lymphocytic choriomeningitis virus, 125
mumps virus, 125
mycoplasma infections, 130–132
poliovirus, 125
polymerase chain reaction. *See* Polymerase chain reaction
progressive multifocal leukoencephalopathy, 243
Q fever, 128
rabies virus, 125
rickettsia infections, 127–128
Rocky Mountain spotted fever, 127–128
rubella, 325
spirochetal infections, 128–130
Distemper virus. *See* Canine distemper virus
DNA virus
replication, 26
survival mechanisms, 431
Drugs as antiviral agents, 418–422
adsorption blocking, 419
design, 422
polymerase inhibitors, 421–422
protease inhibitors, 421–422
uncoating blocking, 420–421

E

Ear infection. *See* Deafness, Labyrinthitis
Eastern encephalitis virus
arthropod infection, 113, 115
clinical features of infection, 115
life cycle of, 114–115
Ebola virus, 17
epidemics, 431, 433
hemorrhagic fever with, 109
Echovirus

encephalitis with, 98–99
epidemics, 99
fetal infection, 337
meningitis with, 97–98
nonpolio manifestations of, 96–97
receptor, 25
Reye's syndrome, association with, 215
seasonal distribution of infection, 96–97
serotypes, 93
specimens for isolation and diagnosis, 125
Eclipse phase of infection, 24
Ecological cycle
California encephalitis virus, 119–120
Eastern encephalitis virus, 114–115
Japanese encephalitis virus, 122–123
rabies, 170–173
St. Louis encephalitis virus, 116–117
Western encephalitis virus, 115–116
Ectromelia virus, history of study, 37
Electron microscopy
negative staining, 13
shadow casting, 13
virus structure studies, 13–14
Encephalitis. *See also* specific viruses
arboviruses, 110–112
California encephalitis virus. *See* California encephalitis virus
clinical features of, 88–89
coxsackie virus, 98–99
cytomegalovirus, 166
Eastern encephalitis virus. *See* Eastern encephalitis virus
epidemiology of encephalitis, 112
Epstein–Barr virus, 200
etiological agents, 89–90, 92, 98–100
herpetic
atypical forms of, 149
clinical presentation of, 144–145
diagnosis, 145–146
differential diagnosis, 125, 148
pathogenesis of, 140–144
sequelae of, 148–149
treatment of, 146–149
incidence of, 88
influenza virus, 199–200
Japanese encephalitis virus. *See* Japanese encephalitis virus
measles, subacute encephalitis with immuno-suppression, 234–235
mumps, 199
Murray Valley encephalitis virus, 124
St. Louis encephalitis virus St. Louis encephalitis virus

Encephalitis (*contd.*)
seasonal distribution of, 91–93
Sindbis virus. *See* Sindbis virus
tick-borne, 121–122
transmission of, 87–88
varicella–zoster virus, 156–157
Venezuelan equine encephalitis virus. *See*
Venezuelan equine encephalitis virus
Von Economo encephalitis, 372–373, 430
West Nile virus. *See* West Nile virus
Western encephalitis virus. *See* Western
encephalitis virus
Encephalitis virus, history of, 6
Encephalomyelitis
acute disseminated encephalomyelitis. *See*
Postinfectious encephalomyelitis
postinfectious encephalomyelitis. *See* Postinfectious encephalomyelitis
rabies vaccine-induced encephalomyelitis,
178–179, 183–185
Viliusk encephalomyelitis, 261–262
Encephalomyocarditis virus
demyelination in infection, 187–189
strains of, 188
English sweating disease, epidemics, 430
Enteroviruses
characteristics, 93
classification, 93–94
Coxsackie virus. *See* Coxsackie virus
Echovirus. *See* Echovirus
epidemiology, 94
Poliovirus. *See* Poliovirus
rodent enteroviruses in human disease, 100
seasonal distribution of infection, 94–95
serotypes, 93
specimens for isolation and diagnosis, 125
Theiler's virus, 187
Envelope, structure in viruses, 12–13
Environmental control, virus spread, 412–414
Epstein–Barr virus. *See also* Burkitt's lymphoma,
Mononucleosis, infectious
cerebral tumor, association with, 383–384
chronic fatigue syndrome, association with,
221–223
culture of, 161
diseases associated with, 134
epidemiology, 161
Guillain–Barré syndrome, association with,
205–206
latency, 136, 164
neurologic complications from, 163–164
postinfectious encephalomyelitis, 200
receptor, 25

recovery in multiple sclerosis, 255–256
Reye's syndrome, association with, 215
specimens for isolation and diagnosis, 125
T cell activity during primary infection, 192
Equine infectious anemia virus
discovery of, 265
features of disease, 282–283
Experimental allergic neuritis
demyelination in, 183
histologic findings of, 186
latency, 183
Experimental autoimmune encephalitis
antigens in induction, 182
demyelination mechanisms, 190
discovery of, 181
histologic findings of, 185
latency, 182
species susceptibility to, 183
Eye infection. *See* Retinitis

F

Feline immunodeficiency virus, features of disease, 283–284
Feline panleukopenia virus, cerebellar hypoplasia
with, 342
Fetus
cerebral malformations, virus-induced animal
models, 340–345
cytomegalovirus infection, 320, 325–329
human immunodeficiency virus infection, 320,
329–334
malformations, relating to viral infections,
347–348
mechanisms of viral injury, 317–319
organogenesis, virus-induced animal models,
340
rare viral infections, 337–339
rubella infection, 319–325
varicella–zoster virus infection, 335–337
Filoviridae
distinguishing features in, 17
morphology of, 15, 20
Flaviviridae
distinguishing features in, 19
Japanese encephalitis virus. *See* Japanese
encephalitis virus
morphology of, 15, 20
Murray Valley encephalitis virus, 124
St. Louis encephalitis virus. *See* St. Louis
encephalitis virus
tick-borne encephalitis viruses. *See* Tick-borne
encephalitis viruses
Yellow fever, 411–412

Foscarnet, cytomegalovirus treatment, 329

G

Ganciclovir, cytomegalovirus treatment, 329,
    418–419
Gastrointestinal tract, viral entry barrier, 38
Genome
    classification of viruses, 14–15
    nature of viruses, 11–12
    structure in viruses, 12–13
German measles. *See* Rubella
gp41
    astrocytic membrane protein homology, 308
    neurotoxicity of, 306
gp120
    neuroleukin homology, 308
    neurotoxicity of, 306
Granulocyte, characteristics of, 64
Growth factors, synthesis and effects, 67
Guanarito virus, 105
Guillain–Barré syndrome
    axonal neuropathies with, 208–209
    brachial neuritis with, 209
    clinical features of, 203
    cytomegalovirus, association with, 165
    demyelination mechanisms, 192
    diagnosis, 203
    discovery of, 202
    histologic findings of, 186
    immunologic studies of, 204–205
    incidence, 202
    nosology, 202
    outcome, 203–204
    treatment, 204
    vaccine-associated disease, 207–208
    viruses associated with, 205–207

H

Hantaviruses, 17
Hearing loss. *See also* Deafness, Labyrinthitis
Hematogenous spread
    blood–brain barrier, virus permeability, 46–47,
        49–50
    blood–cerebrospinal fluid barrier, structure, 50
    extraneural multiplication of viruses, 47–48
    induction by rabies neural tissue vaccine,
        178–179
    steps in CNS invasion, 50–53
    viremia, maintenance of, 48
    viruses utilizing, 43
Hemorrhagic fever
    arenaviruses in, 105, 107–108
    filoviruses in, 109

Hepadnaviridae
    hepatitis B virus. *See* Hepatitis B virus
    morphology of, 15, 20
    distinguishing features in, 16
Hepatitis, Guillain–Barré syndrome association,
    205–206
Hepatitis B virus, vasculitis, 406–407
Herpes simplex virus. *See also* Herpes simplex
        virus type 1, Herpes simplex virus type 2
    axonal transport of, 42
    comparison of types, 137
    inflammation and humoral immune response in
        CNS, 80
    neonatal infection, 334–335, 348
    neuroinvasion, 40–44
    neurovirulence, 57, 59
    receptor, 25
    recovery in multiple sclerosis, 255–256
    retinitis with, 389
    Reye's syndrome, association with, 215
    treatment of neonates, 335
Herpes simplex virus type 1
    activation of, 138, 140
    diseases associated with, 134
    encephalitis
        atypical forms of, 149
        clinical presentation of, 144–145
        diagnosis, 145–146
        differential diagnosis, 125, 148
        pathogenesis of, 140–144
        sequelae of, 148–149
        treatment of, 146–149
    epidemiology, 137–138, 144
    hydrocephalus in infection, 345
    latency, 136–140, 143, 149
    localization in brain, 141–143
    mutant studies of neuroinvasiveness and neu-
        rovirulence, 143–144
    olfactory bulb infection, 141–142
Herpes simplex virus type 2
    activation of, 150
    clinical features, 150
    diseases associated with, 134
    encephalitis from, 150–151
    epidemiology, 150
    latency, 137
Herpes zoster
    epidemiology, 152–153
    neurological complications of, 153, 156–159
    pathogenesis, 153–154
    clinical features, 155–156
    postherpetic neuralgia with, 159
    virus. *See* Varicella–zoster virus

Herpesviruses
    cytomegalovirus. *See* Cytomegalovirus
    diseases associated with infection, 133–135
    distinguishing features in, 16
    Epstein–Barr virus. *See* Epstein–Barr virus
    herpes simplex virus. *See* Herpes simplex virus
    human herpesvirus. *See* Human herpesvirus 6,
        Human herpesvirus 7
    immunodeficiency, association with, 83–84
    latency, 136–140, 143, 149, 154, 164, 168
    morphology of, 15, 20
    portals of entry, 39
    receptors, 25
    replication, 135–136
    structure, 135
    vaccination against, 416
    varicella–zoster virus. *See* Varicella–zoster virus
Hog cholera virus, 344
Host defense. *See* B cell, Immune system,
        Immunoglobulin, T cell
Human herpesvirus 6
    chronic fatigue syndrome, association with,
        222–223
    diseases associated with, 134
    neurologic diseases from, 167
    recovery in multiple sclerosis, 255–256
Human herpesvirus 7
    chronic fatigue syndrome, association with,
        222–223
    diseases associated with, 134
    neurologic diseases from, 167–168
Human immunodeficiency virus. *See also*
        Acquired immunodeficiency syndrome
    animal models of infection, 309–311
    blood supply screening, 289, 413
    clinical syndromes of congenital infection,
        331–332
    dementia with, 297–299, 302
    diagnosis of congenital infection, 333
    genome and genes, 288
    glycoproteins of, 288
    Guillain–Barré syndrome, association with,
        205–206
    history of, 8, 287, 329
    maternal transmission rate, 329–331
    mutation of, 287
    myopathies in infection, 301–302
    neuroinvasiveness of, 303
    neurologic diseases from, 296–297
    neurotoxicity, indirect mechanisms, 305–309
    neurotropism of, 303–305
    neurovirulence of, 58–59, 305
    pathogenesis, 292–293, 313, 330–331

    peripheral neuropathies with, 300–301
    prevalence of infection, 290–291, 313
    primary infection of nervous system, 295–296
    protease inhibitor therapy, 312–313, 421–422
    quantitation by polymerase chain reaction, 23
    receptor, 25, 288
    replication of, 288, 292–293
    strains, 291, 302
    susceptibility of cell types to infection,
        291–292, 303–305
    transmission, 288–290, 294, 331
    zidovidine therapy, 294, 311–312, 333–334
Human respiratory synctial virus, 17
Human spumavirus, chronic fatigue syndrome
        association, 223
Human T cell lymphotropic viruses. *See also*
        Human T cell lymphotropic virus type I,
        Human T cell lymphotropic virus type II
    comparison of types, 276–277
    history of, 8
    neurovirulence of, 59
Human T cell lymphotropic virus type I
    associated leukemia, lymphoma, and myelopa-
        thy, 269–270
    discovery of, 268–269
    epidemiology, 270–271
    eye involvement, 275
    myelopathy, clinical manifestations of,
        271–272
    pathologic findings of infection, 272–275
    polymyositis, association with, 275
    recovery in multiple sclerosis, 255, 257
    transmission of, 271
    treatment, 276
Human T cell lymphotropic virus type II
    chronic fatigue syndrome, association with,
        223
    discovery of, 276
    diseases associated with, 276
Hybridization, nucleic acids in virus detection,
        22, 37
Hydrocephalus, virus induction in animals,
        345–347

I

Idoxuridane, history of herpetic encephalitis treat-
        ment, 146–147
Immune system
    cellular activation in, 64–66
    cerebrospinal fluid defenses, 76–78
    clearance of virus from CNS, 82–84
    complement in viral defense, 73–74
    cytokine network of, 66–68

differentiation and maturation of cell populations, 62–64
immunoglobulins in viral defense, 69–73
inflammatory response of, 78–80, 82
memory of, 61–62
viral antigens, 68–69
virus infected cells, immune attack, 74–76
Immunization. *See* Vaccine
Immunocytochemistry, detection of viruses, 37
Immunoglobulin
  in cerebrospinal fluid, 76–77, 80, 82
  classification, 69–70
  extracellular virus, interaction with, 72, 74
  genes, 63
  half-life of, 62, 70
  infected cell destruction, 74–75
  overview of functions, 70
  structure of, 70–71
  viral antigens, 68–69
Immunosuppression
  acquired immunodeficiency syndrome. *See* Acquired immunodeficiency syndrome, Human immunodeficiency virus
  adenoviruses and, 83–84
  bovine immunodeficiency virus. *See* Bovine immunodeficiency virus
  feline immunodeficiency virus. *See* Feline immunodeficiency virus
  measles virus and, 83–84
  papovaviruses and, 83–84
  poliovirus and, 83–84
  simian immunodeficiency virus. *See* Simian immunodeficiency virus
  subacute measles encephalitis with, 234–235
Inclusions, viral
  cytomegalic inclusion disease, 326–327
  inclusion body myositis, 404–405
Infant. *See* Neonate
Infectious cycle. *See* Virus–cell infectious cycle
Inflammation, response in CNS, 78–82
Influenza
  fetal infection, 338, 340, 345, 347
  postinfectious encephalomyelitis with, 199–200
  receptor for virus, 25
  Reye's syndrome, association with, 214–215
  myositis, association with, 404
  virus survival mechanisms, 431
Interference, virus–virus interactions in, 28
Interferons
  effects, 66–67
  virus treatment, 419
  synthesis, 66

Interleukins, synthesis and effects, 66–67

J
Japanese encephalitis virus
  arthropod infection, 113, 122–123
  clinical features of infection, 123–124
  epidemiology, 122
  hydrocephalus in infection, 346–347
  inflammation and humoral immune response in CNS, 80
  life cycle of, 122–123
  vaccination against, 122, 124
JC virus
  cerebral tumor, association with, 381–382
  fetal infection, 339
  progressive multifocal leukoencephalopathy, association with, 242, 245–248
Junin virus, Argentinean hemorrhagic fever, 105, 108

K
Koch's postulates
  overview of, 426
  retrovirus considerations, 428–429
  slow infection considerations, 427–428
  viruses as exception, 426–427
Kozhevnikov's epilepsy, virus involvement, 258–259
Kuru
  cannibalism, association with, 356
  disease description, 354–355
  epidemiology, 353–354
  history of, 353–354
  incubation period, 356
  transmission, 355–356, 364

L
Laboratory diagnosis. *See* Diagnosis
Labyrinthitis
  clinical features of, 400
  pathogenesis, 396–397
  virus types, 395
La Crosse virus, 113, 118–120, 344
Lamivudine, human immunodeficiency virus treatment, 312
Lassa fever
  sudden acquired deafness, 399
  virus, 105, 107
Latency
  dynamic latency, 136
  experimental autoimmune encephalitis, 182
  herpesviruses, 136–140, 143, 149, 154, 164, 168

Latency (*contd.*)
    static latency, 136
Lentiviruses
    bovine immunodeficiency virus. *See* Bovine
        immunodeficiency virus
    caprine arthritis–encephalitis virus. *See*
        Caprine arthritis–encephalitis virus
    classification of, 279
    equine infectious anemia virus. *See* Equine
        infectious anemia virus
    feline immunodeficiency virus. *See* Feline
        immunodeficiency virus
    human immunodeficiency virus. *See* Human
        immunodeficiency virus
    neurologic diseases with infection, 279–280
    simian immunodeficiency virus. *See* Simian
        immunodeficiency virus
    species specificity of, 279
    visna virus. *See* Visna virus
Leptospirosis
    antibiotic therapy, 130
    clinical features of infection, 129
    epidemiology, 129
Leukemia. *See* Human T cell lymphotropic virus
    type I, Murine leukemia virus
Leukoencephalitis. *See* Acute hemorrhagic
    leukoencephalitis
Leukoencephalopathy. *See* Progressive multifocal
    leukoencephalopathy
Liposome, drug delivery, 422
Lyme disease
    clinical features of infection, 130
    epidemiology, 130
Lymphocyte. *See* B cell, T cell
Lymphocytic choriomeningitis virus, 105
    cerebellar hypoplasia in rats, association with,
        342
    clinical manifestations, 106–107
    epidemiology, 105–106
    fetal infection, 338
    hemorrhagic fevers, association with, 107–108
    noncytopathic effects in infection, 31
    prevalence of infection in meningitis, 105
    specimens for isolation and diagnosis, 125
Lysis, cells in viral infection, 30

M

Machupo virus, Bolivian hemorrhagic fever, 105,
    108
Macrophage
    characteristics of, 64
    neurotoxicity of activation factors, 307
    pericytes, 77

Malignant catarrhal fever disease, cerebrovascular
    disease, 407–408
Marburg virus, hemorrhagic fever, 109
Measles
    epidemics, 430
    history of, 7, 430
    migration, 432
    postinfectious encephalomyelitis with, 184,
        192, 194–196, 212
    subacute measles encephalitis with immuno-
        suppression, 234–235
    subacute sclerosing panencephalitis. *See* Suba-
        cute sclerosing panencephalitis
    sudden acquired deafness with, 398–400
    treatment, 239
Measles virus
    immunodeficiency, association with, 83–84
    receptor, 25
    recovery in multiple sclerosis, 255, 257
    replication of, 237–239
    retinitis, association with, 391
    Reye's syndrome, association with, 215
    T cell activity during primary infection, 192
    vaccination against, 412
Memory cell, life span, 62
Ménière's disease, viral involvement, 400
Meningitis
    acquired immunodeficiency syndrome with,
        296–297
    coxsackie virus and, 97–98
    echovirus and, 97–98
    clinical features of, 88
    etiological agents, 89–90, 92, 97–98, 100
    history of, 4
    incidence, 88
    lymphocytic choriomeningitis virus. *See* Lym-
        phocytic choriomeningitis virus
    Mollaret's meningitis
        features of, 259–260
        virus involvement, 260
    seasonal distribution, 91–93
    transmission, 87–88
Mink. *See* Aleutian mink disease virus
Molecular mimicry, virus-induced demyelination,
    190–191, 208
Mollaret's meningitis
    features of, 259–260
    virus involvement, 260
Mononuclear cells. *See* B cell, Macrophage, T
    cell
Mononucleosis, infectious
    clinical features, 161–162
    diagnosis, 162

epidemiology, 161
neurologic complications, 163–164
viruses causing, 160, 164
Morbillivirus. *See* Measles virus
Mouse hepatitis virus, demyelination in infection, 187–188
Mouse polyoma virus, cerebral tumor induction, 381
Mouse sarcoma virus, cerebral tumor association, 381–382
Multiple sclerosis
    antiviral antibodies, serologic studies, 253–254
    demyelination, morphological studies, 254–255
    epidemics, 251
    evidence for viral involvement, 248–249, 251–258
    familial aggregation, 250–251
    geographic distribution of, 249–250
    migration studies, 250
    virus involvement, 7–8, 255–258
Mumps virus
    characteristics of, 100
    clinical manifestations of infection, 101
    CNS infections, 101–102
    epidemiology, 100–101
    fetal infection, 339
    hydrocephalus induction, 345–347
    postinfectious encephalomyelitis with, 199
    specimens for isolation and diagnosis, 125
    sudden acquired deafness with, 399
    vaccination against, 100, 102, 412
Murine leukemia virus
    budding, 277–278
    cellular localization, 278–279
    incubation period, 277
Murine paramyxovirus, hydrocephalus in infection, 347
Murray Valley encephalitis virus, 124
Mutation, rates in RNA viruses, 28–29
Mycoplasma infections
    clinical features of, 131
    differential diagnosis from acute viral CNS infections, 130–132
    epidemiology, 130–131
Myelin. *See* Demyelination
Myelitis. *See also* Poliomyelitis
    B virus and, 151
    postinfectious encephalomyelitis
        acute hemorrhagic leukoencephalitis, 201–202
        and chickenpox, 193, 197
        demyelination mechanisms, 192
        and Epstein–Barr virus, 200

histologic findings, 185
and influenza, 199–200
localized syndromes, 200–201
and measles, 184, 192, 194–196
and mumps, 199
nosology, 192
and rubella, 193, 198–199
transverse myelitis, postinfectious syndrome, 200–201
varicella–zoster virus and, 157
Myositis
    coxsackie virus in, 403–404
    immune response in pathogenesis, 405
    inclusion body myositis, 404–405
    influenza virus in, 404
Myxoviridae, receptors, 25

N
Neonate
    herpes simplex virus infection, 320, 334–335
    human immunodeficiency virus infection, 331
    prenatal viral infections. *See* Fetus
Neural growth factors, synthesis and effects, 66
Neuroinvasiveness
    and axonal transport, 42–43
    definition of, 36
    hematogenous route, 46–51, 53
    human immunodeficiency virus, 303
    neural pathway, 40–43
    olfactory route, 44–46
Neurotropism
    definition of, 36
    human immunodeficiency virus, 303–305
    size of virus, relationship to CNS extracellular space, 53–54
    spreading of virus, 53–55
    vulnerability of cell populations, 55
Neurovirulence
    definition of, 36, 56
    dependence of viral strains, 56–58
    human immunodeficiency virus, 305
Newcastle disease virus
    fetal effects in chicks, 340
    postinfectious encephalopathy, 212
Nucleocapsid, structure in viruses, 12–13
Nucleoside analogs, as antiviral agents, 421–422

O
Olfactory spread
    anatomic factors in, 44–45
    evidence of viruses utilizing, 46
    history of study, 44
    viruses utilizing, 43

Olfactory spread (*contd.*)
Oncogenesis. *See* Cancer
Orbivirus. *See* Bluetongue virus, Colorado tick
    fever virus
Orthomyxoviridae
    distinguishing features in, 17
    influenza. *See* Influenza
    morphology of, 15, 20

P

Panencephalitis
    progressive rubella panencephalitis
      clinical features of, 240
      epidemiology, 239–240
      history of study, 239, 241
      pathogenesis, 240
    subacute sclerosing panencephalitis
      clinical manifestations of, 232–233
      history of study, 231–232
      host response abnormalities in pathogenesis,
        235–236
      incidence, 232
      pathologic findings of, 233
      recovery of measles virus, 233–234
      replication defect in measles virus, 237–239
      second-agent hypothesis in pathogenesis,
        236–237
      subacute measles encephalitis with immuno-
        suppression, 234–235
Papovaviruses
    BK virus. *See* BK virus
    cerebral tumor, association with, 381–386
    distinguishing features in, 16
    immunodeficiency, association with, 83–84
    JC virus. *See* JC virus
    morphology of, 15, 20
    recovery in progressive multifocal leukoen-
      cephalopathy, 242–243, 245
Parainfluenza virus, Reye's syndrome, association
    with, 215
Paramyxoviridae
    distinguishing features in, 17
    measles. *See* Measles virus
    mumps. *See* Mumps virus
    morphology of, 15, 20
    parainfluenza. *See* Parainfluenza virus
Parkinson's disease, virus, possible roles, 372–373
Parvoviruses
    clinical features of infection, 104
    CNS complications of, 104
    distinguishing features in, 16
    morphology of, 15, 20
    receptors, 25
    replication of, 104

vasculitis and parvovirus B19, 407
Pathogenesis of CNS infections, 35–59
    entry of viruses, 38–40
    experimental approaches, 36–38
    hematogenous route of viral spread, 46–53
    neural route of virus spread, 40–44
    neurovirulence, 56–59
    olfactory route of viral spread, 44–46
    spread of virus within CNS, 53–56
    vulnerability of cell populations, 55
Penetration
    blocking by drugs, 419
    mechanisms in virus infection, 26
Peripheral nerve, virus spread to CNS, 40–43,
    387
Persistence, viruses in CNS
    anatomic factors in, 229
    immunologic factors in, 229–231
    viral mutation in, 230–231
Picornaviridae
    distinguishing features in, 19
    enterovirus. *See* Enteroviruses
    morphology of, 15, 20
    receptors, 25
Placenta
    maternal and fetal blood relationship,
      316–317
    virus transmission, 316–317
Poliomyelitis. *See also* specific viruses
    clinical features of, 88–89
    epidemics, 95–96
    etiological agents, 89–90, 92
    postpolio syndrome. *See* Postpolio syndrome
    seasonal distribution of, 91–93
    transmission, 87–88
    vaccination against, 95–96, 412
Poliovirus
    culture of, 424–425
    immunodeficiency, association with, 83–84
    neuroinvasion of, 40, 43–44
    neurotropism of, 55
    neurovirulence of, 56–57
    receptor, 25
    serotypes, 93
    specimens for isolation and diagnosis, 125
Polymavirus. *See* BK virus, JC virus, Simian
    virus 40
Polymerase chain reaction
    applications in virology, 424
    cytomegalovirus detection, 328
    detection of viruses, 22–23, 37, 126, 220
    Epstein–Barr virus detection, 162
    herpes simplex virus detection, 145–146
    human herpesvirus 6 detection, 167

human immunodeficiency virus detection, 310, 330, 333
principles of, 22
quantitation of viruses, 22–23
rubella virus detection, 325
specificity of, 23
varicella–zoster virus, 153
Population, impact on viral spread, 432–434
Postherpetic neuralgia
  amitryptyline therapy, 160
  clinical features of, 159
  incidence of, 159
Postinfectious encephalomyelitis
  acute hemorrhagic leukoencephalitis, 201–202
  and chickenpox, 193, 197
  demyelination mechanisms, 192
  and Epstein–Barr virus, 200
  histologic findings, 185
  and influenza, 199–200
  localized syndromes, 200–201
  and measles, 184, 192, 194–196
  and mumps, 199
  nosology, 192
  and rubella, 193, 198–199
Postpolio syndrome
  clinical features of, 217–218
  epidemiology, 217
  history of, 211, 216
  mechanisms of, 218–220
  progression of, 218
Poxviridae
  distinguishing features in, 16
  morphology of, 15, 20
  smallpox. *See* Smallpox
  vaccinia. *See* Vaccinia virus
Prevention and therapy of infections, 411–422
  environmental control, 412–414
  vaccines, 414–417
  antiviral drugs, 418–422
Prion. *See* Bovine spongiform encephalopathy, Creutzfeldt–Jakob disease, Kuru, Scrapie
Progressive multifocal leukoencephalopathy
  diagnosis of, 243
  epidemiology, 242
  histopathologic findings in, 241–243
  immunocompromised patients, 248
  papovavirus recovery, 242–243, 245
  pathogenesis, 245–248
  treatment, 248
Progressive rubella panencephalitis
  clinical features of, 240
  epidemiology, 239–240
  history of study, 239, 241
  pathogenesis, 240

Q

Q fever, differential diagnosis from acute viral CNS infections, 128
Quantitation of viruses
  dose assays, 21
  hybridization of nucleic acids, 22
  plaque-forming unit assays, 21
  polymerase chain reaction, 22–23
Quarantine, environmental control, 176–177, 412

R

Rabies vaccine-induced encephalomyelitis
  Guillain–Barré syndrome induction, 178–179, 185
  histologic findings of, 185
  time of onset, 183–184
Rabies virus
  antigenically-similar viruses, 170
  axonal transport of, 42
  clinical manifestations of disease, 175
  control of infected animals, 176–177, 413
  culture of, 170
  history of, 3–4, 36–37, 169
  human transmission, 173
  immune serum therapy, 178
  incubation period, 175
  mortality from, 170, 176
  neurotropism of, 54–55
  neurovirulence of, 58–59
  noncytopathic effects in infection, 31–32
  pathogenesis, 173–174
  pathologic findings, 176
  portals of entry, 39
  postexposure prophylaxis, 177–178
  postinfectious encephalopathy, 212
  receptor, 25
  specimens for isolation and diagnosis, 125
  sylvatic hosts, 170–172
  transmission efficiency from bites, 174–175
  vaccination against, 178–179, 183–184
  variants of, 172
Rasmussen's disease, virus involvement, 259
Rat virus, retinitis with, 393
Recombination of viruses, 29
Release. *See* Budding
Reoviruses
  bluetongue virus. *See* Bluetongue virus
  Colorado tick fever virus. *See* Colorado tick fever virus
  distinguishing features in, 18
  hydrocephalus in infection, 345
  morphology of, 15, 20
  neurovirulence of, 57
  orbivirus. *See* Orbivirus

Reoviruses (*contd.*)
  Reye's syndrome, association with, 215
Replication
  blocking by drugs, 421–422
  DNA viruses, 26
  effects of virus replication on cells, 29–33
  RNA viruses, 26–27, 266
Respiratory syncytial virus, Reye's syndrome
    association, 215
Retinitis
  animal virus induction, 392–394
  cytomegalovirus in, 389–390
  herpes simplex virus in, 389
  measles virus in, 391
  pathogenesis, 388–389
  rubella virus in, 391–392
  varicella–zoster virus in, 390–391
Retroviruses
  cerebral tumor, association with, 381–383
  classification, 267–268
  distinguishing features in, 18
  genome of, 267
  human immunodeficiency virus. *See* Human
      immunodeficiency virus
  human spumavirus. *See* Human spumavirus
  human T cell lymphotropic viruses. *See* Human
      T cell lymphotropic viruses
  Koch's postulates, modification of, 428–429
  latency, 267
  morphology of, 15, 20, 267
  replication of, 26–27, 266–267
Reye's syndrome
  aspirin, association with, 211, 216
  clinical manifestations, 213–214
  epidemiology, 213
  histologic findings of, 214
  history of, 211–213
  mortality from, 214
  viruses associated with, 214–216
Rhabdoviridae
  distinguishing features in, 17
  morphology of, 15, 20, 169
  rabies. *See* Rabies virus
  receptors, 25
Ribavirin, antiviral therapy, 418, 422
Rickettsia infections, differential diagnosis from
    acute viral CNS infections, 127–128
Rift Valley fever virus, 17, 344
RNA viruses
  replication, 26–27, 266
  survival mechanisms, 431
Rocio virus, 124
Rocky Mountain spotted fever
  clinical features of, 128

differential diagnosis from acute viral CNS
    infections, 127–128
  epidemiology, 127–128
Roseolovirus. *See* Human herpesvirus 6, Human
    herpesvirus 7
Ross River virus, demyelination in infection, 187,
    189
Rubella
  congenital rubella syndrome features, 322–325,
      348
  deafness with, 397–398
  epidemics, 319
  fetal age effects on infection rate, 320–321
  German measles, 319
  pathogenesis of fetal anomalies, 320–322,
      324–325
  postinfectious encephalomyelitis, 193,
      198–199
  prenatal diagnosis, 325
  progressive rubella panencephalitis
    clinical features of, 240
    epidemiology, 239–240
    history of study, 239, 241
    pathogenesis, 240
  retinitis with, 391–392
  vaccination against, 319, 325, 412
Rubeola. *See* Measles virus
Rubivirus. *See* Rubella virus

S
Sabiá virus, 105
St. Louis encephalitis virus
  clinical features of infection, 117–118
  epidemics, 117
  hydrocephalus in infection, 347
  life cycle of, 116–117
  mortality, 118
Schizophrenia
  genetics, 374
  seasonality of births, 374
  virus, possible roles, 373–374
Sclerosis. *See* Amyotrophic lateral sclerosis, Mus-
    cular sclerosis
Scrapie
  comparison to visna, 227–228
  forms of prion protein, 352–353
  history of, 7, 349–350
  knockout mice studies, 353, 426
  onset in sheep, 350
  pathogenesis, 350–351
  physical-chemical properties of agent,
      351–352
  recovery in multiple sclerosis, 255, 257
  retinitis with, 394

Reye's syndrome, association with, 215
slow infection prototype, 227–228
transmission, 364
Seasonal distribution, acute neurologic diseases,
91–97
Semliki Forest virus, demyelination in infection,
187, 189
Shingles. *See* Herpes zoster
Simian immunodeficiency virus
cellular localization of, 285–286
features of disease, 284
neuropathologic findings, 284–285
origin of, 284
Simian sarcoma virus, cerebral tumor association,
381–382
Simian virus 40
cerebral tumor, association with, 381–385
demyelination in infection, 186–187
progressive multifocal leukoencephalopathy,
association with, 245–248
Sindbis virus
clearance from CNS, 83
inflammation and humoral immune response in
CNS, 79, 81
Sindbis virus, neurovirulence, 58
Skin, viral entry barrier, 38
Slow infection. *See also* Chronic neurologic diseases
Koch's postulates, modification of, 427–428
prototypes of, 227–228
scrapie. *See* Scrapie
visna. *See* Visna
Smallpox, eradication, 411
Spirochetal infections, differential diagnosis from
acute viral CNS infections, 128–130
Spread of virus
environmental control, 412–414
hematogenous spread
blood–brain barrier, virus permeability,
46–47, 49–50
blood–cerebrospinal fluid barrier, structure,
50
extraneural multiplication of viruses, 47–48
induction by rabies neural tissue vaccine,
178–179
steps in CNS invasion, 50–53
viremia, maintenance of, 48
viruses utilizing, 43
neurotropism, 53–55
olfactory spread
anatomic factors in, 44–45
evidence of viruses utilizing, 46
history of study, 44
viruses utilizing, 43

peripheral nerve, virus spread to CNS, 40–43,
387
population effects, 432–434
travel effects, 432–433
Structure of viruses, 12–14
Subacute sclerosing panencephalitis
clinical manifestations of, 232–233
history of study, 231–232
host response abnormalities in pathogenesis,
235–236
incidence, 232
pathologic findings of, 233
recovery of measles virus, 233–234
replication defect in measles virus, 237–239
second-agent hypothesis in pathogenesis,
236–237
subacute measles encephalitis with immunosuppression, 234–235
Sudden acquired deafness. *See* Deafness
Susceptibility of cell types to infection, 35–36
human immunodeficiency virus, 291–292,
303–305
Swine influenza vaccine, Guillain–Barré syndrome association, 207–208

T
T cell
activation of, 64–66
activity in virus-induced demyelination, 192
categories of action against viruses, 72–73
in cerebrospinal fluid, 77
cross-reactivity of antigens, 73
differentiation and maturation of, 62–64, 67
infected cell destruction, 74–76
surface markers for, 63, 65
viral antigens, 69
Tat, neurotoxicity, 306–307
Taxonomy, viruses, 14–15
Temperature, viral entry effects, 38–39
Teratogenesis. *See* Fetus
Theiler's virus, demyelination in infection, 187
Tick-borne encephalitis viruses
clinical features of infection, 121–122
epidemiology, 121–122
Tobacco mosaic virus, discovery of, 5
Togaviridae
alphavirus. *See* Alphaviruses and Arboviruses
distinguishing features in, 18
flavivirus. *See* Arboviruses and Flaviviruses
morphology of, 15, 20
rubivirus. *See* Rubella virus
Transformation
cell properties, 379
efficiency of virus types, 380

Transformation (*contd.*)
  pathogenesis of, 379–380
  viral induction, 30–31, 379–380
Transgenic mouse
  applications in virology, 425–426
  knockout studies of scrapie, 353, 426
Transverse myelitis, postinfectious syndrome,
    200–201
Travel, effect on virus spread, 432–433
Tumor necrosis factors
  neurotoxicity, 307–308
  synthesis and effects, 66, 68

U

Uncoating
  blocking by drugs, 420–421
  mechanisms in virus infection, 26
Uveoencephalitis syndrome. *See* Vogt–
    Koyanagi–Harada syndrome

V

Vaccine
  active immunization, 414–417
  attenuated vaccine development, 415
  bluetongue virus, fetal cerebral effects of vac-
    cine, 342–343
  chickenpox, 159
  Guillain–Barré syndrome, vaccine-associated
    disease, 178–179, 185, 207–208
  hematogenous spread, induction by rabies
    neural tissue vaccine, 178–179
  herpesvirus, 416
  Japanese encephalitis virus, 122, 124
  killed vaccine, 415–416
  measles, 412
  mumps, 100, 102, 412
  neurologic complications, 414–415
  passive immunization, 417
  poliomyelitis, 95–96, 412
  rabies, 178–179, 183–184
  recombinant vectors, 417
  rabies vaccine-induced encephalomyelitis
    Guillain–Barré syndrome induction,
      178–179, 185
    histologic findings of, 185
    time of onset, 183–184
  rubella, 319, 325, 412
  swine influenza vaccine, Guillain–Barré syn-
    drome association, 207–208
  synthetic vaccines, 416–417
Vaccinia virus, 16
  eradication of, 411
  hydrocephalus in infection, 346
  and postinfectious encephalomyelitis, 192–194

Varicella–zoster virus. *See also* Chickenpox, Her-
    pes zoster
  activation of, 154
  encephalitis with, 156–157
  diseases associated with, 134
  epidemiology, 152–153
  fetal infection, 335–337
  history of study, 151–152
  immunocompromised patients, risks, 156, 158,
    160
  immunotherapy, 160
  latency, 154
  lesions associated with, 158
  myelitis with, 157
  neurological complications, 153, 156–159
  retinitis with, 390–391
  Reye's syndrome, association with, 214–215
  sudden acquired deafness with, 399
Variola virus. *See* Smallpox
Vasculitis
  cerebrovascular disease in animals,
    407–409
  hepatitis B virus in, 406–407
  parvovirus B19 in, 407
  pathogenesis of, 405–406
Venezuelan equine encephalitis virus
  clinical features of infection, 120–121
  demyelination in infection, 187, 189
  epidemiology, 120
  fetal infection, 337, 344
Vesicular stomatitis virus, demyelination in infec-
    tion, 187, 189
Vidarabine
  herpetic encephalitis treatment, 147, 418
  immunocompromised patient treatment, 160
Viluisk encephalomyelitis
  features of, 261
  virus involvement, 261–262
Viremia. *See* Hematogenous spread
Virion
  definition of, 13
  morphology of, 13
Virology
  history of, 5, 11
  taxonomy, 14–15
Virus–cell infectious cycle
  assembly and release, 27
  attachment, 24–26
  blocking by drugs, 419–422
  duration of cycle, 23–24
  overview of steps, 23–24, 420
  penetration and uncoating, 26
  replication, 26–27
  susceptibility of cell types, 35–36

Visna
  comparison to scrapie, 227–228
  epidemiology, 261
  features of, 281
  pathogenesis, 282–293
  slow infection prototype, 227–228
Visna virus
  cellular localization, 281
  demyelination in infection, 187
  mutation of, 287
Vogt–Koyanagi–Harada syndrome
  features of, 261
  virus involvement, 261
Von Economo encephalitis
  epidemics, 372, 430
  parkinsonism, association with, 373

W
Wesselsbron virus, 344
West Nile virus, 124
Western encephalitis virus
  clinical features of infection, 117
  life cycle of, 115–116

Y
Yellow fever, eradication attempts, 411–412

Z
Zidovidine
  human immunodeficiency virus treatment, 294,
    311–312, 333–334, 419
  myopathy induction, 301–302
Zoster. *See* Herpes zoster